MW01043125

BAKERMAN'S ABC's OF ADULT AND PEDIATRIC DRUG THERAPY

Paul Bakerman, M.D.
Seymour Bakerman, M.D., PhD.

Published by
Interpretive Laboratory Data, Inc.
Post Office Box 7066
Greenville, NC 27835-7066
0-700-ABC-BOOK

ISBN 0-945577-05-2

INTERPRETIVE LAB DATA
P.O. BOX 2250
MYRTLE BEACH, SC 29578
803-448-3055

PREFACE

This book was started because there is a need for a clear, concise pocket-sized paperback textbook covering adult and pediatric drug therapy and emphasizing the clinical applications of these drugs.

The format in the text is uniform throughout. Drugs are listed alphabetically by generic name for rapid reference. Trade names are listed in the index. Individual drug listings include the following headings: generic name, select brand names, uses, mechanism of action, dosage forms, dosage in various conditions, pharmacokinetics, adverse effects, contraindications, and drug interactions. At times, one or several of these sections are not included when this information seemed less important. We have not attempted to cover all adverse effects, but to emphasize more important aspects due to the frequency, seriousness, or uniqueness of the effects. <u>The strength of this book is the clinical application of drug therapy</u>.

We wish to acknowledge the contributions of many people who made suggestions that improved the text of this book; these include Dr. Amy Beiter, Dr. David Beyda, Dr. Alan Frechette, Dr. Gerald Gong, Dr. Joanne Gordon, Dr. Kent Haverkamp, Dr. Judith Hunt, Dr. Rodney Ohmart, Dr. John Stock, Dr. David Tellez, Dr. Kristine Thomas, and Dr. Rebecca Wood. Dr. Karen Lewis made helpful suggestions and Dr. Karen Gerdes provided moral support. Other suggestions came from many other attending physicians and residents at Phoenix Children's Hospital and Maricopa Medical Center. Dr. Steven Curry and Dr. Paul Liu reviewed the text extensively and made many helpful suggestions. Dr. H.G. Adams provided a systematic approach to antimicrobial agents that was used throughout the text. The entire text was reviewed by clinical pharmacists Debra Cipolletti and Chrys Jallo and their suggestions have strengthened this book considerably. Dr. Paul Peckar provided reviews of psychiatric drugs, as well as inspiration to complete this project.

Phyllis Broughton and Ruth Carson helped draw figures and provided technical support for this work. Janine Jones Tripp spent countless hours above and beyond scheduled work time typing the text. Marvin Alligood, Jr. has done an outstanding job proofreading the text. Janine and Marvin have held this project together and have ensured that each revision was as near perfection as possible, down to the smallest detail.

This work could not have been completed without tremendous support from the wife of one of the authors (S.B.) the mother of another (P.B.), and the president of the publishing company, Winona Bakerman. Christina, Molly and Edward provided psychological, physical, and intellectual support throughout this project. Beth and John Bakerman provided technical support. Please contact me if you have any questions, comments or suggestions that would improve this text; my telephone number is (602) 239-3563. Paul Bakerman M.D.

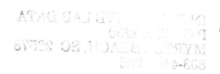

DEDICATION

This book is dedicated to the memory of Seymour Bakerman. It began as a collaboration between father and son, and although he was unable to see it in its final form, we hope he would be proud. Seymour Bakerman was an exceptional man and not just his family felt this way, he was deeply loved by his students, staff and friends. As a person he approached life with overt enthusiasm that was infectious. He treated everyone equally, and with fairness. As a physician, Seymour Bakerman would want to be remembered as a teacher. When you walked into his classroom the first day, you knew immediately that something was different. He treated everyone with respect. He taught with organization, dedication, and enthusiasm, but at the same time was always listening to the students to see if they were learning. The honor he cherished most was repeatedly winning the Golden Caduceus Award for outstanding teacher until it was renamed the Seymour Bakerman Award.As his family, there was never any question that we came first in his life. He was the kind of father every child should have and the husband every woman dreams of. As a family, we have completed this project as a tribute to Seymour Bakerman, teacher and physician; our father, husband and friend.

TABLE OF CONTENTS

Drugs in this book are arranged alphabetically by generic name. Brand names are listed in the index. The following general topics are covered in this text:

TABLE OF CONTENTS (Cont.) Page

The authors have extensively reviewed the drug dosage schedules to ensure that the recommendations are consistent with current practice. In an individual situation these recommendations should not be considered absolute. Clinical practice is constantly evolving; current standards should be dictated by medical literature and specialists in various areas. The manufacturer's product information insert should be consulted prior to prescribing or administering any drug. Uses of drugs at times may not be approved by the Food and Drug Administration (FDA). If use of a drug is controversial or dosage recommendations vary, references are provided. This book is meant to provide information for teaching purposes. It is not meant to be a complete drug information source, and standard references should be consulted for more detailed information. It is the responsibility of the physician to assess the suitability of a particular drug and dosing schedule in individual situations. Dosage recommendations in this book are compiled from current literature, when cited, and from the following general sources:

1. Package inserts for individual products.

2. American Hospital Formulary Service Drug Information 1991, McEvoy, G.K. et al., eds., Bethesda, American Society of Hospital Pharmacists Inc., 1991.

3. Harriet Lane Handbook 12th edition, Greene, M.G., ed., St. Louis, Mosby Year Book, 1991.

4. Benitz, W.E. and Tatro, D.S. The Pediatric Drug Handbook 2nd edition, Chicago, Year Book Medical Publishers, Inc. 1988.

ACETAMINOPHEN

(Tylenol, Tempra, Datril, Liquiprim, Neopap, Paracetamol)

USES: Uses of acetaminophen are given in the next Table:

Uses of Acetaminophen
Pain (Analgesic)
Fever (Antipyretic)

Acetaminophen is used in the treatment of pain and fever; it does not have obvious anti-inflammatory activity. Acetaminophen is the preferred alternative to aspirin for those with a history of peptic ulcer and those with a coagulation disorder such as hemophilia. There is no relationship between acetaminophen and Reye's syndrome. Acetaminophen, in combination with oral doses of an opiate, (eg, codeine, oxycodone) produces greater analgesic effect than that produced by either acetaminophen or higher doses of the opiate alone. Acetaminophen and aspirin are equally effective as antipyretics.

DOSAGE FORMS: Tabs: 80, 160, 325, 500, 650mg; Drops: 100mg/ml; Elixir: 120mg/5ml, 160mg/5ml, 325mg/5ml; Supp: 120, 125, 325, 650mg.

Acetaminophen inhibits the action of endogenous pyrogen on the hypothalamic heat regulator centers; it also inhibits prostaglandin synthetase.

DOSAGE: Acetaminophen is usually administered orally but if necessary, may be administered rectally; dosage orally or rectally, based on age, for pain and fever is given in the next Table:

Dosage, Orally or Rectally, of Acetaminophen for Pain and Fever

Age	Dosage
Children	10-15mg/kg every 4-6 hours orally or rectally.
Adults Children >11 years	325-650mg every 4-6 hours orally or rectally. Do not exceed 4g daily. Dosage in adults for long term therapy should not exceed 2.6g daily.

PHARMACOKINETICS: Absorption: Rapid from the upper GI tract; Peak: 10-60 minutes. Therapeutic Range: 10-25mcg/ml(10-25mg/L); Time to Peak Plasma Level: 0.5-1.0 Hours; Half-Life: 1 to 3 hours; Plasma Protein Binding: 30-50% Excretion: Conjugated with glycine, sulfuric acid and cysteine. Time to Steady State: 10 to 20 hours; Toxic Range: 100-250mcg/ml.

ADVERSE EFFECTS: Unlike aspirin, acetaminophen has no significant effect on platelet aggregation. Adverse effects include rash, urticaria, neutropenia thrombocytopenia and renal tubular necrosis.

This drug may cause hepatic failure. Hepatic toxicity may appear 3-5 days after ingestion of a toxic dose. Most of the acetaminophen is normally metabolized in the liver to sulfate and glucuronide conjugates; a small amount is metabolized by the P-450 system to a potentially toxic intermediate, acetimidoquinone, which is metabolized by reaction with glutathione. Acetimidoquinone arylates vital nucleophilic macromolecules within hepatocytes, resulting in hepatic necrosis. Serious toxicity is likely to occur if the ingested dose is more than 140mg/kg. Blood specimens are collected about 4 hours and 8 hours after ingestion.

A nomogram of plasma or serum acetaminophen concentration versus time since ingestion is shown in the next Figure (Rumack, B.H. and Peterson, R.G., Pediatr. Supp. 62, 898-903, 1978):

Nomogram of Plasma or Serum Acetaminophen Concentration versus Time Since Acetaminophen Ingestion

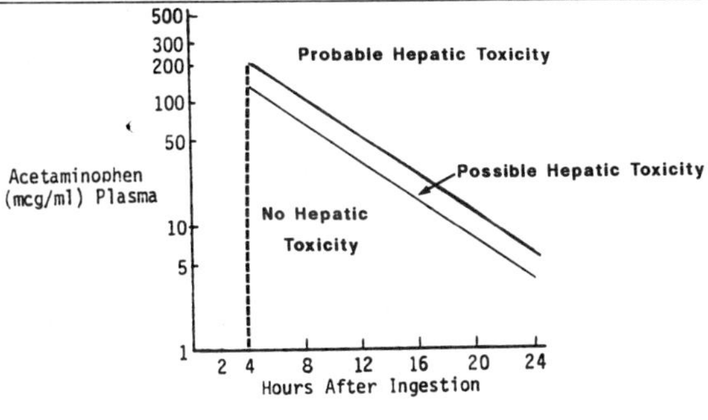

ACETAMINOPHEN (Cont.)
The half-life for acetaminophen elimination is 2 to 4 hours. The first sample is used to determine whether therapy with N-acetylcysteine (Mucomyst) should be started. Treatment should begin within 24 hours of ingestion. If the concentration of acetaminophen in the specimen collected 4 hours after ingestion is greater than 150mcg/ml, therapy should be begun using N-acetylcysteine. N-acetylcysteine is believed to prevent hepatotoxicity because its sulfhydryl groups act as a glutathione substitute, binding to the metabolite. N-acetylcysteine (Mucomyst, Mead Johnson), available as a 20 percent solution, is administered orally, diluted 1:4 with a soft drink or grapefruit juice to mask its taste (Smilkstein, M.J. et al., N. Engl. J. Med. 319, 1557-1562, 1988). The most common side effect of N-acetylcysteine therapy is vomiting; if vomiting occurs within one hour of administration of a dose, repeat dose. Liver function tests should be done to follow the patient. Contact the Rocky Mountain Poison Center, Denver, Colorado (1-800-525-6115) for the most recent information on acetylcysteine therapy. (Prescott, L.F. and Critchley, J.A., Ann. Rev. Pharmacol. Toxicol. 23, 87-101, 1983).

An algorithm for the treatment of acetaminophen overdose is given in the next Figure;(Hall,A. and Rumack, B., Amer. Family Phys.33,(5),110, 1986):

Treatment for Acetaminophen Overdose

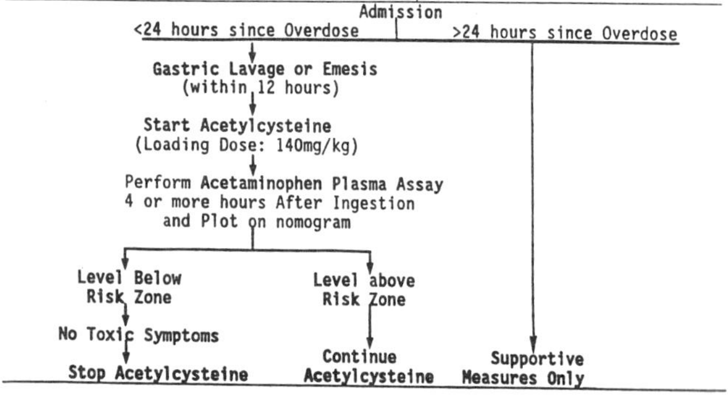

ACETAMINOPHEN/CODEINE

(Tylenol/Codeine [McNeil]; Capital/Codeine [Carnrick]; Empracet/Codeine [Burroughs-Wellcome]; Phenaphen/Codeine [Robins]; also available as generic)

USES: **Acetaminophen/codeine** is used to relieve **mild to moderate pain.** Acetaminophen with codeine produces greater analgesic effect than that produced by either acetaminophen or higher doses of codeine alone.

DOSAGE FORMS: Dosage forms of selected acetaminophen/codeine drugs are given in the next Table:

Dosage Forms of Selected Acetaminophen/Codeine Drugs

Drug	Acetaminophen(mg)	Codeine Phosphate (mg)
Tylenol/Codeine (McNeil) #1,tabs	300	7.5
Tylenol/Codeine (McNeil) #2,tabs	300	15
Tylenol/Codeine (McNeil) #3,tabs	300	30
Tylenol/Codeine (McNeil) #4,tabs	300	60

DOSAGE: Adults: 1-2 of #1, #2, #3, or 1 of #4 every 4 hours as needed. Not recommended for children under 3 years. Dosage of codeine by weight, 0.25-1.0mg/kg/dose. See CODEINE for dosage in various conditions.
Elixir(McNeil): Codeine phosphate 12mg, acetaminophen 120mg per 5ml; alcohol 7%. Adults: 15ml every 4 hours as needed. Children: Under 3 years, not recommended. 3-6 years, 5ml; 7-12 years, 10ml, both 3-4 times daily.

PRECAUTIONS: Use with caution in head injury, increased intracranial pressure, acute abdominal conditions, impaired renal, hepatic, thyroid or adrenocortical function, prostatic hypertrophy or urethral stricture.

ADVERSE EFFECTS: Dizziness, sedation, nausea, vomiting, constipation, urinary retention, rash, respiratory depression, hepatoxicity with overdose.

DRUG INTERACTIONS: Effects are potentiated with alcohol, CNS depressants, monoamine oxidase inhibitors, tricyclic antidepressants, and anticholinergics.

ACETAZOLAMIDE
(Diamox)

USES: Acetazolamide is a **carbonic anhydrase(CA) inhibitor** as illustrated in the next reaction: $CO_2+H_2O \xrightleftharpoons{(CA)} HCO_3+H^+$; uses are given in the next Table:

Uses of Acetazolamide (Diamox)
Glaucoma: Acetazolamide decreases aqueous humor
Open-Angle (Non-Congestive, Chronic Simple)
Secondary Glaucoma
Short-Term Preoperative Therapy to lower Intraocular Pressure in Angle-Closing (Obstructive, Narrow-Angle) Glaucoma when delay of surgery is desired.
Epilepsy: Adjunct to other anticonvulsants
Edema: Secondary to congestive heart failure or drug therapy
Hydrocephalus
Acute High Altitude Sickness:

Acute High Altitude Sickness: When acetazolamide is given before and for a short time after acute exposure to high altitude, the incidence and severity of acute mountain sickness may be reduced. Acetazolamide does not prevent acute altitude sickness, but shortens the time of acclimatization. Acetazolamide is indicated in those who are susceptible to acute mountain sickness and in those who must ascend rapidly. It does not prevent the development of pulmonary or cerebral edema. It has little, if any, effect after symptoms have developed.

DOSAGE FORMS: Tabs: 125, 250mg; Caps: (Sustained Release): 500mg; Vials (Sodium): 500mg/5ml for IV

DOSAGE: Acetazolamide is administered orally; acetazolamide sodium is preferably administered by direct IV injection. Dosage of acetazolamide is given in the next Table:

Dosage of Acetazolamide

Condition	Age	Route	Dosage
Glaucoma(Dec. Aqueous Humor) Open-Angle Glaucoma	Adults	Oral	250mg, 1-4 times daily. or 500mg or extended-release capsules once or twice daily
Secondary Glaucoma and Preoperatively in Adults with Acute Angle-Closure Glaucoma	Adults	Oral	250mg every four hours or 250mg, twice daily or 500mg initially, followed by 125-250mg every four hours
	Adults	IV or IM	500mg; repeat, if necessary in 2-4 hours
Glaucoma	Children	Oral	8-30mg/kg or 300-900mg/m^2 daily in 3 divided doses
Acute Glaucoma	Children	IV or IM	5-10mg/kg every 6 hours
Seizures(Adjunct to other Anticonvulsants)	Children & Adults	Oral	8-30mg/kg daily in 1-4 divided doses; max. 1g/day
Edema (Secondary to CHF)	Children	Oral, IV	5mg/kg or 150mg/m^2, once daily in the A.M.
	Adults	Oral	250-375mg daily in the A.M.
Hydrocephalus	Children	Oral	20-25mg/kg/day orally in 2 or 3 divided doses
Acute High Altitude Sickness	Adults	Oral	250mg every 8-12 hours or 500mg every 24 hours as extended-release caps. Begin 24-48 hours before and continue during ascent; continue at high altitude, as necessary.

ADVERSE EFFECTS: Adverse effects are dose related; GI: Nausea, vomiting, diarrhea; CNS: Drowsiness, paresthesias, muscle weakness; Hematologic: Bone marrow depression; Renal and Metabolic: Dysuria, renal calculi, elevated serum uric acid.

PHARMACOKINETICS: Following oral administration, peak in 1-3 hours; excreted unchanged by kidney.

DRUG INTERACTIONS: Predisposes to salicylate toxicity. Salicylates greatly increase acetazolamide levels. Excretion of procainamide, quinidine, and possibly tricyclic antidepressants may be decreased.

ACETYLCYSTEINE
(Mucomyst)

USES: Uses of acetylcysteine are given in the next Table:

Uses of Acetylcysteine
Antidote for Acetaminophen Overdose
Mucolytic Agent in Adjunctive Treatment of Acute and Chronic Bronchopulmonary Disorders
Meconium Ileus Equivalent in Cystic Fibrosis

Acetylcysteine is a derivative of the amino acid, L-cysteine and is a reducing agent.

DOSAGE FORMS: Oral Inhalation, Intratracheal Instillation and Oral Sol'n: 10% (100mg/ml) and 20% (200mg/ml)

DOSAGE: As an antidote for acetaminophen overdose, acetylcysteine is administered orally as a 5% solution; dilute 20% solution with 1 part 20% solution and 3 parts cola soft drink, Fresca, other soft drinks, grapefruit juice or orange juce. If administered via a gastric tube or Miller-Abbott tube, water may be used as diluent.

As a mucolytic agent, acetylcysteine, as a 10-20% solution, is usually administered by nebulization, direct application, or by intratracheal instillation.

Dosage of acetylcysteine is given in the next Table:

Dosage of Acetylcysteine

Condition	Age	Route	Dosage
Antidote for Acetaminophen Overdose	Adults or Children	Oral or Nasogastric Tube	140mg/kg followed by 70mg/kg every 4h for a total of 18 doses. Example: 10kg child; Loading Dose: 28ml of 5% sol'n; Maintenance Dose: 14ml of 5% sol'n every 4h (Smilkstein, M.J. et al., NEJM 319, 1557-1562, 1988).
Mucolytic Agent	Adults or Children	Nebulizer	3-5ml of 20% sol'n or 6-10ml of 10% sol'n, 3 or 4 times daily or 1-10ml of 20% sol'n or 2-20ml of the 10% sol'n, every 2-6h.
		Closed Tent	Heavy mist may require up to 300ml of 10% or 20% sol'n.
		Direct Instillation.	1-2ml of 10-20% sol'n, as often as every hour
		Intratracheal Instill.	1-2ml of 10-20% sol'n, every 1-4 hrs.
Meconium Ileus Equivalent	Children	Oral or Rectal	5-30ml, given 3-6x per day orally or rectally

ADVERSE EFFECTS: Toxicity: nebulized or intratracheal installation: local irritation; may cause bronchospasm, stomatitis, rhinorrhea, nausea. Hemoptysis may occur with prolonged use. Oral administration: nausea, vomiting, diarrhea, dyspepsia, and skin rashes.

ACNE, TREATMENT

Treatment of acne is given in the next Table(Buxton, P.K., Brit. Med.J. 296, 41-45, 1988; Murphy, G.M. and Greaves, M.W., Brit. Med. J. 296, 546-548, 1988):

Treatment of Acne
First Line:
"Facial sauna"
Topical Treatment
Benzoyl peroxide
Salicylic acid
Tetracycline by mouth for several months
Second Line:
Topical vitamin A acid
Topical antibiotics
Ultraviolet light
Third Line:
Oral retinoids for 3-4 months

Acne vulgaris, the common type of acne, occurs most often during puberty, affecting 30-40% of boys peaking between the ages of 18 and 19 years, and slightly less common in females, peaking between the ages of 16 and 18 years. In most adolescents, acne clears spontaneously with minimal scarring.

"Facial Sauna": The patient should hold a hot wet towel on the face, followed by gentle washing with a plain soap.

Topical Treatment: There are topical preparations, benzoyl peroxide, salicylic acid, which act as keratolytics, dissolving the keratin plug of the comedone.

Tetracycline: The mainstay of treatment is oral tetracycline; tetracycline is given for the first week, 1g daily, then 500mg (250mg,twice daily) on an empty stomach. Minocycline or doxycycline are alternative drugs for therapy. Improvement may not be apparent for several months.

Erythromycin is an alternative to tetracycline, and co-trimoxazole can be used for gram-negative folliculitis.

The growth of the bacteria, Propionobacterium acnes is inhibited by these antibiotics.

Topical Vitamin A: Vitamin A, as a cream or gel, is helpful in some patients.

Topical Antibiotics: Erythromycin, topical tetracycline in N-desylmethyl-sulfoxide, meclocycline sulfosalicylate, clindamycin lotion (1%) have been used topically.

Ultraviolet light: Ultraviolet light therapy is less effective than natural sunlight but is helpful for extensive acne.

Retinoids: For severe cases resistant to other treatment, the synthetic vitamin A derivative, isotretinoin, is very effective and clear most cases in a few months. Isotretinoin is teratogenic so must not be given in pregnancy. Isotretinoin reduces the size of sebaceous glands by 90% in the first month of treatment.

ACQUIRED IMMUNODEFICIENCY SYNDROME (AIDS); TREATMENT OF OPPORTUNISTIC INFECTIONS

Opportunistic Infections: The majority of morbidity and mortality seen in AIDS patients is primarily related to overwhelming infection that is primarily of protozoal, viral, mycobacterial and fungal origin; bacterial infections are much less frequent except in children. Opportunistic infections in AIDS and typical syndrome(s) are given in the next Table: (Lotze, M.T., AIDS Research 2, No. 2, 141-148,1986):

Opportunistic Infections in AIDS

Agent	Typical Syndrome(s)
Viruses	
Cytomegalovirus	GI Bleeding and Perforation, Diarrhea, Proctitis, Enteritis, Chorioretinitis, Hepatitis, Lymphadenopathy
Epstein-Barr Virus	Lymphadenopathy, Lymphoma(?)
Hepatitis B & Non-A, Non-B Hepatitis	Hepatitis
Herpes Virus, Hominis	Mucosal and Cutaneous Ulcers (especially Perirectal) Localized
Herpes Zoster	Disseminated Skin Lesions
Bacteria	
Salmonella Shigella Campylobacter Chlamydia Neisseria Gonorrheae Treponema Pallidum	Gay Bowel Syndrome (Proctocolitis): Extensive Diarrhea and Local Bleeding
Mycobacteria	
Avium-Intracellulare	Hepatosplenomegaly, Lymphadenopathy, Enterocolitis, Weight Loss & Debilitation Pneumonitis
Tuberculosis	Pneumonia, Draining Lesions
Fungi	
Candida Albicans	Stomatitis, Esophagitis, Enterocolitis, GI Bleeding
Cryptococcus Neoformans	Meningitis, Peritoneal Masses and Peritonitis
Histoplasma Capsulatum	Hepatosplenomegaly
Protozoa	
Pneumocystis Carinii	Pneumonia
Cryptosporidium	Enterocolitis, Gay Bowel Syndrome
Entamoeba Histolytica	Gay Bowel Syndrome (Proctocolitis)
Giardia Lamblia	Gay Bowel Syndrome (Proctocolitis)
Toxoplasma Gondii	Encephalitis, Chorioretinitis, Lymphadenopathy

ACQUIRED IMMUNODEFICIENCY SYNDROME (AIDS) (Cont.)

Diarrhea is one of the main symptoms of AIDS and can be related to numerous pathogens.

Mycobacterium avium-intracellulare(MAI) is the most common bacterial complication.

The parasite, P. carini pneumonia develops in 60 to 85 percent of AIDS patients.

The most common fungal infection in AIDS is candidiasis; cryptococcus neoformans is the most common central nervous system fungal pathogen.

More than 90% of patients with AIDS die within 12 months of their first major AIDS-related opportunistic infection.

Opportunistic infections in AIDS, arranged by syndrome, are given in the next Table; (Adler, M.W., Brit.Med.J. 294, 1145-1147, May 2,1987):

Opportunistic Infections in AIDS

Syndrome (Features)	Protozoa	Viruses	Bacteria	Fungi
Lung (Cough, shortness of breath, fever, hypoxia; chest X-ray infiltrates)	P. carinii pneumonia	Cytomegalovirus Herpes simplex virus	Mycobacteria* Str. pneumoniae H. influenzae M. catarrhalis Group B streptococcus	Cryptococcus
Central Nervous System(CNS) (Meningitis/ encephalitis or focal signs)	Toxoplasma	Cytomegalovirus Herpes simplex virus Progressive multifocal leucoencephalopathy(papovavirus)	Mycobacteria*	Aspergillus Crytococcus Candida
Gut (Dysphagia High Volume diarrhea Bloody diarrhea/ colitis	Crytosporidium Isospora belli Microsporidia	Cytomegalovirus Herpes simplex virus	Mycobacterium avium intracellulare M. tuberculosis Salmonella	Candida
Pyrexia of undetermined origin (Fever, Weight Loss ± lymphadenopathy		Consider all pathogens & focal or disseminated infection		

*M tuberculosis and atypical mycobacteria.

ACQUIRED IMMUNODEFICIENCY SYNDROME (AIDS) (Cont.)

TREATMENT: See Zidovudine for treatment of HIV.

Treatment of infectious organisms complicating HIV infection involves the organisms listed in the next Table:

Treatment of Infectious Organisms
Protozoa
Viruses
Fungi
Bacteria

Protozoa Infections: Treatment of protozoa infections is given in the next Table; (Weller, I.V.D., Brit. Med. J. 295, 200-203, July 18, 1987):

Treatment of Protozoal Infections

Infection	Drug	Dosage	Side Effects
Pneumocystis Carinii Pneumonia	Trimethoprim-sulfamethoxazole	Based on 20mg/kg/day of Trimethoprim; I.V. divided into 3 or 4 doses, then oral, Duration: 14-21 days.	Nausea, vomiting, headche, fever, rash, marrow suppression with neutropenia or both, nephritis, Stephens-Johnson syndrome, hyperbilirubinemia
	Pentamidine isethionate	4mg/kg/day; I.V. as slow single daily, infuse over 1-2 hrs. Duration: 14-21 days.	Hypotension, hypoglycemia, renal failure, hepatitis, marrow suppression with neutropenia, thrombocytopenia or both
	Pentamidine mesylate (Not available in U.S.A.)	2-5mg/kg/day; Infusion Duration: 14-21 days	
	Trimetrexate with Leucovorin rescue (Experimental)	30mg per sq. meter, IV bolus daily, Duration: 21 days; 20 mg per sq. meter, IV bolus or orally every six hrs. Duration: 23 days	Minimal toxicity with transient neutropenia or thrombocytopenia and transaminase.
Toxoplasmosis	Sulfadoxine plus Pyrimethamine	100mg/kg daily in 4 divided doses; Oral, Duration: indefinitely. 25mg daily; Oral, Duration: Indefinitely	As for sulphonamides
	Clindamycin	500mg four times daily; Oral, Duration: Indefinitely	
Isosporiasis	Trimethoprim-Sulfamethoxazole: 16mg Trimethoprim, 80mg Sulfamethoxazole	2 tablets four times daily; Oral, Duration: indefinitely	As for sulphonamides

ACQUIRED IMMUNODEFICIENCY SYNDROME (AIDS) (Cont.)

Pneumocystis Carinii Pneumonia(PCP): The most common cause of death in patients with AIDS is PCP. Drugs used in the treatment of PCP are given in the next Table; (Hughes, W.T., N. Engl. J. Med. 317, 1020-1023, Oct. 15, 1987):

Drugs Used in Treatment of Pneumocystis Carinii Pneumonia(PCP)	
Usual:	Trimethoprim-sulfamethoxazole
	Pentamidine isethionate
Investigational:	Trimetrexate with leucovorin rescue
	Pyrimethamine-sulfadoxine (Fansidar)
	Dapsone (Diaminodiphenylsulfone) alone or in combination with Trimethoprim
	Difluoromethylornithine (ornithine decarboxylase inhibitor eflornithine hydrochloride)

Prophylaxis: The management of AIDS should include prophylaxis since about 75% of patients with AIDS will acquire PCP, 25% will die and 30% to 40% of those who recover will have one or more recurrent episodes.

For prophylaxis, give trimethoprim-sulfamethoxazole one double-strength tablet twice daily on three consecutive days per week (Hughes, W.T. et al., N. Engl. J. Med. 316, 1627-1632, 1987). Trimethoprim-sulfamethoxazole is cheaper and more convenient than pentamidine, and may be effective prophylaxis against other infections (Wormser, G.P. et al., Arch. Intern. Med. 151, 688-692, 1991). For those who cannot take trimethoprim-sulfamethoxazole, inhalation of pentamidine, which avoids systemic toxicity should be considered (Montgomery, A.B. et al., Lancet 2, 480-483, 1987). Pentamidine is effective for both primary and secondary prophylaxis of PCP in patients with AIDS (Hirschel, B. et al., N. Engl. J. Med. 324, 1079-1083, 1991; Leoung, G.S. et al., N. Engl. J. Med. 323, 769-775, 1990). Fansidar (pyrimethane-sulfadoxine) is similar to trimethoprim-sulfamethoxazole and has been effective (Gottlieb, M. et al., Lancet 2, 398-399, 1984). Dapsone is effective prophylactically (Metroka, C.E. et al., Third International Conference on AIDS, Wash.,D.C., June 1-5, 1987, abstract).

Treatment of PCP: The two drugs in general use are trimethoprim-sulfamethoxazole and pentamidine isethionate; these drugs are equally effective.

I.V. trimethoprim-sulfamethoxazole is usually given for three weeks; however, if after 1-2 weeks fever and symptoms abate and blood gas values improve, then give trimethoprim-sulfamethoxazole by mouth. Side effects may occur, typically after seven to 10 days; decrease in dosage of sulfamethoxazole did not result in a decrease in side-effects (McLean, I. et al., Lancet 2, 858, Oct. 10, 1987). Folinic acid (15mg on alternate days) is used to prevent cytopenia.

Pentamidine: If side effects of trimethoprim-sulfamethoxazole are severe, use pentamidine; give pentamidine by slow I.V. infusion, avoid hypotension and painful intramuscular sterile abscesses.

An aerosol preparation of pentamidine is being developed. The aerosol preparation delivers the drug to the lung with only one percent absorbed by the body thus eliminating systemic toxic side effects (Montgomery, A.B., et al., Lancet 2, 480-483, 1987; Conte, J.E., Ann. Intern. Med. 101, 495, Oct. 1987).

Dapsone-Trimethoprim: Patients with mild first episodes of PCP were treated with oral dapsone,100mg/day, plus oral trimethoprim 20mg/kg/day, given for 21 days; the control group received oral trimethoprim-sulfamethoxazole. Both treatments were equally effective (>90%), and dapsone-trimethoprim was better tolerated (Medina, I. et al., Program and Abstracts of the Interscience Conference on Antimicrobial Agents and Chemotherapy 27, 261, Oct. 1987). The major adverse effects of dapsone-trimethoprim have been methemoglobinemia and anemia (Leoung, G.S. et al., Ann. Intern. Med. 105, 45, 1986). Dapsone may cause fatal hemolysis in G6PD deficient patients.

Trimetrexate with leucovorin rescue has shown initial promise in treating PCP infections in patients with AIDS (Allegra, C.J., N. Engl. J. Med. 317, 978-985, Oct. 15, 1987). The NIH soon will begin a year-long study to compare trimetrexate against the standard treatment.

Prophylaxis After First Attacks of Pneumocystis Carinii: Use low dose trimethoprim-sulfamethoxazole or pyrimethamine-sulfadoxine (Fansidar) one tablet weekly (Gottlieb, M. et al., Lancet 2, 398-399, 1984; Flanegan, T. et al., N. Engl. J. Med. 317, 1155, Oct. 29, 1987), but sulphonamide sensitivity may occur with both drugs. Pentamidine inhaled once every two weeks after an induction phase of 5 doses over 14 days is effective secondary prophylaxis (Montaner, J.S.G. et al., Ann. Intern. Med. 114, 948-953, 1991).

ACQUIRED IMMUNODEFICIENCY SYNDROME (AIDS) (Cont.)

Toxoplasmosis: Cerebral toxoplasmosis is the most common manifestation of toxoplasma infection.

Sulphadiazine plus pyrimethamine:The combination of sulphadiazine plus pyrimethamine is effective if treatment is started early. Sulfadoxine (100mg/kg daily, max. 6g daily in 4 divided doses) plus pyrimethaprim (75mg on day 1, 50mg on day 2, 25mg daily thereafter) continue treatment indefinitely.

Prophylaxis: Pyrimethamine-sulfadoxine (Fansidar)

Clindamycin: Clindamycin has been substituted for sulphadiazine plus pyrimethamine.

Dexamethaxone: Dexamethasone has been used to reduce cerebral edema.

Isosporiasis: Isosporiasis is treated with trimethoprim-sulfamethoxazole; relapses occur in half of all cases.

Cryptosporidiosis: Responses have been obtained with spiramycin 1g orally, 4 times daily and interleukin-2. Other drugs that have been used are 2-difluoromethyl ornithine and oral bovine transfer factor.

Codeine phosphate, loperamide and other drugs may be given for symptomatic relief.

Viral Infections: Treatment of viral infections is given in the next Table; (Weller, I.V.D., Brit. Med. J. 275, 200-203, July 18, 1987):

Treatment of Viral Infections

Infection	Drug	Dosage	Side Effects
Herpes Simplex	Acyclovir	5-10mg/kg/8 h; IV, 10-14 days	Minimal
	Acyclovir	200mg/5 times daily; Oral, 10-14 days	Minimal
	Prophylaxis	200mg/4 times daily (lower frequency possible); Oral, Duration:? Indefinite	Minimal
Varicella Zoster	Acyclovir	10mg/kg/8 h; I.V, 10 days	Minimal
	Acyclovir	400mg/4 times daily; Oral, 10 days	Minimal
		800mg/4 times daily being evaluated	
	Vidarabine (Adenine Arabinoside)	10mg/kg daily; I.V., 5 days	G.I.; CNS; Hematologic
Cytomegalovirus	Ganciclovir	7.5mg/kg daily in 3 divided doses.	Thrombocytopenia, Azotemia, Marrow Suppression with Neutropenia

Herpes Simplex: Acyclovir is the drug of choice for the treatment of severe mucocutaneous and systemic infections with herpes simplex.

Prophylaxis: Prophylaxis is used after severe infection and in patients with chronic HIV infection and increasing severity and frequency of recurrences.

Varicella-Zoster: Acyclovir or vidarabine are used to treat varicella-zoster infections.

Cytomegalovirus: Ganciclovir is used to treat cytomegalovirus infections.

ACQUIRED IMMUNODEFICIENCY SYNDROME (AIDS) (Cont.)

Fungal Infections: Treatment of fungal infections is given in the next Table:

Treatment of Fungal Infections

Infection	Drug	Dosage	Side Effects
Dermatophytic	Imidazole Creams		
Oral Candida	Nystatin	500,000 units to 1 cup water, 4 times daily; Rinse mouth as long as possible, Duration: 48 h. after symptoms or culture neg.	G.I., Diarrhea, nausea, vomiting
Esophageal Candidiasis	Ketoconazole	200-400mg once daily; Oral, Long-term	Monitor liver function
Cryptococcus Neoformans	Amphotericin B plus Flucytosine	0.25 to 1mg/kg daily; I.V., >6 wks. plus 50-110mg/kg daily; Oral, >6 wks.	Common and potentially dangerous
Histoplasmosis, Disseminated	Amphotericin B	0.25 to 1mg/kg daily; I.V., >6 wks.	Common and potentially dangerous
Aspergillus Species	Amphotericin B	0.25 to 1mg/kg daily; I.V., >6 wks.	Common and potentially dangerous

Oral Candida: Oral candida is often asymptomatic in its early stages and treatment may not be required. In more severe infections, mystatin rinse is effective.

Esophageal Candidiasis: Ketoconazole may be the drug of choice for esophageal candidiasis.

Cryptococcus Neoformans: Cryptococcal and other systemic fungal infections require treatment with amphotericin, 0.25mg/kg daily increasing to 0.5mg/kg daily and finally to 1mg/kg daily if necessary for at least 6 weeks with flucytosine.

Histoplasmosis: Initially, amphotericin B is used followed by ketoconazole suppression to prevent relapse.

Aspergillus Species: Use amphotericin B.

See **ANTIFUNGAL DRUGS** and individual agents, including **AMPHOTERICIN B, FLUCONAZOLE, FLUCYTOSINE, KETOCONAZOLE AND NYSTATIN.**

Bacterial infections: Treatment of bacterial infections is given in the next Table:

Treatment of Bacterial Infections

Infection	Drug
Bacterial pneumonia	Conventional Antibiotics
Skin infections	Conventional Antibiotics
Salmonella infections	Conventional Antibiotics
Mycobacterium Tuberculosis	Triple Drug Therapy: Isoniazid, Rifampin, and Ethambutol
Mycobacterium Avium-Intracellulare(MAI)	Ansamycin; Clofazamine and Cycloserine. Ethionamide and Ethambutol are effective only at high concentrations. Resistant to isoniazid and Rifampin.
Gum and Periodontal Disease	Metronidazole

Bacterial Pneumonias and Skin Infections: Use conventional antibiotics.

Mycobacterium Tuberculosis: Use conventional therapy.

Mycobacterium Avium Intracellulare: These organisms are resistant to conventional therapy.

Gum and Periodontal Disease: Gum and periodontal disease respond to local treatment with antibacterial mouthwashes or oral metronidazole.

ACQUIRED IMMUNODEFICIENCY SYNDROME (AIDS) (Cont.)

Summary of Drugs Used in Treating Infectious Complications of AIDS: Drugs used in infectious complications of AIDS are listed in the next Table; (Ratafia, M. and Scott, F.I., American Clinical Products Review, pgs. 26-29, May, 1987):

Summary of Drugs Used in Treating Infectious Complication of AIDS

Aspergillus
- Amphotericin
- Flucytosine

Candida albicans
- Disseminated disease
  - Amphotericin
- Esophagitis
  - Ketoconazole
- Oral thrush
  - Clotrimazole
  - Nystatin
- Transient fungemia
  - Amphotericin

Coccidioides immitis
- Amphotericin
- Ketoconazole

Cryptococcus neoformans
- Meningeal
  - Amphotericin
  - Flucytosine
- Nonmeningeal
  - Ketoconazole

Cryptosporidium
- Spiramycin

Cytomegalovirus
- Acyclovir

Giardia lamblia
- Metronidazole
- Quinacrine hydrochloride

Herpes simplex virus
- Acyclovir
- Vidarabine

Herpes Zoster
- Acyclovir
- Vidarabine

Histoplasma capsulatum
- Amphotericin

Isospora belli
- Trimethoprim

Mycobacterium avium-intracellulare
- Ansamycin
- Capreomycin
- Clofazimine
- Cycloserine
- Ethambutol hydrochloride
- Ethionamide
- Isoniazid
- Pyrazinamide
- Pyridoxine hydrochloride
- Rifampin
- Streptomycin

Pneumocystis Carinii Pneumonia(PCP)
- Trimethoprim-sulfamethoxazole (TMP-SMZ)
- Pentamidine isethionate

Petriellidium boydii
- Miconazole

Toxoplasma gondii
- Sulfadiazine
- Pyrimethamine

ACYCLOVIR
(Zovirax)

USES: **Acyclovir** is a **synthetic purine nucleoside** analog with antiviral activity; uses are given in the following Table:

Uses of Acyclovir
Mucosal and Cutaneous Herpes Simplex (HSV-1 and HSV-2)
Treatment of Initial Episode
Treatment of Recurrent Episodes
Herpes Simplex Encephalitis
Varicella Zoster Infections
Treatment of Initial Episode (Chickenpox)
Treatment of Recurrent Episodes (Herpes Zoster)
CMV Prevention
EBV Infections (?)

Mechanism of Action: Acyclovir interferes with viral DNA synthesis and inhibits viral replication.

DOSAGE FORMS: Caps: 200mg; Susp: 200mg/5ml; Parenteral: 500mg, 1gm; Topical: 5% ointment.

DOSAGE: Dosage of acyclovir for treatment of Herpes Simplex Virus and Varicella-Zoster Virus is given in the next Table (The Medical Letter 32, 73-78, August 10, 1990; CDC, "1989 Sexually Transmitted Diseases Treatment Guidelines," MMWR 38(S-8), 1-40, Sept. 1, 1989):

Dosage of Acyclovir

Condition	Age	Route	Dosage
Genital Herpes-First Episode	Adult	Oral, Topical, IV	Usual (moderate symptoms): 200mg orally 5x daily for 10 days; Mild symptoms: 5% ointment 0.5 inch ribbon/4 sq. inch every 3 hours up to 6x daily for 7 days - apply with glove; Severe symptoms: 5mg/kg IV every 8 hours for 5 days.
Genital Herpes-Recurrence	Adult	Oral	200mg orally 5x daily or 800mg orally 2x daily for 5 days.
Genital Herpes-Suppressive Therapy for Frequent Recurrence	Adult	Oral	200mg orally 2-5x daily or 400mg orally 2x daily for 1 yr or longer (Kaplowitz, L.G. et al., JAMA 265, 747-751, February 13, 1991).
Herpes Proctitis-First Episode	Adult	Oral	400mg orally 5x daily for 10 days.
Mucocutaneous Herpes-Immunocompromised Host	Adult	Oral, Topical	Moderate symptoms: 400mg orally 5x daily for 7 days; Mild symptoms: 5% ointment 0.5 inch ribbon/4 sq. inch every 3 hours up to 6x daily for 7 days - apply with glove;
	Adult Children	IV	Severe symptoms: 5mg/kg IV every 8 hours for 7 days.
Herpes Simplex Encephalitis	Children	IV	10mg/kg every 8 hours for 10-21 days.
Herpes Simplex Neonatal	Neonate	IV	10mg/kg every 8 hours for 10 days.
Varicella-Immunocompromised	Adult Children	IV	500mg/sq. meter every 8 hours for 7 days.
Herpes Zoster Immunocompromised	Adult Children	IV	10mg/kg every 8 hours for 7 days.
Herpes Zoster Normal Host	Adult	Oral	800mg 5x daily for 7-10 days.

Acyclovir has been used successfully for the prevention of cytomegalovirus (CMV) infection in immunocompromised hosts following renal and bone marrow transplants (Balfour, H.H. et al., NEJM 320, 1381-1387, 1989; Meyers, J.D. et al., NEJM 318, 70-75, 1988). Efficacy of acyclovir for treatment of Epstein-Barr Virus (EBV) infections is unproven. Acyclovir treatment of chronic fatigue syndrome did not show benefit over placebo (Straus, S.E. et al., NEJM 319, 1692-1698, 1988).

ACYCLOVIR (Cont.)
PHARMACOKINETICS: Absorption: 15-30% of oral dose is absorbed. Peak: 1.5-2.5 hours after oral dose. Distribution: Widely distributed, CSF levels are 50% of serum concentrations. Half-Life: initial phase, 0.34 hours; terminal phase, 2.1-3.5 hours. Excretion: Primarily excreted unchanged in the urine. Dosage adjustment necessary in renal failure.
ADVERSE EFFECTS: GI: Nausea, vomiting, diarrhea (oral therapy); CNS: Headache (13%), encephalopathy (lethargy, confusion, seizures, coma) occurs rarely; Renal: Impaired renal function (5-10%) - frequency minimized by slow IV infusion (over 1 hour). May progress to acute renal failure. Adequate hydration is needed to prevent renal tubular crystallization. Extravasation may cause severe local reactions.

ADENOSINE
(Adenocard)
USES: **Adenosine** is an **endogenous nucleoside;** uses are given in the following Table:

Uses of Adenosine
Acute Termination of Supraventricular Tachycardia (SVT)
Differentiating SVT with Aberration from Ventricular Tachycardia (VT)

Adenosine has recently been released in the United States for treatment of SVT. Adenosine triphosphate (ATP) has been available in Europe for several years and is considered the drug of choice for treatment of SVT; the pharmacologically active metabolite is adenosine. Adenosine has similar efficacy to that of Verapamil when used to treat SVT (approx. 90%) but onset of action is faster and adverse reactions are minor and of short duration (DiMarco, J.P. et al., "Adenosine for Paroxysmal Supraventricular Tachycardia: Dose Ranging and Comparison with Verapamil," Ann. Intern. Med. 113, 104-110, July, 1990).
Mechanism of Action: Inhibits sinus node automaticity, depresses atrioventricular nodal conduction and refractoriness, with lengthened PR interval.
DOSAGE FORMS: Injection: 3mg/ml, 2ml vials.
DOSAGE: Adenosine is administered by rapid intravenous bolus. Dosage is given in the next Table (Pinski, S.L. and Maloney, J.D., Cleveland Clinic J. of Med. 57, 383-388, June, 1990; Overholt, E.D. et al., Amer. J. Cardiol. 61, 336-340, 1988):

Dosage of Adenosine

Age	Dosage
Adults	6mg IV bolus. If no response in 30 seconds, increase dosage to 9mg then 12mg.
Children	37.5 micrograms/kg IV bolus. If no response in 30 seconds, increase dosage by 37.5 micrograms/kg; maximum dosage: 375 micrograms/kg.

PHARMACOKINETICS: Metabolism: actively transported into cells and degraded; Half-Life: less than 10 seconds.
DRUG INTERACTIONS: Theophylline: blocks the effects of adenosine (competitive antagonist of adenosine receptors; Dipyridamole enhances effects of adenosine (blocks uptake into cells by binding surface receptors).
ADVERSE EFFECTS: Mild to moderate symptoms including facial flushing, chest pressure, chest pain or dyspnea occur in 36% of patients. Hypotension is rare (mild to moderate, 0.8%; severe, none). Arrhythmias may occur including ventricular ectopy (33%), sinus bradycardia (5%), and atrioventricular block (3%). SVT recurs in 9% (DiMarco, J.P. et al., Ann. Intern. Med. 113, 104-110, July, 1990).

ALBUMIN, HUMAN

(Normal Serum ALbumin)

USES: Uses of albumin are given in the next Table:

Uses of Albumin
Hypovolemia
Hypoproteinemia
Severe Burns
Hyperbilirubinemia and Erythroblastosis Fetalis

Hypovolemia: Albumin is used to expand plasma volume and maintain cardiac output in treatment of shock or impending shock (surgery, hemorrhage, trauma, burns).

Hypoproteinemia: In hypoproteinemia, albumin can temporarily compensate for protein deficiencies until the underlying condition is corrected. Conditions associated with hypoproteinemia are as follows: acute nephrotic syndrome, acute hepatic cirrhosis or coma, premature infants, toxemia of pregnancy, anuria, postoperative and T.B. patients. Do not use in chronic nephrosis, chronic cirrhosis or undernourishment.

Severe Burns: Albumin may be used in conjunction with IV infusion solutions and other measures to prevent hemoconcentration and counteract protein deficit created by loss of albumin in exudates.

Hyperbilirubinemia and Erythroblastosis Fetalis: Albumin is used as an adjunct to exchange transfusions; its bilirubin binding capacity reportedly reduces the number of transfusions.

DOSAGE FORMS: Injection; 5% (5g/dl; 0.18mEqNa/ml): 50, 250, 500ml bottles; 25% (25g/dl; 0.15mEq Na/ml): 20, 50, 100ml bottles.

DOSAGE: Albumin solutions are administered by IV infusion. Dosage is given in the next Table:

Dosage of Albumin

Condition	Adult	Dosage
Hypoproteinema	Children or Adults	0.5-1gm/kg/dose. Repeat every 1-2 days as calculated to replace ongoing losses. Administer 5% at <5-10ml/min. Administer 25% at <2ml/min.
Hypovolemic Shock	Children or Adults	0.5-1gm/kg/dose, repeated PRN. Max. dose: 6gm/kg/day. Administer 5% at <2-3ml/min. Administer 25% at <1ml/min.
Hyperbilirubinemia	Children or Adults	4ml(1g) per kg of 25% Albumin 1-2 hours before transfusion

ADVERSE EFFECTS: Adverse effects of albumin occur infrequently. Adverse reactions are caused by allergy or protein overload. Hypotension may occur.

ALBUTEROL

(Proventil, Ventolin)

USES: Uses of albuterol are given in the next Table:

Uses of Albuterol
Bronchodilator: Relief of Bronchospasms
Bronchial Asthma
Chronic Reversible Obstructive Airway Disease
Exercise-Induced Bronchospasm

Albuterol is used as a bronchodilator for relief of bronchospasm in bronchial asthma and chronic reversible obstructive airway disease; albuterol is used to prevent exercise-induced bronchospasm.

Albuterol stimulates beta-adrenergic receptors (relaxation of bronchial and uterine muscles, vasodilation of the arterioles that supply the skeletal muscles, increased heart rate and contractiblity) and has little or no effect on alpha-adrenergic receptors. Albuterol has a greater stimulating effect on bronchial, uterine, and vascular smooth muscles (beta-2 receptors) than on the heart (beta-1 receptors).

The bronchodilator effects of albuterol, compared to that of an anti-cholinergic agent (ipratropium bromide), given by aerosol alone or in sequence in patients with chronic obstructive pulmonary disease, are about equipotent in maximal doses (Easton, P.A. et al., N. Engl. J. Med. 315, 735-739, 1986).

DOSAGE FORMS: Oral Inhalation, Aerosol (Albuterol): 90mcg/dose; Oral Sol'n (Albuterol Sulfate): 2mg/5ml; Tabs: 2, 4mg; Solution for nebulization (Albuterol): 0.5% (5mg/ml).

DOSAGE: Albuterol is administered by oral inhalation; albuterol sulfate is administered orally. Dosage is given in the next Table:

Dosage of Albuterol

Route	Age	Dosage
Inhalation	Adults & Children >12 years	180mcg(2 inhalations) every 4-6 hrs.; 1 minute lapse between inhalations.
Exercise-Induced Bronchospasm	Adults & Children >12 years	180mcg(2 inhalations) 15 minutes before exercise.
Status Asthmaticus (Nebulization)	Adults & Children >12 years	2.5mg (0.5ml) 3 or 4 times daily, dilute to final volume of 3ml; may require 5 or 10mg doses; more frequent doses as needed.
	5-12 years	2.5-5mg (0.5-1.0ml) every 4-6 hours; more frequent doses as needed.
	<5 years	1.25-2.5mg (0.25-0.5ml) every 4-6 hours; more frequent doses as needed.
	By weight	Dose based on weight is 0.15mg/kg (max. 5mg) up to every 20 minutes as needed for acute bronchospasm (Schuh, S. et al., Pediatrics 83 513-518, 1989).
Orally	Adults & Children >12 years	2 or 4mg, 3 or 4 times daily;increase dosage if necessary to a max. of 8mg, 4 times daily
	6-11 years	2mg, 3 or 4 times daily; increase dosage, if necessary to a max. of 24mg daily in divided doses
	2-6 years	0.1mg/kg,3 times daily (not to exceed 2mg, 3 times daily); increase dosage if necessary to a maximum of 0.2mg/kg, 3 times daily (not to exceed 4mg, 3 times daily).
	Geriatric	2mg, 3 or 4 times daily; dosage may be gradually increased to 8mg, 3 or 4 times daily

ADVERSE EFFECTS: Some of the principal adverse effects relate to beta-1 stimulation: tachycardia, palpitation, peripheral vasodilation, tremor and nervousness. Muscle cramps may occur.

ALLOPURINOL
(Zyloprim, Lopurin)

USES: Uses of allopurinol are given in the next Table:

Uses of Allopurinol
Gout
Myeloproliferative Disorders e.g.. Polycythemia Vera, Leukemia, Lymphoma or Secondary to Treatment of these Disorders
Recurrent Calcium Oxalate Renal Calculi

Allopurinol is a competitive inhibitor of the enzyme, xanthine oxidase and thus blocks conversion of hypoxanthine to xanthine and xanthine to uric acid; serum uric acid concentration is decreased.

Gout: Allopurinol is indicated in patients with frequent disabling attacks of gout. Allopurinal is the preferred drug in the treatment of chronic tophaceous gout. The drug is not recommended for the management of asymptomatic hyperuricemia because of possible adverse effects. Allopurinol is used for the management of gout when uricosurics cannot be used because of adverse effects, allergy, or inadequate response; when there are visible tophi or radiographic evidence of uric acid deposits and stones; or when serum urate concentrations are greater than 8.5-9.0mg/dl and a family history of tophi and low urate excretion exists. It is also used for the management of primary or secondary gouty nephropathy with or without secondary oliguria. Allopurinol does not have analgesic or anti-inflammatory activity; thus it has no value in treatment of acute gout attacks.

During the early stages of treatment with allopurinal, the frequency of attacks of gouty arthritis may increase; therefore, colchicine or a nonsteroidal anti-inflammatory drug should be given prophylactically during the initial months of therapy.

Allopurinol is used in genetic disorders of purine metabolism.

Myeloproliferative Disorders: Allopurinol is used prophylactically to reduce uric acid in myeloproliferative neoplastic disorders, especially after cancer chemotherapy or radiation therapy.

Recurrent Calcium Oxalate Renal Calculi: Allopurinol is used in the management of recurrent calcium oxalate renal calculi in males whose urinary urate excretion exceeds 800mg daily and in females whose urinary urate excretion exceeds 750mg daily.

DOSAGE FORMS: Tabs: 100, 300mg

DOSAGE: Allopurinol is administered orally, usually in a single daily dose, preferably after meals. Fluid intake should be sufficient to yield a daily urine output of at least 2 liters and to maintain a neutral or preferably, alkaline urine. Dosage is given in the next Table:

Dosage of Allopurinol

Condition	Age	Dosage
Gout	Adults	100mg once daily; inc. by 100mg at weekly intervals until serum urate conc. falls to 6mg/dl or less or until max. dose of 800mg/dl daily. Usually: mild gout, 200-300mg daily, moderate, 400-600mg daily. Minimum conc. of serum uric acid in 1-3 wks
Myeloproliferative Disorders	Adults	600-800mg daily for 2-3 days beginning 1-2 days before initiating chemotherapy
	<6 years	150mg daily, 50mg 3 times a day for 2-3 days beginning 1-2 days before initiating chemotherapy.
	6-10 yrs.	300mg daily, 100mg, 3 times a day for 2-3 days beginning 1-2 days before initiating chemotherapy.
	Adults or Children	10mg/kg/day, three times a day. Max. dose 600-800mg/day
Recurrent Calcium Oxalate Renal Calculi in Patients with Hyperuricosuria		200-300mg daily; adjust dosage depending on 24-hour urinary urate excretion.

ALLOPURINOL (Cont.)

Dosage based on creatinine clearance is given in the next Table:

Creat. Clear(ml/min)	Maintenance Dosage
0	100mg every 3 days
10	100mg every 2 days
20	100mg Daily
40	150mg Daily
60	200mg Daily
80	250mg Daily

Dosage Based on Creatinine Clearance

PHARMACOKINETICS: Absorption: 80-90%; Metabolism: Allopurinal is metabolized by xanthine oxidase to oxypurinol; oxypurinal also inhibits xanthine oxidase; Half-Life: The half-life of allopurinol is 1-3 hours and that of oxypurinol is 20-30 hours. The long half-life of oxypurinol accounts for the long duration of action of allopurinol; this permits administration of allopurinol once daily. Excretion: Oxypurinal is excreted by the kidney.

ADVERSE EFFECTS: A toxic reaction associated with hypersensitivity may occur; this reaction may be manifested by a diffuse, erythematous, desquamating skin rash, fever, eosinophilia, hepatic and renal dysfunction. Death has occurred in patients with this reaction.

Occasional reactions include nausea, vomiting, diarrhea, abdominal discomfort, metallic taste, drowsiness and headache.

Hepatotoxicity, hematologic and nervous system effects may occur.

Hypoxanthine stones may occur, especially in patients with renal disease.

INTERACTIONS: Allopurinol inhibits the oxidation of mercaptopurine; reduce mercaptopurine to one-third to one-fourth the usual amount. Also, mercaptopurine is a metabolite of azathioprine.

Allopurinal inhibits drugs metabolizing coumarin; give coumarin in lower doses.

LABORATORY: Monitor serum uric acid and serum creatinine and urine output.

ALPRAZOLAM

(Xanax)

USES: Alprazolam is a benzodiazepine that has antianxiety and sedative-hypnotic actions. Uses are given in the next Table:

Uses of Alprazolam
Situational Anxiety
Generalized Anxiety Disorder
Panic Disorder
Agoraphobia (abnormal fear of public places)
Possible use in Major Depressive Episodes

DOSAGE FORMS: Tabs: 0.25, 0.5, 1 and 2mg

DOSAGE: Alprazolam is administered orally; dosage is given in the next Table:

Dosage of Alpazolam

Condition	Age	Dosage
Anxiety	Adults	0.25 to 0.5mg, three times daily; max. daily dose, 4mg
	Elderly or Debilitated	0.25mg, two or three times daily
Panic Disorder or Agoraphobia	Adults	0.5mg three times daily after meals for two days. The dose is increased by adding 0.5 mg to one of the existing doses every two days until 2mg three times daily is given. Increase in dosage is stopped when significant improvements or excessive sedation is observed.

PHARMACOKINETICS: Absorption: Rapid; Time-to-Peak: One to two hours; Protein Binding: 70%; Half-Life: Young males, 11 hours; elderly males, 19 hours. Steady State: 2-5 days when given 3 times daily.

ADVERSE EFFECTS: Frequent: Drowsiness, ataxia. Occasional: Confusion; amnesia; paradoxical excitment; dizziness; withdrawal symptoms, including convulsions on abrupt discontinuance; rebound insomnia or excitement. Rare: Hypotension, blood dyscrasias, jaundice, allergic reactions, paradoxical rage reactions, stuttering. When discontinuing therapy, dosage of the drug should be decreased by no more than 0.5mg every 3 days to prevent withdrawal.

ALUMINUM HYDROXIDE
(Amphojel, AlternaGel and Other brands)

USES: Uses of alumninum hydroxide are given in the next Table:

Uses of Aluminum Hydroxide
Relief of Peptic Ulcer Pain
Promote Healing of Peptic Ulcers
Relief of Acid Indigestion, Heart Burn, and "Sour" Stomach
Esophageal Reflux
Decrease GI Bleeding
Reduce Serum Phosphorus:
Hyperparathyroidism Secondary to Chronic Hemodialysis
Calcinosis Universalis
Prevent Recurrent Phosphate Renal Calculi

Peptic Ulcer: The clinical use of antacids, such as aluminum hydroxide, is based on their ability to increase the pH of gastric secretions from pH 1.3 to pH3.0-pH3.5. Antacid-induced increases in gastric pH inhibit the proteolytic action of pepsin, an effect which is particularly important in patients with peptic ulcer disease.

Aluminum hydroxide is slowly solubilized in the stomach and reacts with hydrochloric acid to form aluminum chloride plus water; other aluminum derivatives are formed. About 17-30% of the aluminum chloride is absorbed and then excreted rapidly by the kidney.

Reduce Serum Phosphate: Aluminum containing antacids combine with dietary phosphate in the intestine forming insoluble, nonabsorbable aluminum phosphate which is excreted in the feces. Note that aluminum carbonate binds phosphate more than aluminum hydroxide.

DOSAGE FORMS: Caps: 475, 500mg; Gel Susp.: 320, 450, 600, 675/5ml; Tabs: 300, 600mg.

DOSAGE: Aluminum hydroxide is administered orally. Duration of action is 20-60 minutes on an empty stomach. If administered 1 hour after meals, acid neutralizing effects may persist up to 3 hours. Dosage is given in the next Table:

Dosage of Aluminum Hydroxide

Condition	Age	Dosage
Peptic Ulcer	Children	5-15ml every 3-6 hours or 1 and 3 hours after meals and just before sleep
	Adults	15-45ml every 3-6 hours or 1 and 3 hours after meals and just before sleep
Prophylaxis of GI Bleeding	Infants	2-5ml/dose every 1-2 hours per nasogastric tube
	Children	5-15ml/dose every 1-2 hours per nasogastric tube
	Adults	30-60ml/dose every hour per nasogastric tube
Hyperphosphatemia (plus Dietary Restriction)	Adults	30-40ml, 3 or 4 times daily
	Pediatric	50-150mg/kg/day, 4-6 times daily to maximum adult dose

ADVERSE EFFECTS: Most common adverse effect is constipation. With prolonged administration, aluminum-containing antacids can cause phosphorus depletion accompanied by extensive calcium loss (Spencer, H. & Kramer, L., J. Nutr. 116, 316-319, 1986).

ALUMINUM HYDROXIDE WITH MAGNESIUM HYDROXIDE
(Maalox, etc.)

USES: Uses of aluminum hydroxide with magnesium hydroxide are given in the next Table:

Uses of Aluminum Hydroxide with Magnesium Hydroxide
Relief of Peptic Ulcer Pain
Promote Healing of Peptic Ulcers
Relief of Acid Indigestion, Heart Burn, and "Sour" Stomach
Esophageal Reflux
Decrease GI Bleeding
Reduce Serum Phosphorus:
Hyperparathyroidism Secondary to Chronic Hemodialysis
Calcinosis Universalis
Prevent Recurrent Phosphate Renal Calculi

Peptic Ulcer: The clinical use of antacids, such as aluminum hydroxide with magnesium hydroxide, is based on their ability to increase the pH of gastric secretions from pH 1.3 to pH 3.0-pH 3.5. Antacid-induced increases in gastric pH inhibit the proteolytic action of pepsin, an effect which is particularly important in patients with peptic ulcer disease.

Aluminum hydroxide with magnesium hydroxide is slowly solubilized in the stomach and reacts with hydrochloric acid to form aluminum chloride plus water; other aluminum derivatives are formed. About 17-30% of the aluminum chloride is absorbed and then excreted rapidly by the kidney.

Reduce Serum Phosphate: Aluminum containing antacids combine with dietary phosphate in the intestine forming insoluble, nonabsorbable aluminum phosphate which is excreted in the feces. Note that aluminum carbonate binds phosphate more than aluminum hydroxide.

DOSAGE FORMS: Many preparations available.

DOSAGE: Aluminum hydroxide with magnesium hydroxide is administered orally. Duration of action is 20-60 minutes on an empty stomach. If administered 1 hour after meals, acid neutralizing effects may persist up to 3 hours. Dosage is given in the next Table:

Dosage of Aluminum Hydroxide with Magnesium Hydroxide

Condition	Age	Dosage
Peptic Ulcer	Children	5-15ml every 3-6 hours or 1 and 3 hours after meals and just before sleep.
	Adults	15-45ml every 3-6 hours or 1 and 3 hours after meals and just before sleep.
Prophylaxis of GI Bleeding	Infants	2-5ml/dose every 1-2 hours per nasogastric tube.
	Children	5-15ml/dose every 1-2 hours per nasogastric tube.
	Adults	30-60ml/dose every hour per nasogastric tube.
Hyperphosphatemia (plus Dietary Restriction)	Adults	30-40ml, 3 or 4 times daily.

ADVERSE EFFECTS: Most common adverse effect is constipation. With prolonged administration, aluminum-containing antacids can cause phosphorus depletion accompanied by extensive calcium loss (Spencer, H. & Kramer, L., J. Nutr. 116, 316-319, 1986).

AMANTADINE

(Symmetrel)

USES: **Amantadine** is used as **prophylaxis** and **symptomatic treatment** of respiratory infections caused by **influenza A** virus strains; it may prevent illness when administered before influenza A virus invades tissue. Prophylaxis should be strongly considered in unvaccinated children and adults at high risk of morbidity and mortality and in infants with life-threatening influenza-associated croup. The drug may be used in conjunction with vaccine.

Amantadine does not protect against influenza B virus infection. Amantadine provides symptomatic relief in Parkinsonian Syndrome. The mechanism of action is unknown but appears unrelated to its action against influenza A.

DOSAGE FORMS: Caps: 100mg; Sol'n: 50mg/5ml

DOSAGE: Amantadine is administered orally preferably in 2 equally divided doses. If insomnia occurs, the last daily dose should be taken several hours before retiring. Dosage is given in the next Table:

Dosage of Amantadine for Prophylaxis and Symptomatic Treatment of Influenza A Infection

Age	Dosage
1-9 Years	4.4-8.8mg/kg daily(max. 150mg daily)
10-64 years	200mg daily
>64 years	100mg daily

Prophylaxis: Institute amantadine prior to or as soon as possible after contact with individual with influenza A virus infection; continue for at least 10 days. If inactivated influenza A virus vaccine is unavailable or contraindicated, continue for up to 90 days if repeated and uncontrolled exposure to influenza A occurs. When amantadine is used in conjunction with inactivated influenza A virus vaccine, the drug is given for 10-21 days after the vaccine is given.

Symptomatic: Continue therapy for 24-48 hours after disappearance of symptoms.

Dosage in Parkinson's Disease: 100mg once or twice daily.

Dosage in Renal Impairment: Maintenance dosage as a function of creatinine clearance is given in the next Table:

Maintenance Dosage and Creatinine Clearance

Creatinine Clearance(ml/min per 1.73m^2)	Maintenance Dosage
> 80	100mg twice daily
60-80	200mg/100mg on alternate days
40-60	100mg once daily
30-40	200mg twice daily
20-30	100mg 3 times daily
10-20	200mg/100mg alternating every 7 days

ADVERSE EFFECTS: Insomnia, nervousness, irritability, fatigue, mental depression, pychoses, orthostatic hypotension and urinary retention. Livedo reticularis occurs in 1-5% of patients receiving amantidine for Parkinsonian Syndrome.

AMIKACIN
(Amikin)

USES: Amikacin is an **aminoglycoside antibiotic** that is often effective for treatment of infections caused by gram-negative strains including some strains of Pseudomonas aeruginosa resistant to other aminoglycosides, e.g., kanamycin, gentamicin, tobramycin and netilmicin. It should generally be reserved for treatment of serious infections caused by susceptible gram-negative strains known or suspected to be resistant to these drugs.

The spectrum of activity is given in the next Table:

Spectrum of Activity of Amikacin
Gram Neg. Bacteria: Pseudomonas, E. Coli, Proteus, Providencia, Klebsiella, Enterobacter, Serratia, Citrobacter
Nocardia Asteroides
Mycobacterium Avium-Intracellulare
Gram Pos. Bacteria: Staphylococci but not Pneumococci, Streptococci, or Neisseria
Not Anaerobes

Prior to and during therapy, the causative organism should be cultured and in-vitro susceptibility tests conducted.

DOSAGE FORMS: Injection: (IM or IV) 50mg/ml; 250mg/ml

DOSAGE: Amikacin sulfate is administered by IM injection or IV infusion. For adults, IV infusions are prepared by adding 500mg of amikacin to 100-200ml of IV infusion fluid such as 0.9% sodium chloride or 5% dextrose; infuse over 30-60 minutes. For pediatric patients, the volume of infusion depends on the patient's needs; infuse over 1-2 hours in infants or 30-60 minutes in older children. See Aminoglycosides for calculation of loading dose and maintenance dose.

Dosage is given in the next Table:

Dosage of Amikacin, Normal Renal Function

Age		Dosage
Neonate <28 wks,	0-7 Days	7.5mg/kg/dose every 24 hours
	>7 Days	7.5mg/kg/dose every 18 hours
Neonate 28-34 wks,	0-7 Days	7.5mg/kg/dose every 18 hours
	>7 Days	7.5mg/kg/dose every 12 hours
Neonate term	0-7 Days	7.5mg/kg/dose every 12 hours
	>7 Days	7.5mg/kg/dose every 8 hours
Children and Adults		5mg/kg/dose every 8 hours; Max dose: 1.5g daily.

Premature infants should have individualized dosing. Check trough level prior to second dose, give dose only if trough is appropriate.

For children & adults, daily dosage should not exceed 1.5g.

Dosage in Renal Impairment: Initial dose, 7.5mg/kg. For subsequent doses, give 7.5mg/kg at intervals (in hours) calculated by multiplying the patient's steady-state serum creatinine (in mg/dl) by 9. Alternately, dosing may be based on adjusted creatinine clearance, as described in aminoglycosides section.

MONITOR:

Specimen: Red top tube, separate serum and freeze. Obtain serum specimens as follows:

(1) 24-48 hours after starting therapy if loading dose is not given.
(2) 5 to 30 minutes before I.V. amikacin (trough).
(3) 30 min. following complet. of a 30 min. I.V. infusion of amikacin(peak)
Do not use heparinized collection tubes.

Therapeutic Range: 15-25mcg/ml; Toxic Level, Peak: >30mcg/ml; Toxic Level, Trough: >5mcg/ml; Half-Life: 2-3 hours; Time to Steady State: Adults, 5-35 hours; Children, 3.5-15 hours; varies with dosage; may be significantly prolonged in patients with renal dysfunction.

Draw Samples as Follows: Peak: 60 minutes post I.M. injection (normal renal function). Peak: 30 minutes after end of 30 I.V. infusion; directly after 60 minute I.V. infusion (normal renal function). Trough: Immediately prior to next dose. Sampling is often done prior to attainment of steady state to help prevent toxicity and to ensure therapeutic efficacy.

AMIKACIN (Cont.)

High concentrations of beta-lactam antibiotics (penicillins, cephalosporins) inactivate aminoglycosides (gentamicin, streptomycin, amikacin, tobramycin and kanamycin); to reduce this interaction, specimens containing both classes of antibiotics should either be assayed immediately using a rapid method or stored frozen.

The first serum level of amikacin is obtained when amikacin has reached steady-state serum concentrations; steady-state is reached in 5 to 13 hours (adults) and 3.5 to 15 hours (children) after starting therapy if the patient has not received a loading dose (steady state = 5-7 drug half-lives; half-life of amikacin is 2 to 3 hours). The following times should be recorded on the laboratory requisition form and on the patient's chart:

Trough Specimen Drawn ____(Time) (5 to 30 minutes before Amikacin)
Amikacin Started ________(Time)
Amikacin Completed _______(Time) (30 min. I.V. Infusion)
Peak Specimen Drawn ______(Time) (30 min. after I.V. Amikacin)

ADVERSE EFFECTS: The three main toxic side effects of amikacin are ototoxicity(2-10%), nephrotoxicity(3-10%), and neuromuscular blockage; it is important to control the dose given by monitoring peak and trough levels of the drug, particularly in patients with any degree of renal failure. As renal function declines, drug half-life increases. To minimize risk of toxicity, it has been recommended that peak levels not exceed 30mcg/ml and that trough levels should fall below 5mcg/ml.

Amikacin is eliminated exclusively by renal excretion; excessive serum concentrations may occur and lead to damage to the renal proximal tubules; damage is usually reversible if discovered early.

Ototoxicity is usually due to vestibular damage and is often not reversible.

Other adverse effects include hypersensitivity reactions, hematologic effects, central nervous system effects and gastrointestinal disturbances.

AMILORIDE

(Midamor; with Hydrochlorothiazide: Moduretic)

USES: **Amiloride** is a **potassium-sparing diuretic;** amiloride is similar to triamterene, but differs from spironolactone in that amiloride does not inhibit aldosterone. Amiloride acts directly on the distal renal tubules, thereby producing increased sodium excretion and decreased potassium excretion. Bicarbonate excretion is increased and calcium excretion is decreased. Since most sodium is reabsorbed in the proximal renal tubules, amiloride is relatively ineffective when administered alone, and concomitant administration of a diuretic (such as a thiazide diuretic, ethacrynic acid, or furosemide) which blocks reabsorption of sodium proximal to the distal portion of the nephron, is required for maximal diuretic effects. The uses of amiloride are given in the next Table:

Uses of Amiloride
Edema: Congestive Heart Failure, Nephrotic Syndrome, Cirrhosis of the Liver
Hypertension: Usually Combined with Other Diuretics
Hypokalemia, Diuretic-Induced

DOSAGE FORMS: Tabs(Midamor): 5mg; Combined with Hydrochlorothiazide (Moduretic): Amiloride, 5mg, plus Hydrochlorothiazide, 50mg.

DOSAGE: Amiloride is administered orally; dosage is given in the next Table:

Dosage of Amiloride

Condition	Age	Dosage
Usual	Adult	5-10mg daily; higher doses have been used occasionally (max. 40mg daily)
	Children	0.625mg/kg daily up to adult doses.

Amiloride is often administered with hydrochlorothiazide. Generally, dosage requirements for each drug should be adjusted independently prior to initiating therapy with a fixed combination. For further discussion of combination preparation, see HYDROCHLOROTHIAZIDE AND AMILORIDE section.

PHARMACOKINETICS: Absorption: 50%; 30% with food; Onset of Action: 2 hrs.; Peak Effect: 3-4 hrs.; Duration of Action: 24 hrs.; Half-Life: 6-9 hrs.; Excretion: Renal, Feces.

ADVERSE EFFECTS: Hyperkalemia may occur. GI(3-8%): nausea, vomiting, anorexia, diarrhea; CNS(3-8%): headache.

AMINOCAPROIC ACID
(Amicar)

USES: Uses of aminocaproic acid are given in the next Table:

Uses of Aminocaproic Acid

- Excessive Fibrinolysis caused by increased Plasminogen (Profibrinolysin) Activation associated with surgical and nonsurgical conditions.
- Prevent or Control attacks of Hereditary Angioedema
- Hemophiliacs prior to and following Tooth Extraction and for other Traumatic Bleeding in the Mouth and Nasopharynx
- Overdose of Streptokinase or Urokinase

Aminocaproic acid is contraindicated in disseminated intravascular coagulopathy (DIC); if aminocaproic acid is used in DIC, it may cause fatal thrombus formation.

Excessive Fibrinolysis: It is necessary to determine whether excess bleeding is due to excessive fibrinolysis or DIC. However, some of the laboratory findings are similar in both conditions: prothrombin time (PT) prolonged; partial thromboplastin time (PTT), prolonged; plasma fibrinogen, decreased; fibrin degradation products (FDP), increased; thrombin time (TT), prolonged. Tests that may help to differentiate DIC and primary fibrinolysis are given in the next Table:

Disseminated Intravascular Coagulopathy (DIC) and Primary Fibrinolysis

Test	DIC	Primary Fibrinolysis
Platelet Count	Reduced	Normal
Protamine Coagulation Test	Positive	Negative
Euglobulin Clot Lysis	Normal or Reduced	Reduced

In primary fibrinolysis, the platelet count is normal, the protamine paracoagulation test is negative, and euglobulin clot lysis is reduced.

Hereditary Angioedema: Aminocaproic acid inhibits C_1 esterase.

Mechanism of Action: Aminocaproic acid is a potent competitive inhibitor of plasminogen activator and inhibits plasmin to a lesser extent. The fibrinolytic system is illustrated in the next Figure:

Fibrinolytic System

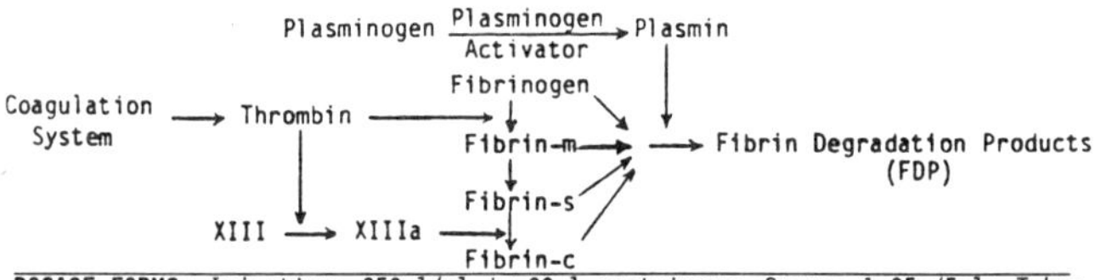

DOSAGE FORMS: Injection: 250ml/ml in 20ml containers; Syrup: 1.25g/5ml; Tabs: 500mg.

DOSAGE: Dosage of aminocaproic acid is given in the next Table:

Dosage of Aminocaproic Acid

Condition	Age	Route	Dosage
Usual	Adults	Oral & IV	Initially, 4-5g orally or by slow IV infusion (in 250ml IV fluid), then 1g (in 50ml of diluent) at hr. intervals or 4-5g every 4 hrs. if renal function is normal (max. 30g/24 hrs.). The dose is reduced to 25% in patients with renal disease or oliguria.
	Children	Oral, IV	Initially, 100mg/kg orally or by slow IV infusion and then 30mg/kg/hr or 100mg/kg every 4-6 hours until bleeding is controlled; max. as for adults.

ADVERSE REACTIONS: The most common adverse effects are nausea, vomiting, and diarrhea. Less common adverse effects are dizziness, pruritus, erythema, rash, hypotension, headache, dyspepsia, inhibition of ejaculation, conjunctival erythema, arrhythmias, fatigue and nasal congestion. Case reports include the following: imflammatory myopathy, generalized thrombosis, liver failure in patients with cirrhosis, cardiac and hepatic necrosis. There is increased risk for thrombosis in women taking oral contraceptives. Free urinary bladder of blood clots when aminocaproic acid is used during surgery.

PHARMACOKINETICS: Oral: Well absorbed; Peak: 2 hrs. after single oral dose; Excretion: Urine, mostly within 12 hrs.

AMINOGLYCOSIDES

Aminoglycosides are used, often in combination with other antibiotics, in the treatment of serious infections; aminoglycosides are used to treat gram-negative infections.

Activities of aminoglycosides (and aztreonam for comparison) are given in the next Table (Pancoast, S.J., Med. Clin. North Am. 72, 581-612, May 1988; Adams, H.G., Personal Communication):

Activities of Aminoglycosides

Aminoglycoside (and Aztreonam)	Gram-positive cocci: S. aureus	Gram-positive cocci: Streptococci	Gram-positive cocci: Strep. entero.	Gram-negative bacilli: H. influenzae	Gram-negative bacilli: PEcK	Gram-negative bacilli: Other Enterics	Gram-negative bacilli: Pseudomonas a.	Anaerobes: B. fragilis	Anaerobes: Res. Anaerobes
Gentamicin	2	▧	▧	3	4	4	3	▧	▧
Tobramycin	2	▧	▧	3	4	4	4	▧	▧
Amikacin	2	▧	▧	3	4	4	4	▧	▧
Aztreonam	▧	▧	▧	4	4	4	4	▧	▧

4=best activity; 3=good activity; 2=some activity; ▧ =little or no activity.
PEcK (Mnemonic)= P. mirabilis, E. coli, Klebsiella; Res.= Resident

Aztreonam (Azactam) has been proposed as a "logical alternative" to aminoglycosides because it is less toxic and does not require monitoring.

There are six aminoglycosides available for clinical use: gentamicin, tobramycin, amikacin, netilmicin, kanamycin and streptomycin. Only the first three are widely used.

Structure: The aminoglycoside antibiotics are amino sugars linked to a central hexose or aminocyclitol nucleus by a glycoside bond.

Mechanism of Action: The aminoglycoside antibiotics penetrate the cell wall and cytoplasmic membrane of susceptible microorganisms, bind to the ribosomes and cause misreading of the genetic code; thus, incorrect amino acids are inserted into the peptide chains. Faulty proteins are produced, which results in death of the microorganisms.

Resistance to Aminoglycosides: Although aminoglycosides inhibit organisms such as Salmonella and Brucella, they are not effective in the treatment of infection caused by these bacteria because aminoglycosides do not enter macrophages or other phagocytic cells (Neu, H.C., Med. Clin. North Am. 71, 1051-1064, Nov. 1987).

Bacteria, such as E. coli, K. pneumoniae and S. marcescens, may develop resistance to aminoglycosides. Resistance develops through plasmid-mediated aminoglycoside modifying enzymes that acetylate, adenylate, or phosphorylate the aminoglycosides rendering them inactive.

DOSAGE: Most aminoglycoside therapy is initiated with a loading dose (usually one-half of the maintenance dose per day) followed by maintenance dose administration adjusted for level of renal performance and the size and body makeup of the patient.

A convenient method for determining aminoglycoside dosage regimens based on patient weight and renal function is as follows:

Loading Dose (LD): Select loading dose in mg/kg (lean body wt.) to provide peak serum levels in the range listed below for desired aminoglycoside.

Lean Body Wt. (Male) = 50kg + 2.3kg for every inch over 5 feet.
Lean Body wt. (Female) = 45kg + 2.3kg for every inch over 5 feet.

AMINOGLYCOSIDES (Cont.)

The usual loading dose for expected peak serum levels is given in the next Table (Sarubbi, F.A. and Hull, J.H., Ann. Int. Med. 39, 617, 1978):

Loading Dosage

Aminoglycoside	Usual Loading Doses	Expected Peak Serum Levels
Tobramycin Gentamicin	1.5 to 2.0 mg/kg	4-10 mcg/ml
Amikacin Kanamycin	5.0 to 7.5 mg/kg	15-30 mcg/ml

Maintenance Dose: Select maintenance dose (as percentage of chosen loading dose) to continue peak serum levels indicated above according to desired dosing interval and patient's creatinine clearance.

$$\text{Creatinine Clearance(Male)} = \frac{\text{Wt. } (140 - \text{age})}{(72)(\text{serum creatinine})}; \quad \text{Wt.=Lean Body Weight}$$

$$\text{Creatinine Clearance(Female)} = \frac{\text{Wt. } (140 - \text{age})}{(72)(\text{serum creatinine})} \times 0.85$$

Percentage of Loading Dose Required For Dosage Interval Selected

C(c)cr(ml/min)	Estimated Half-life* (hrs.)	8hrs.	12hrs.	24hrs.
90	3.1	84%	-	-
80	3.4	80	91%	-
70	3.9	76	88	-
60	4.5	71	84	-
50	5.3	65	79	0
40	6.5	57	72	92%
30	8.4	48	63	86
25	9.9	43	57	81
20	11.9	37	50	75
17	13.6	33	46	70
15	15.1	31	42	67
12	17.9	27	37	61
10**	20.4	24	34	56
7	25.9	19	28	47
5	31.5	16	23	41
2	46.8	11	16	30
0	69.3	8	11	21

*Alternatively, one-half of the chosen loading dose may be given at an interval approximately equal to the estimated half-life.

**Dosing for patients with creatinine clearance 10ml/min should be assisted by measured serum levels.

Example:

58 y/o male, 5 ft. 11 inches, Actual Body Weight = 200lbs.(91kg), Serum Creatinine = 1.6

Lean Body Weight (LBW) = 50kg + 2.3 (11 inches) = 75kg

$$\text{CrCl} = \frac{75(140-58)}{72(1.6)} = 53 \text{ ml/min.}$$

Loading Dose (LD) of Gentamicin = 2mg/kg X 75kg = 150mg

Maintenance Dose = 65% of LD (150mg) q 8hrs.; i.e. 100mg q 8hrs. or
79% of LD (150mg) q 12hrs.; i.e. 120mg q 12hrs.

Then: At steady state, draw trough just prior to dose; draw peak 30 minutes after gentamicin infusion is completed. Recheck serum creatinine every 3-5 days.

ADVERSE EFFECTS: Toxicity and untoward effects are listed in the next Table (Edson, R.S. and Keys, T.F., Mayo Clin. Proc. 58, 99-102, 1983):

Toxicity of Aminoglycosides

Common:
- Renal Toxicity
- Auditory Toxicity
- Vestibular Toxicity

Less Common:
- Neuromuscular Blockade

Minor:
- Hypomagnesemia, Skin Rash, Drug-Induced Fever, Nausea and Vomiting

Rare:
- Peripheral Neuritis

AMINOGLYCOSIDES (Cont.)

Renal Toxicity: Aminoglycosides are eliminated by the kidney and can cause nephrotoxicity by damaging proximal tubular cells; therefore, serum creatinine should be measured as follows: initial specimen before starting therapy and then every 3 days thereafter. Criteria that have been used to detect nephrotoxicity are given in the next Table (Smith, C.R. et al., N. Engl. J. Med. 302, 1106-1109, 1980; Fee, W.E., Laryngoscope 10, (Suppl. 24) 1-19, 1980):

Criteria for Nephrotoxicity of Aminoglycosides

Initial Serum Creatinine	Nephrotoxicity: Rise in Serum Creatinine
<3.0 mg/dl	> 0.5 mg/dl up to 7 days after therapy.
>3.0 mg/dl	> 1.0 mg/dl up to 7 days after therapy. At least one-third above initial value.

Auditory Toxicity: Aminoglycosides can damage cochlear hair cells (sensory hair cells) and thereby produce deafness.

Vestibular Toxicity: Aminoglycosides can damage the vestibular apparatus.

Hypomagnesemia (less than 1.6 mg/dl in almost **40%** of patients) is a frequent early occurrence in patients receiving aminoglycoside therapy; aminoglycosides may produce hypocalcemia and hypokalemia; it may be advisable to monitor serum magnesium for patients receiving aminoglycoside therapy, with use of magnesium replacement therapy when low levels are found (Zaloga, G.P. et al., Surg. Gynecol. Obstet. 158, 561-565, 1984).

Monitoring Aminoglycoside Levels (Bakerman, S., ABC's of Interpretive Laboratory Data, 2nd Ed., Interpretive Laboratory Data, Inc. P.O. Box 7066, Greenville, N.C. 27835-7066).

SPECIMEN: Red top tube, separate serum and freeze. Obtain serum specimens as follows:

(1). 24-48 hours after starting therapy if loading dose is not given.
(2). 5 to 30 minutes before I.V. (trough).
(3). 30 minutes following completion of a 30 minute I.V. infusion of peak.
Do not use heparinized collection tubes.

Draw Samples as Follows: Peak: 60 minutes post I.M. injection (normal renal function). Peak: 30 minutes after end of 30 minute I.V. infusion; directly after 60 minute I.V. infusion (normal renal function). Trough: Immediately prior to next dose. Sampling is often done prior to attainment of steady state to help prevent toxicity and to ensure therapeutic efficacy.

High concentrations of beta-lactam antibiotics (penicillins, cephalosporins) inactivate aminoglycosides (gentamicin, streptomycin, amikacin, tobramycin and kanamycin); to reduce this interaction, specimens containing both classes of antibiotics should either be assayed immediately using a rapid method or stored frozen.

METHOD: RIA; EMIT; SLFIA (Ames); Fluorescence Polarization (Abbott).

The first serum level of aminoglycoside is obtained when aminoglycoside has reached steady state serum concentrations: steady-state is reached in 4-5 half-lives. The following times should be recorded on the laboratory requisition form and on the patient's chart:

Trough Specimen Drawn___(Time) (5 to 30 minutes before dose)
Amikacin Started_____(Time) (30 min. I.V. infusion)
Amikacin Completed____(Time) (30 min. I.V. infusion)
Peak Specimen Drawn___(Time) (30 min. after I.V. or 1hr. after an IM dose).

AMINOPHYLLINE

USES: Aminophylline is theophylline ethylene diamine; aminophylline and other theophylline salts can be given orally or parenterally. Theophylline can be given only orally.

Aminophylline formulations vary in their equivalence to anhydrous theophylline from 79% to 86%.

Uses of aminophylline as a bronchodilator are given in the next Table:

Uses of Aminophylline as a Bronchodilator
Relief of Acute Asthmatic Symptoms
"Prophylactic" Agent for Controlling the Symptoms and Signs of Chronic Asthma
Control Apnea of Infancy

Theophylline is the most widely prescribed bronchodilator in the United States for maintenance therapy in patients with chronic asthma.

Theophylline stimulates the central nervous system at the medullary level and is used to treat apnea of prematurity.

The mechanism of action is not clear. It has been thought that theophylline inhibits the enzyme phosphodiesterase which metabolizes cyclic 3', 5' AMP. This compound acts as a "second messenger" in the cell, and its action upon smooth muscle is to decrease tension or motility. However, the concentration of theophylline necessary to inhibit phosphodiesterase in-vitro would be toxic in-vivo [Svedmyr, N., "The Role of the Theophyllines in Asthma Therapy," Scand. J. Respir. Dis. (Suppl.) 101, 125-137, 1977]. Other theories relate to the effects on intracellular calcium (Brisson, G.P., Malaise-Lagge, F. and Malaise, W.J., "The Stimulus-Secretion Coupling of Glucose-Induced Insulin Release VII, A Proposed Site of Action for Adenosine 3', 5' Cyclic Monophos- phate", J. Clin. Invest. 51, 232-241, 1972) and prostaglandin antagonism (Horrobin, D.F., Manku, M.S., Franks, D.J. and Hamet, P., "Methylxanthines Phosphodiesterase Inhibitor Behave as Prostaglandin Antagonists in a Perfused Rat Mesenteric Artery Preparation", Prostaglandins 13, 33-40, 1977).

In addition to its bronchodilator effect, theophylline has positive cardiac, inotropic effect (increase in strength of contraction of the heart), vasodilatory and diuretic actions. It also stimulates diaphragmatic contraction action in normal subjects(Aubier, M., DeTroyer, A., Sampson, M., Macklem, P.T., and Roussos, C., "Aminophylline Improves Diaphragmatic Contractility." N. Engl. J. Med. 305, 249-252, 1981) and in patients with chronic obstructive pulmonary disease, theophylline improves the contractile properties of the diaphragm and prevents the occurrence of diaphragmatic fatigue.

Effects of theophylline on different systems are given in the next Table:

Effects of Theophylline on Different Systems
Respiratory System:
Relaxation of Smooth Muscle with Bronchodilation: Relief of bronchospasm and increased flow rates and vital capacity; dilates pulmonary arterioles, reduces pulmonary hypertension, and reduces alveolar carbon dioxide tension and increases pulmonary blood flow.
Nervous System:
Stimulates all Levels of the CNS but to a lesser extent than does caffeine. In the medulla, lowers the threshold of the respiratory center to carbon dioxide but significant increases in rate & depth of respiration occur only if respiration is depressed. Alleviation of neonatal apnea and apnea of Cheyne-Stokes Respiration may be caused by direct stimulation of the medullary respiratory center.
Cardiovascular System:
In doses larger than those required for bronchodilation, produces inotropic effect (increase in strength of contraction of the heart) and a positive chronotropic effect at the sinoatrial node (increase in heart rate)
Renal Effects: Diuretic effect is usually mild

AMINOPHYLLINE (Cont.)

DOSAGE FORMS: IV: 25mg/ml (19.7mg Theophylline)(79%); Liquid (Oral): 105mg/5ml (90mg Theophylline)(Somophylline)(85% Theophylline); Tablets: 100mg (78.9mg Theophylline), 200mg (157.8mg Theophylline)(79%); Tablets (Extended-Release): 225mg (177.5mg Theophylline)(79%), Others.

DOSAGE: Theophyllines are usually administered orally. For faster absorption of theophyllines, take conventional dosage forms with a full glass of water on an empty stomach 30-60 minutes before meals or 2 hours after meals.

To minimize local GI irritation, oral theophyllines may be taken with meals or immediately after meals,with a full glass of liquid or with antacids.

Extended-release theophylline preparations are indicated in patients with relatively continuous or frequently recurring asthma symptoms.

Aminophylline may be administered undiluted by slow IV injection or preferably, in large volume parenteral fluids by slow IV infusion.

IM injection of aminophylline causes intense local pain and is not recommended.

Choice of Drugs for Asthma

- Aminophylline infusion or Oral Theophylline*
- Beta-2 Agonist
- Cromolyn
- Corticosteroids

***IV aminophylline in the acute management of asthma may not provide additional bronchodilatation compared to beta-adrenergic agents alone and side effects may be increased (Siegel, D. et al., Ann. Rev. Respir. Dis. 132, 283-286, 1985). Many clinicians no longer use this therapy for acute asthma.**

Dosage of Aminophylline for Acute Therapy: For acute therapy, an intravenous loading dose of about 6mg/kg aminophylline, if ideal body weight, will usually yield a serum concentration in the range 10 to 15mcg/ml in patients who have previously taken no theophylline. The intravenous loading dose should be infused over a period of at least 30 minutes to minimize the probability of serious arrhythmias.

A protocol for aminophylline therapy for acute asthmatic attack is given in the next Figure (Hendeles, L. and Weinberger, M. in Individualizing Drug Therapy, Vol. I, Taylor, W.J. and Finn, A.L., eds., Gross, Townsend and Frank, Inc., N.Y., N.Y., 1981, pgs. 32-65):

Aminophylline Therapy for Asthma

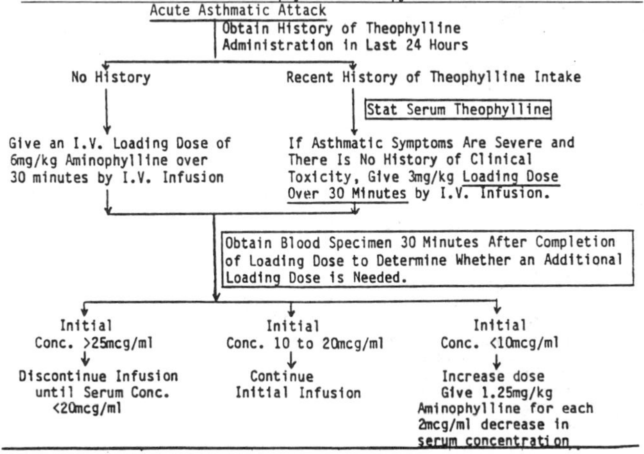
Acute Asthmatic Attack
Obtain History of Theophylline Administration in Last 24 Hours
No History
Recent History of Theophylline Intake
Stat Serum Theophylline
Give an I.V. Loading Dose of 6mg/kg Aminophylline over 30 minutes by I.V. Infusion
If Asthmatic Symptoms Are Severe and There Is No History of Clinical Toxicity, Give 3mg/kg Loading Dose Over 30 Minutes by I.V. Infusion.
Obtain Blood Specimen 30 Minutes After Completion of Loading Dose to Determine Whether an Additional Loading Dose is Needed.
Initial Conc. >25mcg/ml
Initial Conc. 10 to 20mcg/ml
Initial Conc. <10mcg/ml
Discontinue Infusion until Serum Conc. <20mcg/ml
Continue Initial Infusion
Increase dose Give 1.25mg/kg Aminophylline for each 2mcg/ml decrease in serum concentration

AMINOPHYLLINE (Cont.)
Blood Specimen: (Loading Dose in Hospital) A blood sample for aminophylline assay should be drawn prior to loading dose if the patient has a history of theophylline therapy; then obtain a blood specimen 30 minutes after completion of loading dose.
Maintenance Dose: The aminophylline infusion rate necessary to attain a serum level of 10mcg/ml for different conditions is as follows (Powell, R., School of Pharmacy, Univ. N.C.):

Aminophylline Infusion Rate

Adults:

Characteristic	0.5mg/kg/hr x Factor	Aminophylline Infusion Rate
Nonsmoker	0.5mg/kg/hr x 1 =	0.5 (mg/kg/hr)
Smoker (within last 3 mos > 1 pack/day) Plus ages 10-16	0.5mg/kg/hr x 1.6 =	0.8 (mg/kg/hr)
CHF (edema, x-ray)	0.5mg/kg/hr x 0.4 =	0.2 (mg/kg/hr)
Pneumonia, Viral Respiratory Infection	0.5mg/kg/hr x 0.4 =	0.2 (mg/kg/hr)
Cirrhosis	0.5mg/kg/hr x 0.4 =	0.2 (mg/kg/hr)
Severe hepatic obstruction (PEER < 100L/min or PCO_2 > 45mmHg)	0.5mg/kg/hr x 0.8 =	0.4 (mg/kg/hr)

Example. The aminophylline infusion rate in a 60kg male who smokes 2 packs of cigarettes per day and currently has signs and symptoms of CHF: Aminophylline infusion rate = 0.5mg/kg/hr · 60kg · 1.6 · 0.4 = 19.2mg/hr
Premature Infants and Neonates: Aminophylline Infusion Rate = 0.19mg/kg/hr
Infants 4 to 52 Weeks:Aminophylline Infusion Rate=0.37 + (0.012 x Age in Wks)
Children (1 to 9 Years of Age): Aminophylline Infusion Rate = 1.0mg/kg/hr.
Interindividual and intraindividual differences or changes in theophylline clearance in children necessitates frequent therapeutic drug monitoring (Kubo, M., et al., J. Pediatr. 108, 1011-1015, 1986).
Blood Specimen (Inpatient Maintenance Dose): Obtain a blood specimen 4 to 8 hours after start of maintenance I.V. infusion and 18 to 30 hours after starting the infusion and at 12 to 24 hour intervals thereafter for possible adjustment of the infusion rate until the infusion is discontinued. As a function of results, the dose may be altered appropriately.
Outpatient Maintenance Dose: Maintenance dose to achieve a peak level of 10 to 20mg/L is given in the next Table (Powell, R.):

Maintenance Dose of Theophylline or Aminophylline (mg/kg/day) Ideal Body Wt.

	Theophylline (mg/kg/day)	Aminophylline (mg/kg/day)
Adult - Nonsmoker	10	12
Smoker	15	19
Cirrhotic	4	5
Children (1-8)	12-24	15-30
Children (9-12)	10-20	12.5-25
Children (12-16)	8-18	10-22.5

MONITOR: Blood Specimens (Outpatient Maintenance Dose): Blood specimens should be obtained at about 3 day intervals and at the time of peak concentration or about 2 to 4 hours after a scheduled dose depending on the product formulation.
Concentrations of 5 to 10 mcg/ml may be effective for some patients, particularly children.
ADVERSE EFFECTS: Adverse effects usually are seen when serum levels rise above 20mg/liter. Early signs of toxicity are nausea, vomiting and headache. Toxic reactions are listed in the next Table:

Toxic Reactions of Theophylline

Gastrointestinal: Abdominal Pain, Nausea, Vomiting
Cardiovascular: Tachycardia, Arrhythmias
Blood Pressure: Elevated
Central Nervous System: Agitation, Irritability, Insomnia, Tremor, Seizures, Convulsions, Coma.
Occasionally: Hyperthermia, Diuresis, Ketosis, Hyperglycemia

An acute oral overdose should be treated by induced emesis, followed by oral administration of activated charcoal (repeat every two hours). Obtain blood for assay of electrolytes, glucose, urea, arterial gases and theophylline; repeat every six hours. Correct dehydration and hypokalemia. Treat seizures with intravenous benzodiazepines. Theophylline-induced seizures are very difficult to control; animal data suggests that phenobarbital but not phenytoin might be useful for prevention of seizures in patients with toxic serum theophylline levels (Blake, K.V. et al., Ann. Emerg. Med. 17, 1024-1028, 1988). Monitor with ECG. Correct hypokalemia, acidosis and hypoxia. Consider hemodialysis or hemoperfusion.

AMIODARONE

(Cordarone)

USES: Amiodarone, a class III antiarrhythmic drug, is used to treat life-threatening ventricular arrhythmias that are refractory to other anti-arrhythmic drugs. The high incidence of side effects limits the usefulness of amiodarone. Uses of amiodarone are given in the next Table:

Uses of Amiodarone
Suppress Recurrences of:
Ventricular arrhythmia
Supraventricular arrhythmia
Atrial Flutter or Fibrillation
A-V Nodal Reentrant Tachycardia

Amiodarone prolongs refractoriness in both the A-V node and accessory pathways and slows A-V nodal conduction; thus, it is particularly useful in patients with reciprocating tachycardia or atrial flutter and fibrillation associated with the Wolff-Parkinson-White syndrome.

Amiodarone is useful in preventing both supraventricular and ventricular arrhythmias in patients with hypertrophic cardiomyopathy.

Amiodarone may control the tachycardia in patients with the bradycardia-tachycardia syndrome; because it may worsen bradycardia, a permanent pacemaker should be in place.

Amiodarone has a slow onset of action and the full therapeutic response may not be evident for one week to three months. After the drug is discontinued, effects may persist for months.

Mechanism of Action: Amiodarone is a class III antiarrhythmic drug. It prolongs the duration of the action potential 50% to 90%, prolongs the effective refractory period and decreases phase 4 depolarization. There is little or no depression of phase 0. Sinus node and junctional automaticity are decreased and PR, QT, and QRS durations are prolonged.

DOSAGE FORMS: Tabs: 200mg.

DOSAGE: Amiodarone is given orally; dosage for treatment of ventricular and supraventricular arrhythmias is given in the next Table (Am. J. Cardiol. 53, 1564-1569, 1984):

Dosage of Amiodarone

Condition	Daily Dose: Loading	Daily Dose: Adjustment	Daily Dose: Maintenance
Refractory Ventricular Arrhythmias	800-1,600mg for 1-2 weeks Children: 10-15 mg/kg or 600-800mg/1.73m^2 daily for 4-14 days	600-800mg for about 1 month	200-600mg Children: 5mg/kg or 200-400mg/1.73m^2 daily for several weeks. Reduce to lowest effective level.
Supraventricular Arrhythmias	600mg for 1 week Children: same dose as for ventricular arrhythmias	200-400mg	200mg every other day to 200mg daily. Children: same dose as for ventricular arrhythmias
Bradycardia-Tachycardia Syndrome with Pacemaker in Place	400mg		200-600 mg

Rapid loading: 800-2000mg, 2 or 3 times daily; IV: Research only.

ADVERSE EFFECTS: The high incidence of adverse effects limits the usefulness of amiodarone; adverse effects occur in 50% of patients causing 10% to discontinue the drug. Adverse effects are given in the next Table (Kreeger, R.W. and Hammill, S.C., Mayo Clin. Proc. 62, 1033-1050, 1987):

Adverse Effects of Amiodarone

	Adverse Effects	Percent(%)
Cardiac Toxicity:	Proarrhythmia	2
	Bradycardia (necessitating pacing)	4
	Congestive heart failure	4
Noncardiac Toxicity:	Photosensitivity	20
	Sleep disturbance	10
	Nausea and anorexia	10
	Tremor, ataxia, neuropathy	10
	Headache	5
	Pulmonary toxicity	5
	Thyroid disorder or Hepatotoxicity	<3

AMIODARONE (Cont.)

Amiodarone-induced pulmonary toxicity is potentially fatal and reportedly occurs in 5.8% of patients. Pulmonary toxicity occurs more frequently with advanced age, higher maintenance doses, higher levels of amiodarone metabolite, and pretreatment pulmonary diffusion abnormalities (Dusman, R.E. et al., Circulation 82, 51-59, 1990).

DRUG INTERACTIONS: Drug interactions necessitate reduction of dosage of warfarin, digoxin, procainamide, quinidine, phenytoin, flecainide, mexiletine.

PHARMACOKINETICS: GI Absorption: Poor and variable (bioavailability of 22 to 50%); Onset; Oral: 4-6 hours; I.V. 5-10 minutes; Metabolism: Liver; Half-Life: 53 to 61 days after long-term therapy. Protein-Binding: Strong.

AMITRIPTYLINE

(Elavil, Endep, Generic)

USES: Amitriptyline is a **heterocyclic antidepressant** used to treat **depression** and **anxiety.** Uses of amitriptyline in patients with **depression** are given in the next Table:

Uses of Amitriptyline in Depression
Major Depressive Episodes of Major Depression
Mixed Bipolar Disorder
Depressed Bipolar Disorder
Depressive Periods of Dysthymic Disorder
Panic Disorder
Phobic Disorder
Atypical Depression
Other Proposed Uses:
Abnormal Eating Behavoir in Bulimic Patients
Prophylaxis of Migraine Headache
Some Patients with Chronic Muscle-Contraction Headache unresponsive to Analgesic Therapy

Amitriptyline is as effective as imipramine in the treatment of the first three conditions listed in the previous Table.

Mechanism of Action: Amitriptyline, like other heterocyclic antidepressants, act by blocking the reuptake of norepinephrine and serotonin by the presynaptic nerve terminals within the central nervous system.

DOSAGE FORMS: Tabs:10, 25, 50, 75, 100 and 150mg; Sol'n (IM): 10mg/ml in 10ml containers.

DOSAGE: Amitriptyline is administered orally or intramuscularly. Dosage is given in the next Table:

Dosage of Amitriptyline

Age	Route	Dosage
Adults	IM	20-30mg, four times a day; substitute oral route as soon as possible
Adults (Hospitalized)	Oral	Initially, 100mg daily in divided doses increased gradually to 200mg daily if necessary.
Adults (Outpatients)	Oral	25mg twice daily for three days, 50mg twice daily for three days. After 2-3 weeks of therapy, a single daily dose is given at bedtime; if limited benefit is observed by the third week, the daily dose is increased weekly (max. 300mg daily) until satisfactory response is obtained. Maintenance: use lowest dose 75-100mg to maintain remission.
Elderly and Adolescents	Oral	25-50mg daily, increase slowly as above but use a maximum of 100mg daily in divided doses.

PHARMACOKINETICS: Absorption: almost complete; Metabolism: The main metabolite of amitriptyline is nortriptyline which is also active; Half-Life: The half-life of amitriptyline is 15 hours and for nortriptyline 27 hours; Onset of Therapeutic Effects: 1-4 weeks.

AMITRIPTYLINE (Cont.)

ADVERSE EFFECTS: Adverse effects of amitriptyline are mediated through blockage of histamine(H_1), muscarinic acetylcholine, and alpha-1 adrenergic receptors; the clinical manifestations of blockage of these receptors by amitriptyline are given in the next Table (Richelson, E., J. Clin. Psychiatry 43:11 [Sec.2], 4-11, 1982):

Adverse Effects of Amitriptyline

Blockage of Histamine (H_1) Receptors	Blockage of Muscurinic Acetylcholine Receptors	Blockage of Alpha-1-Adrenergic Receptors
Sedation, Drowsiness	Blurred vision	Postural hypotension
Weight gain	Dry mouth	Dizziness
Hypotension	Sinus tachycardia	Reflex tachycardia
	Constipation	
	Urinary retention	
	Memory dysfunction	

In addition, amitriptyline is a potent blocker of serotonin uptake; this blockage is associated with postural hypotension.

DRUG INTERACTIONS: Drug interactions of amitriptyline are given in the next Table:

Drug Interactions of Amitriptyline

Property (Blockage)	Drug Interaction
Norepinephrine	Blockage of the antihypertensive effects of: guanethidine (Ismelin and Esimil) clonidine (Catapres) alpha-methyldopa (Aldomet) Augmentation of pressor effects of sympathomimetic amines (concomitant use can be fatal).
Histamine (H_1) Receptors	Potentiation of central depressant drugs.
Alpha-1-Adrenergic Receptors	Potentiation of the antihypertensive effect of Prazosin (Minipress).

AMITRIPTYLINE, PERPHENAZINE

(Triavil, Etrafon)

USES: The commercial products, Triavil and Etrafon, contain perphenazine, an antipsychotic drug and amitriptyline (see write-up on Amitriptyline). This combination is used in patients with **anxiety** or **psychosis** associated with **depression.**

DOSAGE FORMS: The dosage forms of Triavil and Etrafon (tablets) are given in the next Table:

Dosage Forms of Triavil and Etrafon

Triavil	Etrafon	Perphenazine(mg)	Amitriptyline(mg)
2-25	2-25	2	25
4-25	4-25	4	25
4-50		4	50
2-10	2-10	2	10
4-10	4-10	4	10

DOSAGE: These drugs are not recommended for children. Dosage is given in the next Table:

Dosage of Combination Amitriptyline and Perphenazine

Condition	Dosage
Initially, Elderly and Adolescents	One 4-10 tab, 3-4 times daily
Psychoneurotics	One 2-25 or 4-25 tab, 3-4 times a day or one 4-50, 2 times daily.
Psychosis	Two 4-25 tabs, 3-4 times daily.

Max. 4 tabs of 4-50 or 8 tabs of other strengths daily. The dosage should be reduced as symptoms improve.

ADVERSE EFFECTS: (see write-up on Amitriptyline). Tardive dyskinesia, extrapyramidal reactions, hyperthermia, arrhythmias, drowsiness, anticholinergic effects, blood dyscrasias, jaundice, hypotension, retinopathy, may mask emetic signs of disease, lowered seizure threshold, rash.

PRECAUTIONS: Cardiovascular, respiratory or renal disease, epilepsy, glaucoma, hyperthyroidism, pregnancy, lactation, suicidal tendencies, urinary retention, electroshock therapy, exposure to extreme heat.

CONTRAINDICATIONS: Coma, bone marrow or CNS depression, liver damage, during or within 14 days of MAOIs, acute myocardial infarction.

MONOTOR: Blood, liver, renal and ocular function.

AMMONIUM CHLORIDE

USES: Uses of ammonium chloride are given in the next Table:

Uses of Ammonium Chloride

- **Metabolic Alkalosis** resulting from Chloride Loss following Vomiting, Gastric Suction, Gastric Fistula Drainage and Pyloric Stenosis
- Increased Calcium Ionization in Alkalotic Tetany
- Alkalosis from excessive use of Alkalinizing Drugs
- Diuretic-Induced Chloride Depletion
- Promoting Diuresis, Particularly in Edematous Conditions Associated with Hypochloremia
- Treatment of Premenstrual Tension and Meniere's Syndrome via its Diuretic Effect
- Increase Solubility of Calcium and Phosphate Ions in Management of Patients with Phosphatic Calculi in Urinary Tract
- Urine Acidification as Adjunct to Treatment of Urinary Tract Infection

When ammonium chloride is given for only three or four days at a time, it merely produces a mild symptomatic acidosis. When it is given continuously for weeks, it can cause a severe acidosis.

Ammonium chloride has been used in the treatment of metabolic alkalosis, due to vomiting or gastric suction. However, in these patients, potassium loss is also present. For this reason, solutions containing saline and potassium chloride may be preferable.

Ammonium chloride is valuable in the treatment of metabolic alkalosis due to diuretics such as thiazides, furosemide, and ethacrynic acid.

Mechanism of Action: The acid-forming properties of ammonium chloride is based on the dissociation of ammonium chloride to ammonium cation and a chloride anion ($NH_4Cl \rightarrow NH_4^+ + Cl^-$). The ammonium ion is converted to ammonia by the liver releasing a hydrogen ion; the hydrogen ion produces an acidosis. The reaction is as follows: $NH_4^+ \rightarrow NH_3 + H^+$. The ammonia is later converted to urea and excreted. Part of the chloride is also excreted by the kidneys along with sodium and water; thus, the chloride acts as a diuretic.

DOSAGE FORMS: Tabs: 300, 500mg; 1gm; Caps: 300, 500mg; Sol'ns/Syrup: 500mg/5ml; Inject: 0.4mEq/ml (2.14%); 4.0mEq/ml (21.4%); 5.0mEq/ml (26.75%)

DOSAGE: Acidifying Agent: Administer orally or by slow IV infusion. Diuretic: Administer orally. Dosage is given in the next Table:

Dosage of Ammonium Chloride

Condition	Age	Route	Dosage
Usual	Adults	Oral or IV	4-12g daily in divided doses every 4-6 hrs. Max. dose 6gm/day IV or 12gm/day orally.
Usual	Children	Oral or IV	75-300mg/kg daily in 4 divided doses. Max. dose 6gm/day.
Diuretic	Adults	Oral	4-12g daily in divided doses every 4-6 hrs. for 3-4 days followed by a rest period of a few days after which therapy is resumed.
Meniere's Syndrome	Adults	Oral	3g given 3 times daily with meals for 3 days; omit drug for 2 days and the cycle is repeated indefinitely.
Premenstrual Edema	Adults	Oral	3g daily in 3 divided doses for 4-5 days prior to menstruation.

ADVERSE REACTIONS: Safety and efficacy of ammonium chloride concentration for injection in children have not been established.

Large doses of ammonium chloride may cause metabolic acidosis secondary to hyperchloremia. Do not use in patients with severe hepatic dysfunction, since ammonia toxicity may occur; do not use in patients with renal insufficiency.

Ammonium chloride may cause gastric irritation.

AMOBARBITAL
(Amytal)

USES: Amobarbital is an intermediate acting barbituate (4-8 hours). Uses are given in the next Table:

Uses of Amobarbital
Hypnotic (Inducing Sleep) for **Insomnia**
Sedative (Calming; Reducing Excitement) Preoperatively
Control **Status Epilepticus;** Acute Seizures; Acute Episodes of Agitated Behavior in Psychoses
Narcoanalysis, Narcotherapy and Diagnostic Aid in Schizophrenia

Amobarbital is a barbituate that is used principally as a hypnotic in the short-term treatment for periods up to 2 weeks in duration of insomnia; it is also used for routine sedation preoperatively.

Amobarbital sodium may be used IV or IM to control status epilepticus or acute seizures resulting from meningitis, poisons, eclampsia, tetanus, or chorea.

DOSAGE FORMS: Tabs: 30mg; Caps: 200mg; Injection: 250, 500mg vials.

DOSAGE: Amobarbital is administered orally. Amobarbital sodium may be administered orally or by deep IM or slow IV injection. IV administration of the drug should usually be reserved for emergency treatment of acute seizure states or acute episodes of psychotic behavior. IV injection rate should not exceed 100mg/minute (1ml of a 10% conc. or equivalent) for adults or 60mg/m^2 per minute (0.6ml of a 10% conc. or equivalent) for children. Dosage is given in the next Table:

Dosage of Amobarbital

Condition	Age	Route	Dosage
Sedation	Adults	Oral	30-50mg, 2 or 3 times daily
	Children	Oral	2mg/kg daily or 70mg/m^2 daily in 4 equally divided doses
Preoperatively for Sedation	Adults	Oral	200mg, 1 to 2 hours before surgery
Labor		Oral	200-400mg; additional doses of 200-400mg may be given at 1- to 3-hr. intervals up to a max. of 1g.
Hypnotic	Adults	Oral	65-200mg at bedtime; limit 2 weeks
	Adults	IM	65-200mg: Max. dose 500mg.
	Children	IM	2-3mg/kg
Anticonvulsant	(>6 yrs)	IV	3-5mg/kg; inject slowly IV
	Adults	IV	65-500mg; do not exceed 1g

ADVERSE EFFECTS: Barbituates have the following disadvantages: dependence, unnatural sleep, hangover and hepatic enzyme induction; barbituates have been largely replaced by benzodiazepines.

Therapeutic Range: 5-14mcg/ml; Toxic: over 30mcg/ml; Half-life: 8-42 hours. Barbituates are one of the leading causes of accidental poisoning death in children and adults and are a leading mode of suicide attempt. The majority of barbituate overdose cases have involved the use of phenobarbital, pentobarbital and secobarbital. The symptoms of acute barbituate intoxication affect primarily the central nervous system and the cardiovascular system. The fatal plasma concentration is greater in the long-acting barbituates than in the short-acting barbituates. The depth and severity of coma in barbituate poisoning are graded; the grading system is given in the next Table:

Grading of Coma in Barbituate Poisoning

	Characteristics		
Grade	Deep Tendon Reflexes	Painful Stimuli	Vital Signs
I	Intact	Withdraws	
II	Intact	No Response	
III	Reduced or Absent	No Response	
IV	Absent	No Response	Respiratory Depression and/or Circulatory Instability

A flat EEG and abnormal reflexes may occur during acute intoxication; these findings do not necessarily indicate structural damage to the CNS. Electrolytes and serum levels of calcium should be followed; it may be advisable to monitor pulmonary wedge pressure.

AMOXICILLIN

(Amcill, Amoxil, Larotid, Trimox, Utimox, Wymox)

USES: The **aminopenicillin** group include: amoxicillin, ampicillin, bacampicillin, cyclacillin, hetacillin. Amoxicillin is used like the other aminopenicillins and is used principally for the treatment of infections caused by susceptible **gram-negative** and **gram-positive** bacteria. Activities of amoxicillin are given in the next Table (Parry, M.F., Med. Clin. No. Am. 71, 1093-1112, 1987; Adams, H.G., Personal Comm.):

Activities of Amoxicillin

	Gram-positive cocci			Gram-negative bacilli						Anaerobes	
	S. aureus	Streptococci	Strep. entero.	H. influenzae	P. mirabilis	E. coli	Klebsiella	Other Enterics	Pseudomonas a.	B. fragilis	Res. Anaerobes
Amoxicillin	4*	4	4	4*	4	2	▩	▩	▩	2	3

4=best activity; 3=good activity; 2=some activity; ▩=little or no activity; Res.= Resident; *Beta-lactamase negative.

The usual susceptible bacteria are given in the next Table:

Usual Spectra of Activity of Amoxicillin

Gram-Negative Bacteria	Gram-Positive Bacteria
Haemophilus Influenza (Beta-Lactamase Negative)	Streptococcus Pneumoniae
Proteus Mirabilis	Enterococci
Escherichia Coli	Nonpenicillinase-Producing Staphylococci
Neisseria Gonorrhoeae (Beta-Lactamase Negative)	Listeria
Salmonella	

Amoxicillin, like other aminopenicillins, generally should not be used for the treatment of streptococcal or staphylococcal infections when a natural penicillin (penicillin G and penicillin V) would be effective.

DOSAGE FORMS: Chewable Tabs:125, 250mg; Caps:250, 500mg; Drops:50mg/ml(15ml); Susp: 125mg/5ml, 250mg/5ml (80, 100, 150ml)

Amoxicillin has activity essentially identical to ampicillin. However, amoxicillin is better absorbed, plasma levels are higher, and it has a longer duration of action. Adverse effects are similar to ampicillin although diarrhea is much less frequent with amoxicillin because of better absorption.

DOSAGE: Amoxicillin, which is available as the trihydrate, is administered orally without regard to meals; dosage is given in the next Table:

Dosage of Amoxicillin

Condition	Age	Dosage
Upper Respiratory Tract Infections (Including Otitis Media and Sinusitis);	Adults and Children >20kg	250mg every 8 hours or if necesary, 500mg every 8 hours. Continue for at least 10 days or 2-3 days after eradication of infection.
Genito-Urinary Tract Infection; Skin and Skin-Structures	>1 month	20-40mg/kg daily in divided doses every 8 hours. Continue for at least 10 days or 2-3 days after eradication of infection. Higher doses (40-100mg/kg daily) have been used as follow-up to IV therapy in more serious infections.
Acute, Uncomplicated Urinary Tract Infections in Non-pregnant Women	Non-Pregnant Women	Single 3g oral dose.

AMOXICILLIN (Cont.)

Condition	Age	Dosage
Lower Respiratory Tract Infection	Adults and Children >20kg	500mg every 8 hours; continue for at least 10 days or 2-3 days after eradication of infection.
	<20kg	40mg/kg daily in divided doses every 8 hours; continue for at least 10 days or 2-3 days after eradication of infection. Higher doses (40-100mg/kg daily) have been used as follow-up to IV therapy in more serious infections.
Gonorrhea, Acute Uncomplicated (Susceptible strains)*	Adults and Children >45kg	Single 3g oral dose plus 1g of oral probenecid; follow amoxicillin by multiple-day doxycycline or tetracycline in adults & children >8 yrs. to treat chlamydial and mycoplasmal infections.
	Children <45kg	Single 50mg/kg dose plus 25mg/kg (up to 1g) of oral dose of probenecid. Note that probencid is contraindicated in Children younger than 2 years of age.
Gonococcal Infections, Disseminated (Gonococcal Arthritis-Dermatitis Syndrome) (Susceptible strains)	Adults	Single 3g dose of amoxicillin plus single 1g dose of probenecid followed by 500mg of amoxicillin given orally every 6 hours for at least 7 days.
Gonococcal Infections, Disseminated (Susceptible strains)*	Adults	IV Penicillin G Potassium or Sodium (10 million units daily) for 3 days or until improvement occurs and then 500mg of amoxicillin given orally every 6 hours to complete at least 7 days of therapy.
Gardnerella Infect., Non-Specific Vaginitis	Adults	Alternative to metronidazole; amoxicillin, 500mg 4 times daily, 7 days.
Prophylaxis of Bacterial Endocarditis: GI, Biliary, Genitourinary Tract Surgery or Instrumentation in Low-Risk Patients and Minor or Repetitive Procedures	Adults and Children >27kg	Am. Heart Assoc.(AHA) recommendation: 3g amoxicillin orally 1 hour prior to the procedure and 1.5g orally 6 hours later.
	Children <27kg	Am. Heart Assoc.(AHA) recommendation: Amoxicillin, 50mg/kg orally 1 hour prior to the procedure and a dose of 25mg/kg orally 6 hours later.

*Amoxicillin or penicillin is no longer recommended for empiric therapy for gonococcal infections due to the spread of penicillinase-producing Neisseria gonorrhoeae; recommendations are for beta-lactamase negative strains (1989 STD Treatment Guidelines, Morbidity and Mortality Weekly Report 38, S-8, September 1, 1989).

ADVERSE REACTIONS: Amoxicillin is contraindicated in patients who are hypersensitive to any penicillin.
Toxicity: Anaphylaxis, rash, fever, diarrhea, superinfection; Interactions: antagonized by tetracyclines and chloramphenicol. Elimination by renal excretion; T 1/2 hour = 1 hour.

AMOXICILLIN/CLAVULANIC ACID
(Augmentin)

USES: Amoxicillin is an **aminopenicillin**, active against a wide variety of **gram-positive** and **gram-negative** bacteria. Activities of amoxicillin/clavulanic acid are given in the next Table (Parry, M.F., Med. Clin. No. Am. 71, 1093-1112, 1987; Adams, H.G., Personal Comm.):

Activities of Amoxicillin/Clavulanic Acid (Augmentin)

	Gram-positive cocci			Gram-negative bacilli						Anaerobes	
	S. aureus	Streptococci	Strep. entero.	H. influenzae	P. mirabilis	E. coli	Klebsiella	Other Enterics	Pseudomonas a.	B. fragilis	Res. Anaerobes
Amoxicillin/Clavulanic Acid	4	4	4	4	4	3	4	3	XXX	4	4

4=best activity; 3=good activity; 2=some activity; XXX=little or no activity.
Res. = Resident.

Clavulanic acid, a beta-lactamase inhibitor, extends the activity to include **beta lactamase-producing strains** of H. influenzae, H. ducreyi, Neisseria gonorrhoeae, Staphlococcus aureus and Moraxella (Branhamella) catarrhalis, E. coli, Klebsiella, Proteus and Citrobacter diversus.

Bacteroides fragilis and Legionella pneumophilia are also sensitive to amoxicillin/clavulinic acid.

Amoxicillin/clavulinic acid is not active against Pseudomonas aeruginosa and Serratia and many strains of Enterobacter, Morganella and Providencia.

Uses of amoxicillin/clavulanic acid are given in the next Table:

Uses of Amoxillin/Clavulanic Acid

Acute Otitis Media and Acute Sinusitis caused by H. influenzae and Moraxella (Branhamella) catarrhalis
Mild to Moderate Lower Respiratory Infections caused by beta-lactamase-producing H. influenzae and Moraxella (Branhamella) catarrhalis
Primary and Recurrent Urinary Tract Infections caused by E. coli. and other bacteria.
Skin and Soft Tissue Infections
Chancroid caused by beta-lactamase-producing H. ducreyi.
Human and Animal Bite Wounds

Amoxicillin/clavulinic acid is the drug of first choice for the treatment of Moraxella (Branhamella) catarrhalis (The Medical Letter 30, 33-40, March 25, 1988).

DOSAGE FORMS: Amoxicillin/clavulinic acid is available for oral administration in fixed combination as the commercial product Augmentin; fixed combinations are given in the next Table:

Fixed Combinations of Amoxicillin/Clavulinic Acid (Augmentin)

Product	Amoxicillin(mg)	Clavulinic Acid(mg)
Augmentin 250 Tablets	250	125
Augmentin 500 Tablets	500	125
Augmentin 125 Oral Susp.	125	31.25
Augmentin 250 Oral Susp.	250	62.5
Augmentin 125 Chewable	125	31.25
Augmentin 250 Chewable	250	62.5

AMOXICILLIN/CLAVULANIC ACID (Cont.)

DOSAGE: Dosage of amoxicillin/clavulanic acid as Augmentin is given in the next Table:

Dosage of Amoxicillin/Clavulanic Acid as Augmentin

Condition	Age	Dosage (Augmentin)
Usual	Adults and Child.> 40kg	One Augmentin 250 tablet every eight hours.
	Child.< 40kg	20mg/kg daily based on amoxicillin component in divided doses every eight hours.
Severe Infections and Infections of Respiratory Tract Otitis Media, Sinusitis Lower Respiratory Tract Infections and Other Infections	Adults and Child.> 40kg	One Augmentin 500 tablet every eight hours.
	Child.< 40kg	40mg/kg daily based on amoxicillin component in divided doses every eight hours.

ADVERSE REACTIONS: Diarrhea/loose stools (9% or more), nausea (3%), skin rashes and urticaria (3%), vomiting (1%), and vaginitis (1%).

Other adverse effects include abdominal discomfort, flatulence, headache, dizziness and moderate increases in serum transaminase; pseudomembraneous colitis has been reported in two cases.

Do not use in patients who are allergic to penicillin.

AMPHOTERICIN B
(Fungizone)

USES: Amphotericin B is an **antifungal** and **antiprotozoal antibiotic;** it is the most effective treatment for most systemic mycoses. Systemic uses are given in the next Table:

Systemic Uses of Amphotericin B
Antifungal: Aspergillus fumigatus; Paracoccidioides brasilienses; Blastomyces dermatitidis; Candida albicans, C.guilliermandi and C. tropicalis; Coccidioides immitis; Cryptococcus neoformans; Histoplasma capsulatum, Mucor mucedo, Rhodotorula spp., and Sporothrix schenckii
Antiprotozoal: Leishmania braziliensis, L. mexicana and L. donovani, Naegleria species, variable activity against Acanthamoeba castellani and A. polyphagia
Other Organisms: Not active against bacteria, rickettsiae or viruses

Amphotericin B is used topically to treat cutaneous and mucocutaneous candidal infections.

Mechanism of Action: Amphotericin B exerts its antifungal activity by binding to sterols in the fungal cell membrane. The drug is not active against organisms, such as bacteria, that do not contain sterols in their cell membranes. When amphotericin B binds to cell membranes of fungal cells, the membranes become more permeable and cellular constituents are lost. Mammalian kidney and erythrocytes contain sterols, and these cells may be damaged by amphotericin B.

DOSAGE FORMS: Injection: 50mg vials; Cream: 3%; Lotion: 3%; Ointment: 3%

DOSAGE: Amphotericin B is administered by slow IV.

An initial test dose of amphotericin is given: 1mg, dissolved in 50 to 150ml of 5% dextrose in water(D5W) and infused over at least 20 to 30 minutes. Monitor therapy with blood pressure, pulse, temperature and respiratory rate every 30 minutes for 4 hours to assess patient response to the drug.

If this test dose is tolerated, on the next day a dose of 0.25mg/kg is given by slow I.V. infusion over 6 hours at a concentration not greater than 0.1mg/ml in 5% dextrose. The daily dose is then increased gradually (usually in 5mg-10mg increments) on each subsequent day, to a maximum of 0.5 to 1.0mg/kg/day, or up to 1.5mg/kg/day given every other day.

The duration of therapy varies with the nature and severity of the infection. Usually, several months of therapy are necessary for an adequate response; relapse may occur if therapy is discontinued prematurely. Histoplasmosis, cryptococcosis, or blastomycosis may be adequately treated with a total IV dose of 2-4g. Total doses of 35mg/kg have been given for the treatment of chronic pulmonary histoplasmosis and 40mg/kg for disseminated histoplasmosis.

There is evidence that to successfully treat a systemic fungal infection, serum amphotericin B concentration should be maintained at twice the in-vitro MIC for the infecting fungus.

Cutaneous and Mucocutaneous Candidal Infections: For the treatment of cutaneous and mucocutaneous candidal infections, amphotericin B may be applied topically as a 3% cream, lotion or ointment to affected areas 2-4 times daily for 1-4 weeks. To prevent self-reinfection from the GI tract in the treatment of chronic or recurrent cutaneous or mucocutaneous monilial infections, 500,000 units of nystatin, oral tablets, 3 times daily may be administered.

ADVERSE EFFECTS AND LABORATORY STUDIES FOR PATIENTS WITH AMPHOTERICIN B: Adverse effects and laboratory studies on amphotericin B are given in the next Table;(Hermans, P.E. & Keys, T.F., Mayo Clin. Proc. 58,223-231, 1983):

Amphotericin B: Adverse Effects and Laboratory Studies

Adverse Effects	Laboratory Studies
Nephrotoxicity (very common - 80% or more)	Serum Creatinine; alternate days until an increase occurs;then daily level. A serum creatinine value of up to 3mg/dl is acceptable.
Hypomagnesium	Serum magnesium, weekly
Anemia	Hemoglobin, Hematocrit, weekly
Leukopenia (rare)	Leukocyte Count, weekly
Hypokalemia (common)	Serum potassium, daily to weekly; dec. secondary to nephrotoxicity
Thrombocytopenia (rare)	Platelet count, weekly
Hepatic Dysfunction(rare)	Serum glutamic-oxalacetic transaminase(SGOT); and serum alkaline phosphatase (weekly)

Other adverse effects include anaphylactic reaction (rare); anorexia, nausea, vomiting, headaches, fever, chills, malaise, muscle and joint pain are commonly associated with IV infusion, and may be treated with non-steroidal anti-inflammatory agents or steroids when necessary.

AMPICILLIN

(Omnipen, Polycillin, Principen, Totacillin)

USES: Ampicillin is an **aminopenicillin;** the aminopenicillins include: amoxicillin, ampicillin, bacampicillin, cyclacillins, hetacillin. Ampicillin is used like the other aminopenicillins and is used principally for the treatment of infections caused by susceptible **gram-negative** and **gram-positive bacteria.** Activities of ampicillin are given in the next Table (Parry, M.F., Med. Clin. No. Am. 71, 1093-1112, 1987; Adams, H.G., Personal Comm.):

Activities of Ampicillin

	Gram-positive cocci			Gram-negative bacilli						Anaerobes	
	S. aureus	Streptococci	Strep. entero.	H. influenzae	P. mirabilis	E. coli	Klebsiella	Other Enterics	Pseudomonas a.	B. fragilis	Res. Anaerobes
Ampicillin	4*	4	4	4*	4	2	▩	▩	▩	2	3

4=best activity; 3=good activity; 2=some activity; ▩=little or no activity; Res.= Resident; *Beta-lactamase negative.

The usual susceptible bacteria are given in the next Table:

Usual Spectra of Activity of Ampicillin

Gram-Negative Bacteria	Gram-Positive Bacteria
Escherichia Coli	Streptococcus Pneumoniae
Neisseria Gonorrhoeae (Beta-Lactamase Negative)	Enterococci
Haemophilus Influenza (Beta-Lactamase Negative)	Nonpenicillinase-Producing Staphylococci
Proteus Mirabilis	Listeria
Salmonella	

Ampicillin, like other aminopenicillins, generally should not be used for the treatment of streptococcal or staphylococcal infections when a natural penicillin (penicillin G and penicillin V) would be effective.

DOSAGE FORMS: Caps: 250mg, 500mg; Chewable Tabs: 125mg; Susp. 125mg/5ml, 250mg/5ml, 500mg/5ml; Drops: 100mg/ml; Injection: 125, 250, 500mg, 1, 2, 10g

Ampicillin is an inhibitor of bacterial cell wall synthesis.

DOSAGE: Ampicillin is commercially available as anhydrous ampicillin or ampicillin trihydrate for oral administration, and as the sodium salt for IM or slow IV injection or IV infusion. Maximum oral absorption is achieved 1 hour before or 2 hours after meals. Direct IV injections should be made slowly over 10-15 minutes. For intermittent IV infusion, infusion rate should be adjusted so that the dose of the drug is administered before 10% or more of the drug is inactivated in the IV solution.

Dosage for adults is usually the same for both parenteral and oral routes.

For most infections, except gonorrhea, therapy should be continued for at least 48-72 hours after eradication of infection.

Dosage of ampicillin in different conditions is given in the next Table:

Dosage of Ampicillin in Different Conditions

Condition	Age	Route	Dosage
Meningitis/ Septicemia *	Neonate <7 days	IV	100-150mg/kg/day divided every 12 h.
	7-28 days	IV	150-200mg/kg/day divided every 6-8 h.
	Infants & Children	IV	200-300mg/kg/day divided every 6 h.
	Adults & >40kg	IV	8-14g or 150-200mg/kg/day divided every 3-4 h.

* Ampicillin should be used in combination with either an aminoglycoside or a cephalosporin (i.e. Cefotaxime or Ceftazidime) for initial empiric therapy for neonatal meningitis. Infants and children may receive either ampicillin and chloramphenicol or cephalosporin (i.e. Cefotaxime or Ceftazidime) alone (ampicillin must be added to cephalosporin therapy up to 6-8 weeks of life to cover Listeria and enterococcus as causative agents). (Committee on Infectious Diseases, Treatment of Bacterial Meningitis, Pediatrics 81, 904-907, 1988).

Dosage of Ampicillin in Different Conditions (Cont.)

Condition	Age	Route	Dosage
Respiratory Tract, Skin or Skin Structure Infections	Adults and >40kg	Oral or Parenteral	250-500mg every 6 h.
	<40kg	Parenteral	25-50mg/kg daily in eqully divided doses every 6 h.
GI or Urinary Tract Infections	Adults and >40kg	Oral or Parenteral	500mg every 6 hours
	<40kg	Oral or Parenteral	50-100mg/kg daily in equally divided doses every 6 hours.
Gonorrhea, Uncomplicated, Nonpenicil-linase-Producing Neisseria Gonorrhoeae #	Adults, >45kg	Oral	Single 3.5g ampicillin plus 1g oral probenecid, plus multiple-day doxycycline or tetracycline in adults and children older than 8 years for coexisting chlamydial and mycoplasmal infections.
Gonorrhea, Disseminated (Gonococcal-Arthritis-Dermatitis Syndrome) (Susceptible strains)#	Adults	Oral	Single 3.5g ampicillin plus 1g oral probenecid followed by 500mg ampicillin every 6h for at least 7 days. or IV penicillin G potassium or sodium (10 million units daily) for 3 days or until improvement occurs and then 500mg ampicillin orally every 6 h. for at least 7 days.

Ampicillin or penicillin is no longer recommended for empiric therapy for gonococcal infections due to the spread of penicillinase-producing Neisseria gonorrhoeae; recommendations are for beta-lactamase negative strains (1989 STD Treatment Guidelines, Morbidity and Mortality Weekly Report 38, S-8, September 1, 1989).

Condition	Age	Route	Dosage
Gardnerella Infections (Nonspecific Vaginitis)	Adults	Oral	Alternate to metronidazole; ampicillin, 500mg 4 times daily for 7 days.
Prophylaxis of Bacterial Endocarditis (Dental Procedures or Minor Upper Respiratory Tract Surgery or Instrumentation) Low Risk Patients (Oral agents often preferred	Adults; Children >27kg	IM or IV	Am. Heart Assoc.(AHA)Recommendation: 2g ampicillin IM or IV 30 minutes prior to procedure then IM or IV ampicillin 1g or oral amoxicillin 1.5g 6 h. after initial dose.
	<27kg	IM or IV	Am. Heart Assoc.(AHA)Recommendation: 50mg/kg ampicillin IM or IV 30 min. prior to procedure then IM or IV ampicillin 25mg/kg or oral amoxi-cillin 25mg/kg 6 h. after initial dose.
Prophylaxis of Bacterial Endocarditis (GI, Biliary or Genito-urinary Tract Surgery or Instrumentation)	Adults Children >27kg	IM or IV	Am. Heart Assoc.(AHA)Recommendation: 2g ampicillin IM or IV and 1.5mg/kg (max. 80mg) of gentamicin IM or IV 30 minutes prior to procedure and again 8h. later. Alternatively, follow up dose may be oral amoxicillin 1.5g 6h. after initial dose.
	<27kg	IM or IV	Am. Heart Assoc.(AHA)Recommendation: 50mg/kg ampicillin, IM or IV and 2mg/kg gentamicin IM or IV, 30 min. prior to the procedure and half doses 8 h. later. Alternatively, follow up dose may be oral amoxi-cillin 25mg/kg 6h. after initial dose.

AMPICILLIN (Cont.)

Dosage in Renal Failure: Dosage of ampicillin in renal failure is given in the next Table:

Dosage of Ampicillin in Renal Failure

Glomerular Filtration Rate(GFR)	Age	Dosage
10-50mg/min.	Adults	Usual dose of ampicillin every 6-12 h.
<10ml/min.	Adults	Usual dose of ampicillin every 12-16 h

PHARMACOKINETICS: Absorption: 50%; absorption is delayed by food. Peak: 1-2 hours; Protein Binding: 15-25%; Half-Life: Adults, 1-1.3 hours; neonates, 2 hours; anuria, 10-20 hours; chronic liver disease, 2 hours. Half-life is significantly prolonged by probenecid; penicillinase sensitive; dialysable; Excretion: 35% of oral dose active in urine; 70% of IM dose active in urine.

ADVERSE EFFECTS: Ampicillin is contraindicated in patients who are hypersensitive to any penicillin. Toxicity: Anaphylaxis(rarely), rash(7%-10%), fever, diarrhea, superinfection, nausea and vomiting.

INTERACTIONS: When ampicillin is used with the bacteriostatic antibiotics, erythromycin and tetracyclines, its effectiveness may be decreased or destroyed.

AMPICILLIN PLUS SULBACTAM
(Unasyn)

USES: Sulbactam is a beta-lactamase inhibitor; the addition of sulbactam to ampicillin extends the antibacterial spectrum of ampicillin. Activities of ampicillin/sulbactam are given in the next Table (Parry, M.F., Med. Clin. No. Am. 71, 1093-1112, 1987; Wright, A.J. and Wilkowske, C.J., Mayo Clin. Proc. 62, 806-820, 1987; Adams, H.G., Personal Comm.):

Activities of Ampicillin/Sulbactam (Unasyn)

	Gram-positive cocci: S. aureus	Gram-positive cocci: Streptococci	Gram-positive cocci: Strep. entero.	Gram-negative bacilli: H. influenzae	Gram-negative bacilli: P. mirabilis	Gram-negative bacilli: E. coli	Gram-negative bacilli: Klebsiella	Gram-negative bacilli: Other Enterics	Gram-negative bacilli: Pseudomonas a.	Anaerobes: B. fragilis	Anaerobes: Res. Anaerobes
Ampicillin/Sulbactam	4	4	4	4	4	3	4	3	▩	3	4

4=best activity; 3=good activity; 2=some activity; ▩ =little or no activity;
Res.= Resident.

The spectrum of antibacterial activity of Unasyn is given in the next Table (Wright, A.J. and Wilkowske, C.J., Mayo Clin. Proc. 62, 806-820, 1987; Parry, M.F., Med. Clin. No. Am. 71, 1093-1112, 1987):

Antibacterial Activity of Ampicillin plus Sulbactam

Gram-Positive: Cocci	Gram-Positive: Bacilli	Gram-Negative: Enteric Bacilli	Gram-Negative: Cocci
Staph. Aureus	Listeria	P. mirabilis	**Neisseria Gonorrhoeae**
Streptococcus		E. coli	**Moraxella (Branhamella)**
Pneumoniae		**K. pneumoniae**	**Catarrhalis**
(Pneumococcus)		Salmonella	
Enterococcus			
		Other Bacilli	
		H. Influenzae	
		Anaerobic Bacilli	
		Bacteroides fragilis	

The bacteria that are typed in bold are those that are normally resistant to ampicillin alone but are susceptible to ampicillin plus sulbactam.

DOSAGE FORMS: Ampicillin and sulbactam are supplied together in a 2:1 ratio (1g of ampicillin and 0.5g of sulbactam).

DOSAGE: Ampicillin plus sulbactam (Unasyn) is administered intramuscularly and intravenously. Dosage is given in the next Table:

Dosage of Ampicillin plus Sulbactam (Unasyn)

Route	Dosage
Intramuscular	1.5g (1g ampicillin plus 0.5g sulbactam) every 6 hours.
Intravenous	1.5-3g every 6 hours.

Dosage in children is based on ampicillin component.

AMPICILLIN PLUS SULBACTAM (Cont.)

ADVERSE EFFECTS: Adverse reactions are mainly due to the ampicillin; the combination drug may cause more gastrointestinal symptoms than ampicillin alone. The adverse effected shared by all penicillins are given in the next Table (Wright, A.J. and Wilkowski, C.J., Mayo Clin. Proc. 62, 806-820, 1987):

Adverse Effects Shared by All Penicillins
Allergic reactions (rarely anaphylactic)
Skin rashes
Diarrhea
Neuromuscular irritability, including seizures associated with large doses or renal failure.
Hematologic changes such as neutropenia and anemia (at times hemolytic)
Drug-induced fever
Nephropathy (as component of serum sickness-type reaction) or interstitial nephritis.

Adverse effects associated specifically with ampicillin are skin rashes, diarrhea ad pseudomembranous colitis.

PHARMACOKINETICS: Half-Life: One hour for both drugs; Excretion: Excretion in urine is equal.

AMRINONE LACTATE

(Inocor)

USES: Amrinone lactate is a cardiac inotropic agent and peripheral vasodilator; it differs in structure and mode of action from catecholamines and digoxin. Amrinone acts by inhibition of type III phosphodiesterase resulting in increased cAMP in cardiac muscle and vascular smooth muscle. Amrinone increases the force and velocity of myocardial contraction and causes peripheral vasodilatation without increasing myocardial oxygen demand in patients with severe congestive heart failure. Peripheral arteriolar vasodilatation reduces left ventricular systolic wall stress which negates the increase in myocardial oxygen consumption resulting from the enhanced contractile state (Baim, D.S., Am. J. Cardiol. 63, 23A-26A, 1989).

DOSAGE FORMS: Parenteral injection: 5mg/ml.

DOSAGE: Optimal dosage of amrinone has not been determined. The manufacturers suggest 0.75mg/kg IV loading dose over 2-3 minutes, followed by maintenance dosage rate of 5-10mcg/kg/min. A second dose of 0.75mg/kg may be administered after 30 minutes if necessary. A safer way to administer the loading dose is over a longer period of time (5-60 minutes), particularly in patients with cardiovascular stability or on other inotropic agents. Other recommendations include 0.75mg/kg IV loading dose over 5-10 minutes, followed by 2.5-20mcg/kg/min (Marcus, R.H. et al., Amer. J. Cardiol. 66, 1107-1112, November, 1990) or 1-3mg/kg load over 2-3 minutes, followed by 5-20mcg/kg/min (Hines, R., J. of Cardiothoracic Anesthesia 3, 24-32, 1989). Suggested dosage in infants is 3-4.5mg/kg by slow IV infusion in divided doses, followed by 10mcg/kg/min infusion; neonates may receive a similar loading dose, followed by infusion of 3-5 mcg/kg/min (Lawless, S. et al., Critical Care Med. 17, 751-754, 1989), but a smaller loading dose (eg, 0.75mg/kg) is commonly used to minimize the risk of hypotension.

ADVERSE EFFECTS: Hypotension (particularly during administration of loading dose), arrhythmias, thrombocytopenia (in up to 15% of patients), hepatotoxicity, hypersensitivity reactions.

MONITOR: Blood pressure, heart rate, central venous pressure, fluids and electrolytes.

PHARMACOKINETICS: Onset of effects: 2-5 minutes, peak within 10 minutes after a single IV dose. Half-life: adults, 2.6-8h.; infants, 6.8h. (mean); neonates, 22.2h. (mean). Excretion: urine.

ANAEROBIC INFECTIONS, TREATMENT

Drugs for anaerobic infections are given in the next Table (Hill, M.K. and Sanders, C.V., Infect. Dis. Clin. No. Am. 2, 57-83, Mar. 1988):

Drugs for Anaerobic Infections

Generic (Trade)	Adult Dosage (IV)	CNS Coverage
Pen G	10-20 million units/day	Yes
Piperacillin	3-4g every 4-6 hrs.	Yes
Cefoxitin (Mefoxin)	1-2g every 4-6 hrs.	No
Metronidazole (Flagyl)	1g loading, then 500mg every 6 hrs.	Yes
Clindamycin (Cleocin)	900mg every 8 hrs.	No
Chloramphenicol (Chloromycetin)	500mg to 1g every 6 hrs.	Yes but erratic penetration into abscess cavities and development of resistant species.
Imipenem/Cilistatin (Primaxin)	500mg to 1g every 6 hrs.	Not yet studied.
Ticarcillin/Clavulanate (Timentin)	3.1g every 4 hrs.	Not yet studied.
Ampicillin/Sulbactam (Unasyn)	2g every 6 hrs.	Not yet studied.

Activities of major classes of antibiotics against anaerobic pathogens are given in the next Table (Styrt, B. and Gorbach, S.L., N. Engl. J. Med. 321, 298-302, 1989):

Activities of Antibiotics Against Anaerobes

	B. Fragilis	B. Melaninogenicus	Fusobacterium	Clostridium	Propionibacterium Actinomyces	Peptostreptococcus
Pen G	0-1	0-3	2	1-2	3	3
Antipseudomonal PCN	2-3	1-3	3	3	3	3
Cefoxitin	2	3	2-3	0-2	3	3
Imipenem/Cilistatin (Primaxin)	3	3	2	3	3	3
Beta-lactam and Beta-lactamase inhib	3	3	3	3	3	3
Clindamycin	2-3	3	3	2	3	3
Chloramphenicol	3	3	3	3	3	3
Metronidazole	3	3	3	3	0	2-3

3 = best activity; 2 = good activity; 1 = some activity; 0 = no activity.

Anaerobic infections may occur at many sites, including: CNS (abscess), head and neck (chronic sinusitis or otitis, gingivitis, odontogenic or oropharyngeal infections), lungs (pneumonia, abscess, empyema), GI tract (peritonitis, intraabdominal or liver abscess), female genital tract (tubo-ovarian abscess, salpingitis, septic abortion, endometritis, Bartholin's gland abscess, bacterial vaginosis), skin and soft tissue (cellulitis, necrotizing fasciitis, myonecrosis, decubitus ulcers, diabetic foot ulcers, bite wounds) (Styrt, B. and Gorbach, S.L., N. Engl. J. Med. 321, 240-246, 1989). Treatment is usually based on expected antibiotic sensitivities; synergistic combinations of antibiotics may be useful in serious anaerobic infections, particularly Bacteroides species and Clostridium species (Brook, I., Pediatr. Infect. Dis. J. 6, 332-335, 1987).

ANTIARRHYTHMIC DRUGS

Treatment of common arrhythmias is given in the next Table (Keefe, L.D. et al., Drugs 22, 363-400, 1981; Textbook of Advanced Life Support, American Heart Association, 1987):

Treatment of Common Arrhythmias

Arrhythmia	Acute Therapy First-line [Alternatives]	Chronic Therapy & Prophylaxis First-line [Alternatives]
Supraventricular Arrhythmias		
Asystole	Epinephrine [Atropine]	
Sinus Tachycardia	Treat underlying cause	Propranolol
with Heart Failure	Treat underlying cause	Digitalis
Atrial Premature Contractions (PAC's)	Seldom require therapy	Quinidine [Procainamide Verapamil, Beta-adrenergic blocking agents, diltiazem]
Paroxysmal Supraventricular Tachycardia (formerly Atrial Tachycrdia).	Vagal maneuvers, facial immersion (water temp. 5-18 C) cardioversion (0.25-2 W-s/kg). [Verapamil, Adenosine, Digitalis, Propranolol]	Digoxin, Propranolol, Verapamil [Quinidine, Disopyramide, Procainamide. Amiodarone].
Atrial Flutter	DC cardioversion [Digitalis, Verapamil, Beta-blockers, Overdrive Pacing].	Quinidine, Procainamide.
Atrial Fibrillation	Digitalis, Quinidine, Propranolol, DC cardioversion.	Digitalis, Verapamil (prophylaxis-same as for other atrial arrhythmias) [Beta-blockers].
Wolff-Parkinson-White Syndrome	DC cardioversion	Amiodarone [Quinidine, Beta-blockers, Kent bundle resection].
Ventricular Tachyarrhythmias		
Premature Ventricular Complexes(PVCs) eg, Acute Myocardial Infarction.	Lidocaine [Procainamide, Bretylium].	Quinidine [Procainamide, Disopyramide].
Ventricular Tachycardia	DC cardioversion or Lidocaine	Quinidine, Amiodarone [Beta-blockers, Procainamide, Disopyramide, Apridine, Mexilitine, Ventricular resection].
Ventricular Fibrillation and Flutter	Electrical defibrillation. Cardiopulmonary resuscitation. [Adjuncts: Lidocaine, Bretylium].	Amiodarone, Bretylium [Implantable defibrillator].
Torsades de pointes	Magnesium [pacemaker, isoproterenol]	
Other		
Digitalis - Induced	See Discussion: Discontinue K^+ replacement, Lidocaine, Phenytoin, Atropine, Digoxin Immune Fab	
Sinus Bradycardia	Oxygen, Atropine, Temporary Pacing [Isoproterenol]	Permanent Pacing
AV Conduction Defects		
First Degree	None	
Second Degree Type I	None Atropine; Discontinue drug, Pacemaker	
Type II	Pacemaker	
Third Degree	Pacemaker except for congential.	

ANTIARRHYTHMIC DRUGS (Cont.)

ASYSTOLE: The guidelines for treatment of asystole is given in the next Figure (JAMA 255, 2933, 1986):

Guidelines for Treatment of Asystole: Adults, Children

If rhythm is unclear and possibly ventricular fibrillation, defibrillate as for ventricular fibrillation; if asystole is present (confirmed by two leads), then

Continue CPR

↓

Establish IV access

↓

Epinephrine, 1:10,000, 0.5-1.0mg IV push;
(Peds: 0.01mg/kg = 0.1ml/kg);
repeat epinephrine every 5 minutes.

↓

Intubate (as soon as possible)

↓

Atropine, 1.0mg IV push (repeat in 5 minutes)
(Peds: 0.02mg/kg, minimum: 0.1mg)

↓

(Consider bicarbonate; the value of bicarbonate is questionable during cardiac arrest, and it is not recommended for the routine cardiac arrest sequence; give 1mEq/kg; half of original dose may be repeated every 10 minutes if it is used.

↓

Consider pacing

SINUS TACHYCARDIA: Sinus tachycardia in adults is defined as a heart rate faster than 100 beats/min. that is caused by rapid impulse formation by the normal pacemaker; conditions causing sinus tachycardia are given in the next Table:

Conditions Causing Sinus Tachycardia
Fever, Exercise, Emotion, Pain
Anemia
Shock
Congestive Heart Failure
Certain Drugs; Thyrotoxicosis

Treatment: It may be a beneficial physiologic response to a demand for a higher cardiac output. The underlying cause should be diagnosed and treated appropriately. Medical therapy is usually not indicated.

A beta-adrenergic blocking agent (eg, propranolol [Inderal]) may be useful if heart failure is not present. Beta blockers slow a rapid sinus rate resulting from enhanced sympathetic tone or increased levels of circulating catecholamines.

Digitalis may control sinus tachycardia associated with congestive heart failure (CHF) but is not useful when the increased sinus rate is due to other causes.

PREMATURE ATRIAL COMPLEXES (PAC's): A premature atrial complex is an electrical impulse that originates in the atria outside of the sinus node. It is premature, occurring before the next expected sinus beat. Premature atrial complexes often occur without apparent cause; conditions causing premature atrial complexes are given in the next Table:

Conditions Causing Premature Atrial Complexes
Stimulants: Caffeine, tobacco, alcohol
Sympathomimetic drugs
Hypoxia
Elevation of atrial pressure
Digitalis intoxication

Acute Therapy: None necessary.

Chronic Therapy and Prophylaxis: Premature atrial complexes are usually benign and do not require therapy. However, if they are symptomatic or trigger paroxysmal supraventricular tachycardias, they may require suppression. The drug of choice is quinidine. Other drugs that can be tried include procainamide, verapamil, beta-adrenergic blocking agents, and diltiazem. Flecainide and amiodarone can also suppress PAC's but their potentially serious side effects preclude their use for PAC's.

ANTIARRHYTHMIC DRUGS (Cont.)

PAROXYSMAL SUPRAVENTRICULAR TACHYCARDIA(PSVT) (formerly Atrial Tachycardia): PSVT is one of the most common arrhythmias seen in the emergency department. It is characterized by repeated episodes (i.e. paroxysms) of atrial tachycardia with an abrupt onset lasting from a few seconds to many hours.

Treatment: Approach to treatment depends on whether the patient is stable or unstable. Treatment strategies are given in the next sections (Adult Advanced Cardiac Life Support, JAMA 255 2933-2954, 1986; Brown D.D. et al., Patient Care pgs. 26-48, Sept. 15, 1987; Textbook of Advanced Cardiac Life Support, American Heart Association, 1987).

Stable Patients: The treatment of stable adult patients with PSVT is given in the next Table:

Paroxysmal Supraventricular Tachycardia: Stable Adult

Vagal Maneuvers (gentle Carotid Sinus Massage on one side for a few seconds).

↓

Adenosine*

↓

Verapamil, 5mg IV over 5 minutes.
- Contraindications: History of severe bradycardia, hypotension, congestive heart failure or concomitant acute use of IV beta blockers.
- Give calcium chloride (10ml, 10%, over 5-8 minutes before verapamil to decrease the hypotensive effect)
- If no effect from verapamil may repeat in 30 minutes.

↓

Repeat Verapamil 10mg after 15-20 min.

↓

Cardioversion (see next page)

or Digoxin, IV (0.75-1mg IV loading)(see DIGOXIN)

or Edrophonium (Tensilon), IV, 2-5mg, over 60 seconds. If no response in 5 minutes, may give additional 2-5mg (Max. total dose: 10mg).

or Propranolol, IV, 1-3mg at rate of ≤ one mg/min. Stop injection as soon as heart rate slows down (may use atropine for excessive bradycardia or when blood pressure decreases significantly. If tachycardia continues, may repeat IV propranolol after 5 minutes, but do not exceed a total dose of 5mg. Propranalol and Verapamil generally should not be administered IV within a few hours of each other due to risk of severe depression of myocardial contractility.

*Adenosine is considered by many clinicians to have replaced verapamil as the drug of choice for acute termination of PSVT (Rankin, A.C. and McGovern, B.A., Ann. Intern. Med. 114, 513-515, 1991).

Vagal maneuvers may be helpful in converting patients with PSVT. The most commonly employed vagal maneuvers are carotid massage (unless cerebrovascular disease or a carotid bruit is present), the Valsalva maneuver, head-down tilt with deep inspiration, and/or activation of the "diving reflex" by ice water facial immersion (unless ischemic heart disease is suspected).

Stable pediatric patients with PSVT are treated initially with vagal maneuvers (usually, ice wrapped in a washcloth is applied to the face for 20-30 seconds). Digitalization using age-appropriate divided doses over 12-24 hours is usually the next step. Verapamil (0.1-0.2mg/kg) should only be used by a cardiologist experienced with calcium channel blockers in pediatrics, since cardiovascular collapse has been reported with verapamil in neonates and infants. Propranalol (0.01-0.2mg/kg) has also been used, but concommitant use with calcium channel blockers is contraindicated. Transesophageal atrial pacing has been used successfully to terminate SVT in children (Dick, M. et. al., "Acute Termination of Supraventricular Tachyarrhythmias in Children by Transesophageal Atrial Pacing," Amer. J. Cardiol. 61, 925-927, 1988).

ANTIARRHYTHMIC DRUGS (Cont.)

Unstable Patients: The treatment of unstable adult patients with PSVT are given in the next Figure:

Cardioversion Procedure for Paroxysmal Supraventricular Tachycardia in the Unstable Adult Patients

1. Use short-acting barbiturate or IV diazepam to induce amnesia.
2. IV line in place; monitor ECG continuously.
3. Administer supplemental oxygen.
4. Synchronous cardioversion.

Give first shock: 75-100 J
↓
If necessary, give 2nd shock: 200 J
↓
If necessary, give 3rd shock: 360 J
↓
Correct Underlying Abnormalities; Pharmacological Therapy

Synchronize the defibrillator to prevent the electrical shock from being applied during repolarization of the ventricles (T wave) and causing ventricular fibrillation.

Unstable pediatric patients with PSVT are treated by synchronous cardioversion using 0.2J/kg then 0.4J/kg then 1.0J/kg. If unsuccessful, correct the underlying abnormalities and use pharmacological therapy.

ATRIAL FLUTTER: Atrial flutter is defined as rapid atrial rate generally around 280-340 beats/minute with varying degrees of atrioventricular block.

In atrial flutter, the impulse is conducted around some area of the atrium in a circular motion, arriving back at the same point at a rapid rate.

Atrial flutter may be associated with sick sinus syndrome, hypoxia, pericarditis, valvular heart disease and less commonly, acute myocardial infarction. There is usually a 2:1 AV block and a ventricular rhythm of about 150 beats/min. This arrhythmia is uncommon in pediatric patients and has been strongly associated with congenital heart disease, repaired or palliated: D-transposition of the great arteries (20.5%); complex congenital lesions (17.8%); ASD (12.1%); Tetralogy of Fallot (7.9%); Normal (6.3%); Other causes (35.4%)(Garson, A., et al., "Atrial Flutter in the Young: A collaborative Study of 380 Cases," JACC 6, 871-878, 1985).

Acute Therapy: If the patient is hypotensive, having ischemic pain, or in severe congestive heart failure, synchronized cardioversion at low energy levels is the treatment of choice. The procedure for cardioversion is given in the next Figure (Ferri, F.F., Practical Guide to the Care of the Medical Patient, C.V. Mosby Co., Wash. D.C., 1987, pg. 132):

Cardioversion Procedure for Atrial Flutter: Adult

1. Use short-acting barbiturate or IV diazepam to induce amnesia; have anesthesiologist in attendance.
2. IV line in place; monitor ECG continuously.
3. Synchronous cardioversion

Give first shock: 20-25 J
↓
If necessary, give 2nd shock: 50 J
↓
If necessary, give 3rd shock: 100 J
↓
If necessary, give 4th shock: 200 J

Synchronize the defibrillator to prevent the electrical shock from being applied during repolarization of the ventricles (T wave) and causing ventricular fibrillation.

If the patient is only mildly symptomatic, then an attempt might be made to control the rate with pharmacological therapy. The strategy for drug

ANTIARRHYTHMIC DRUGS (Cont.)
treatment of atrial flutter is given in the next Figure (Pritchett, E.L.C. and Anderson, J.L., Am. J. Cardiol. 62, ID-2D, Aug. 25, 1988):

Drug Treatment of Atrial Flutter

To Slow Ventricular Rate	To Maintain Sinus Rhythm
Digitalis	Type IA Antiarrhythmics:
Calcium Channel Blockers:	Quinidine
Verapamil (Calan, Isoptin)	Procainamide
Diltiazem (Cardizem)	Disopyramide
Nifedipine (Procardia, Adalat)	
Beta-Blockers:	
Atenolol (Tenormin)	
Metoprolol (Lopressor)	
Nadolol (Corgard)	
Pindolol (Visken)	
Propranolol (Inderol)	
Timolol (Blocadren)	

First, the ventricular rate can be slowed with digitalis, a calcium channel blocker such as verapamil or beta-blocking drugs. Verapamil and beta-blockers may exacerbate bradycardia and/or congestive heart failure.

Once the ventricular rate is controlled, the patient can be placed on a Type I antiarrhythmic drug such as quinidine or procainamide.

Chronic Therapy and Prophylaxis: Prophylaxis against recurrent paroxysmal atrial flutter may be achieved by the drugs used for acute therapy.

ATRIAL FIBRILLATION: Atrial fibrillation is defined as totally chaotic atrial activity caused by simultaneous discharge of multiple atrial foci. The atrium is frequently firing between 350 and 700 times per minute. Conduction through the AV node is markedly irregular; the ventricular rate is usually between 120 and 200 per minute.

Atrial fibrillation may be associated with sick sinus syndrome, hypoxia, increased atrial pressure, pericarditis and other conditions. In acute ischemic heart disease, increased left atrial pressure secondary to congestive heart failure is the most common cause. This arrhythmia is rare in pediatric patients, and therapy is similar to that for adults.

Acute Therapy: The therapy of atrial fibrillation is given in the next Table

Treatment of Acute Atrial Fibrillation
Drug Therapy
Digoxin
Digoxin plus quinidine (if necessary)
Propranolol
Cardioversion

Digoxin: Give digoxin, 0.5mg IV loading dose (slow), then 0.25mg IV every 4-8 hrs until the ventricular rate is controlled or until patient receives a full digitalizing dose (adults: 10-15mcg/kg lean body weight); maintenance dose is 0.125-0.25mg orally daily (decrease dosage in patients with renal insufficiency and elderly patients). The success rate is only 15%-20% of patients.

Quinidine: In those patient who do not respond to digoxin, quinidine is added to help convert the patient to normal sinus rhythm; administer quinidine sulfate, 300mg every 6 hours. Quinidine should never be used alone to control ventricular response in atrial fibrillation since in the absence of digoxin, quinidine will increase ventricular response-a situation that is potentially dangerous (Internal Medicine Alert 10, 80, Oct. 31, 1988). Quinidine increases digoxin levels which may lead to toxicity.

Propranolol: Propranolol may be used when acute atrial fibrillation does not respond to digoxin. The dosage of propranolol is as follows: 0.5mg IV (slowly) followed by IV boluses of 1mg every 5 min. to a total of 5mg.

Cardioversion: Cardioversion in atrial fibrillation (success rate 90%) is indicated under the conditions listed in the next Table:

Indications for Cardioversion in Atrial Fibrillation
Ventricular rate >140 beats/min. and the patient is symptomatic (eg., acute myocardial infarction, chest pain, dyspnea, congestive heart failure).
Lack of conversion to normal sinus rhythm after 3 days of therapy with digoxin and quinidine.

Prepare patient for cardioversion as follows (Ferri, F.F., "Practical Guide to the Care of the Medical Patient" C.V. Mosby Co., Wash. D.C., 1987):

ANTIARRHYTHMIC DRUGS (Cont.)

Quinidine: Start quinidine at least 24 hrs before cardioversion to help maintain normal sinus rhythm once it is achieved.

Left Atrium: If the left atrium is 4.5cm, the probability of achieving or maintaining normal sinus rhythm is minimal.

Digoxin: Do not give digoxin on the morning of the cardioversion; determine digoxin level.

Food-Intake: No food intake for 8 hours before cardioversion.

Anticoagulation: Anticoagulation may be advisable for 3 weeks before and 3 weeks after cardioversion, especially in patients with mitral valve disease or a history of thromboembolism.

The procedure for cardioversion is given in the next Figure:

Cardioversion Procedure for Atrial Fibrillation: Adult

1. Use short-acting barbiturate or IV diazepam to induce amnesia; have anesthesiologist in attendance.
2. IV line in place; monitor ECG continuously.
3. Give first shock: 100 J
   ↓
   If necessary, give 2nd shock: 200 J
   ↓
   If necessary, give 3rd shock: 300 J
   ↓
   If necessary, give 4th shock: 360 J
4. Synchronize the defibrillator to prevent the electrical shock from being applied during repolarization of the ventricles (T wave) and causing ventricular fibrillation.

WOLFF-PARKINSON-WHITE(WPW) SYNDROME: The WPW syndrome is a disorder of conduction of the electrical impulses of the heart, in which normally formed sinoatrial impulses are conducted to the ventricles both by way of the atrioventricular (A-V) node and by an abnormal conductive pathway (usually the bundle of Kent). The syndrome is defined electrocardiographically as shown in the next Figure (Hospital Medicine, pgs 102-103, Oct. 1988):

Electrocardiograph of Wolff-Parkinson-White Syndrome

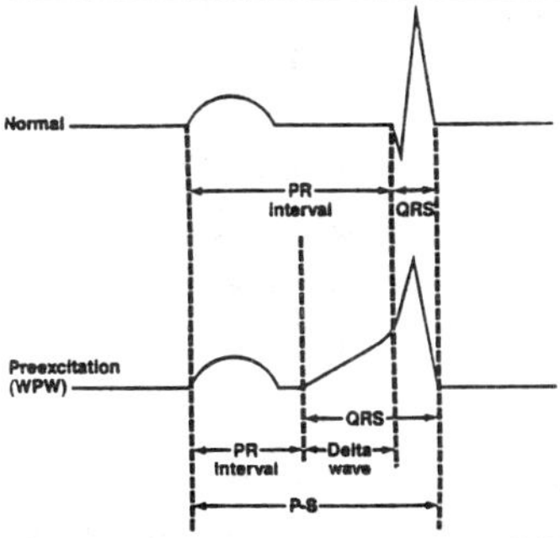

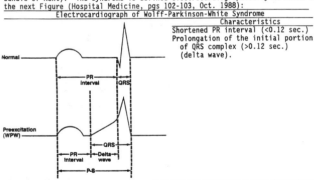

Characteristics

Shortened PR interval (<0.12 sec.)
Prolongation of the initial portion of QRS complex (>0.12 sec.) (delta wave).

Acute Therapy: Cardioversion is probably the treatment of choice as acute therapy for tachyarrhythmias associated with the WPW syndrome. Verapamil is also used in acute therapy. Adenosine may soon become the drug of choice in this condition due to its effectiveness with less severe side effects than verapamil.

Chronic Therapy and Prophylaxis: Amiodarone is very effective in preventing recurrences. Amiodarone lengthens the effective refractory period of the accessory pathway for both anterograde and retrograde conduction.

Other drugs that may be effective are quinidine and beta-blockers.

ANTIARRHYTHMIC DRUGS (Cont.)

VENTRICULAR TACHYARRHYTHMIAS: The ventricular tachyarrhythmias are listed in the next Table:

Ventricular Tachyarrhythmias
Premature Ventricular Complexes (PVCs)
Ventricular Tachycardia
Ventricular Flutter and Fibrillation

Lidocaine is the drug of choice for prevention or immediate control of serious ventricular arrhythmias especially when these occur in association with acute myocardial infarction; lidocaine acts rapidly, usually does not depress A-V conduction or myocardial contractility.

PREMATURE VENTRICULAR COMPLEXES (PVCs): PVCs are a common occurence after **acute myocardial infarction.**

A premature ventricular complex is a depolarization that arises in either ventricle prior to the next expected sinus beat, i.e., prematurely.

Acute Therapy: Suppressive therapy with lidocaine or, if it is unsuccessful, with procainamide is indicated, followed by bretylium.

Chronic Therapy: Quinidine, procainamide or disopyramide may be used. Encainide and flecainide were started 6 to 60 days after acute myocardial infarction and continued for one year. Treated patients had a higher mortality rate than untreated patients, so these drugs are not indicated for routine treatment of PVCs (The Cardiac Arrhythmia Pilot Study (CAPS) Investigators, Am. J. Cardiol. 61, 501-509, 1988).

VENTRICULAR TACHYCARDIA: When three or more beats of ventricular origin occur in succession at a rate in excess of 100 per minute, ventricular tachycardia is present. The rhythm is usually regular.

Therapy: The symptomatic patient with ventricular tachycardia requires emergency treatment. The presence or absence of pulse determines the therapy as given in the next Figure (Textbook of Advanced Cardiac Life Support. American Heart Association, 1987):

Treatment of Sustained Ventricular Tachycardia (VT): Adult

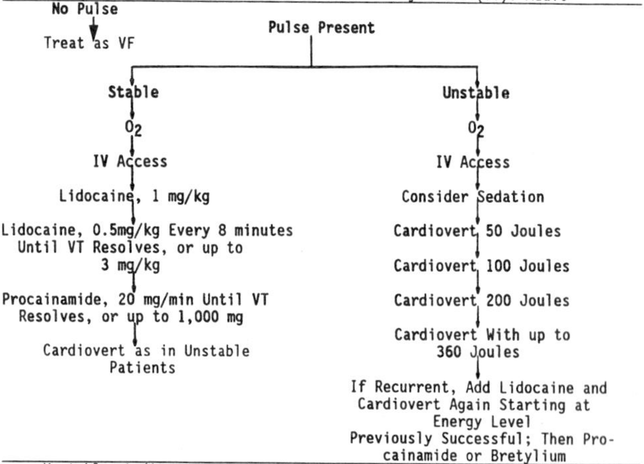

Unstable indicates symptoms, eg., chest pain or dyspnea, hypotension (systolic blood pressure <90 mm Hg), congestive heart failure, ischemia, or infarction.

If hypotension, pulmonary edema, or unconsciousness is present, unsynchronized cardioversion (defibrillation) should be done to avoid delay associated with synchonization.

ANTIARRHYTHMIC DRUGS (Cont.)

VENTRICULAR FIBRILLATION (VF): In ventricular fibrillation, the ventricles do not contract in a synchronous manner and on gross observation, the ventricular myocardium appears to be quivering. There is no cardiac output. Patients with acute myocardial infarction are at particular risk of ventricular fibrillation during the first day or two after infarction, and a proportion of the episodes of VF will be fatal even if defibrillation facilities are available.

Treatment: Treatment of ventricular fibrillation is basic life support and electrical defibrillation; lidocaine, epinephrine and sodium bicarbonate may be given if necessary; details are given in the next Figure (Chamberlain, D., Brit. Med. J. 292, 1068-1070, 1986; Textbook of Advanced Cardiac Life Support, American Heart Association, 1987):

Treatment of Ventricular Fibrillation: Adult

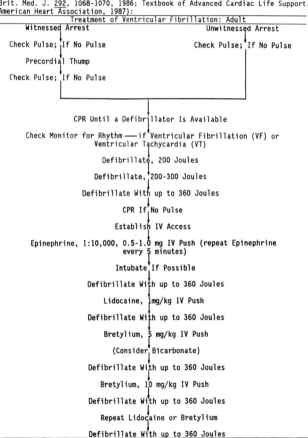

Witnessed Arrest	Unwitnessed Arrest
↓	↓
Check Pulse; If No Pulse	Check Pulse; If No Pulse
↓	↓
Precordial Thump	
↓	
Check Pulse; If No Pulse	

↓

CPR Until a Defibrillator Is Available

↓

Check Monitor for Rhythm — if Ventricular Fibrillation (VF) or Ventricular Tachycardia (VT)

↓

Defibrillate, 200 Joules

↓

Defibrillate, 200-300 Joules

↓

Defibrillate With up to 360 Joules

↓

CPR If No Pulse

↓

Establish IV Access

↓

Epinephrine, 1:10,000, 0.5-1.0 mg IV Push (repeat Epinephrine every 5 minutes)

↓

Intubate If Possible

↓

Defibrillate With up to 360 Joules

↓

Lidocaine, 1mg/kg IV Push

↓

Defibrillate With up to 360 Joules

↓

Bretylium, 5 mg/kg IV Push

↓

(Consider Bicarbonate)

↓

Defibrillate With up to 360 Joules

↓

Bretylium, 10 mg/kg IV Push

↓

Defibrillate With up to 360 Joules

↓

Repeat Lidocaine or Bretylium

↓

Defibrillate With up to 360 Joules

Check pulse and rhythm after each shock.

ANTIARRHYTHMIC DRUGS (Cont.)

Treatment of ventricular fibrillation or pulseless ventricular tachycardia in children is similar in principle to treatment in adults; details are given in the next Figure (Drug Therapy in Pediatric Advanced Life Support, American Heart Assoc., 1990):

Treatment of Ventricular Fibrillation: Children

CPR Until a Defibrillator is Available

↓

Check Monitor for Rhythm - if Ventricular Fibrillation (VF) or Pulseless Ventricular Tachycardia (VT)

↓

Defibrillate, 2 J/kg
double; repeat twice if needed

↓

Epinephrine 1:10,000 0.01mg/kg = 0.1ml/kg

↓

Defibrillate, 4J/kg

↓

Lidocaine, 1mg/kg

↓

Defibrillate, 4J/kg

↓

Bretylium, 5mg/kg
double to 10mg/kg and repeat if needed

Check pulse and rhythm after each shock.

DIGITALIS-INDUCED TACHYARRHYTHMIAS: Almost any disorder of cardiac rhythm may occur in patients with digitalis toxicity. The most common arrhythmia are ventricular bigeminy or trigeminy, multiform premature ventricular complexes, nonparoxysmal A-V junctional (nodal) tachycardia, and atrial tachycardia with block. Treatment of digitalis-toxicity-induced tachyarrhythmias is given in the next Table:

Treatment of Digitalis-Toxicity-Induced Tachyarrhythmias

Condition	Treatment
Mild Symptoms	Temporarily discontinue digitalis
Hypokalemia (chronic toxicity)	Potassium replacement
Severe	Lidocaine usually preferred initially Phenytoin (Dilantin)
Second or Third A-V Block	Atropine or temporary pacing (See Figure)
Severe, Life Threatening	Digoxin immune Fab

BRADYCARDIA: The causes of bradycardia are listed in the next Table:

Causes of Bradycardia

- Sinus Bradycardia
- Atrioventricular Block (AV Block)
  - First Degree AV Block
  - Second-Degree AV Block
    - Type I (Wenckebach) Second-Degree Block
    - Type II Second-Degree Block
  - Third-Degree AV Block

SINUS BRADYCARDIA: Bradycardia at a rate of 50 to 60 beats/min. is usually well tolerated; a rate less than 50 beats/min. may be accompanied by hypotension or increased ventricular ectopy such as may occur in patients with acute myocardial infarction.

Sinus bradycardia may be secondary to sinus node diseases, increased parasympathetic tone or drug effects (eg, digitalis, propranolol, or verapamil). Sinus bradycardia, especially in children, is often caused by hypoxia.

ATRIOVENTRICULAR BLOCK (AV Block): AV block is defined as a delay or interruption in conduction between atria and ventricles. It may be due to: (1) lesions along the conduction pathway (eg, calcification, fibrosis, necrosis); (2) increases in the refractory period of some portion of the conduction pathway (such as may occur in the AV node with digitalis); (3) shortening of the supraventricular cycle length with encroachment on the normal refractory period.

ANTIARRHYTHMIC DRUGS (Cont.)

First-Degree AV Block: In first degree AV block, there is simply a delay in passage of the impulse from atria to ventricles. This delay usually occurs at the level of the AV node but may be infranodal. First degree AV block is characterized by prolongation of the PR interval >0.20 sec. (at a rate of 70 beats/min.); the prolongation is constant from beat to beat. This condition may be secondary to ischemia at AV nodes seen particularly in inferior wall myocardial infarction.

Treatment: None.

Second-Degree AV Block: Second degree AV block is characterized by blockage of some (but not all) impluses from the atria to the ventricles.

Type I (Wenckebach) second-degree AV block is defined as progressive prolongation of the PR interval before an impluse is completely blocked; the cycle repeats periodically. In addition, cycle with dropped beat is less than 2 times the previous cycle.

This form of block almost always occurs at the level of the AV node (rarely at His bundle or bundle branch level) and is often due to increased parasympathetic tone or to drug effect (eg, digitalis, propranolol, or verapamil).

Treatment: Treatment of type I is given in the next Table:

Treament of Type I

Condition	Treatment
Transient	None
Dizziness	Atropine, 1mg; may repeat after 5 min; if no response, insert temporary pacemaker. (See Figure)
Block secondary to drugs, eg, digitalis.	Discontinue drug
Associated with anterior wall myocardial infarction.	Insert pacemaker

Type II second-degree AV block is defined as sudden interruption of AV conduction without prior prolongation of the PR interval. This form of AV block occurs below the level of the AV node either at bundle of His (uncommon) or bundle branch level (more common). The possible causes of type II are: degenerative changes in His-Purkinje system; acute anterior wall myocardial infarction; calcific aortic stenosis.

This type of block is usually permanent and often progressess to complete AV block.

Treatment: Treatment of type II is pacemaker insertion.

Third-Degree AV Block: Third-degree AV block is defined as complete blockage of all AV conduction and the atria and ventricles have separate and independent rhythms. It may occur at AV node, bundle of His, or bundle branch level.

Treatment: Immediate pacemaker insertion unless the patient has congenital third-degree AV block and is completely asymptomatic.

Treatment of Bradycardia: Treatment is needed only when bradycardia is associated with symptoms (eg, chest pain, dyspnea, lightheadedness, hypotension, or ventricular ectopy). Supplementary oxygen should be used if available.

Atropine (0.5mg) is usually indicated to increase the sinus rate; however, atropine may cause myocardial ischemia and may precipitate severe ventricular arrhythmias. Temporary pacing may be required in patients unresponsive to atropine.

Isoproterenol (Adult: 2-10mcg/min; Pediatric: 0.05-1.0mcg/kg/min) may be administered by continuous IV infusion if oxygen, atropine, and other measures fail to resolve clinically significant bradycardia.

ANTIARRHYTHMIC DRUGS (Cont.)

The treatment of bradycardia in adults is given in the next Figure (Textbook of Advanced Cardiac Life Support. American Heart Association, 1987):

Treatment of Bradycardia: Adult

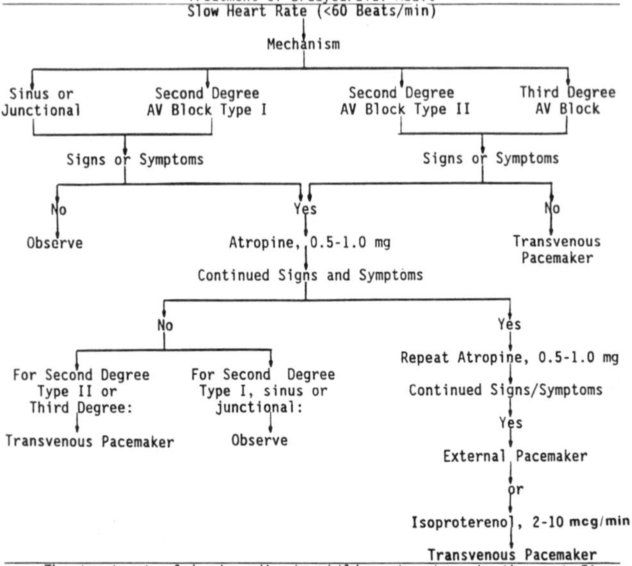

The treatment of bradycardia in children is given in the next Figure (Drug Therapy in Pediatric Advanced Life Support, American Heart Assoc. 1990):

Treatment of Bradycardia: Children

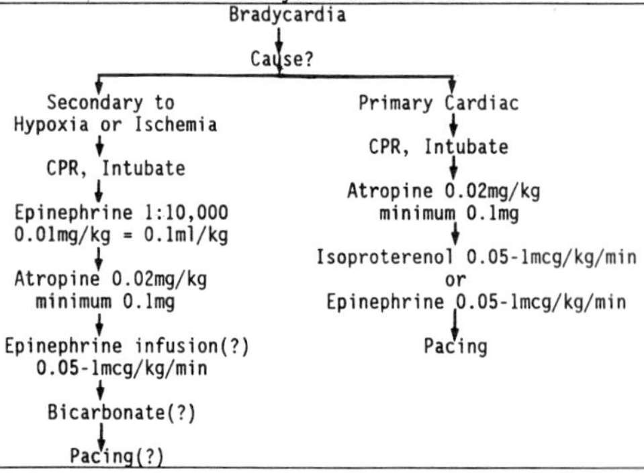

ANTIARRHYTHMIC DRUGS (Cont.)

Classification of Antidysrhythmic Drugs: Antidysrhythmic drugs are grouped on the basis of their effects on the action potential of cardiac cells; action potentials from a ventricular muscle are shown in the next Figure:

Action Potentials from Ventricular Muscle

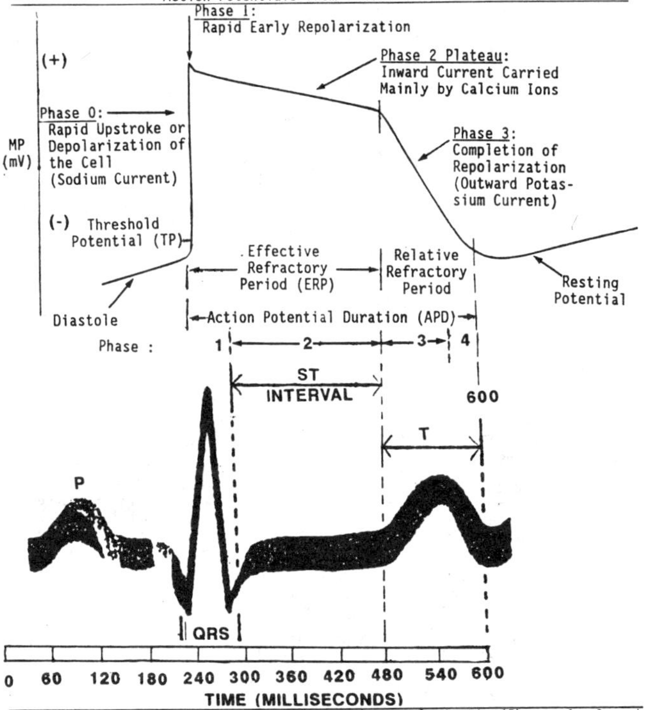

Following rapid depolarization(Phase 0), repolarization(Phases 1, 2 and 3) occurs.

Vertical axis is membrane potential(MP) in millivolts(mV). Cardiac cells have an electronegative resting membrane potential(RMP) which is maintained until a stimulus of sufficient magnitude occurs to lower the RMP to threshold potential(TP) which then results in excitation. Phase 0, or rapid depolarization results from a rapid influx of Na^+ into the intracellular space(ICS). This is followed by three phases of repolarization. The first (phase I) is a short rapid repolarization, followed by a plateau (phase 2) and finally a return to RMP (phase 3).

ANTIARRHYTHMIC DRUGS (Cont.)

The correlation of phase of action potential, action of ventricular muscle and ECG equivalent is given in the next Table:

Correlation: Action Potential and ECG Equivalent

Phase of Action Potential	Action of Ventricular Muscle	ECG Equivalent
0	Instantaneous depolarization	QRS complex
1	Rapid return to 0 mV	-
2	Plateau	ST interval
3	Repolarization	T wave
4	Return to resting potential	Interval between T and P waves.

Antiarrhythmic drugs are classified into five categories, based on their effects on cardiac action potentials, as given in the next Table (Wettrell, G. and Anderson, K.E., Therapeutic Drug Monitoring 8, 59-77, 1986):

Classification of Antidysrhythmic Drugs

Class	Drug	Main Electrophysiological or Pharmacological Effect	Mechanism
IA	Quinidine Procainamide Disopyramide Ajmaline	Depression of Vmax (Prolong refractoriness and slow conduction).	**Local Anesthetic Action** on Nerve and Myocardial Cell Membranes (more sensitive) that slows conduction.
IB	Lidocaine Phenytoin Mexiletine Tocaininde	Depression of Vmax (Shorten duration of refractory period; little effect on conduction in normal tissue).	Same as above
IC	Encainide Flecainide Lorcainide Propafenone	Depression of Vmax (markedly slow conduction but minimal effects on refractoriness).	Same as above
II	Sympathetic Inhibitors, eg, **Beta-Receptor Blockers** Propranolol	Inhibition of Sympathetic Activity on the Heart (Antiadrenergic properties).	Competition with Receptors & Interference with Release of Norepinephrine from Sympathetic Nerves (eg, Guanethidine), or Indirectly by an Action on the Brain, Reducing Outflow of Sympathetic Impulses (eg, Clonidine).
III	Amiodarone Bretylium	Prolongation of Action Potential Duration (Prolong refractoriness).	
IV	Verapamil Diltiazem	Blocking of Slow Inward (Calcium) Current **(Calcium antagonists).**	
V	Alinidine	Selective Anion-Channel Antagonism.	

ANTICOAGULANTS

See also **HEPARIN** and **WARFARIN.**

Anticoagulants; (Heparin and Warfarin) Treatment of Venous Thromboembolic Disease: Guidelines for a regimen of anticoagulant treatment of venous thromboembolism are given in the next Table (Fennerty, A. et al., Brit. Med. J. 297, 1285-1288, Nov. 19, 1988):

Anticoagulant Treatment of Venous Thromboembolic Disease

Day	Action
1-5 inclusive	Blood specimen for activated partial thromboplastin time (PTT) and prothrombin time (PT).
	Heparin infusion: 5000 units followed by 1400 units/hour. Check PTT after 4-6 hours of infusion and daily thereafter, adjusting infusion rate to keep the PTT 1.5-2.0 times the control or 1.5-2.5 times the patients admission PTT.
3 (5 P.M.)	Induction dose of warfarin, 10mg (5-15mg/day).
4 (9-10 A.M.)	Blood specimens for PTT and PT (little change expected).
(5 P.M.)	Warfarin, 10mg
5 (9-10 A.M.)	Blood specimens for PTT and PT (mild change).
(5 P.M.)	Warfarin, 10mg
6 (9-10 A.M.)	Blood specimen for PT. Suggested maintenance dose of warfarin will depend on this result.
(5 P.M.)	Maintenance dose (usually 5 to 7.5mg) depending on PT.
7 onwards	PT stabilized at 16 to 20 seconds, 1.3-1.5 times control value. Blood specimens for PT taken as usual at 9:00 A.M. and warfarin dose adjusted accordingly. Monitor PT twice during second week and weekly until maintenance dose established. Warfarin is given for four weeks (or longer if there are persisting risk factors). A patient with a single recurrence is treated for three months; those with repeated thromboembolic episodes receive longer treatment(sometimes life-long).

Heparin is normally given for 5 days to maintain a PTT between 1.5 and 2.0 times the control value or 1.5 to 2.5 times the patient's admission PTT.

Warfarin requires about three days to begin acting and is often started on the third or fourth day of heparin therapy. However, some physicians start warfarin on day 1 or day 2 of heparin administration if the PTT is within the therapeutic range; this helps to avoid prolonged IV therapy and hospitalization necessitated by a delayed start of oral anticoagulant. Early warfarin administration has two important effects: reduction of risk of heparin-induced thrombocytopenia and cost of treatment (Gallus, A. et al., Lancet 2, 1293-1296, 1986). However, some evidence suggests that the recurrence of thromboembolism is decreased with a longer course of heparin therapy.

Warfarin is started with the aim of maintaining the PT at 1.3-1.5 times the control values. Warfarin produces an anticoagulant effect in 2-3 days and antithrombotic effects in 5-6 days.

A new approach to the measurement of PT has been introduced because the traditional assay varies from laboratory to laboratory. The rabbit brain thromboplastins that are currently used are highly variable. The World Health Organization has developed a new measurement, the International Normalized Ratio (INR). Each lot of reagent is assigned a sensitivity index to make it equivalent to pure human brain thromboplastin. For example, a PT ratio of 1.3 based on rabbit brain thromboplastin and a control of 12 seconds is equivalent to an INR of 2.0.

When the predicted dose is given, the patient may be discharged. Consensus on the duration of warfarin therapy has not been obtained; it is usually recommended that warfarin should be continued for three months after the first episode of pulmonary embolism or deep vein thrombosis in the absence of underlying risk factors: recurrent deep vein thrombosis (two episodes), prolonged immobilization, malignancy, or congenital deficiency of antithrombin III, protein C, or protein S. Lifelong therapy may be recommended for the latter group.

However, some clinicians recommend a much shorter duration of therapy: four to six weeks in patients with no persisting risk factors (Petiti, O.B. et al., Am. J. Med. 81, 255-259, 1986; Fennerty, A.G. et al., Clin. Lab. Haematol. 9, 17-21, 1987); three months for patients with a repeat thromboembolic event; and lifelong treatment in patients with repeated episodes or with a continuing risk factor, eg, malignancy or antithrombin III deficiency (Fennerty, A. et al., Brit. Med. J. 297, 1285-1288, Nov. 19, 1988; Hyers, T. et al., Chest 95 Supple, February, 1989).

ANTICOAGULANTS (Cont.)

Following hospitalization, monitor change in drugs and diet, especially relating to vitamin K. If PT becomes prolonged, subcutaneous vitamin K reverses the anticoagulant effect within 6-24 hours. On an outpatient basis, maintain a PT ratio 1.3 to 1.5 times the control value (INR, 2-3). Patients with mechanical prosthetic valves or recurrent systemic embolism require more intensive anticoagulation to maintain a PT ratio 1.5 to 2.0 times the control value (INR, 3-4.5)(Hirsh, J. et al., Chest 95 Supple, 1989). The PT should be obtained once to twice weekly for two weeks and then once every two weeks if results are in the therapeutic range; then, once a month will usually be sufficient.

Thrombolytic Drugs and Treatment of Pulmonary Emboli: Thrombolytic drugs (streptokinase, tissue plasminogen activator (t-Pa)) clear pulmonary emboli more rapidly than anticoagulants (heparin, warfarin); however, they have not been shown to reduce mortality. They are generally reserved for life threatening massive pulmonary embolism (Hall, R., Thorax 40, 729-733, 1985; Goldhaber, S.Z. et al., Lancet 2, 886-888, 1986; Goldhaber, S.Z. et al., Lancet, 294-298, 1988).

Thrombolytic Drugs and Treatment of Myocardial Infarction: see **MYOCARDIAL INFARCTION, TREATMENT.**

ANTIDEPRESSANTS

The pharmacology of antidepressants is given in the next Table (Richelson, E., J. Clin. Psychiatry 43: 11 (Sec.2), 4-11, 1982; Rudorfer, M. and Potter, W., Drugs 37, 713-738, 1989; Peckar, Paul J., Personal Communication 1988):

Pharmacology of Antidepressants

	Potency; Blockage of		Adverse Effects; Blockage of Receptors to		
ANTI-DEPRESSANT	Serotonin Uptake	Norepinephrine (NE)Uptake	Histamine (H_1)	Muscurinic Acetylcholine	Alpha-1 Adrenergic
Fluoxetine (Prozac)	3+ to 4+	0 to 1+	Min.	Min.	Min.
Amitrip. (Elavil)	2+ to 4+	1+ to 2+	Max.	Max.	Max.
Imipramine (Toframil)	1+ to 4+	1+ to 2+	Intermed. to Min.	Intermed.	Min.
Trazadone (Desyrel)	1+ to 3+	1+	Min.	Min.	Max. to Intermed.
Nortrip. (Pamelor)	1+ to 3+	2+	Intermed. to Min.	Intermed. to Min.	Intermed. to Min.
Protrip. (Vivactil)	3+	3+	Min.	Max.	Min.
Desipramine (Norpramin)	0 to 3+	4+	Min.	Min.	Min.
Doxepin (Sinequan)	3+	1+	Max.	Intermed.	Max.
Amoxapine (Asendin)	0 to 2+	2+ to 3+	Intermed. to Min.	Min.	Intermed.
Trimipramine (Surmontil)	1+	1+	Max.	Intermed.	Max.
Maprotoline (Ludiomil)	0 to 1+	2+	Intermed.	Min.	Min.

Fluoxetine is a new antidepressant which is putatively a "pure" serotonin uptake blocker; it has a long half-life so that once-a-day(20mg) is effective in most patients. Furthermore, fluoxetine dose not promote weight gain.

Blockage of Neurotransmitter(Serotonin, Norepinephrine) Uptake by Antidepressants: Neurotransmitters(serotonin and norepinephrine) are synthesized and released by neurons to communicate with other cells. The uptake of these chemical messengers back into the nerve ending from which they are released is a means of terminating neurotransmission at the synapse. Antidepressants block the sites of serotonin and norepinephrine uptake into the presynaptic nerve endings, increasing the time that the neurotransmitter is in contact with its receptor (Richelson, E., J. Clin. Psychiatry 43: 11 (Sec. 2), 4-11, 1982).

There is a biogenic amine hypothesis of affective illness which states that a deficiency of certain biogenic amines, e.g., norepinephrine, at functionally important synapses causes depression, while an excess produces mania (Maas, J.W., Arch. Gen. Psychiatry 32, 1357-1361, 1975).

Adverse Effects of Antidepressants: Adverse effects of antidepressants are medicated through blockage of serotonin, norepinephrine, histamine (H_1), muscurinic acetylcholine, and alpha-1 adrenergic receptors; the clinical manifestations of blockage of these receptors are given in the next Table (Richelson, E., J. Clin. Psychiatry 43: 11 [Sec, 2], 4-11, 1982):

Adverse Effects of Antidepressants

Property	Possible Clinical Consequence
Blockade of norepinephrine uptake at nerve endings.	Blockade of the antihypertensive effects of guanethidine (Ismelin and Esimil), Clonidine(Catapres), and alpha-methyldopa (Aldomet). Augmentation of pressor effects of sympathomimetic amines.
Blockade of serotonin uptake at nerve endings.	Postural hypotension.
Blockade of histamine H_1 receptors.	Potentiation of central depressant drugs. Sedation, drowsiness, weight gain, hypotension.
Blockade of muscarinic acetylcholine receptors.	Blurred vision, dry mouth, sinus tachycardia, constipation, urinary retention, memory dysfunction.
Blockade of alpha-1-adrenergic receptors.	Potentiation of the antihypertensive effect of prazosin (Minipress). Postural hypotension, dizziness, reflex tachycardia.

ANTI-DIARRHEA DRUGS

Anti-diarrhea drugs are listed in the next Table:

Anti-Diarrhea Drugs

Drug	Dosage
Kaolin and Pectin (Kaopectate, Pargel)	Non-prescription. Children 3-6 years: 15-30ml/dose; children 6-12 years: 30-60ml/dose; Adults: 60-120ml/dose. Use after each bowel movement or every 3-4 hours as needed
Bismuth Subsalicylate (Pepto-Bismol)	Non-prescription. Note: contains salicylates
Opioid Preparations:	
Diphenoxylate Hydrochloride with Atropine Sulfate (Lomotil) Dosage Forms: Syrup: 2.5mg diphenoxylate and 25mcg atropine/5ml Tab: 2.5mg diphenoxylate and 25mcg atropine	Adults: 1-2 tablets or 5-10 ml, 3-4 times daily for 24-48 hours initially to control diarrhea (max. 8 tabs daily); then 1 tablet or 5ml 2-3 times per day if necessary. Children: Diphenoxylate 0.3-0.4mg/kg/day divided tid-qid or 2-5 years 4ml 3 times daily. 5-8 years 4ml 4 times daily. 8-12 years 4ml 5 times daily. Not recommended under 2 years of age.
Loperamide Hydrochloride (Imodium) Dosage Forms: Cap 2mg. Liquid: 1mg/5ml.	Adults: 4mg initially, then 2mg as necessary to a max. of 16mg daily. Children: 0.4-0.8mg/kg/day in 2-4 divided doses (Max.: 7 days).
Paregoric Dispense 30 or 60ml	Adults: 5 to 10ml, 1-4 times daily until diarrhea is controlled. Children: 0.25 to 0.5ml/kg, 1-4 times daily.
Opium Tincture	Adults: 0.6ml (range, 0.3 to 1ml) 4 times daily; max. 6ml daily. Children: 0.005-0.01mg/kg/dose every 2-4 hrs. to a max. of 6 doses in 24 hrs.
Kaolin-Pectin Combinations:	Non-prescription
Kaolin-Pectin and Paregoric (Parepectolin) Each 30ml of suspension contains opiuim 15mg (Paregoric equivalent 3.7ml) pectin 162mg, and kaolin 5.5g (alcohol 0.69%).	
Kaolin-Pectin and Belladonna Alkaloids (Donnagel)	Non-prescription
Donnagel PG Each 30ml of suspension contains kaolin 6g, pectin 142.8mg, hyoscyamine sulfate 0.1037mg, atropine sulfate 0.0194mg, scopolamine hydrobromide 0.0065mg and opium 24mg.	Non-prescription Adults: 30ml initially, then 15ml every 3 hrs Max: 4 doses daily. Children: 10lb: 2.5ml/dose 20lb: 5ml/dose 30lb: 5-10ml/dose
Codeine Sulfate or Phosphate Codeine Sulfate: 15,30 and 60mg. Codeine Phosphate: Sol'n for Injection: 15, 30, 60mg/ml. Tabs: 15, 30 and 60mg.	Adults: Oral: 15 to 60mg every 4-8 hours. IM: 15-30mg every 2-4 hours. Children: Not recommended.

Generally, anti-diarrheal agents should be avoided in children, particularly preparations containing opioids or codeine. These agents may produce side effects and mask signs of more serious illness.

ANTIEMETICS FOR CANCER PATIENTS

Drugs used as antiemetics are listed in the next Table (The Medical Letter 29, 2-4, Jan. 1 1988):

Antiemetics for Cancer Patients

Generic (Trade) Name	Available Preparations	
	Oral	Parenteral
Cannabinoids:		
Nabilone (Cesamet)	X	
Dronabinol (Marinol)	X	
Dopamine Antagonist:		
Metoclopramide (Reglan)	X	X
Antipsychotic Drugs:		
Phenothiazines, eg, Prochlorperazine (Compazine), Promethazine (Phenergan)	X	X
Butyrophenones eg, Haloperidol (Haldol)	X	X
Serotonin ($5\text{-}HT_3$) Receptor Antagonist:		
Ondansetron (Zofran)		X
Corticosteroids:		
Dexamethaxone (Decadron)	X	X
Methylprednisolone (Solu-Medrol)		X
Combinations:		
I.V. Metoclopramide with I.V. Dexamethasone		X
I.V. Metoclopramide with I.V. Methylprednisolone		X
Nabilone with Dexamethasone		

Mechanism of Action: Emesis, induced by cancer chemotherapeutic drugs, is thought to occur following stimulation of the vomiting center for neurotransmitters, such as dopamine, 5-hydroxytryptamine ($5HT_3$; serotonin), or opiate-endorphins; antiemetics block these receptors.

Drugs: The cannabinoids, nabilone or dronabinol, may relieve nausea and vomiting caused by drugs other than cisplatin; however, the cannabinoids can cause disturbing CNS effects.

Metoclopramide or prochlorperazine in high doses can be highly effective. Intravenous corticosteroids are also effective in many patients.

Suggested doses for selected agents are as follows:

Drug	Dosage
Nabilone (Cesamet)	Adults: 1-2mg orally every 12 hours
Metoclopramide (Reglan)	Adults: 2mg/kg orally or IV before therapy then every 4 hours.
Prochlorperazine (Compazine)	Adults: 5-10mg orally, rectally, IM or IV, 3-4 times daily. Children: 0.4mg/kg daily in 3-4 divided doses orally, rectally, IM or IV. Not recommended in children less than 2 years.
Promethazine (Phenergan)	Adults: 12.5-25mg orally, rectally, IM or IV; repeat doses every 4 hrs as needed (Max. 100mg/day). Children: 0.25-0.5mg/kg/dose orally, rectally, IM or IV 4-6 times daily.
Haloperidol (Haldol)	Adults: 3-5mg orally 2 or 3 times daily. Use lower doses in geriatric or debilitated patients (0.5-2mg orally 2-3 times daily). Higher doses may be required. Children: 0.01-0.15mg/kg orally in 2 or 3 divided doses.
Ondansetron (Zofran)	Adults and Children: 0.15mg/kg IV 30 min before chemotherapy and at 4 and 8 hours.
Dexamethasone (Decadron)	Adults: 10-20mg IV before chemotherapy, additional (usually lower) doses for 1-3 days.

ANTIFUNGAL DRUGS

Indications for use of antifungal drugs for treatment for deep-seated mycoses are given in the next Table (Terrell, C.L. and Hermans, P.E., Mayo Clin. Proc. 62, 1116-1128, 1987):

Indications for Use of Antimicrobial Drugs in Deep-Seated Mycoses

Indication	Amphotericin B	Flucytosine (5-FC)*	Ketoconazole	Miconazole
Candidiasis				
Candidemia, if dec. host resistance	Yes	Synergy with amphotericin B	...	...
Disseminated	Yes(with 5-FC)		Yes(?)	?
Persistent urinary	Yes(with 5-FC)		...	...
Histoplasmosis	Yes	Resistant	Yes	?
Blastomycosis	Yes	Resistant	Yes(?)	?
Coccidioidomycosis (severe primary pulmonary, progressive pulmonary disseminated)	Yes	Resistant	Yes(?)but relapses are common; not in meningitis	Yes-but relapses are common
Cryptococcosis				
Pulmonary, if decr. host resistance	Yes	Synergy with amphotericin B	Yes(?)	...
Progressive pulmonary	Yes		Yes(?)	...
Disseminated(including meningitis)	Yes(with 5-FC)		No	...
Aspergillosis		Almost always resistant		
Invasive pulmonary	Yes		No	No
Disseminated	Yes		No	...
Sporothrix infections**				
Disseminated	Yes	Resistant	No	...
Mucormycosis	Yes	Resistant	No	No
Paracoccidioidomycosis	Yes	No	Yes	Yes
Pseudallescheria boydii	No	No	Yes(?)	Yes

* 5-FC=5-fluorocytosine; **Cutaneous and lymphangitic infections should be treated with orally administered iodide solutions.

Fluconazole is indicated for the treatment of oropharyngeal, esophageal, and systemic (eg, urinary tract, pneumonia, peritonitis) candidiasis and for treatment of cryptococcal meningitis (as an alternative)(see **FLUCONAZOLE**)

Itraconazole is indicated for treatment of paracoccidiodomycosis; its use in patients with other fungal infections is not completely established. Itraconazole is not currently available in the U.S.A.

Dosages of antifungal drugs (general guidelines) for treatment for deep-seated mycoses are given in the next Table (Terrell, C.L. and Hermans, P.E., Mayo Clin. Proc. 62, 1116-1128, 1987):

Dosages of Antimicrobial Agents for Deep-Seated Mycoses

Drug (Trade Name)	Route of Administration	Daily Dose	Total Dose or Duration
Amphotericin B (Fungizone)	Intravenous (conc. 0.1mg/ml in D5W only)	0.6-1.0mg/kg of body weight. Usual adult dose: 50mg. Increase dosage slowly from 0.25mg/kg.	3 to 4g
Fluconazole (Diflucan)	Oral or intravenous	200-400mg	Depends on condition. Min. 2-4 weeks; up to 3-4 mo. or longer.
Flucytosine (Ancobon)	Oral	150mg/kg of body weight	Up to 90 days
Ketoconazole (Nizoral)	Oral	200-400mg (higher doses have been used)	Probably 6 mo. or longer
Miconazole (Monistat)	Intravenous	600-3600mg* daily or 20-40mg/kg/day in 3 divided doses given over 30-60min.	Probably 60 days or longer
Itraconazole	Oral	200-400mg	Unknown

*For specific dosage, review package insert.

ANTIFUNGAL DRUGS (Cont.)

Some of the adverse effects and drawbacks of antifungal drugs are given in the next Table (Dismukes, W.E., Ann. Intern. Med. 109, 177-179, 1988):

Adverse Effects and Drawbacks of Antifungal Drugs

Drug	Adverse Effects
Amphotericin B	Fever, chills, headache and myalgias; bone marrow and renal toxicity; poor penetration into CSF.
Fluconazole	Headache, rash, nausea, vomiting, diarrhea, transaminase elevation.
Flucytosine	Bone marrow suppression; hepatic dysfunction; diarrhea.
Miconazole(I.V.)	Toxic to skin, heart and hematologic system.
Ketoconazole	Poor penetration into CSF; hepatotoxicity; inhibition of testosterone and adrenal corticosteroid synthesis.

ANTIHEMOPHILIC FACTOR VIII

(Humate-P, Hemofil, Profilate, Koate-HT, Monoclate)

USES: Antihemophilic factor(AHF) is used in the treatment of hemophilia A in patients with a deficiency in factor VIII and in some patients with acquired factor VIII inhibitors.

DOSAGE: Antihemophilic factor is administered by slow IV injection or by IV infusion. Use plastic syringes to administer AHF by IV injection. The approximate level of AHF necessary to achieve hemostasis in different conditions is given in the next Table:

Approximate Antihemophilic Factor(AHF) VIII to Achieve Hemostasis in Different Conditions

Condition	Approximate AHF VIII Level (% of Normal)
Hemorrhage	30%
Hemarthrosis	5%-10%
Minor Surgical Procedures	30%-50%
Major Surgical Procedures	80%-100% initially, then 30-50% for 10-14 days postop.

The approximate percentage increase in plasma antihemophilic factors (AHF) levels expected from a given dose is given in the next equation:

$$\text{Expected Factor VIII Increase (in \% of normal)} = \frac{\text{Units Administered}}{\text{Body Weight (kg)}} \times 2$$

The dose required to achieve a particular percentage increase in the plasma antihemophilic factor(AHF) level is given in the next equation:

Units Required = Body Weight(kg) x 0.5 x Desired Factor VIII Increase (in % of normal)

ANTIHEMOPHILIC FACTOR VIII (Cont.)

The approximate dosage of antihemophilic factor(AHF) VIII is given in the next Table:

Dosage of Antihemophilic Factor(AHF) VIII

Condition	Dosage
Prophylactic Management	<50kg, 250 units daily in the morning; >50kg, 500 units daily in the morning. If bleeding occurs too frequently, increase dose appropriately to maintain AHF level of 15%.
Joint Hemorrhages, no Aspiration	5-10 units/kg at 8-12 hr. intervals for 1 or more days.
Joint Hemorrhage, with Aspiration	8 units/kg given just before the procedure; 8 units/kg given 8 hrs. later and repeated as necessary.
Hemarthrosis, Fully Developed	25 units/kg to obtain AHF level of 50%
Hemorrhages into Skeletal Muscle:	
Non-Vital Areas, Minor	8-10 units/kg daily, 2 or 3 days or until pain and swelling are relieved
Non-Vital Areas, Serious	8 units/kg at 12 hour intervals for 2 days; then once daily for 2 more days, if necessary
Near Vital Organs, e.g. Neck or Subperitoneum	15 units/kg; then 8 units/kg every 8 hrs. for 48 hrs.; after 48 hrs., 4 units/kg may be given every 8 hrs. for another 48 hrs. or longer
Overt Bleeding	15-25 units/kg followed by 8-15 units/kg every 8-12 hrs. for 3-4 days as necessary
Bleeding from Massive Wounds or Hemorrhage into Vital Tissues, e.g., CNS	40-50 units/kg followed by 20-25 units/kg every 8-12 hrs. as necessary to achieve AHF level of 80-100% of normal
Major Surgical Procedures	26-30 units/kg before surgery followed by 15 units/kg every 8 hrs. after surgery. Maintain factor VIII level above 30% and increase dosage if necessary. The level should 'e approximately 60% just after administration of a dose. Continue therapy for 10-14 days postoperatively.

PHARMACOKINETICS: Half-Life: 12 hrs. (4-24 hrs.).

ADVERSE EFFECTS: The incidence of acute adverse effects are directly related to the rate of infusion; acute adverse effects are as follows: headache, flushing, tachycardia, paresthesia, nausea, vomiting, back pain, hypotension, somnolence, lethargy, loss of consciousness, disturbance of vision, constriction in the chest, and rigor.

Other effects include fever, chills, urticaria, and mild allergic reactions.

There are two serious and life-threatening conditions transmitted by antihemophilic factor(AHF) VIII; these are human immunodeficiency virus(HIV), the cause of acquired immunodeficiency syndrome(AIDS) and non-A, non-B hepatitis. Heat-treating preparations of AHF destroys HIV. However, 15,000 of the 20,000 hemophiliacs that were treated with non-heat-treated preparations are infected with HIV; it may be that all of these patients will develop AIDS.

Non-A, non-B hepatitis permeates our blood supply and heat-treatment does not destroy this virus. How many AHF deficiency patients will develop chronic cirrhosis is not known. Newer methods of factor VIII preparation such as treatment with organic solvent and detergent may be more effective in inactivating viruses including HIV, hepatitis B and non-A, non-B hepatitis.

ANTIHISTAMINES

The formula of histamine and the action of histamine on receptors is given in the next Figure (Naclerio, R.M. et al., Ped. Infect. Dis. 7, No. 3, 215-224, 1988):

Formula of Histamine and Action of Histamine on Receptors

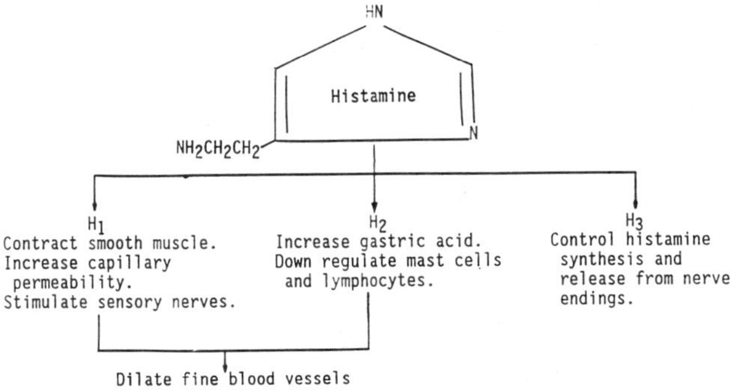

Histamine acts on receptors, H_1, H_2, and H_3. Two major classes of drugs block histamine receptors: antihistamines and H_2 antagonists. Antihistamines have various clinical effects, as listed in the following Table (Naclerio, R.M., et al., Ped Infect. Dis. 7, No. 3, 215-224, 1988):

Effects of Antihistamines
Competitively Antagonize H_1 Receptors
Inhibit Cholinergic Stimulation
Local Anesthetic Properties
Sedation
Prevent IgE Dependent Release of Histamine From Mast Cells and Basophils
Do Not Block Gastric Acid Secretion

USES: Clinical uses of antihistamines vary according to the specific properties of a particular agent. Clinical uses of antihistamines are given in the following table:

Uses of Antihistamines
Rhinitis-Allergic or Infections
Allergic Dermatoses (eg, Pruritis and Urticaria)
Transfusion Reactions
Prevention and Treatment of Nausea, Vomiting and Vertigo
Sedation (Sleep Aid)
Antitussive

Whereas histamine is an ethylamine with a primary amino group and a nitrogen-containing heterocyclic ring, H_1 blockers (antihistamines) generally have a tertiary amino group, and two aromatic substituents separated from the ethylamine core by substitution of carbon, nitrogen, or oxygen; this

ANTIHISTAMINES (Cont.)
latter substitution accounts for the classification and properties of antihistamines, as given in the following Table:

Properties of Antihistamines
Ethylenediamine Derivatives: Weak CNS effects, but drowsiness may occur; Adverse GI effects common.
Ethanolamine Derivatives: CNS Depression Common; Drowsiness in 50%; Adverse GI effects uncommon; Antiemetic (Dimenhydrinate and Diphenhydramine); Anticholinergic.
Propylamine Derivatives: CNS stimulation, drowsiness uncommon.
Phenothiazine Derivatives: Most Phenothiazines used as antipsychotics; Antihistamine, Antipruritic, Antiemetic Properties
Piperazine Derivatives: CNS depression may occur; Antipruritic, Antiemetic Properties; Treatment of motion sickness.
Piperidine Derivatives: Highly selective for H1 receptors; nearly devoid or anticholinergic effects; poor penetration into CNS; low incidence of side effects.

Examples of more commonly used antihistamines are given in the following Table:

Classification of Antihistamines
Ethylenediamine Derivatives
Antazoline (Arithmin)
Pyrilamine
Tripellennamine (PBZ)
Ethanolamine Derivatives
Carbinoxamine (Rondec, others)
Clemastine (Tavist)
Dimenhydrinate (Dramamine, others)
Diphenhydramine (Benadryl, others)
Doxylamine (Sleep 2-Nite, Unisom, others)
Propylamine Derivatives
Brompheniramine (Dimetapp and others)
Chlorpheniramine (Chlor-Trimeton, Contac, Triaminic, others)
Triprolidine (Actidil, AllerAct, Actifed, others)
Phenothiazine Derivatives
Methdilazine (Jacaryl)
Promethazine (Phenergan)
Trimepramine (Temaril)
Piperazine Derivatives
Hydroxyzine (Atarax, Vistaril, others)
Meclizine (Antivert, others)
Piperidine Derivatives
Terfenadine (Seldane)
Astemizole (Hismanal)
Others
Cyproheptadine (Periactin)
Azatadine (Optimine)
Diphenylpyraline (Hispril)
Phenindamine (Nalahist)

Note: Some brand names may contain combinations of agents.

ANTIHISTAMINES (Cont.)

A list of oral antihistamines is given in the next Table:

Oral Antihistamines

Classifications and Generic Name	Trade Name	Adult Dosage	Dosage Forms
Alkylamines			
Brompheniramine maleate	Dimetane	4mg every 4-6 h	Tabs: 4mg; Liquid
	Dimetane Extentabs	8-12mg every 8-12 h	Tabs: 8,12mg
Chlorpheniramine	Chlor-trimeton	4mg every 4-6 h	Tabs: 4mg; Liquid
	Chlor-trimeton Repetabs	9-12mg every 8-12 h	Tabs: 8,12mg; capsules
Dexchlorpheniramine	Polaramine	2mg every 4-6 h	Tabs: 2mg; Liquid
	Dexchlor	4-6mg every 8-10 h	Tabs: 4,6mg
	Polaramine Repetabs	4-6mg every 8-10 h	Tabs: 4,6mg
Triprolidine	Actidil	2.5mg every 4-6 h	Tabs: 2.5mg; Liq.
Ethanolamines			
Carbinoxamine	Clistin	4-8mg every 6-8 h	Tabs: 4mg
Clemastine	Tavist	2.68mg every 12 h	Tabs: 2.68mg; Liq.
	Tavist-1	1.34mg every 12 h	Tabs: 1.34mg
Diphenhydramine	Benadryl	25-50mg every 4-6 h	Tabs: Capsules, Liquid: 25,50mg
Ethylenediamines			
Pyrilamine		25-50mg every 6-8 h	Tabs: 25mg
Tripelennamine	PBZ	25-50mg every 4-6 h	Tabs:25,50mg; Liq.
	PBZ-SR	100mg every 8-12 h	Tabs: 100mg
Phenothiazines			
Promethazine	Phenergan	12.5mg every 12 h or 25mg at bedtime	Tabs: 12.5,25mg; Liquid
Piperazines			
Hydroxyzine	Atarax, Vistaril	25mg every 6-8 h	Tabs: 25mg
Meclizine	Antivert	25-50mg once daily	Tabs: 25, 50mg
Piperidines			
Terfenadine	Seldane	60mg every 12 h	Tabs: 60mg
Astemizole	Hismanal	10mg daily	Tabs: 10mg
Others			
Azatadine	Optimine	1-2mg every 12 h	Tabs: 1mg
Cyproheptadine	Periactin; Pyrohep	4mg every 6-8 h	Tabs: 4mg; Liquid
Diphenylpyraline	Hispril	5mg every 12 h	5mg "spansules"
Phenindamine	Nolahist	25mg every 4-6 h	Tabs: 25mg

The antihistamine now most commonly prescribed in the United States is terfenadine (Seldane); it is claimed that terfenadine does not cause sedation.

The antihistamine that is the second most commonly prescribed is Tavist-D; a tablet of Tavist-D contains 1.34mg of clemastine plus 75mg of phenylpropanolamine. Phenylpropanolamine is a sympathomimetic, which acts as a nasal decongestant.

Consultants to the Medical Letter recommend chloropheniramine as an inexpensive first choice for antihistamine treatment of allergic rhinitis; terfenadine, which is claimed to be nonsedating, may be a useful daytime alternative for some patients.

ADVERSE EFFECTS: CNS depression may occur and impair the patient's ability to perform potentially hazardous tasks, especially with ethanolamine derivatives. Alcohol may potentiate these effects. Some patients, especially children, may have paradoxial CNS stimulation. GI effects include pain, anorexia, nausea, vomiting, diarrhea or constipation. Cholestasis and hepatitis occur rarely. Anticholinergic effects including dry mouth, thickened bronchial secretions, urinary retention, vertigo, blurred vision, nervousness and other symptoms may occur, especially with ethanolamines. Hematologic and sensitivity reactions occur rarely. Geriatric patients are particularly susceptible to adverse effects, including dizziness, sedation, and hypotension.

CAUTIONS: Use with caution or not at all in patient with underlying diseases potentially adversely affect by anticholinergic side effects: angle-closure glaucoma, bladder obstruction, pyloroduodenal obstruction, acute asthmatic attack, severe hypertension, coronary artery disease.

DRUG INTERACTIONS: Within 14 days of MAO's, may cause hypertensive crisis. Sympathomimetics potentiated, CNS depressants, eg, alcohol potentiates sedation.

ANTILYMPHOCYTIC GLOBULIN (LYMPHOCYTE IMMUNE GLOBULIN)
(Atgam, Antithymocyte Globulin)

USES: Antilymphocytic globulin (lymphocyte immune globulin) is an immunoglobulin G(IgG) prepared from plasma or serum of healthy horses hyperimmunized with human thymus lymphocytes; it is a selective immunosuppressant that reduces the number of circulating, thymus-dependent lymphocytes (T-cells) that are partly responsible for graft rejection. It has little effect on B-cells. Uses are given in the next Table:

Uses of Antilymphocytic Globulin (Lymphocyte Immune Globulin)
Renal Transplant Patients
Aplastic Anemia

Renal Transplant Patients: Antilymphocytic globulin is used to minimize allograft rejection in renal transplant patients; when antilymphocytic globulin is administered at the time of rejection, resolution of the acute episode is enhanced.

Aplastic Anemia: Antilymphocytic globulin is used in patients with moderate to severe aplastic anemia in patients who are unsuitable for bone marrow transplantation; partial to complete hematologic remission may be induced.

Antilymphocytic globulin is not useful in patients with aplastic anemia secondary to neoplastic disease, storage disease, myelofibrosis, or Fanconi's syndrome or in patients exposed to myelotoxic agents or radiation.

DOSAGE FORMS: 50mg IgG per ml.

DOSAGE: Antilymphocytic globulin is administered by slow IV infusion.

Intradermal sensitivity testing is done prior to administration of antilymphocytic globulin. The skin test procedure consists of intradermal injection of 0.1ml of a 1:1000 dilution of the concentrate for injection in 0.9% sodium chloride injection (5mEq of equine IgG); use only freshly diluted drug. A control dose of 0.9% sodium chloride is administered; sites are observed 1 hour, positive test is greater than 10mm erythema or wheal.

A dose should not be infused in less than four hours. Dosage is given in the next Table:

Dosage of Antilymphocytic Globulin (Lymphocyte Immune Globulin)

Condition	Age	Dosage
Prevention of Renal Allograft Rejection	Adults or Children	Give first dose within 24 hrs. before or after transplantation. 15mg/kg daily for 14 days followed by alternate-day therapy with the same dosage for another 14 days (a total of 21 doses in 28 days).
Treatment of Acute Renal Allograft Rejection	Adults or Children	On diagnosis, start 10-15mg/kg daily for 14 days; if necessary, follow by alternate-day therapy with the same dosage for up to another 14 days (up to a total of 21 doses in 28 days).
Aplastic Anemia	Adults	10-20mg/kg daily for 8 to 14 days; additional alternate-day therapy up to a total of 21 doses may be administered.

PHARMACOKINETICS: Half-Life: 6 days (1.5-12 days).

ADVERSE EFFECTS: Common adverse effects (10-50%): Chills, fever, leukopenia, thrombocytopenia and dermatologic reactions(rash, pruritis, urticaria, wheal and flare).

Other reactions (1-5%): Arthralgia, chest or back pain, headache, nausea and/or vomiting, diarrhea, peripheral thrombophlebitis, stomatitis, dyspnea, hypotension, night sweats, pain at infusion site. Rarely(<1%): Anaphylaxis, serum sickness, tachycardia, laryngospasm, pulmonary edema, herpes simplex virus reactivation, local and systemic infections or myalgias. Severe leukopenia, hemolysis, and thrombocytopenia may occur necessitating RBC or platelet transfusions.

MONITOR: Complete blood count(CBC) including platelets.

ANTIMIGRAINE DRUGS

Drugs used for the treatment of migraine are listed in the next Table:

Drugs Used in the Treatment of Migraine

Generic Name	Trade (Product) Name
Ergotamine Tartrate	Ergomar, Ergostat, Medihaler Ergotamine
Ergotamine Tartrate plus Caffeine	Cafergot, Wigraine
Ergotamine Tartrate, Caffeine, Belladonna Alkaloids, Pentobarbital	Cafergot-PB
Dihydroergotamine mesylate	D.H.E. 45
Propranolol	Inderal
Isometheptene, Dichloralphenazone, Acetaminophen	Midrin
Methysergide Maleate with Tartrazine	Sansert

ANTITUBERCULOUS AGENTS

Drugs recommended for initial treatment of tuberculosis are given in the next Table (Van Scoy, R.E. and Wilkowske, C.J., Mayo Clin. Proc. 62, 1129-1136, 1987; The Medical Letter 30, 43-44, April 8, 1988):

Drugs Recommended for Initial Treatment of Tuberculosis*

Drug	Daily Dose(mg/kg)** Children	Daily Dose(mg/kg)** Adults	Maximal daily doses in children and adults	Twice weekly dose(mg/kg) Children	Twice weekly dose(mg/kg) Adults
Isoniazid (INH and Others)	10-20, p.o. or I.M.	5, p.o. or I.M.	300mg	20-40; max. 900mg	15; max. 900mg
Rifampin (Rifadin, Rimactane)	10-20, p.o. IV form available	10, p.o. IV form available	600mg	10-20: max. 600mg	10; max. 600mg
Strepto-mycin ***	20-40, I.M.	15,*** I.M.	1g	25-30, I.M.	25-30, I.M
Ethambutol# (Myambutol)	15-25, p.o.	15-25, p.o.	2.5g	50	50
Pyrazina-mide	15-40, p.o.	15-40, p.o.	2g	50-70	50-70

*I.M.= intramuscularly; p.o. = orally.
**Doses based on weight should be adjusted as weight changes.
***Streptomycin doses should be adjusted to estimated creatinine clearance. Levels should be measured in patients with renal insufficiency.
#Not recommended in children <5 years of age.

Treatment Regimens: Regimens for treatment of tuberculosis are given in the next Table (The Medical Letter 30, 43-44, April 8, 1988):

Regimens for Treatment of Tuberculosis

Status	Treatment
Initial treatment of uncomplicated pulmonary and extrapulmonary tuberculosis.	Isoniazid and rifampin daily for six months with pyrazinamide added during first two months.
	or Isoniazid and rifampin without pyrazinamide for nine months.
	or Twice-a-week supervised therapy with isoniazid and rifampin for nine months (following several weeks of daily doses).
Disseminated tuberculosis, tuberculous meningitis, tuberculosis in patients with AIDS	Isoniazid, rifampin and ethambutol (or pyrazinamide) are given initially; when isoniazid, rifampin and ethambutol are used, pyrazinamide is often added during the first two months (Am. Rev. Respir. Dis. 134, 355, 1986).
Prophylaxis	Isoniazid; Adults: 300mg daily as single dose; Children: 10mg/kg daily (max. 300mg daily).

ANTIVIRALS

Clinical indications of antiviral drugs are given in the next Table (Reines, E.D. and Gross, P.A., Med. Clin. No. Am. 72, 691-715, 1988):

Clinical Indications of Antiviral Drugs

	Herpes Simplex	Varicella-Zoster	Respiratory Syncytial Virus	Influenza A	AIDS	Cytomegalovirus
Acyclovir (Zovirax)	Y	Y				
Ribavirin (Virazole)			Y			
Amantadine (Symmetrel)				Y		
Idoxuridine	Y					
Zidovudine (AZT)(Retrovir)					Y	
Ganciclovir						Y

Y = Yes

Recommended dosages and indications for **antiviral agents** available for clinical use are given in the next Table (Hermans, P.E. and Cockerill, F.R., Mayo Clin. Proc. 62, 1108-1115, December 1987; Reines, E.D. and Gross, P.A., Med. Clin. No. Am. 72, 691-715, 1988; "Antiviral Chemotherapy" in Infect. Dis. Clin. No. Am. 1, 311-499, June, 1987):

Recommended Dosages and Indications for Antiviral Drugs for Clinical Use

Generic(Trade) Name	Dosage and Route*	Indications
Acyclovir (Zovirax)	Topical: 5% cream 6 times/day for 10 days	Initial episode of **genital herpes**
	5% cream 6 times/day for 5 days	Recurrent episodes of genital herpes
	Oral: 200mg 5 times/day for 10 days	Initial episode of genital herpes
	200mg 5 times/day for 5 days	Recurrent episodes of genital herpes
	200mg 2 or 3 times/day for up to 6 mo.	Suppression of recurrent genital herpes
	Intravenous: 5mg/kg of body weight 3 times/day for up to 10 days	Severe initial episode of genital herpes; mucocutaneous herpes simplex in immunocompromised patients
	10mg/kg of body weight 3 times/day	Herpes simplex encephalitis
	7.5-10mg/kg of body weight 3 times/day	**Varicella-zoster virus** infections in immunocompromised patients
Ribavirin (Virazole)	Aerosol therapy with a 20mg/ml solution 12-18 h./day	Severe lower respiratory tract infection due to **respiratory syncytial virus** in infants and young children
	Aerosol therapy with a 20mg/ml solution 12-18 h./day	Influenza A and B (not FDA approved)
	Intravenously, up to 60mg/kg/day	**Lassa fever** (not FDA approved)
	Orally, up to 1g/day, divided into 4 doses	Lassa fever (not FDA approved)
Amantadine (Symmetrel)	100mg 2 times/day orally	**Influenza A** prophylaxis and treatment
Rimantadine	200mg, once a day orally	Same as for amantadine but not FDA approved
Idoxuridine (Stoxil, Herplex, Dendrid)	Eyedrops every h. during the day and every 2 h. during the night	Topical therapy for superficial keratitis due to **herpes simplex virus**

ANTIVIRALS (Cont.)
(Table continued)

Generic(Trade) Name	Dosage and Route*	Indications
Vidarabine (adenine arabinoside)(Vira-A)	Eyedrops 5 times/day at 3 h. intervals	Same as Idoxuridine
	15-30mg/kg of body weight/day intravenously given over 12 h.	Disseminated **herpes simplex and zoster** and herpes simplex encephalitis (Acyclovir has become drug of choice)
Zidovudine(AZT) (Retrovir)	200mg every 4 h. orally, around the clock or 6-12mg/kg/day in divided doses every 4 hrs IV.	**Acquired immune deficiency syndrome (AIDS)**
Ganciclovir	Intravenously 10mg/kg/day in 2-3 divided doses.	**Cytomegalovirus** infection in patients with liver or kidney transplant. (Only temporary remission in most patients with bone marrow transplant or with AIDS).

* Dosages may need adjustment in patients with renal or hepatic insufficiency and in cases of drug interactions.

Acyclovir: Acyclovir has antiviral activities against certain members of the herpes virus family: herpes simplex types 1 and 2, varicella zoster virus and Epstein-Barr virus, but not against cytomegalovirus (Reines, E.D. and Gross, P.A., Med. Clin. No. Am. 72, 691-715, May, 1988). Acyclovir is the most effective drug for the treatment of **herpes simplex** and **varicella-zoster infection.**

Ribavirin: Ribavirin has been approved by the FDA for treatment of **respiratory syncytial virus infections** that occur in infants and young children (Rodriquez, W.J. and Parrott, R.H., Infect. Dis. Clin. No. Am. 1, 425-439, June, 1987). It has been used to treat influenza A and B and Lassa fever.

Amantadine: Amantadine is the preferred antiviral drug for the prophylaxis **of influenza A** and may be beneficial therapeutically when used early in the course of the disease. Amantadine is active only against influenza A viruses (Tominack, R.L. and Hayden, F.G., Infect. Dis. Clin. No. Am. 1, 459-478, June, 1987; Reines, E.D. and Gross, P.A., Med. Clin. No. Am. 72, 691-715, May 1988).

Rimantadine: Rimantadine is a structural analogue of amantadine with the same spectrum of activity, mechanism of action and clinical indications. Rimantadine and amantadine have similar toxicities, but with rimantadine, there is an increased incidence of gastrointestinal complaints but less central nervous system toxicity (Bektimirov, T.A. et al., Bull. Who 63, 51, 1985).

Idoxuridine: Idoxuridine is used only in the treatment of **herpetic keratitis.**

Vidarabine: Vidarabine, previously the drug of choice in the treatment of severe **herpetic infections,** has been replaced by the more effective acyclovir.

Zidovudine [Azidothymidine(AZT)](Retrovir): Retrovir has been approved by the FDA for certain HIV infected adult patients who have a history of cytological confirmed Pneumocystis carinii pneumonia or an absolute CD4(T4-helper/inducer) lymphocyte count of less than 200 per mm^3 in the peripheral blood before therapy is begun. Retrovir has improved the quality of life and prolonged the life of some patients with AIDS (Bakerman, S., Understanding AIDS, Interpretative Lab. Data, Inc., P.O. Box 7066, Greenville, NC 27835-7066).

Ganciclovir: Ganciclovir is used to treat **cytomegalovirus** infections in patients who have undergone kidney or liver transplantation; its effects are only temporary in patients who have undergone bone marrow transplantation and patients with acquired immunodeficiency syndrome (AIDS) who have cytomegalovirus infections (Reines, E.D. and Gross, P.A., Med. Clin. No. Am. 72, 691-715, May 1988; McKinlay, M.A. and Otto, M.J., Infect. Dis. Clin. No. Am. 1, 479-493, June 1987).

ANXIETY, TREATMENT

For treatment of anxiety, the **benzodiazepines** are the drugs of choice; all benzodiazepines are effective against both anxiety and insomnia. The most widely used benzodiazepines in treatment of anxiety are given in the next Table (Brown, C.S. et al., Arch. Intern. Med. 151, 873-884, 1991):

Treatment of Anxiety

Generic Name	Trade Name	Half-Life(hrs)*	Adult Dosage
Alprazolam	**Xanax**	6-20	**0.25-6mg/day in 3 doses**
Lorazepam	**Ativan**	10-20	**0.5-6mg/day in 2-3 doses**
Clorazepate	**Tranxene**	36-200	**7.5-90mg/day in 3 doses**
Oxazepam	**Serax**	4-15	**30-120mg/day in 3-4 doses**
Chlordiazepoxide	**Librium**	36-200	**25-200mg/day in 3-4 doses**
Prazepam	**Centrex**	36-200	**20-60mg/day in 2-3 doses**
Diazepam	**Valium**	20-200	**2-40mg/day in 3-4 doses**
Halazepam	**Paxipam**	36-200	**20-160mg/day in 3-4 doses**
Clonazepam	**Klonopin**	20-80	**0.5-6mg/day in 3 doses**

*Includes active metabolites.

In the treatment of anxiety, alprazolam (Xanax) is the drug that is most often prescribed. Alprazolam, lorazepam and oxazepam have intermediate half-lives, ranging from 5 to 20 hours. The others have very slow rates of elimination or major active metabolites with long half-lives of 1-3 days.

Adult anxiety disorders are listed in the next Table (Diagnostic and Statistical Manual of Mental Disorders, Edition 3 (revised), Washington, D.C., American Psychiatric Assoociation, 1987):

Adult Anxiety Disorders
Panic Disorder
Generalized Anxiety Disorder
Obsessive-Compulsive Disorder
Post-Traumatic Stress Disorder
Atypical Anxiety Disorder
Phobic Disorders

ARTHRITIS

OSTEOARTHRITIS: Drugs used in the treatment of osteoarthritis to relieve pain are given in the next Table:

Drugs Used in Treatment of Osteoarthritis
Aspirin
Acetaminophen
Nonsteroidal Anti-Inflammatory Drugs (NSAIDs)
Local Anti-Inflammatory Therapy with Intraarticular Instillation of Corticosteroids

Aspirin: Aspirin is often regarded as the drug of choice for the treatment of osteoarthritis. Recommended doses of aspirin (as many as 12, 325mg tablets a day) produce analgesic and antipyretic effects. Anti-inflammatory effect is achieved when a minimal salicylate blood level of 20mg/dl has been reached which occurs if 12 or more 325mg aspirin tablets are taken for an average of four days.

Acetaminophen: Acetaminophen is an effective antipyretic analgesic with no anti-inflammatory properties.

Non-Steroidal Anti-inflammatory Drugs: When exacerbations of osteoarthritis occur, local anti-inflammatory therapy, eg, intralesional steroid injections or a NSAID can be temporarily used instead of acetaminophen to provide relief of pain and inflammation. The NSAIDs may be used during the inflammatory episodes of osteoarthritis; these drugs are as effective as aspirin and may be better tolerated, however adverse reactions may occur.

Local Anti-Inflammatory Therapy with Intraarticular Instillation of Corticosteroids: Intraarticular instillation of corticosteroids may be used for short-term treatment of acute joint inflammation, with symptomatic improvement in 24 hours, maximal effect within 3 days.

ARTHRITIS (Cont.)
RHEUMATOID ARTHRITIS: Drugs used in the treatment of rheumatoid arthritis are given in the next Table:

Drugs Used in Treatment of Rheumatoid Arthritis
Aspirin
Nonsteroidal Anti-Inflammatory Drugs (NSAIDs)
Steroids
Antimalarials (eg, hydroxychloroquine)
Gold
Penicillamine
Methotrexate
Azathioprine
Sulfasalazine
Immunosuppressants (eg, cyclosporine, cyclophosphamide)

The traditional approach to patients with rheumatoid arthritis involves the stepwise use of drugs with careful assessment of risk vs. benefits. The first step in drug therapy utilizes nonsteroidal anti-inflammatory drugs including salicylates. For patients with early rheumatoid arthritis who can tolerate the drug, aspirin is a good first choice of therapy. Nonsalicylate NSAIDs are better tolerated in some patients; choice should be based on potential toxicity. If one agent in this class is not effective after 2-3 weeks, it should be replaced with another from a different chemical class of NSAIDs.

The second step in drug therapy involves the use of disease-modifying anti-rheumatic drugs (DMARD's). This step often utilizes antimalarial agents or gold salts.

Antimalarials: Hydroxychloroquine is the most commonly used agent because retinopathy occurs less frequently than with other antimalarials. Mechanism of action is unknown, but may involve inhibition of various enzymes, including collagenases. Eye examinations should be performed frequently roughly at 3-month intervals (Rosenberg, A.M., J. Pediatr. 114, 171-178, 1989).

Gold Salts: Gold salts modify the disease process in rheumatoid arthritis. Gold compound are listed in the next Table:

Gold Compounds
Auranofin
Aurothioglucose
Gold Sodium Thiomalate (Aurothiomalate)

Auranofin is administered orally whereas aurothioglucose and gold sodium thiomalate are given by injection.

Gold salts suppress the function of the immune system by reducing the activity of macrophages (Symposium: Am. J. Med. 75, 1-91, 1983) and lymphocytes. In addition, aurothiomalate reduces the numbers of circulating lymphocytes, and auranofin inhibits the release of prostaglandin(PG), PGE_2 from synovial cells and release of leukotriene (LT), LTB_4 and LTC_4 from polymorphonuclear leukocytes (Barrett, M.L. and Lewis, G.P., Agents Actions 19, 109-115, 1986).

The next drugs that are typically considered include penicillamine, methotrexate, and azathioprine.

Penicillamine: Although the exact mechanism of action is unknown, penicillamine may act by reducing circulating immune complexes, including rheumatoid factor. This drug has potentially serious side effects, including an anti-vitamin B_6 effect, hematologic (leukopenia, thrombocytopenia) and renal (proteinuria, hematuria) side effects.

Methotrexate: Methotrexate probably acts as an anti-inflammatory agent rather than an immunosuppressive agent in the doses used to treat rheumatoid arthritis. Side effects may be significant, including GI, hematologic, hepatic and pulmonary effects.

Azathioprine: Azathioprine is a purine analog that is converted to 6-mercaptopurine. Immunosuppression results and inhibition of inflammation may be a result of monocyte inhibition (Rosenberg, A.M., J. Pediatr. 114, 171-178, 1989).

Steroids are used in several different situations. Low-dose oral corticosteroids are used to treat intermittent exacerbations of the disease process ("flares") or as "bridge" therapy following NSAIDs while initiating DMARD therapy (Roth, S.H., J. Rheum. 16, 1408-1409, 1989). Intra-articular steroids may be useful for localized severe joint involvement.

Other therapies that have been used include sulfasalazine cyclosporine and cyclophosphamide.

Some rheumatologists suggest that a more aggressive approach to therapy may be desirable; earlier treatment with DMARD therapy may be beneficial in certain patients (Wilske, K.R. and Healey, L.A., J. Rheum. 16, 565-567, 1989; Roth, S.H., J. Rheum. 16, 1408-1409, 1989).

ASPIRIN

[Acetylsalicylic Acid(ASA)]

USES: Aspirin exhibits analgesic, antipyretic, anti-inflammatory activity, and inhibits platelet aggregation; uses are given in the next Table:

Uses of Aspirin

Pain: Treatment of mild to moderate pain.

Fever

Anti-Inflammatory: Rheumatoid Arthritis, Juvenile Rheumatoid Arthritis, Osteoarthritis, Polyarthritic Conditions (eg, Psoriatic Arthritis, Reiter's Syndrome, Ankylosing Spondylitis), Systemic Lupus Erythematosus, Nonarticular Inflammation, Rheumatic Fever, and Mucocutaneous Lymph Node Syndrome (Kawasaki's Disease)

Inhibits Platelet Aggregation: Treatment of Arterial and possibly Venous Thrombosis.

Osteoarthritis: Aspirin is often regarded as the drug of choice for the treatment of osteoarthritis; aspirin is used to relieve pain and is used during inflammatory episodes of osteoarthritis. Recommended doses of aspirin (as many as 12,325mg tablets a day) produce analgesic and antipyretic effects. Antiinflammatory effect is achieved when a minimal salicylate blood level of 20mg/dl has been reached which occurs if 12 or more 325mg aspirin tablets are taken daily for an average of four days.

Rheumatoid Arthritis: Aspirin is used as a Step 1 drug in the treatment of rheumatoid arthritis.

Rheumatic Fever: Salicylates are considered to be the drugs of choice for the symptomatic treatment of patients with rheumatic fever who have only polyarthritis or those who develop mild carditis without cardiomegaly or congestive heart failure(CHF).

Thrombosis: Aspirin inhibits platelet aggregation via platelet cyclooxygenase inhibition and has been used to prevent arterial thrombosis. Aspirin has been shown to reduce the risk of recurring transient ischemic attack(TIAs) and stroke or death in men who have had single or multiple TIAs; it has not been established that aspirin prevents stroke.

Aspirin alone reduced the five-week mortality rate following acute myocardial infarction by 23%; when both aspirin and streptokinase were used in combination, reduction in the five-week mortality was 42% (ISIS-2 Study, Lancet 2, 349-360, 1988).

Aspirin, taken the evening before surgery, reduces the incidence of thrombosis following radial-artery catheterization, and may reduce the incidence of thrombosis following coronary, iliac, femoral, popliteal or tibial artery percutaneous transluminal angioplasty.

Aspirin or dipyridamole, used in conjunction with an oral anticoagulant, has been used to reduce the incidence of thrombosis in patients with prosthetic heart valves.

Mucocutaneous Lymph Node Syndrome (Kawasaki's Disease): Aspirin is the drug of choice for the treatment of mucocutaneous lymph node syndrome (Kawasaki's Disease) because of anti-inflammatory and potential antithrombic effects.

Mechanism of Action: All cells, except nonnucleated erythrocytes, are capable of synthesizing prostaglandins which are released in response to trauma of any kind. The pathological release of prostaglandins which contribute to inflammation, fever, and pain is inhibited by aspirin. The synthesis of prostaglandins and the inhibition by aspirin is illustrated in the next Figure (Vane, J. and Botting, R., FASEB J. 1, 89-96, 1987):

Synthesis of Prostaglandins and Inhibition by Aspirin

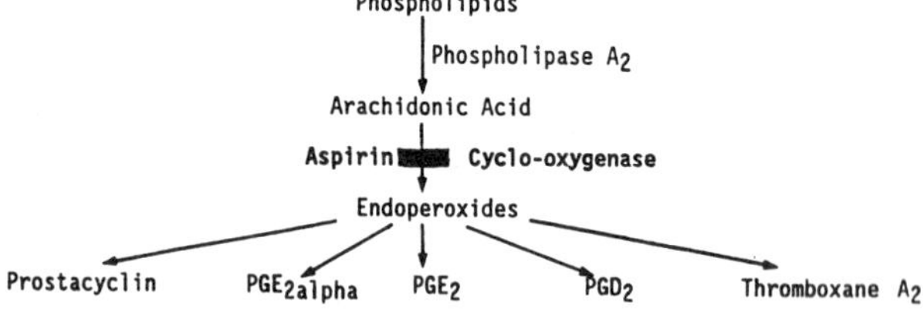

ASPIRIN (Cont.)

Aspirin irreversibly aceylates and inactivates cyclooxygenase, an enzyme which catalyzes the formation of prostaglandin precursors (endoperoxides) from arachidonic acid.

PGE_2 may be especially important in the inflammatory process.

In the development of fever, endogenous pyrogen is released from leukocytes and acts directly on the thermoregulatory center in the hypothalamus. This effect is associated with a rise in prostaglandins in the brain. Aspirin prevents the temperature-rising effects of pyrogens and the rise in brain prostaglandin levels.

The action of prostaglandins on platelets and blood vessels is given in the next Table:

Action of Prostaglandins on Platelets and Blood Vessels

Prostaglandin	Cell Source	Effect on Platelets	Effect on Blood Vessels
Thromboxane A_2	Platelets	Aggregation	Vasoconstriction
Prostacyclin (Prostaglandin I_2)	Vascular Endothelium	Inhibits Aggregation	Vasodilation

Aspirin (up to 1g daily) blocks the synthesis of thromboxane A_2 and thus inhibits platelet aggregation; it is used to prevent and treat arterial thrombosis (Hirsh, J., Arch. Intern. Med. 145, 1582, 1985).

DOSAGE FORMS: Tabs: 65, 75, 200, 300, 325, 500, 600, 650mg; Chewable Tabs: 65, 81mg; Caps: 325mg; Suppositories: 60, 65, 130, 150, 195, 200, 300, 325, 600mg and 1.2g

DOSAGE: Aspirin is usually administered orally, preferably with food or a large quantity(240ml) of water or milk to minimize gastric irritation. Aspirin tablets should not be administered rectally. Dosage of aspirin is given in the next Table:

Dosage of Aspirin

Condition	Age	Route	Dosage
Analgesia or Antipyresis	Adults >11 yrs.	Oral or Rectal	325-650mg every 4 h. as necessary; higher single doses (e.g. 975mg or 1 gram) for analgesia in some patients
	2-11 yrs.	Oral or Rectal	60-80mg/kg daily, in 4-6 divided doses, Max. total daily dose 3.6g.
	<2 years	"	Must be individualized
Inflammatory Diseases: Rheumatoid Arthritis; Osteoarthritis; or other Polyarthritic or conditions	Adults	Oral	Initial: 2.4-3.6g daily, in divided doses; when necessary, increase dosage by 325mg to 1.2g daily no more frequently than at weekly intervals. Maintenance: 3.6-5.4g daily; higher doses may be necessary.
Juvenile Rheumatoid Arthritis	<25kg	Oral	Initial: 60-90mg/kg daily in divided doses. When necessary, increase dosage by 10mg/kg daily no more frequently than at weekly intervals. Maintenance: 80-100mg/kg daily; up to 130mg/kg daily
	>25kg	Oral	Initial:2.4-3.6g daily in divided doses. When necessary, inc. dosage by 10mg/kg daily; no more frequently than at weekly intervals. Maintenance: 80-100mg/kg daily; up to 130mg/kg daily.

ASPIRIN (Cont.)

Dosage of Aspirin (Continued)

Condition	Age	Route	Dosage
Rheumatic Fever	Adult	Oral	4.9-7.8g daily in divided doses every 4-6 hours for up to 1-2 weeks, then decrease to 60-70mg/kg daily for 1-6 weeks or as long as necessary and then gradually withdraw over 1-2 weeks.
	Children	Oral	90-130mg/kg daily in divided doses every 4-6 hours for up to 1-2 weeks, then decrease to 60-70mg/kg daily for 1-6 weeks or as long as necessary and then gradually withdraw over 1-2 weeks.
Rheumatic Fever with Carditis, Cardiomegaly or Congestive Heart Failure Treated with Corticosteroids		Oral	Aspirin therapy is usually initiated as steroid therapy is gradually withdrawn. 60mg/kg daily in divided doses for 2-4 weeks. If relapse, reinstitute for 3-4 additional weeks.
Thrombosis: TIAs	Adult	Oral	1.3g daily in 2-4 divided doses
Prevent Recurrent Myocardial Infarction	Adult	Oral	300-325mg once daily
Mucocutaneous Lymph Node Syndrome (Kawasaki's Syndrome)			During Febrile Period: 80-120mg/kg daily in divided doses. When Fever Subsides: Decrease dosage; if disease uncomplicated, continue aspirin for 6-10 weeks.

ADVERSE EFFECTS: Repeated administration of high doses of aspirin produces drug accumulation; adverse reactions of aspirin are given in the next Table:

Adverse Reactions of Aspirin
Gastrointestinal Reactions
Inhibition of Platelet Aggregation and Hemostasis
Central Nervous System Effects
Analgesic Nephropathy
Liver Function Abnormalities
Allergic Reactions
Drug-Drug Interactions
Salicylate Toxicity

Aspirin may cause gastric distress and G.I. bleeding.

Salicylates must not be used in children with varicella infections or influenza-like illnesses because use of salicylates in these conditions has been associated with an increased risk of developing Reye Syndrome. Salicylates should generally be avoided in children unless there are specific indications such as juvenile rheumatoid arthritis, rheumatic fever, or mucocutaneous lymph node syndrome due to the risk of Reye Syndrome.

CONTRAINDICATIONS: Use with caution in patients with platelet and bleeding disorders. Aspirin may precipitate urticaria, angioedema, bronchospasm, rhinitis or shock in some patients.

PHARMACOKINETICS: Absorption: Rapid from stomach and small intestine. Therapeutic level: 15-30mg/dl; Half-Life(Adults): 2-4 hours; Half-Life(Children): 2-3 hours; Time to Peak Plasma Level: 1-2 hours; Time to Steady State, Adults: 10.0-22.5 hours; Time to Steady State, Children: 10-15 hours. Toxicity may appear in the range of 20-30mg/dl. At >30mg/dl, toxicity will definitely occur. Aspirin is lethal at levels >70mg/dl. Salicylate blood levels do not correlate well with degree of intoxication in chronic salicylism.

MONITOR: Therapeutic levels: 15-30mg/dl. Follow serum levels when high doses are used for prolonged lengths of time.

In acute salicylate toxicity, the Done nomogram (Done, A.K., Pediatrics 26, 800-807, 1960) can be used to predict severity of intoxication from a single determination of serum salicylate, provided that the time of ingestion is known and sufficient time has elapsed between ingestion and sampling of blood (six hours). This nomogram has many shortcomings - it applies only to acute poisonings, one-time ingestion in patients who have had no aspirin in the previous 24 hours. It does not apply to patients who have ingested enteric coated or liquid preparations, or patients who have pre-existing acidosis or hypoalbuminemia. Aspirin levels are assumed to have peaked. As with other ingestions, local poison control center should be contacted (eg, Rocky Mountain Poison Center 1-800-332-3073). The Done nomogram is shown in the next Figure:

Serum Salicylate Concentration and Expected Severity of Intoxication at Varying Intervals of Time Following Ingestion

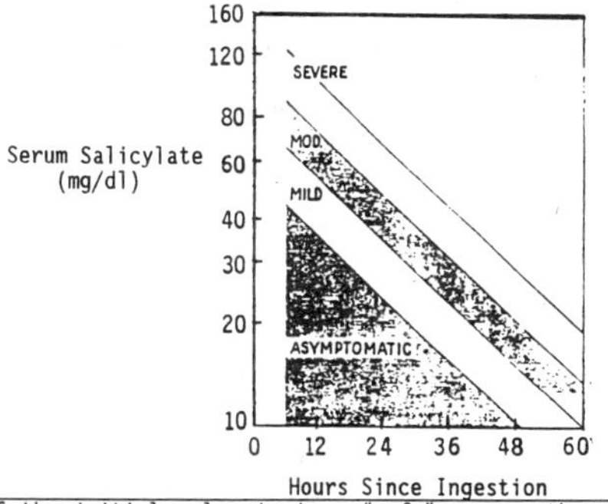

If the initial value is in a "safe" range, the determination of serum salicylate should be repeated in two to four hours; then, if the serum salicylate does not rise between tests, the child is considered not to be at risk for serious intoxication. Laboratory data suggestive of aspirin are a positive urine by clinitest (reducing substances) and a negative glucose oxidase and positive ferric chloride test on boiling urine.

Laboratory tests, other than serum salicylate levels, that should be used to monitor complications of salicylate toxicity are given in the next Table:

Laboratory Tests to Monitor Possible Complications of Salicylate Toxicity

Tests	Monitor Complications
Arterial Blood Gases (pH. PCO_2, HCO_3^-)	Respiratory alkalosis; metabolic acidosis; hypermetabolism
Serum Electrolytes (Na^+, K^+, Cl^-, CO_2 Content)	Anion gap increased; $(Na^+)-(Cl^-+CO_2$ content): due to increased lactic acid, ketones and salicylic acid. Inappropriate fluid retention: detect the effects of bicarbonate diuresis following therapy with bicarbonate for acidosis
Serum and Urine Osmolality	Inappropriate secretion of antidiuretic hormone
Blood Glucose	Blood glucose may be low, normal or elevated; Blood glucose should be maintained at elevated levels to ensure adequate supply of glucose to brain.
Prothrombin Time (PT)	If prolonged, vitamin K therapy indicated

Following acute ingestion, children quickly pass through the state of pure respiratory alkalosis and present with some degree of metabolic acidosis. The toxic properties of salicylates result principally from direct stimulation of the respiratory center (respiratory alkalosis) and influence on metabolic pathways (metabolic acidosis).

Symptoms of hypocalcemic tetany, secondary to alkalosis, may develop.

Reference: Temple, A.R., Pediatr. Supp. 62, 873-876, Dec. 1978; Atwood, S.J., Ped. Clin. N. Am. 27, 871-879, 1980.

ASPIRIN WITH CODEINE

(Empirin with Codeine)

USES: Empirin with codeine is used to relieve mild to moderate pain.

DOSAGE FORMS: Dosage forms of selected aspirin/codeine drugs are given in the next Table:

Dosage Forms of Selected Aspirin/Codeine Drugs

Drug	Aspirin (mg)	Codeine Phosphate (mg)
Aspirin/Codeine (BW) #2, tabs	325	15
Aspirin/Codeine (BW) #3, tabs	325	30
Aspirin/Codeine (BW) #4, tabs	325	60

DOSAGE: Adults: 1-2 tabs of #2 or #3 or 1 tab. of #4 every 4 hours as needed. Not recommended for children.

PRECAUTIONS: Use with caution in the following conditions: Asthma, gastritis, head injury, increased intracranial pressure, acute abdominal conditions, impaired renal, hepatic, thyroid, or adrenocortical function, prostatic hypertrophy or urethral stricture.

CONTRAINDICATIONS: Severe bleeding or coagulation disorders, peptic ulcer, last trimester of pregnancy.

ADVERSE EFFECTS: Dizziness, sedation, allergic reactions, gastric upset, nausea, vomiting, constipation, urinary retention, prolonged bleeding time, respiratory depression, overdose.

INTERACTIONS: Potentiation with alcohol, CNS depressants, anticoagulants, hypoglycemics, tricyclic antidepressants, anticholinergics, alcohol, NSAIDs; corticosteroids increase risk of GI bleeding. May antagonize uricosurics.

ASTEMIZOLE

(Hismanal)

USES: **Astemizole** is a specific, selective, **histamine antagonist** of the **H-1 histamine receptor.** Astemizole is a piperidine antihistamine, related to terfenadine (Seldane); sedation does not occur as often as with other antihistamines because astemizole does not cross the blood brain barrier. Uses are given in the next Table:

Uses of Astemizole
Seasonal Allergic Rhinitis, eg, Hay Fever
Chronic Idiopathic Urticataria

DOSAGE FORMS: Tabs: 10mg.

DOSAGE: Astemizole is administered orally. Dosage is given in the next Table:

Dosage of Astemizole

Age	Dosage
Adults and Children >12 years	**10mg** once daily OR **30mg** on the first day, 20mg on the second day, then 10mg once daily.

PHARMACOKINETICS: Rapidly absorbed; absorption reduced by 60% when taken with meals; Peak: 1 hour; Metabolism: Extensive first pass metabolism and subsequent hepatic metabolism; Half-Life: Distribution phase, 20 hrs.; Elimination phase, 7-11 days; Excretion: Feces.

ADVERSE EFFECTS: Astemizole, compared to classical antihistamines, has much less frequent incidence of CNS and anticholinergic side effects. Since experience with this drug is limited, the adverse effects have not been fully described. The most frequent adverse effects are related to the CNS (2-7%): drowsiness, fatigue, appetite increase, weight gain, nervousness, and dizziness. Adverse GI effects including nausea, diarrhea, and abdominal pain do not occur more frequently than with placebo. Dry mouth is reported in 5% of patients.

ASTHMA

The four major groups of antiasthmatic drugs used in the treatment of asthma are given in the next Table:

Major Groups of Antiasthmatic Drugs
Sympathomimetic Drugs (Beta-Agonists)
Cromolyn
Xanthines, eg, Theophylline
Corticosteroids
Anticholinergics

Mechanism of Action: The mechanisms of action of sympathomimetics and methylxanthines (eg, theophylline), on smooth muscle cells, and of cromolyn and corticosteroids on mast cells are illustrated in the next Figure:

Mechanisms of Action of the Bronchodilators on Smooth Muscle and Mast Cells

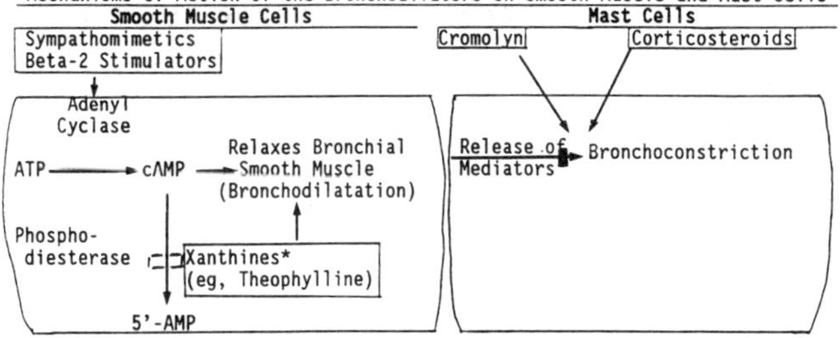

*The mechanism of action of theophylline is not limited to phosphodiesterase inhibition and other mechanisms may be more important in relieving bronchospasm.

Sympathomimetics Drugs: The sympathomimetics stimulate beta-2 receptors, which then activate the plasma membrane enzyme adenyl cyclase; this enzyme catalyzes the formation of cyclic AMP from ATP. Cyclic AMP acts to relax bronchial smooth muscle leading to bronchodilatation.

Characteristics of sympathomimetic drugs are listed in the next Table (Hiller, F.C. and Wilson, F.J., Med. Clin. N. Amer. 67, 669-684, May 1983):

Adrenergic Bronchodilators

Drug	Alpha	Beta-1	Beta-2	Effective Given Orally	Subcut. Inject.	Oral Dose	Metered Dose Inhaler	Nebulizer Sol.	Duration of Action (hr)
Ephedrine	+	+	+	+	+	+			
Epinephrine	+	++	++	0	+		+	+	1.5-2
Isoproterenol		++	++	0			+	+	1.5-2
Isoetharine		+/-	++	0			+	+	1.5-2
Metaproterenol		+	++	++		+	+	+	4-6
Terbutaline		+/-	++	++	+	+			4-6
Albuterol		+/-	++	++		+	+		4-6
Fenoterol		+/-	++	++					4-6

Sympathomimetic drugs directly stimulate alpha; beta-1 and/or beta-2 adrenergic receptors in effector tissue, or they indirectly stimulate these receptors by affecting intact intraneural norepinephrine stores. Stimulation of receptors produce effects as follows: beta-2 receptors: dilation of bronchioles; beta-1 receptor stimulation is responsible for cardiac side effects, that is, increase in both heart rate and force of contractions; alpha receptors are involved in bronchoconstriction and cause a rise in blood pressure. The ideal drug for bronchodilatation would stimulate beta-2 receptors only. Note that ephedrine and epinephrine stimulate alpha, beta-1 and beta-2 receptors while isoproterenol and metaproterenol stimulate both beta-1 and beta-2 receptors.

Oral sympathomimetic agents work similarly to inhaled agents but require much larger doses, have a higher incidence of side effects and slower peak effects.

Patients using sympathomimetic drugs by inhalation are often advised to pause for a few minutes between puffs, instead of taking two puffs rapidly.

ASTHMA (Cont.)
When a child is free of acute attacks and maintenance drug therapy is required, two puffs of terbutaline (0.25mg/puff) taken rapidly is as effective as two puffs taken three or ten minutes apart. However, during wheezing episodes, a ten minute pause between puffs produces better bronchodilation than rapid inhalation (Pederson, S., J. Allergy Clin. Immunol. 77, 505-509, 1986).
Cromolyn: Cromolyn blocks the release from mast cells of the chemical mediators that cause bronchospasm; since it is not a bronchodilator and has no anti-inflammatory or antihistaminic action, it can only be used prophylactically and not in an acute attack.

Cromolyn is used in long-term prophylactic therapy, particularly in those patients in whom allergens have been incriminated or in those patients whom asthmatic attacks are induced by exercise. Cromolyn may not have an immediate effect on bronchial reactivity (except in exercise-induced bronchospasm) and several months of therapy may be necessary before its efficacy can be determined.

Cromolyn is administered by an inhaler. For children over 5 years old and adults, the usual dose is 20mg qid-tid; begin with a qid schedule and decrease slowly as tolerated. It may be mixed with a sympathomimetic for use in a jet nebulizer.
Xanthines: The xanthines, eg, theophylline, relax bronchial smooth muscle. Xanthines inhibit phosphodiesterase, but this mechanism does not entirely account for the bronchodilating properties of theophylline. The mechanism of action of theophylline is not completely understood.

Theophylline is a methylxanthine derivative; various derivatives of theophylline have been prepared in an attempt to increase its water solubility (aminophylline; oxtriphylline and theophylline sodium glycinate). Aminophylline is theophylline ethylene diamine; oxtriphylline is the choline salt of theophylline. Dyphylline is a neutral xanthine derivative that is not converted to theophylline; theophylline levels cannot be measured when this drug is used.

Different oral theophylline preparations are listed in the next Table (Petty, T.L., "Airway obstruction: consider two possibilities," Diagnosis, 92-97, Sept. 1986):

Oral Theophylline Preparations

Dosing Interval	Preparations
tid or qid	Aminophyllin; Choledyl; Theophylline (Generic)
bid	Respbid; Slo-bid; Theo-Dur
once daily	Theo-24; Uniphyl

Theophylline is used primarily as oral maintenance therapy for patients chronic or prolonged seasonal symptoms. Stable serum concentrations are achieved with twice-daily administration of slow-release preparations. Children may require three times daily dosing. Once-a-day preparations may be associated with more erratic serum concentrations than the twice-a-day preparations. Serum levels should be monitored and maintained in the range of 10 to 20 microgram/ml. Below 10 microgram/ml, bronchodilator effects fall off. The half-life is shortened in cigarette smokers.
Corticosteroids: Corticosteroids inhibit the release from mast cells of the chemical mediators that cause bronchospasm, inflammatory reactions and edema.

Short courses of prednisone (0.5-2.0mg/kg/day) given orally are used in the management of moderate to severe asthma; this therapy (Dose: Prednisone 40mg on first day, decrease by 5mg/day), has been demonstrated to decrease the relapse rate following acute therapy in the emergency room (Chapman, K.R. et al., N. Engl. J. Med. 324, 788-794, March 1991) hydrocortisone or methylprednisolone is given I.V. in the treatment of an acute severe asthmatic attack. Maintenance therapy with oral corticosteroids is associated with the risks of adrenal suppression and development of Cushing's syndrome and should only be used as a last resort.

ASTHMA (Cont.)

Corticosteroid Aerosols for Asthma: Corticosteroid aerosols for asthma are given in the next Table:

Corticosteroid Aerosols for Asthma	
Drug	Dosage
Beclomethasone (Vanceril or Beclovent)	Adults: 2 inhalations tid Children(Ages 6-12): 1 or 2 inhalations tid
Flunisolide (AeroBid)	Adults and Children(Ages 6-15): 2 inhalations bid
Triamcinolone Acetonide (Azmacort)	Adults: 2 inhalations tid Children(Ages 6-12): 1 or 2 inhalations tid

Inhaled corticosteroids are useful adjuncts to maintenance therapy for patients with severe asthma and may allow tapering or discontinuation or oral corticosteroids. Corticosteroid aerosols may cause systemic effects and adrenal suppression but physical changes of hypercortisolism have not been reported. Oropharyngeal candidiasis is a common adverse effect of oral aeroso treatment. Bronchodilators should always be used in conjunction with corticosteroids.

Anticholinergics: Anticholinergic agents, atropine and ipatropium bromide have been used in the management of acute asthma. Cholinergic nerves and muscarinic receptors are located in the larger central airways; stimulation of these receptors result in smooth-muscle contraction and increased secretions, and anticholinergic agents inhibit these effects. In general, anticholinergic agents are less effective than beta-agonists in producing bronchodilation but may be a useful adjunct to other bronchodilator therapy (Gross, N.J., N. Engl. J. Med. 319, 486-494, 1988).

Aerosols: The sympathomimetic drugs, cromolyn and steroids can be delivered as aerosols; the aerosol is delivered by a hand-bulb nebulizer, a pump-driven nebulizer, a metered-dose inhaler (MDI) or an IPPB machine.

Aerosols are more advantageous as compared to systemic administration, in that the effects of the drugs are more rapid, and side effects are decreased.

The metered dose inhaler (MDI) produces an aerosol for high-energy release at the nozzle, following containment in a pressurized chamber. The solution or suspension to be delivered contains the active drug, along with a propellant, stabilizers, and flavoring agents. The inhaler should be held four to six inches from the patient's mouth. The patient inhales slowly, pausing at the end of inhalation for five to ten seconds, facilitating gravitational sedimentation of the aerosol, and finally slowly exhaling against pursed lips to promote deposition.

Treatment of Acute Asthmatic Attack (George, R.B. and Owens, M.W., Disease-a-Month 37, 183-186, March, 1991): Initial management of acute asthma is inhaled sympathomimetic **beta-2 agonists.** These drugs may be administered by metered dose inhaler (MDI) or, in sicker patients, by hand-held nebulizer. Oral or subcutaneous routes may be preferred in certain situations. These drugs are very effective bronchodilators with a rapid onset of action.

Corticosteroids should usually be added, particularly in sicker patients; the parenteral route is usually used in sicker patients, but oral therapy is also effective. Dosage recommendations vary; suggestions for adults include: hydrocortisone 200mg IV every 6 or 8 hours or methylprednisolone 40mg IV every 6 or 8 hours and for children, methylprednisolone 0.5-1mg/kg IV every 6 hours. Duration of therapy will depend on severity of asthmatic episode. Patients who are not receiving steroids on a chronic basis or repeated steroid "bursts" may have the drug abruptly discontinued after 3-5 days. Oral therapy following IV treatment may be at a lower dose and may require weaning off the drug. Inhaled steroids should be avoided in the acute setting, since the inhaled route may cause bronchial irritation.

Aminophylline (IV theophylline) has traditionally been used as a bronchodilator in acute management of asthma (see **AMINOPHYLLINE** section). Goal is to maintain levels in the therapeutic range (10-20mg/liter). Recent data suggests that IV aminophylline may not provide additional bronchodilatation compared to treatment with beta-adrenergic agents alone and that side effects may be increased (Siegel, D. et al., Am. Rev. Respir. Dis. 132, 283-286, 1985).

Anticholinergic agents may be useful adjuncts to beta-adrenergic therapy; some patients may respond more than others, and the exact role of these agents has not been fully defined (Gross, N.J. et al., N. Engl. J. Med. 319, 486-494, 1988).

ASTHMA (Cont.)

Complications of Bronchial Asthma: Complications of bronchial asthma are given in the next Table (Siegel, S.C. and Rachelefsky, G.S., J. Allergy Clin. Immunol. 76, 1-14, 1985):

Complications of Bronchial Asthma
I. Infections
A. Otitis Media
B. Sinusitis
C. Bronchitis
D. Pneumonitis
II. Atelectasis
III. Pneumomediastinum and Pneumothorax
IV. Growth Complications
A. Linear Growth
B. Thoracic Deformities
V. Psychologic Problems
VI. Bronchopulmonary Aspergillosis
VII. Respiratory Failure

ATENOLOL

(Tenormin)

USES: Atenolol is a beta-1 selective adrenergic blocking agent; the uses of atenolol are given in the next Table:

Uses of Atenolol
Treatment of Angina
Antihypertensive Agent
Myocardial Infarction

Treatment of Angina: Atenolol inhibits myocardial beta-1 adrenergic receptors. There is a decrease in the rate of sinoatrial(SA) node discharge and an increase in recovery time. There is a decrease in myocardial contractility and heart rate; this leads to a reduction in myocardial oxygen consumption accounting for the effectiveness of the drug in stable chronic angina.

Antihypertensive Agent: The precise mechanism of atenolol's hypotensive effect is not clear. It is thought that atenolol reduces blood pressure by decreasing cardiac output, decreasing sympathetic outflow from the CNS and/or by decreasing renal renin release. Treatment of hypertension with atenolol is given in the next Table (The 1988 Report of the Joint National Committee on Detection, Evaluation, and Treatment of High Blood Pressure, Arch. Intern Med. 148, 1023-1038, 1988):

Treatment of Hypertension with Atenolol

Step 1: Nonpharmacologic Approaches (see **HYPERTENSION**)

↓

Step 2: **Diuretic** or **Beta Blocker** or **Calcium Antagonists** or **ACE Inhibitor** **(eg Atenolol)**

↓ Observe up to 6 months; if atenolol ineffective then,

Step 3: If atenolol chosen as first drug, increase the dosage.
or Add a second drug of a different class
or Substitute another drug

↓

Step 4: If atenolol choosen as first drug, add a second drug
or Add a third drug of a different class
or Substitute

↓

Step 5: Consider further evaluation and/or referral
or Add a third or fourth drug

"Step-Down": For patients with mild hypertension, after 1 year of control, consider decreasing or withdrawing atenolol and other hypotensive drugs.

Myocardial Infarction: Use of beta-blockers following myocardial infarction in hemodynamically stable patients reduces mortality rate by 13% (see **MYOCARDIAL INFARCTION, TREATMENT**).

ATENOLOL (Cont.)

DOSAGE FORMS: Oral: 25, 50, 100mg; IV: 0.5mg/ml.

DOSAGE: Atenolol is administered orally or IV. Safety and efficacy of atenolol in children have not been established. Dosage is given in the next Table:

Dosage of Atenolol

Condition	Route	Dosage
Hypertension	Oral	25-50mg once daily, alone or combination with a diuretic. If combination therapy required, do not use commercially available preparations containing atenolol in combination with chlorthalidone initially. Adjust dosage by administering each drug separately. Full hypotensive effect may not be seen for 1-2 weeks. Dosage may be increased to 200mg daily.
Angina	Oral	50-100mg once daily. Adjust according to clinical response and to maintain a resting heart rate of 55-60 beats/min.
Myocardial Infarction	IV	5mg over 5 minutes, followed 10 min. later by 5mg over 5 min. Give 50mg orally 10 min. after second IV dose; maintenance: 100mg once daily or divide into 2 doses. Reduce to 50mg daily if necessary.
Renal Failure	Oral	If creatinine clearance 15-35ml/min per 1.73m^2, then max. dosage 50mg daily. If creatinine clearance <15ml/min per 1.73 m^2, then max. dosage 50mg every other day.

PHARMACOKINETICS: Absorption: 50-60%; Onset: 1 hr. (heart rate); Duration: 24 hrs.(heart rate);24 hrs.(antihypertensive);Half-Life:6-7 hrs.;Protein-Binding: 10%; Excreted Unchanged in Urine: 85%.

ADVERSE EFFECTS: Cardiovascular: Bradycardia (3%); profound hypotension; second-or third-degree atrioventricular(AV) block; congestive heart failure (CHF). Treatment of cardiovascular(CV) complications of atenolol therapy are given in the next Table:

Treatment of Cardiovascular(CV) Complications of Atenolol Therapy

Complication	Treatment
Bradycardia	IV atropine
AV Block	Isoproterenol or a transvenous cardiac pacemaker
Hypotension	Vasopressors
Congestive Heart Failure	Digitalis and diuretic

Coldness of extremities; postural hypotension (2-4%); leg pains.

CNS Effects:Dizziness; fatigue; mental depression; lethargy; drowsiness, unusual dreams, insomnia, lightheadedness; vertigo; visual disturbances, hallucinations, disorientation; short-term memory impairment, emotional lability, sexual dysfunction

GI Effects:Diarrhea and nausea (2-4%).

Respiratory: Bronchospasm Other: Masking of symptoms of hypoglycemia, hypertriglyceridemia, decreased HDL cholesterol

CONTRAINDICATIONS: Sinus bradycardia, sick sinus syndrome, A-V block greater than first degree; cardiogenic shock; overt cardiac failure; asthma, chronic obstructive pulmonary disease; use with caution in insulin-treated diabetic patients and patients with peripheral vascular disease; should not be discontinued abruptly in patients with ischemic heart disease.

DRUG INTERACTIONS: Drug interactions are given in the next Table:

Drug Interactions of Atenolol

Drug	Interaction
Cimetidine	May reduce bioavailability of beta-blockers
Drugs Metabolized by liver, eg, Lidocaine, Coumarin Chlorpramazine	Reduces plasma clearance of these drugs
Calcium Channel Blockers	May promote negative inotropic effects on the failing myocardium
Reserpine	Marked bradycardia and syncope

ATENOLOL, CHLORTHALIDONE
(Tenoretic)
USES: Tenoretic is used for the treatment of hypertension. It consists of two hypotensive agents, atenolol, a beta-1 selective adrenergic blocking agent and chlorthalidone, which is structurally and pharmacologically similar to thiazide diuretics.

In the treatment of hypertension beta-adrenergic blocking agents often are used concurrently with a diuretic because of their additive effects (step 2). When combination therapy is required, dosage should first be adjusted by administering each drug separately atenolol, chlorthalidone. If it is determined that the optimum maintenance dosage corresponds to the ratio in the commercial combination preparation, then the product (Tenoretic) may be used.
DOSAGE FORMS: The dosage forms (tablets)of Tenoretic are given in the next Table:

Dosage Forms of Tenoretic

Product	Atenolol(mg)	Chlorthalidone(mg)
Tenoretic 50	50	25
Tenoretic 100	100	25

DOSAGE: See Atenolol and Chlorthalidone
ADVERSE EFFECTS: See Atenolol and Chlorthalidone

ATRACURIUM
(Tracrium)
USES: **Atracurium besylate** is a **competitive, nondepolarizing neuromuscular blocking agent** used mainly to produce skeletal muscle relaxation in conditions listed in the next Table:

Uses of Atracurium Besylate
During Surgery after General Anesthesia has been Induced
Increase Pulmonary Compliance during Assisted or Controlled Respirations
Facilitate Endotracheal Intubation
Facilitate Mechanical Ventilation in Intensive Care Settings

Atracurium has minimal cardiovascular side effects and is relatively short acting. Metabolism is by Hofmann elimination (nonenzymatic degradation) and nonspecific esterases; atracurium is useful in patients with impaired renal or hepatic function.
DOSAGE FORMS: IV Injection: 10mg/ml.
DOSAGE: Atracurium besylate is given IV; dosages are the same for adults and children and are given in the next Table:

Dosage of Atracurium Besylate

Route	Dosage
IV bolus	Initially, 0.4-0.5mg/kg followed by 0.08-0.1mg/kg every 20-45 minutes. Use higher doses for more prolonged effects.
IV infusion	Usual: 5-10 micrograms/kg/min (Range: 2-15 micrograms/kg/min).

ADVERSE EFFECTS: Respiratory paralysis will occur; provisions for maintenance of oxygenation and ventilation should be available. Cardiovascular effects are usually minimal and transient. Histamine release may occur at doses greater than 0.5mg/kg.

ATROPINE SULFATE

USES: The uses of atropine sulfate are given in the next Table:

Uses of Atropine Sulfate

Treatment of **Sinus Bradycardia** and **Second and Third Degree AV Block** during **Cardiopulmonary Resuscitation**
Preoperative Medication to Reduce Secretions
Treatment of **Organophosphate Pesticide Toxicity**
Block Muscarinic Effects of **Anticholinesterase agents,** i.e., Neostigmine, Physostigmine, Pyridostigmine
Short-Term **Treatment** of **Bronchospasm**
GI Disorders: Adjunct in **Treatment** of **Peptic Ulcer Disease; Irritable Bowel Syndrome:** Treatment of GI Hypermobility and Diarrhea caused by Reserpine, Guanethidine or Cholinergic Stimulation

Atropine is an **antimuscarinic; antimuscarinics** competitively inhibit the muscurinic effects of acetylcholine. Acetylcholine is an important mediator of nerve conduction. Muscular contraction is mediated by release of acetylcholine from motor nerve terminals and its binding to receptor proteins on muscle. **Atropine blocks the cholinergic receptors in smooth muscles and thus relieves smooth muscle spasms.**

Cardiopulmonary Resuscitation: Atropine sulfate is used in advanced cardiac life support during cardiopulmonary resuscitation for the treatment of sinus bradycardia that is accompanied by severe hypotension or by frequent ventricular ectopic beats. Atropine is also used in the absence of hypotension and ectopic beats if the cardiac rate is less than 50 beats/min. and the cardiac output is reduced. Atropine increases the heart rate by blocking vagal effects.

Preoperative Medication to Reduce Secretions: Atropine sulfate has been used as a preoperative medication to inhibit salivation and excessive secretions of the respiratory tract. However, the commonly used anesthetics, halothane and thiopental and other similar general anesthetics do not tend to stimulate secretion.

Short-Term Treatment of Bronchospasm: Atropine is a potent bronchodilator. Atropine sulfate is used by oral inhalation for the short-term treatment and prevention of bronchospasm associated with bronchial asthma, bronchitis, and chronic obstructive pulmonary disease.

Gastrointestinal(GI) Disorders: Atropine decreases the secretions in the GI tract and inhibits motility.

DOSAGE FORMS: Tabs: 0.4, 0.6mg; Inject: 0.05, 0.1, 0.3, 0.4, 0.5, 0.8, 1.0mg/ml; Oral Inhalation: 0.2, 0.5%

DOSAGE: Atropine sulfate is administered orally or by IM, subcutaneous, or direct IV administration. Atropine sulfate is generally given rapidly IV; slow injection may cause paradoxical slowing of the heart rate. For oral use, atropine is best administered 30 minutes before meals. Dosage is given in the next Table:

Dosage of Atropine

Conditions	Age	Route	Dosage
Cardiopulmonary Resuscitation	Adults	IV	0.5mg; repeat at 3-to 5-minute intervals until desired rate is achieved. Do not exceed 2mg.
	Children	IV	0.02mg/kg, minimum dose 0.1mg
Preoperative Medication to Reduce Secretions	Adults, >20kg	IM or Subcut.	0.4mg (range 0.2-1mg),30-60 min. prior to anticipated time of anaesthesia or at times other preanesthetic medications are administered.
	3kg	IM or Subcut.	0.1mg
	7-9kg	IM or Subcut.	0.2mg
	12-16kg	IM or Subcut.	0.3mg
Hypotonic Radiography of GI Tract(Exam of Duodenum or Colon)	Adults	IM	1mg

ATROPINE SULFATE (Cont.)

Dosage of Atropine			
Condition	Age	Route	Dosage
Block Muscarinic Toxicity of Organophosphate Pesticides	Adults	IV	1-2mg; then 5-60 min. later, 2mg dose IM or IV if necessary. In severe cases, 2-6mg IV; then, 2-6mg IM or IV every 5-60 min.; subsequently, 0.5-1mg orally at intervals of several hours. Up to 50mg in 24 hours.
	Children	IV or IM	0.05mg/kg, repeated every 10-30 min.
Bronchospasm	Adults	Nebulizer	0.025mg/kg, 3 or 4 times daily Maximum dose: 2.5mg
	Children	Nebulizer	0.05mg/kg, 3 or 4 times daily Maximum dose: 2.5mg

PHARMACOKINETICS: Absorption: Atropine is well absorbed from the G.I. tract, following IM administration, oral inhalation, or endotracheal administration; Half-Life: 12-30 hours; Metabolism: Liver: Excretion: Urine.

ADVERSE EFFECTS: Toxic effects are dose related. Therapeutic dose causes dryness of the mouth, and inhibition of sweating. At 1mg, there is definite dryness of the mouth and nose and thirst. At 2mg, there is tachycardia, palpitation and blurring of vision. At 5mg, there is an increase in the above symptoms plus difficulty swallowing, headache, and restlessness. At 10mg, there is an increase in the above symptoms plus ataxia, excitement, disorientation, hallucinations, delirium and coma.

CONTRAINDICATIONS: Glaucoma, obstructive disease of the G.I. tract, obstructive disease of the urinary tract.

AZTREONAM

(Azactam)

USES: Aztreonam is the first approved monobactam antibiotic. Activities of aztreonam are given in the next Table (Neu, H.C., Med. Clin. No. Am. 72, 555-566, May, 1988; Adams, H.G., Personal Comm.):

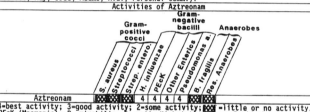

Activities of Aztreonam

	Gram-positive cocci			Gram-negative bacilli				Anaerobes	
	S. aureus	Streptococci	Strep. entero.	H. influenzae	PEcK	Other Enterics	Pseudomonas a.	B. fragilis	Res. Anaerobes
Aztreonam	▩	▩	▩	4	4	4	4	▩	▩

4=best activity; 3=good activity; 2=some activity; ▩ =little or no activity.
PEcK (Mnemonic)= P. mirabilis, E. coli, Klebsiella; Res.= Resident

Aztreonam has excellent activity against aerobic gram-negative bacteria including the bacilli given above plus the cocci, all Neisseria gonorrhoeae (gonococcus), all N. meningitidis(meningococcus), and Moraxella (Branhamella) catarrhalis, both beta-lactamase and nonbeta-lactamase producing strains. It is active against both beta-lactamase and nonbeta-lactamase producing strains of Hemophilus influenzae.

Aztreonam has activity similar to the aminoglycosides; its relative lack of toxicity makes it attractive as an alternative to an aminoglycoside.

Aztreonam has no activity against aerobic gram-positive and anaerobic organisms.

Uses of aztreonam are given in the next Table (Neu, H.C., Med. Clin. No. Am. 72, 555-566, 1988):

Uses of Aztreonam
Urinary Tract Infections (Pyelonephritis and Cystitis)
Lower Respiratory Tract Infections (Bronchitis and Pneumonia)
Septicemia
Skin and Skin Structure Infections (including Wounds or Ulcers and Burns)
Intra-abdominal Infection (including Peritonitis)
Gynecologic Infections (including Endometritis and Pelvic Cellulitis caused by Gram-Negative Bacteria
Bone and Joint Infections

AZTREONAM (Cont.)

DOSAGE FORMS: For injection, 500mg, 1g, 2g.

DOSAGE: Aztreonam is administered by IM or IV injection or infusion; dosage is given in the next Table:

Dosage of Aztreonam

Conditions	Age	Route	Dosage
Urinary Tract Infections	Adults	IV or IM	500mg or 1g every 8 or 12 hrs.
Moderately Severe Systemic Infections	Adults	IV or IM	1g IV or IM or 2g IV every 8 or 12 hours.
Severe System or Life-Threatening Infections	Adults	IV or IM	2g IV every 6 or 8 hours; max. 8g daily.
Cystic Fibrosis	Children	IV or IM	50mg/kg every 6 or 8 hours; max. 8g daily.

The dosage for children has not been established; a dosage schedule for neonates and children 1 month to 15 years of age is as follows: 30-50mg/kg every 6, 8, or 12 hours.

Therapy is continued for at least 48 hours after evidence of eradication of the infection has been obtained. The usual duration of therapy for uncomplicated urinary tract infections is 5-10 days. Patients with more severe infections have received 10-18 days of therapy.

Renal Impairment: Adults with creatinine clearances greater than 30ml/min receive the usual adult dosage; adults with creatinine clearances of 10-30ml/min. should receive an initial dosage of 1 or 2g followed by maintenance doses equal to one-half the usual dose; adults with creatinine clearances of less than 10ml/min should receive the usual initial dosage followed by maintenance doses equal to one-fourth the usual dose.

ADVERSE EFFECTS: Adverse effects have been reported in up to 7% of patients; it was necessary to discontinue the drug in 2%. Adverse effects are given in the next Table:

Adverse Effects of Aztrenam

System (% Incidence)	Effect
Gastro-Intestinal (1-2%)	Diarrhea, nausea, vomiting; pseudomembranous colitis.
Dermatologic and Hypersensitivity Reactions	Rash; immediate hypersensitivity reactions in less than 1% of patients
Hematologic Effects	Transient eosinophilia in up to 11%; leukopenia, neutropenia, thrombocytopenia, pancytopenia, anemia, leukocytosis and thrombocytosis in less than 1% of patients
Hepatic Effects (2-4%)	Transient

PRECAUTIONS: Patients with a hypersensitivity to penicillins and/or cephalosporins may rarely develop a hypersensitive reaction to aztreonam.

PHARMACOKINETICS: IM: Completely absorbed; Protein-Binding: 50-65%; Distribution: Wide tissue distribution including cerebrospinal fluid; Half-Life: 1.7 hours; Excretion: Largely unchanged but some limited biotransformation to a microbiologically inactive metabolite.

BACTERIA

Bacteria			
Gram-Positive		Gram-Negative	
Cocci	Bacilli	Enteric Bacilli	Other Bacilli
Staphylococcus	Bacillus Anthracis (Anthrax)	P. Mirablis	Haemophilus
Aureus	Clostridium	E. Coli	Influenzae
Epidermidis	Perfringens (Welchii)	K. Pneumoniae	Ducreyi (Chancroid)
Streptococcus	Tetani	Campylobacter	Pseudomonas
Pyogenes (Grp.A, and Grps. C,G)	Difficile	Enterobacter	Aeruginosa
Group B	Corynebacterium	Salmonella Typhi	Urinary Tract
Viridans	Diphtheriae	Other Salmonella	Other
Bovis	JK strain	Shigella	Actinobacillus
Enterococcus	Listeria	Bacteroides	Pseudomallei
Anaerobic	Monocytogenes	Oropharyngeal	Bordetella
Pneumoniae (Pneumococcus)		Gastrointestinal	Pertusis (Whooping Cough)
		Providencia	Brucella (Brucellosis)
		Serratia	Gardnerella Vaginalis
		Yersinia	Legionella
Anaerobes		Cocci	Leptotrichia (Vincent's Infection)
Bacteroides Fragilis		Neisseria	Pasteurella
Other Bacteroides		Gonorrhoeae (Gonococcus)	Vibrio Cholerae (Cholera)
Clostridium Perfringens		Neisseria Meningitidis (Meningococcus)	Yersinia Pestis (Plague)
		Moraxella (Branhamella) Catarrhalis	Acinetobacter

BECLOMETHASONE

(Vanceril, Beclovent)

USES: Beclomethasone dipropionate is a **corticosteroid** that is used by oral inhalation; uses are given in the next Table:

Uses of Beclomethasone
Seasonal (Hayfever) or Nonseasonal (Perennial) Rhinitis when Conventional Therapy with Antihistamines or Decongestants are Ineffective
Asthma
Nasal Polyposis

Seasonal (Hayfever) or Nonseasonal (Perennial) Rhinitis: Beclomethasone is used for the treatment of seasonal (hay fever) or nonseasonal (perennial) rhinitis when conventional therapy with antihistamines or decongestants are ineffective. Beclomethasone is as effective as flunisolide, both glucocorticoids producing good to excellent responses (Langrick, A.F., Curr. Med. Res. Opin. 9, 290-295, 1984). These glucocorticoids are more effective than cromolyn and reduce the symptoms of seasonal asthma (Welsh, P.W. et al., Mayo Clin. Proc. 62, 125-134, 1987).

Asthma: Beclomethasone is used with asthma to reduce needs for systemic corticosteroids and thus decrease adverse systemic side effects.

Nasal Polyposis: Intranasal beclomethasone is used in the management of nasal polyposis, principally to prevent recurrence of nasal polyps following surgical removal.

BECLOMETHASONE (Cont.)
DOSAGE FORMS: Aerosol: 200 metered doses; 1 dose = 42 micrograms.
DOSAGE: Beclomethasone dipropionate is administered by nasal inhalation or by oral inhalation. The inhaler delivers about 42 microgram of beclomethasone per metered spray. Dosage is given in the next Table:

Dosage of Beclomethasone Dipropionate by Nasal Spray

Condition	Age	Dosage
Seasonal or Perennial Rhinitis and Management of Nasal Polyposis	Adults & >11 yrs.	Initial: 42 microgram (1 spray) in each nostril 2-4 times daily. Relief in several days and optimum effectiveness in 1-2 weeks. Maintenance: 42 microgram (1 spray) in each nostril 3 times daily.
	6-11 yrs.	Initial: 42 microgram (1 spray) in each nostril 3 times daily. Relief in several days & optimum effectiveness in 1-2 weeks. Maint.: as appropriate

Dosage of Beclomethasone Dipropionate by Oral Inhalation

Condition	Age	Dosage
Asthma	Adults	Initial: 84 micrograms (2 sprays) 3-4 times daily. In severe asthma, higher doses are used. Maximum recommended dose (per manufacturer) is 840 micrograms (20 sprays) daily. Maintenance: Use minimum dose necessary to achieve desired affect.
	6-11 yrs.	Initial: 42-84 micrograms (1-2 sprays) 3 or 4 times daily, maximum of 420 micrograms (10 sprays) daily. Maintenance: Minimum dose necessary.

ADVERSE EFFECTS: Rinse mouth and gargle with water after inhalation; may cause thrush. No systemic affects with doses <1mg/day. Wean cautiously off steroids once inhalant is used. Not recommended for children <6 years.
Large doses associated with prolonged use may cause adrenal suppression; treatment is to decrease dose.

BENZODIAZEPINES see Anxiety, Treatment

BENZTROPINE
(Cogentin)
USES: Benztropine is used to treat both idiopathic and drug-induced **Parkinsonism.**
Benztropine is a competitive antagonist of acetylcholine. It has anticholinergic and antihistaminic effects.
DOSAGE FORMS: Tabs: 0.5, 1,2mg. Injectable: 1mg/ml.
DOSAGE: Benztropine is administered orally or by IM or IV injection. Parenteral administration is reserved for patients who cannot take oral medication or for emergency situations. Dosage is given in the next Table:

Dosage of Benztropine

Condition	Route	Dosage
Arteriosclerotic Idiopathic or Postencephalitic Parkinsonism	Oral	Initially, 0.5-1mg at bedtime. The dosage may be gradually increased in 0.5mg increments at 5-6 day intervals to a max. of 4 to 6mg daily if required and tolerated.
Drug-Induced Extrapyramidal Reactions except Tardive Dyskinesia	Oral, IM, or IV	1 to 4mg once or twice daily. In acute dystonic reactions, initially, 1 to 2mg IM or IV; to prevent recurrence, 1-2mg orally twice daily.

ADVERSE EFFECTS: Adverse reactions to benztropine are mainly anticholinergic and antihistaminic effects. Adverse effects are dose-related and include dry mouth, blurred vision, nervousness, tachycardia, nausea, constipation, drowsiness, decreased sweating, urinary retention .
DRUG INTERACTIONS: Paralytic ileus with phenothiazines, tricyclic antidepressants; antagonizes psychotropics.

BETA-LACTAM ANTIBIOTICS

The beta-lactam antibiotics are listed in the next Table:

Beta-Lactam Antibiotics
Penicillins
Cephalosporins
Carbapenems (Imipenems-Cilastatin) (Primaxin)
Monolactams (Aztreonam) (Azactam)

All have a beta-lactam ring structure as illustrated in the next Figure:

Beta-Lactam Ring Structure

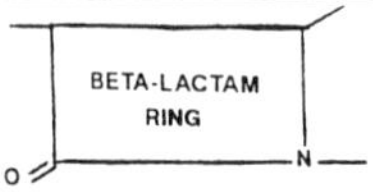

The beta-lactam ring structure, which is essential for antibacterial activity, consists of a four membered ring. The structures of the beta-lactam antibiotics are given in the next Figure:

Structures of Beta-Lactam Antibiotics

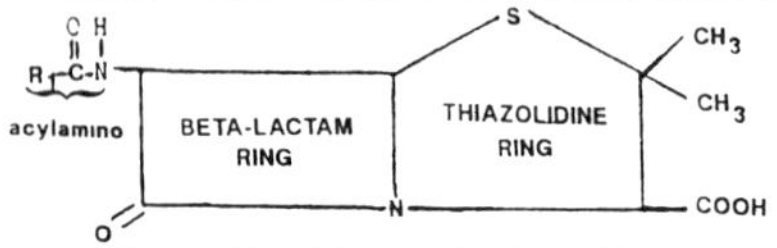

Penicillin(s)

Beta-lactam ring is fused to a five-membered **thiazolidine ring.**

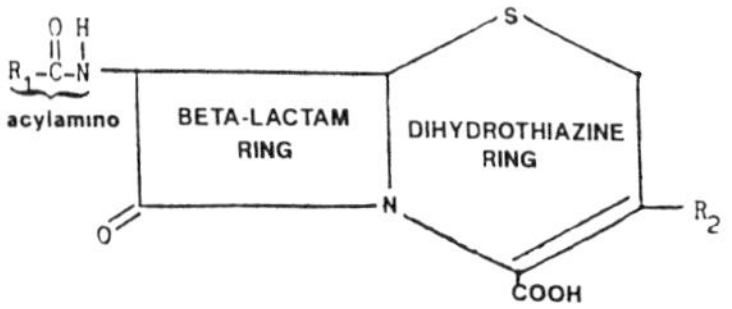

Cephalosporins

Beta-lactam ring is fused to a six-membered **dihydrothiazine ring.**

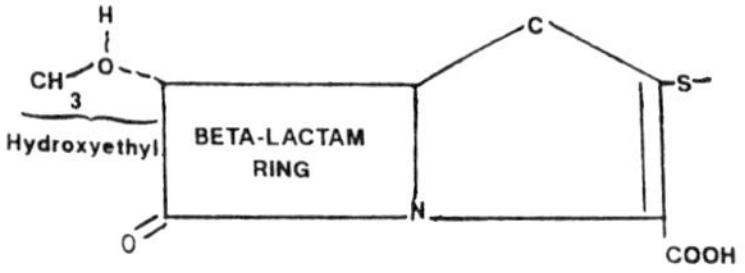

Carbapenems (Imipenems)

Beta-lactam ring is fused to a five-membered ring having a carbon instead of a sulfur and a hydroxyethyl side chain rather than the classic acylamino moiety of penicillins and cephalosporins.

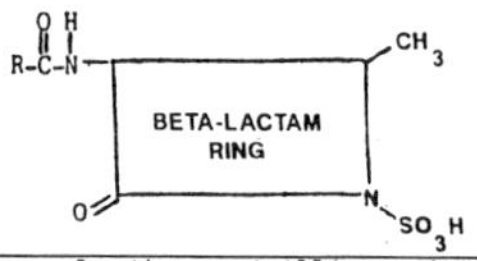

Monolactams (Aztreonam)

The monolactams are compounds in which the bicyclic structure characteristic of other beta-lactams is absent

Penicillins: In the penicillins, the beta-lactam ring is fused to a five-membered thiazolidine ring. **Cephalosporins:** In cephalosporins, the beta-lactam ring is attached to a six-membered dihydrothiazine ring. **Carbapenems (Imipenems):** In the carbapenems, eg, imipenems, the beta-lactam ring fused to a five-membered ring having a carbon instead of a sulfur and a hydroxyethyl side chain rather than the classic acylamino moiety of penicillins and cephalosporins. **Monolactams (Aztreonam):** The monolactams are compounds in which the bicyclic structure characteristic of other beta-lactams is absent.

BETA-LACTAM ANTIBIOTICS (Cont.)

Mechanism of Action of Beta-Lactam Antibiotics: Beta-lactam antibiotics are bactericidal because they inhibit bacterial cell-wall synthesis and may increase breakdown of the cell-wall; the exact mechanism is not completely understood. These antibiotics are believed to inhibit bacterial cell-wall synthesis by inhibiting peptide bond cross-linking of the linear polysaccharide chains which form the supporting structure of the bacterial cell wall. In gram positive bacteria, there is an inhibitor of a cell-wall autolytic enzyme. Beta-lactams decrease the availability of the inhibitor and thus enzymatic breakdown of the cell-wall may occur.

Beta-lactam antibiotics bind to penicillin-binding proteins (PBP's). These proteins are believed to be enzymes that are involved in bacterial cell-wall division, wall elongation, septum formation, and the maintenance of cell shape. PBP's vary in their affinity for different beta-lactam antibiotics, and different bacteria have different numbers of these proteins (S. Aureus: 4; E. coli: 7 or more). Beta-lactam binding to PBP2 and/or PBP3 may cause bacterial cell lysis and the production of long filamentous forms, respectively.

Mechanisms of Bacterial Resistance to Beta-Lactam Antibiotics: The most important mechanism of bacterial resistance to the beta-lactam antibiotics is bacterial production of beta-lactamases, enzymes that hydrolyze the cyclic amide bond of the beta-lactam ring and render it inactive; the action of beta-lactamase on penicillins and cephalosporins is illustrated in the next Figure:

Action of Beta-Lactamase on Penicillins and Cephalosporins

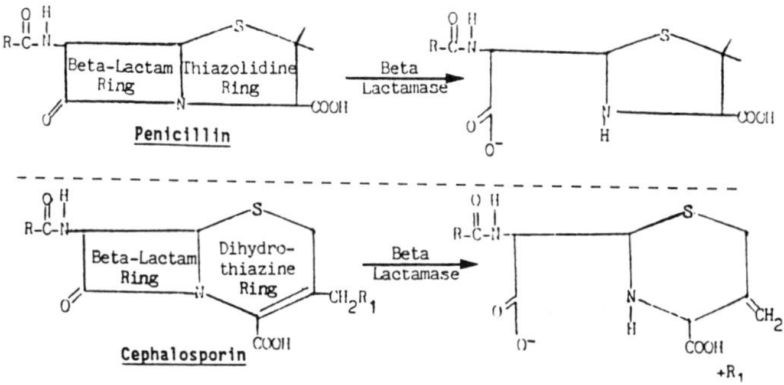

Mechanism of bacterial resistance to the other beta-lactam antibiotics, imipenem and aztreonam, are much less dependent on beta-lactamase production. Imipenem and aztreonam are very resistant to hydrolysis by bacterial beta-lactamases. Bacterial resistance may be due to alterations in outer-membrane proteins or other factors that decrease bacterial permeability to the drug.

Incidence of Beta-Lactamase Production in Bacterial Isolates: The incidence of beta-lactamase production in bacterial isolates is given in the next Table (Neu, H.C., Am. J. Med. 79 (suppl.5B), 2-12, 1985; Doern, G.V. et al., Antimicrob. Agents Chemother. 32, 180-185, 1988; Yogev, R., Adv. Pediatr. Infect. Dis. 3, 181-206, 1988):

Incidence of Beta-Lactamase Production in Bacterial Isolates

	Beta-Lactamase-Producing (%)	
Organism	Hospital Isolates	Community Isolates
Staphylococcus aureus	85	85
Staphylococcus epidermis	80-95	
Moraxella catarrhalis	75	75
Neisseria gonorrhoeae	5-10	
Hemophilus influenzae	20	20
Escherichia coli	20	21
Klebsiella pneumoniae	90	88
Bacteroides fragilis	90	
Pseudomonas aeruginosa	90-100	

BETA-LACTAM ANTIBIOTICS (Cont.)

Classifications, antibacterial spectrum, indications and adverse effects, see: **PENICILLINS, CEPHALOSPORINS, IMIPENEM AND AZTREONAM.**

Cross-Reactions and Other Beta-Lactams: Patients allergic to penicillin occasionally have allergic reactions to cephalosporins and imipenem, a parenteral beta-lactam. However, aztreonam (Azactam), which is also a parenteral beta-lactam, is not associated with allergic reactions due to cross reactivity with penicillin (Saxon, A. et al., Ann. Intern. Med. 107, 204, 1987).

COMBINATIONS OF PENICILLINS WITH BETA-LACTAMASE INHIBITORS: The addition of a beta-lactamase inhibitor (clavulanate or sulbactam) restores amoxicillin, ampicillin and ticarcillin to its original spectra of activity. Beta-lactamase inhibitors resemble penicillin structurally and enhance the in-vitro activity of certain beta-lactam antibiotics by protecting them from hydrolysis by beta-lactamases. They are termed "suicide inhibitors" because they bind to and inactivate beta-lactamases but are destroyed in the process. Examples are given in the next Table:

Combinations of Penicillins with Beta-Lactamase Inhibitors

Combination	Additional Susceptible Bacteria
Ampicillin and Sulbactam (Unasyn)	S. aureus, H. influenzae, Moraxella (Branhamella) catarrhalis, Klebsiella species and Bacteroides fragilis.
Amoxicillin and Clavulanate (Augmentin)	H. influenzae, E. coli, Proteus, K. pneumoniae; S. aureus and S. epidermidis (but not methicillin-resistant strains); M. catarrhalis, N. gonorrhoeae, and Legionella pneumophila.
Ticarcillin and Clavulanate (Timentin)	S. aureus, H. influenzae, N. gonorrhoeae, E. coli, Klebsiella, Providencia and B. fragilis.

The above combinations are the only preparations including a beta-lactamse inhibitor that are currently available.

BETAMETHASONE, TOPICAL
(Valisone, Uticort, Diprolene, Diprosone, Maxivate)

USES: Topical betamethasone is used for the symptomatic relief of inflammatory dermatoses; uses are given in the next Table:

Uses of Topical Betamethasone

Low to Medium Potency:
- **Seborrheic Dermatitis**
- **Atopic Dermatitis**
- **Lichen Simplex Chronicus**
- **Nummular Eczematous Dermatitis**
- **Pruritis Ani**
- **Phototoxic Reactions**
- **Contact Dermatitis due to Allergens, Irritant Chemicals**
- **Mild Psoriasis of the Face and Body Folds**

More Potent Preparation:
- **Psoriasis Affecting the Palms, Soles, Elbows and Knees**
- **Discoid Lupus Erythematosus**
- **Sarcordosis**
- **Necrobiosis Lipoidica Diabeticorum**
- **Hypertrophic Lichen Planus**
- **Lichen Striatus**
- **Familial Benign Pemphigus**
- **Pretibial Myxedema**
- **Alopecia Areata**

DOSAGE FORMS: The potency of betamethasone preparations is given in the next Table:

Potency of Betamethasone Preparations

Potency	Commercial Product	Vehicle	%
High	Diprolene Ointment	Dipropionate	0.05
	Diprosone Cream	Dipropionate	0.05
	Diprosone Ointment	Dipropionate	0.05
	Diprosone Cream	Dipropionate	0.05
	Valisone Ointment	Valerate	0.1
	Maxivate Cream, Ointment, Lotion	Dipropionate	0.05
Intermediate	Benisone Ointment	Benzoate	0.025
	Benisone Cream	Benzoate	0.025
	Diprosone Lotion	Dipropionate	0.02
	Valisone Cream	Valerate	0.1
	Valisone Lotion	Valerate	0.1
	Uticort Cream, Lotion	Benzoate	0.025
Low	Valisone Cream	Valerate	0.01

DOSAGE: Small amounts of the lotion, cream, or ointment is applied gently to the involved areas. Initially, 2-4 applications daily may be required. When satisfactory control is obtained, the frequency of application is reduced to the minimum amount necessary to avoid replapse.

ADVERSE EFFECTS: Adverse reactions to betamethasone are direct by related to the potency, concentration, volume applied, skin condition, duration of use, site and area of application and use of occlusive wraps (Robertson, D.B. and Maibach, H.I., Semin. Dermatol. 2, 238-249, 1983).

Adverse effects are most commonly observed in highly absorptive areas such as face, neck, axilla, perineum and genitals; these effects include epidermal and dermal atrophy resulting in thinning of the skin, striae, telangiectasia and senile-type purpura.

Other adverse effects include rosacea-like dermatoses, perioral dermatitis, acne, folliculitis, nonhealing leg ulcers, hypopigmentation especially in blacks, hypertrichosis, ocular hypertension, allergic contact dermatitis usually caused by vehicle rather than the steroid. FDA pregnancy category C.

Toxicity may occur with high potency betamethasone applied to extensive areas for prolonged periods of time and especially when occlusive dressings are used. Miliaria, bacterial and candidal infections may occur. Bethamethasone may be absorbed in sufficient amounts to suppress pituitary ACTH.

BETHANECHOL

(Urecholine, Urabeth, Duvoid, Myotonachol)

USES: **Bethanechol,** which is structurally and pharmacologically related to **acetylcholine,** is a **cholinergic drug.** It is used in the treatment of acute postoperative and postpartum nonobstructive **urinary retention** and **neurogenic atony of the urinary bladder.**

DOSAGE FORMS: Tabs: 5, 10, 25, 50mg; Inject: 5mg/ml

DOSAGE: Bethanechol chloride is administered orally or by subcutaneous injection only, never by IV or IM. Dosage is given in the next Table:

Dosage of Bethanechol Chloride

Condition	Age	Route	Dosage
Acute Postperative or Postpartum Non-obstructive Urinary Retention or Neurogenic Atony of the Bladder with Retention	Adults	Oral	10-50mg, 2-4 times daily; or 50-100mg, 4 times daily. Min. effective oral dose determined by giving 5 or 10mg initially & repeating that dose at hour intervals until a satisfactory response is obtained. Effects persist up to 6 hours.
	Adults	Sub-Q	2.5-5.0mg. Min. effective subcutaneous dose determined by giving 2.5mg initially and repeating that dose at 15-30 min. to a max. of 4 doses
Chr. Neuro. Bladder	Adults	Sub-Q	7.5-10mg every 4 h. See package insert
Gastroesophageal Reflux	Child	Oral	0.4mg/kg/day in 4 divided doses (ac and hs).

ADVERSE EFFECTS: Flushed skin, sweating, hypotension, bronchospasm, circulatory collapse, abd. cramps, vomiting, diarrhea, bradycardia, cardiac arrest. Adverse effects can be abolished by atropine.

CONTRAINDICATIONS: Asthma, GI or GU obstruction, hypotension or bradycardia, peptic ulcer, hyperthryoidism, epilepsy, vasomotor instability, coronary artery disease, Parkinsonism.

BISACODYL

(Dulcolax, Fleet, and other products)

USES: Bisacodyl is a **laxative;** it is used to evacuate the bowel prior to surgery and prior to radiologic, proctoscopic, or sigmoidoscopic examinations. It is also used in patients with acute or chronic constipation.

Bisacodyl is often combined with the closely related compound, phenolphthalein (both are diphenylmethane laxatives) in numerous laxative preparations.

Mechanism of Action: Bisacodyl stimulates sensory nerves of the colonic mucosa causing reflex peristalsis. In addition, it alters active electrolyte transport and thus affects fluid movement.

DOSAGE FORMS: Tabs: 5mg; Supp.: 10mg; Susp: 10mg/30ml.

DOSAGE: Bisacodyl is administered orally or rectally as a suppository or enema. Bisacodyl tannex is administered rectally as an enema. For occasional use as oral laxative, bisacodyl should be administered the evening before a morning bowel movement is desired. Rectal bisacodyl suppositories and enemas may be administered at the time a bowel movement is desired; usually effective within 15-60 minutes. Tablets should be swallowed whole (not chewed or crushed) and should not be taken within 1 hour of antacids or dairy products. Dosage is given in the next Table:

Dosage of Bisacodyl

Age	Route	Dosage
Adults	Oral	5-15mg
>3 yrs.	Oral	0.3mg/kg or 5-10mg
Adults and >2 yrs.	Rectal	10mg
<2 yrs.	Rectal	5mg

ADVERSE EFFECTS: Abdominal cramps occur occasionally; excessive use can cause rectal irritation.

CONTRAINDICATIONS: Acute surgical abdomen; fecal impaction; intestinal obstruction; abdominal pain of unknown origin; intestinal perforation.

PHARMACOKINETICS: Onset: Orally, 4-8 hours; Rectally, 15 min-1 hour. Metabolism: Absorption is less than 5% by oral or rectal route. Rapidly converted by intestinal and bacterial enzymes to its active desacetyl metabolite.

BLEOMYCIN

(Blenoxane)

USES: Bleomycin is an **antineoplastic** antibiotic that inhibits the incorporation of thymidine into DNA; it also appears to labilize the DNA structure, resulting in scission of both single- and double-stranded DNA. Uses of bleomycin in treatment of cancer are given in the next Table:

Uses of Bleomycin
Lymphomas
Hodgkin's, Non-Hodgkin's
Squamous Cell Carcinomas
Germ Cell Tumors
Testicular Embryonal Cell Carcinoma, Choriocarcinoma, Teratocarcinoma

DOSAGE FORMS: Inj. 15 units per ampule

DOSAGE: Bleomycin sulfate is administered by IV, IM, or subcutaneous injection.

Test Dose: Patients receiving bleomycin may develop an anaphylactoid response, characterized by an exaggerated hyperpyrexic response; this reaction is more likely to occur in lymphoma patients. A test dose of 1-2U is given IM. If no reaction occurs in 2-4 hours, give the regular dose.

Use according to appropriate oncology protocols.

Dosage by IV, IM, or subcutaneous injection is as follows: Weekly or twice weekly doses of 0.25-0.5 units/kg(10-20 units/m^2). Following a 50% regression of tumor size in patients with Hodgkin's disease, a maintenance IV, IM, or subcutaneous dose of 1 unit of bleomycin daily or 5 units weekly can be given. If improvement occurs in patients with Hodgkin's disease or testicular carcinoma, it is usually observed within two weeks; if improvement occurs in patients with squamous cell carcinoma, it is usually observed in three weeks.

Bleomycin may also be given by IV continuous infusion, intrapleurally and intra-arterially.

The dosage should be reduced in patients with impaired renal impairment. See manufacturer's instructions for specific details.

PATIENT INSTRUCTIONS: The patient should be instructed to report any coughing, shortness of breath or wheezing. Hypersensitivity reactions may be indicated by skin rashes, shaking chills or transient high fever. Hyperpigmentation of skin folds, scars or trauma sites should be reported.

PHARMACOKINETICS: The drug is poorly absorbed from the GI tract and skin. The drug must be administered parenterally. The low concentration of bleomycin in bone marrow may be related to the high concentration of the degrading enzyme bleomycin-hydrolase. Half-life: 2 hours with normal renal function.

ADVERSE EFFECTS: Acute Reactions: Fever, anaphylaxis and other allergic reactions. Delayed Reactions: The most serious toxic effect is interstitial pneumonitis (10% of patients) occasionally progressing to pulmonary fibrosis (death in 1% of patients receiving drug). Pulmonary toxicity appears to be dose and age related, occurring most frequently in patients receiving a total dosage of more than 400 units and in patients older than 70 years of age.

The most frequent adverse effect is mucocutaneous toxicity which occurs in at least 50% of patients and is most often observed within 1-3 weeks following start of therapy. Mucocutaneous effects are reversible and dose related and are usually evident after 150-200 units.

Unlike many other antineoplastic agents, bleomycin does not often produce serious bone marrow toxicity.

Other adverse effects include hyperpigmentation and Raynaud's phenomenon.

PARAMETERS TO MONITOR: Assess renal function prior to dosing. Calculate cumulative dose. Monitor temperature initially especially in patients with lymphoma. Pulmonary toxicity is best monitored with CO diffusing capacity and forced vital capacity. X-rays may be helpful in detecting pulmonary fibrosis.

BLOOD COMPONENT THERAPY

The blood components available for transfusion and the indications for the use of these components are given in the next Table:

Blood Components and Indications

Blood Component	Indications
Red Cells	Chronic Anemia; Slow Blood Loss; Acute Blood Loss up to 30% Blood Volume; Exchange Transfusions.
Red Cells: Washed (Leukocyte and Plasma Poor) or Leukocyte Poor	Same as for Red Cells; Leukocyte Poor: Prevent Febrile Reaction Due to Leukocyte Antibodies; Plasma Poor: Prevent IgA Sensitization.
Red Cells, Frozen-Thawed	Same as above plus Autotransfusions and Rare Blood Types.
Whole Blood	Massive Blood Loss
Plasma, Fresh Frozen	Treatment of Bleeding Patients with Multiple Factor Deficiencies
Albumin, 25% (25g/dl)	Burns, Hypoalbuminemia
Albumin, 5% (5g/dl)	Burns, Shock
Platelet Concentrates	Bleeding due to Thrombocytopenia or Platelet Function Abnormality
Granulocyte (Leukocyte) Concentrate	Granulocytopenia with Sepsis
Cryoprecipitate	Factor Deficiency: Hemophilia A, von Willebrand's Disease and Factor XIII Deficiency; Hypofibrinogenemic States
Factor VIII Concentrate	Hemophilia A

Red cell transfusions have largely superceded the use of whole blood. All blood products must be administered through a filter.
Preoperative Crossmatch Guidelines: For patients without preoperative complications undergoing elective surgery, the following guidelines are recommended: Blood is collected from the patient and testing is done for ABO, Rh(D) and antibody screen; cross-match is not recommended. If the patient should require emergency transfusion, blood of the same ABO group and Rh(D) type is selected; on initial spin, crossmatch is performed and the blood released in approxi- mately 10-15 minutes. The standard crossmatch is completed while the patient is being transfused. This approach allows for a reduction in blood inventory and patient costs without sacrificing patient safety. If time allows, a standard crossmatch can be performed prior to transfusion.

The ^{51}Cr-labeled red blood cell survival test has been used to evaluate in-vivo survival of a small sample of donor red blood cells in patients with blood compatibility problems (Pineda, A.A. et al., Mayo Clin. Proc. 59, 25-30, 1984).

RED CELLS: Red blood cells are prepared by centrifugation or sedimentation of a unit of whole blood from a hematocrit of 40% to a hematocrit of 60% to 80%. Red blood cells transfusions are indicated for chronic anemias, slow blood loss, acute blood loss up to 30% blood volume and for exchange transfusions.

Red blood cell transfusions are superior to whole blood transfusions for patients with cardiac disease, chronic anemia and for patients with liver or kidney disease who require restricted sodium or citrate intake.

A unit (hematocrit, 60 to 80%) which contains 200ml of red blood cells, should increase recipients hematocrit about 3% in a 70kg adult. Cells must be administered through a filter; do not exceed 4 hours/unit.

The side effects and hazards of red blood cell transfusion are like that of the transfusion of whole blood.

The number of units of red blood cells required for transfusion to achieve a desired hematocrit in a nonbleeding patient is calculated from the formula:

$$\frac{(\text{Blood vol. x Hct}) + (\text{No. of Units Transfused x 200ml})}{\text{Blood Vol. + No. of Units Transfused X 300ml}} = \text{New Hct.}$$

In this formula, the volume of red blood cells is 300ml and the red cell mass is 200ml. Blood volume(ml) = weight (kg) x .08 (8%) x 1000; Blood volume calculation example: 70kg x .08 x 1000 = 5600ml blood volume. Hct is expressed as a fraction (30% = .30).

BLOOD COMPONENT THERAPY (Cont.)

ADSOL Red Blood Cells: ADSOL red blood cells is a preparation of red blood cells; ADSOL refers to ADditive SOlution system; ADSOL has the following advantages:

(1) This preparation has an improved red blood cell survival with extension of red blood cell shelf life to 42 days.
(2) The infusion rate is similar to whole blood; it is not necessary to add saline at the time of transfusion.
(3) When the product is prepared from the donor, the yield of platelets and plasma factors is increased when these components are separated.

The system is generically called Additive Solution System because it uses a second preservative solution in addition to the anticoagulant solution, citrate phosphate dextrose(CPD) needed for whole blood collection. The additive consists of adenine in 100ml. of normal saline, with a small amount of citrate anticoagulant remaining. The plasma is separated from the red blood cells prior to the addition of the additive solution. Additive solutions differ; AS-1 and AS-5 contain mannitol as a red blood cell stabilizer, whereas AS-3 contains additional citrate and phosphate but does not contain mannitol. Patients with documented mannitol hypersensitivity should not receive AS-1 or AS-5 units.

Because of the small amount of mannitol (AS-1 unit contains 0.75g of mannitol) and the slightly increased volume per unit (60ml.), rare patients with cardiac or renal failure may require volume reduction just prior to transfusion. In these patients, the order must be written as "volume reduced red blood cells." The ADSOL unit of red blood cells will be centrifuged in the Blood Bank just before transfusion and most of the liquid removed, resulting in a product with a hematocrit of about 80% which will not flow nearly as well as the ADSOL units. An order for packed cells without specifying "volume reduced" will be filled with the usual ADSOL RBC's.

A comparison of AS-1 RBC's with CPDA-1 RBC's and CPDA-1 whole blood is shown in the next Table:

Comparison of AS-1 RBC's with CPDA-1 RBC's and CPDA-1 Whole Blood

Parameters Measured After 35 Days Storage	AS-1 RBC's	CPDA-1 RBC's	CPDA-1 Whole Blood
Maximum Storage Period, Days (FDA)	42	35	35
Volume per Unit	310	250	510
Hematocrit, Percent	60	75	40
Viscosity, Relative to Whole Blood	1.2	2.6	1.0
Post-Transfusion Survival (Percent Recovery)	86	78	76
Supernatant Hgb (mg/dl)	112	900	43
Percent of RBC's Lysed During Storage	0.2	0.9	0.2
Supernatant Potassium (mEq/liter)	45	86	27
pH	6.70	6.58	6.72
ATP, Percent of Day Zero	74	52	62
Glucose, Percent of Day Zero	65	15	2

RED CELLS, LEUKOCYTE POOR:

Leukocyte Poor: Leukocyte removal helps to prevent febrile reactions. Recipients who have had multiple transfusions or pregnancies may develop antibodies to HLA or other antigens on leukocytes. Subsequent transfusions with cells carrying these antigens may cause a febrile (non-hemolytic) reaction in 0.5 to 1% of transfusions. Leukocytes may be removed by centrifugation, filtration, or addition of sedimenting agents; the resulting unit contains fewer than 5 x 10^8 white cells (more than 95% removal). Leukocyte poor preparations should be given to patients that require frequent transfusions such as leukemia and aplastic anemia.

BLOOD COMPONENT THERAPY (Cont.)

RED CELLS, WASHED (LEUKOCYTE AND PLASMA-POOR):

Leukocyte Poor: After washing, less than 20% of the leukocytes remain and the unit contains more than 80% of the original red blood cells. Washing is less effective and more expensive than filtration or other means of leukocyte removal and should not generally be used for this purpose alone.

Plasma Poor: Three conditions in recipients are prevented by removing plasma; these are listed in the next Table:

Conditions Prevented by Using Plasma-Poor Red Cells

Component(s) Removed	Condition Prevented
IgA	Anaphylactic Reaction in IgA Deficient Patients: IgA deficient patients develop antibodies to IgA following exposure to IgA in a previous transfusion. Deglycerolized red cells is the component of choice for clinically significant antibodies to IgA.
Complement (C-3)	Hemolytic Episodes in PNH: Patients with paroxysmal nocturnal hemoglobinuria (PNH) have an acquired intrinsic defect in that their red blood cells bind more C-3 than do normal cells.
Electrolytes and Metabolic Products	Electrolyte imbalance

Each unit contains 185ml packed red blood cells in a 200-250ml volume. There are two disadvantages to the use of plasma poor red cells; one is the cost and the other is the shelf-life which is only 24 hours.

IRRADIATED RED CELLS: Certain patient populations are at risk for graft-versus-host disease (GVHD) if they receive unirradiated directed blood donations from HLA-homozygous or partially HLA-identical donors. Patients at risk include neonates and fetuses, patients with congenital immunodeficiency or immunosuppressive chemotherapy, and in other situations. GVHD is caused by T-cells in transfused blood, proliferating and reacting against antigenic sites in the blood recipient. Irradiation destroys lymphocytes and prevents this reaction; granulocytes are not destroyed (Ferrara, J.L.M. and Deeg, H.J., N. Engl. J. Med. 324, 667-674, March, 1991).

DEGLYCEROLIZED RED CELLS (FROZEN-THAWED RED BLOOD CELLS): Red blood cells may be frozen for up to 3 years with glycerol. These preparations are particularly useful for autotransfusions, rare blood types, and clinically significant antibodies to IgA.

WHOLE BLOOD: (Volume 520 ± 45ml, Hct. 40%; smaller volumes for pediatric patients; administer through a filter) (Donor and recipient must be ABO identical crossmatch): Whole blood is given to patients who have had massive blood loss or who are bleeding profusely. Whole blood must be through a filter; transfusion should not be slower than 4 hours/unit. In some centers, whole blood is no longer available; patient may receive a combination of packed red blood cells and fresh frozen plasma.

FRESH FROZEN PLASMA (SINGLE DONOR): Fresh frozen plasma, which may be stored up to one year, is used in the treatment of bleeding patients with multiple clotting factor deficiencies; fresh frozen plasma contains XI, IX, VIII, X, VII, V, II and XIII. Stored whole blood also contains all of these factors but factors V and VIII are unstable in whole blood and are markedly decreased in activity by the second or third day of storage. Infusion of a unit of fresh frozen plasma causes all coagulation factors to rise about 8 percent; fibrinogen level rises about 13mg/dl. Fresh frozen plasma is stored at -20°C or below and requires 30 minutes to thaw in a 37°C water bath.

Fresh frozen plasma is used in the treatment of patients with conditions listed in the next Table:

Conditions Treated with Fresh Frozen Plasma
Disseminated Intravascular Coagulopathy (DIC)
Other Defibrination Syndromes
Liver Disease

BLOOD COMPONENT THERAPY (Cont.)

The disadvantages of the use of fresh frozen plasma are as follows: excessive volume causing circulatory overload, possibility of hepatitis, allergic reactions with chills and fever and blood group antibodies; thus, fresh frozen plasma must be ABO-group specific with the recipients red blood cells.

Deficiency of factor VIII and fibrinogen (factor I) alone should be treated with cryoprecipitated factor VIII concentrates or purified factor VIII concentrates.

Single donor plasma is used instead of pooled plasma because of the high incidence of hepatitis in pooled plasma. The plasma is administered through a filter.

ALBUMIN (25% and 5%): Albumin (25%, 25g/dl) is used in the treatment of burns and other causes of fluid loss to counteract fluid and sodium loss. The dosage is given so as to maintain the circulating plasma level of albumin at 2.5 $\pm$ 0.5g/dl (Tullis, J.L., JAMA 237, 460, 1977).

Albumin (5%, 5g/dl) is used in the treatment of burns and other causes of fluid loss. It may be used in the early treatment of shock due to hemorrhage until blood is available. The usual minimal effective adult dose is 250-500ml. (Borucki, D.T., Blood Component Therapy, Am. Ass. Blood Banks, 3rd Ed., 1981).

PLATELET CONCENTRATES: Platelet concentrates are given to patients who are bleeding due to thrombocytopenia (usually <50,000) or due to abnormal platelet function, or if platelet counts are below 20,000. One platelet concentrate increases the platelet counts of a patient with a 5000ml blood volume by 5,000 per cu mm; the usual dose is six to eight units of platelet concentrates.

ABO and Rh compatibility are desirable because of red blood cell contamination.

Platelet concentrates are not given to patients with thrombocytopenia caused by accelerated platelet destruction, eg, thrombocytopenic purpura (ITP).

Transfusion risks are hepatitis, immunization to HLA and red blood cell antigens, febrile reaction, allergic reactions with urticaria.

Advanced notification when possible is recommended due to short life span of platelets. Life span is 3-5 days depending on type of bag used for storage.

Platelet concentrates may be obtained by use of plateletpheresis; plateletpheresis is the centrifugal separation of platelets from whole blood with either continuous or intermittent return of platelet-poor red blood cells and plasma to the donor. Plateletpheresis involves some risk to the donor.

GRANULOCYTE (LEUKOCYTE) CONCENTRATE: Granulocyte transfusions have been given to patients who are granulocytopenic (<500 neutrophils/cu mm) and have infections, eg, septicemia, that are not responsive to antibiotics or other forms of therapy. Leukocytes are administered daily, usually for 5 days in succession, or until WBC rises above 500 granulocytes. Use of granulocyte transfusions is controversial.

Leukocyte concentrates must be ABO-group compatible and are administered through a blood filter. Transfusion risks include chills, fever, allergic reactions, viral hepatitis, cytomegalic virus infection and in immunodeficient or immunosuppressed patients, graft versus host reaction. CMV seronegative granulocytes are recommended for immunosuppressed CMV-seronegative patients (eg, bone marrow transplant recipients). The presence of red blood cells can result in a hemolytic reaction.

Granulocyte concentrates may be obtained by use of leukapheresis; leukapheresis is the centrifugal separation of leukocytes from whole blood with either continuous or intermittent return of leukocyte-poor cells and plasma to the donor. Leukapheresis involves some risk to the donor.

BLOOD COMPONENT THERAPY (Cont.)

CRYOPRECIPITATE: Cryoprecipitate is a source of Factors VIII, XIII and fibrinogen and is used to treat the conditions listed in the next Table:

Conditions Treated with Cryoprecipitate

- Factor Deficiency
  - Hemophilia A (Factor VIII Deficiency)(Factor VIII Concentrate preferred)
  - von Willebrand's Disease (not responsive to DDAVP)
  - Factor XIII Deficiency
- Hypofibrinogenemic States, eg,
  - Disseminated Intravascular Coagulopathy (obstetrical complications eg, abruptio placenta and amniotic fluid embolism; endotoxin in bacterial sepsis; severe intravascular hemolysis; carcinomatosis)

Cryoprecipitate contains 150mg of fibrinogen, 80 to 100 units of Factor VIII, some Factor XIII and von Willebrand's factor; 1ml of normal plasma contains 1 unit of Factor VIII activity.

A patient with hemophilia A who is bleeding usually has a Factor VIII level of about 2 to 10 percent; the desired therapeutic level is 10 to 100 percent. Cryoprecipitate should be given every 12 hours to a severely bleeding hemophiliac or to a hemophiliac who is about to undergo surgery.

Side effects of cryoprecipitate include viral hepatitis, febrile and allergic reactions.

Cryoprecipitate may be stored for 1 year at -20°C or below and requires 15 minutes to thaw in a 37°C water bath.

FACTOR VIII CONCENTRATE: Factor VIII is indicated for the treatment of hemophilia A patients for the prevention and control of hemorrhagic episodes. In hemophilia, inherited as a sex-linked recessive, there is a deficiency of a part of the Factor VIII molecule, called Factor VIII C. Factor VIII concentrate is obtained from a large number of donors and recipients have developed acquired immunodeficiency syndrome (AIDS). There is also a very high incidence of non-A, non-B hepatitis in patients receiving factor VIII concentrate (Andes, W.A., JAMA 249, 2331, May 6, 1983). These earlier clotting factor concentrates transmitted hepatitis viruses to nearly 100% and human immunodeficiency virus to 60-80% of patients with hemophilia. Newer preparations are much safer and involve heating the preparations for various time periods and under different conditions. Although more longitudinal data is needed, it appears that transmission of HIV has been virtually eliminated and that transmission of hepatitis has been greatly reduced. Hepatitis transmission has been curtailed by use of the hepatitis B vaccine and screening of blood for hepatitis C, as well as the availability of safer concentrate (Epstein, J.S. and Fricke, W.A., Arch. Pathol. Lab. Med. 114, 335-340, 1990).

TRANSFUSION REACTIONS: Transfusion reaction rates are given in the next Table; (Goldfinger, D. and Lowe, C., Transfusion 21, 277, 1981):

Transfusion Reaction Rates

Reaction	Rate (per thousand Units)
Febrile, Nonhemolytic	3.0
Urticarial	1.6
Hemolytic, Delayed	0.7
Hemolytic, Immediate	0.06
	5.36

FEBRILE REACTIONS: Febrile reactions usually occur 1 to 2 hours after the transfusion has been started and lasts for several hours to 24 hours. A febrile reaction is defined as a 2 degree increase in body temperature or a one degree increase in temperature accompanied by shaking chills. The differential diagnosis of febrile reactions to blood transfusion products is given in the next Table:

Differential Diagnosis of Febrile Reactions to Blood Products

- Reactions to:
  - Leukocyte Antigens
  - Platelet Antigens
  - Plasma Proteins
- Hemolytic Reactions
- Bacterial Contamination

BLOOD COMPONENT THERAPY (Cont.)

In the most common cause of a febrile reaction, antibodies in the patient react with antigens present on donor leukocytes.

Signs and symptoms of febrile reactions are as follows: febrile reactions, mild to severe; chills, nausea, vomiting, hypotension, cyanosis, tachycardia, transient leukopenia, chest pain and dyspnea.

Nurses should proceed as follows:

(1) Stop transfusion. Keep I.V. open with slow saline drip.
(2) Recheck patient identification on tie tag and patient arm band, and recheck blood unit numbers.
(3) Notify physician and blood bank.
(4) Send clotted sample and blood container (without removing recipient set) to the blood bank and collect a post-transfusion urine specimen to send to the laboratory marked "Transfusion Reaction Specimen".

Physicians should proceed as follows:

(1) Evaluate patient for possible signs of hemolytic transfusion reaction.
(2) Ordinarily, order the transfusion discontinued.
(3) Administer antihistamine, antipyretics and possibly steroids as indicated.

Prevention: Use washed (leukocyte poor) red cells for subsequent transfusion; use pretransfusion antihistamine in patients who have had previous febrile reactions.

ALLERGIC-ANAPHYLACTOID REACTIONS: Usually, these reactions are mild. Clinical signs and symptoms include pruritis, urticaria, occasional facial and periorbital edema; rarely bronchospasm and anaphylactoid shock. Urticaria is not seen with hemolytic reactions; therefore, a work-up for hemolysis is not necessary.

Usually, the transfusion is discontinued and a antihistamine is administered I.V. (diphenhydramine). If laryngospasm or bronchospasm occur, give epinephrine. If anaphylactoid shock occurs, establish an airway, give I.V. fluid, aminophylline, corticosteroids, and cardio-supportive drugs.

If the reaction is very mild, urticaria only, then slow transfusion rate and administer antihistamines I.V. If there is no clinical improvement, stop transfusion.

Prevention: Patients with a history of allergic transfusion reactions should receive oral diphenhydramine (Benadryl) 30 minutes prior to transfusion. Transfuse packed red blood cells or washed red blood cells instead of whole blood.

Causes: Most of the allergic reactions are probably caused by many different proteins.

Anaphylactoid transfusion reactions are rare; they most often occur in patients with IgA deficiency. About 1 in 850 individuals are deficient in IgA and about 25 percent have IgA antibodies. The diagnosis is made by finding anti-IgA in the recipient plasma and IgA in the donor plasma.

HEMOLYTIC, DELAYED: These reactions usually occur several days after administration of red cells and are most commonly caused by antibody in the recipient reacting with donor red cell antigens. These reactions occur most often in patients who have had multiple transfusions or women previously sensitized to red cell antigens from pregnancy.

The signs and symptoms of delayed hemolytic reaction are: fever, jaundice and occasionally hemoglobinuria; lack of appropriate increase in hematocrit or hemoglobin.

Obtain blood specimens as follows:

Blood Specimens for Delayed Hemolytic Reaction

Specimen	Assay
Purple (EDTA) or Blue (citrate) Top Tube	Direct Coombs Test
Red Top Tube	Antibody Screening Test
Red Top Tube	Antibody Titer
Purple (EDTA) Top Tube	Complete Blood Count (Hgb, Hct, RBC, Indices), Smear
Red Top Tube	Bilirubin, Haptoglobin

The management of delayed hemolytic reaction is supportive; treatment of hypotension or renal failure is similar to acute hemolytic reaction. The usual responsibility of the blood bank is to search for antibody in the recipient.

BLOOD COMPONENT THERAPY (Cont.)

HEMOLYTIC, IMMEDIATE: The most common cause of fatal hemolytic reactions is clerical errors. The most severe hemolytic reactions result from antibody in the recipient reacting with donor cells.

The features are as follows: fever, chills, hypotension, hemoglobinuria, oozing from incisional sites, nausea, anxiety, back pain, tachycardia, oliguria, shock, acute renal failure; death can occur.

Guidelines for evaluation of a suspected immediate hemolytic reaction are as follows:

(1) Stop transfusion immediately; notify and send blood to blood bank; keep I.V. line open with saline.

(2) Recipient: Record and monitor (a) vital signs: temperature, pulse, blood pressure, and respirations; (b) urine output and fluid intake.

(3) Verify that recipient has received proper unit by checking donor numbers against recipient identification bracelet and transfusion request slip.

(4) Return complete I.V. set intact and unused portion of donor unit to blood bank:
- (a) Repeat ABO-Rh typing, antibody screen, compatibility testing
- (b) Bacterial culture

(5) Obtain blood specimens from recipient at a location away from the infusion site:
- (a) Blood Bank: (1 blue (citrate) and red top tube) Repeat ABO-Rh typing, antibody screen, direct Coombs test and donor compatibility testing.
- (b) Hematocrit: Lavender (EDTA) top tube
- (c) Blood Culture: Sterile yellow stoppered tube

(6) Urinalysis for blood assay.

Treatment: Treat shock with vasopressors and appropriate IV fluids. Start fluid balance sheet, charting intake and output. Maintain fluid balance. Maintain renal blood flow with IV furosemide (20-80mg) and/or mannitol. Test for disseminated intravascular coagulation (DIC). Administer appropriate compatible blood components as necessary, i.e., red blood cells, platelets, cryoprecipitate, fresh frozen plasma. Follow status of patient for possible renal failure requiring renal dialysis.

SIDE EFFECTS AND HAZARDS: Side effects associated with transfusion of blood are given in the next Table:

Side Effects Associated with Blood Transfusion

Side Effect	Comment
Hemolytic Transfusion Reactions	Incompatibility between donor red blood cells and recipient plasma.
Transmission of Infectious Disease	Viral hepatitis: Eight percent; mostly non-A Non-B hepatitis. Other diseases that may be transmitted are malaria, brucellosis, trypanosomiasis, Epstein-Barr virus, cytomegalovirus, toxoplasmosis, syphilis in the serological negative phase, Colorado tick fever, AIDS.
Immunization of the Recipient	Recipients who have had transfusions or pregnancies may develop antibodies to HLA or other antigens on leukocytes, or platelets or red blood cells. Subsequent transfusions with cells carrying these antigens may cause a febrile reaction in 0.5% to 1.0% of transfusions; or an anamnestic reaction and a delayed hemolytic reaction (autoimmune hemolytic anemia-like) with a positive direct antiglobulin test.
Allergic Reactions	Urticaria occasionally accompanied by chills and fever; fever; 3% of recipients; may be prevented in patients with known history by premedication with antihistamines. Anaphylactoid Reaction: About 1 in 500 individuals lack IgA and develop anti-IgA antibodies; on subsequent transfusion, an anaphylactoid reaction may occur; treat with adrenalin and corticosteroids.
Other Reactions: Circulatory Overload; Iron Overload; Metabolic Complications	

BLOOD COMPONENT THERAPY (Cont.)

Trisodium citrate is an anticoagulant in blood; one unit of whole blood contains 17mEq of citrate; one unit of packed cells contains 5mEq of citrate. Following transfusions, citrate is metabolized to $[HCO_3^-]$ in equimolar amounts; that is 17mEq of citrate is converted to 17mEq of $[HCO_3^-]$ and 5mEq of citrate is converted to 5mEq of $[HCO_3^-]$. Normally, the $[HCO_3^-]$ load is excreted by the kidney. However, there are certain conditions in which patients receive many units of blood and in which the excretion of $[HCO_3^-]$ by the kidney is compromised; these are given in the next Table:

Blood Transfusions and Compromised Excretion of $[HCO_3^-]$ by the Kidney

Conditions in which many Blood Transfusions may be given:
- Shock
- Trauma
- Sepsis
- Open heart Surgery

Compromised Excretion of $[HCO_3^-]$ by the Kidney:
(Enhanced Renal HCO_3^- Reabsorption)
- ECF Volume Contraction
- Potassium Depletion
- Hypercapnia
- Acute or Chronic Renal Disease
- Oliguria

An example of a consultation request for suspected transfusion reaction is given in the next Figure; (McCord, R.G. and Myhre, B.A., Laboratory Medicine, 9, 39-46, March 1978):

Consultation Request for Suspected Transfusion Reaction

__/__/__ Date ______AM/PM Time ____________ No. of Units ____________ml Vol. Transfused

Clinical Diagnosis Prior to Transfusion____________________

Donor No. of Last Unit Given____________________

PRE TRANSFUSION	POST TRANSFUSION
Temp.________	Temp.________
B/P________	B/P________
Pulse________	Pulse________

CHECK THOSE WHICH APPLY

____Pulse	____Chest Pain	____Back Pain	____Urine Output
____B/P	____Headache	____Jaundice	____Heat at I.V. Site
____Chills	____Dyspnea	____Rash	____Pain at I.V. Site
____Fever	____Hemoglobinuria	____Flushing	____Delirium
____Coma	____Nausea	____Pruritus	____Muscle Tenderness
____Syncope	____Vomiting	____Urticaria	____Petechiae

____Other (Specify)____________________

LIST DONOR NO. FROM ALL SUSPECTED UNITS IN THIS TRANSFUSION SERIES

Donor No.	Date	Time Started	Time Stopped	Amount Given	Whole Blood, Packed cells, Platelets, etc.	Reaction

Complete this portion of the form and return to the TRANSFUSION LABORATORY with post-reaction samples of the patient's urine and blood (clotted). Return the blood bags from all units in this transfusion series.

BLOOD COMPONENT THERAPY (Cont.)

A standard report, used by residents in the Department of Pathology at UCLA School of Medicine, for febrile transfusion reactions and allergic transfusion reactions is as follows:

Standard Consultation Report for Febrile Transfusion Reactions

According to the above information and the chart entry of _/_/_, this age year old man-woman-child experienced chills and a fever (degrees F) during-shortly after the transfusion of a unit of packed cells-whole blood-platelets. There was no complaint of back pain or signs of dyspnea, shock or hemoglobinuria as is often the case in a hemolytic reaction. Furthermore, inspection of pre-transfusion and post-transfusion sera revealed that they were straw-colored, rather than pink or red as one sees with acute intravascular hemolysis. Repeat crossmatch and compatibility testing revealed that compatible blood was administered; vis., ABO, RH type blood was given to a(n) ABO, Rh type recipient. In addition, antibody screening failed to demonstrate the presence of any unexpected antibodies. On the basis of these negative findings, we suspect that the patient experienced a FEBRILE TRANSFUSION REACTION due to pyrogenic material in the unit of blood he-she received. This material usually originates in the granulocytes contained in the blood. With regard to future transfusion of blood to this patient, please read the "Pathology Resident's Note on Febrile Transfusion Reactions" which has been taped into the progress notes.

The appropriate choice of underlined words is selected.

Standard Consultation Report for Allergic Transfusion Reactions

According to the above information and the chart entry of _/_/_, this age year old man-woman-child experienced flushing and pruritis and urticaria during-shortly after the transfusion of a unit of packed cells-whole blood-plasma-cryoprecipitate. There was no complaint of back pain or signs of dyspnea, shock or hemoglobinuria as is often the case in a hemolytic reaction. Furthermore, inspection of a pre-transfusion and post-transfusion sera revealed that they were straw-colored, rather than pink or red as one sees with acute intravascular hemolysis. Repeat crossmatch and compatibility testing revealed that compatible blood was administered; vis., ABO, Rh type blood was given to a(n) ABO, Rh type recipient. In addition, antibody screening failed to demonstrate the presence of any unexpected antibodies. On the basis of these negative findings, we suspect that the patient experienced an ALLERGIC TRANSFUSION REACTION due to allergenic material in the unit of blood he-she received. With regard to future transfusion of blood to this patient, please read the "Pathology Resident's Note on Allergic Transfusion Reactions" which has been taped into the progress notes.

Standard Note on the Causes and Prevention of Febrile Transfusion Reactions

Pathology Resident's Note on Febrile Transfusion Reactions

(If you have not already done so, please see the "Consultation Request for Suspected Transfusion Reaction", which has been inserted into the CONSULTATION section of this patient's chart.)

Granulocytic pyrogenic material can be released in two ways. First, the recipient may have antigranulocytic antibodies (usually leukoagglutinins) in his blood. These antibodies can attach to receptor sites on the granulocyte membrane and, with the aid of the complement system, cause lysis of the granulocyte *in vivo* and concomitant release of pyrogenic substances. Secondly, stored refrigerated granulocytes normally undergo autolysis *in vitro* within 24 hours releasing substances which are pyrogenic. Hence, pyrogenic material can be present in stored blood in the absence of immune lysis.

The problem of febrile reactions due to granulocytic pyrogenic material* can be minimized by giving the patient washed packed erythrocytes. However, washing a fresh unit of packed red cells only removes about 80% of the granulocytes. The remaining cells (if the unit is used immediately) may be subject to immune lysis as described above. If the washed packed cells are stored, the remaining granulocytes will undergo autolysis and again release pyrogenic material.

BLOOD COMPONENT THERAPY (Cont.)

Febrile reactions due to granulocytic pyrogenic material can be eliminated by ordering packed red cells whichhave been refrigerated or frozen. When ordering refrigerated packed red cells, be certain to request that the units be washed. The washing will remove the pyrogenic substance that has been released by granulocyte lysis. In addition, washing will remove any potassium or phosphate that has leaked out of the stored red cells, as well as any lactic acid generated by red cell metabolism. (Washing units of blood introduces the possibility of bacterial contamination, but we feel that the risk is minimal since Federal regulations require that blood be used within 24 hours after thawing and this should preclude significant bacterial growth). If frozen packed red cells are ordered, they will be routinely washed since washing is required to remove the cytoprotective agent, glycerol.

When the administration of whole blood is not vital, the BLOOD BANK recommends the use of frozen packed red cells for the following reasons:

1. These units are extensively washed to remove the glycerol. The pyrogenic material from the lysed granulocytes will be removed during the washing procedure.
2. The process of freezing and thawing destroys many granulocytes which would survive a normal washing procedure.
3. Glycerol is bacteriostatic, therefore greatly decreasing the chance of bacterial growth in the unit of blood.
4. The freezing process is believed to attenuate or even destroy hepatitis virus.

*Administration of platelets may also cause a febrile reaction, but this discussion is limited to correction of anemia only.

Standard Note of the Causes and Prevention of Allergic Transfusion Reactions

Pathology Resident's Note on Allergic Transfusion Reactions

(If you have not already done so, please see the "Consultation Request for Suspected Transfusion Reaction", which has been inserted into the CONSULTATION section of this patient's chart.)

An allergic transfusion reaction is an example of an "immediate-type" hypersensitivity reaction. This kind of reaction is antibody-mediated and occurs within minutes of exposure to an antigen. (This is in contradistinction to the "delayed-type" hypersensitivity reaction which is cell-mediated and occurs within hours or days.) Allergic transfusion reactions (flushing, pruritus, urticaria) are most commonly seen in people who are atopic or who have a congenital lack of IgA antibody; however, they may occur in anyone. Approximately 10% of the population are atopic and are sensitive to a variety of environmental allergens. They experience allergic reactions which are mediated by IgE antibodies. The other type of severe allergic transfusion reaction is the interaction between transfused IgA and anti-IgA antibodies in the recipient's plasma. In this case, the recipient has a congenital lack of IgA and has actually formed IgG antibody against the IgA in the transfused blood. About 1 in 500 recipients lack IgA and could theoretically be at risk.

Prevention of allergic transfusion reactions involves elimination of the offending allergen. When correction of anemia is the only hematologic problem facing the clinician, the BLOOD BANK recommends use of washed packed red cells or frozen reconstituted packed cells. The washing process should remove sufficient allergens (vis., environmental allergens or IgA antibody) to prevent an allergic reaction. In addition, washing removes any potassium or phosphate that has leaked out of the stored red cells, as well as any lactic acid generated by red cell metabolism. If frozen packed red cells are ordered, they will routinely be washed since washing is required to remove the cryoprotective agent, glycerol. (Washing units of blood introduces the possibility of bacterial contamination, but we feel that the risk is minimal since Federal regulations require that blood be used within 24 hours after thawing and this should preclude significant bacterial growth).

When it is absolutely necessary to administer whole blood, plasma or cryoprecipitate to a person who is known to have experienced mild allergic reactions, prophylactic administration of antihistamine should be considered. Furthermore, this patient has a potential risk of development of laryngeal edema. Consequently, it is recommended that a physician be nearby for approximately one half hour post-transfusion; a nurse should continue surveillance for at least 12 hours post-transfusion.

BLOOD COMPONENT THERAPY (Cont.)

When the administration of whole blood is not vital, the BLOOD BANK recommends the use of frozen packed red cells for the following reasons:

1. These units are extensively washed to remove the glycerol. The washing will remove any allergenic material in the unit. (Note: If a patient has ever experienced an anaphylactic reaction due to sensitivity to transfused IgA antibody, then transfusion of frozen red cells is absolutely essential, since routine washing does not remove enough plasma to eliminate the reaction.)
2. Polymorphonuclear leukocyte breakdown produts will also be washed out, thus removing the pyrogenic material responsible for febrile reactions.
3. Glycerol is bacteriostatic, therefore greatly decreasing the chance of bacterial growth in the unit of blood.
4. The freezing process is believed to attenuate or even destroy hepatitis virus.

About two-thirds of all red blood cell transfusions are given in the perioperative period. In the past, it has been rigidly accepted that the criteria for perioperative red blood cell transfusion is a hemoglobin value of 100g/liter (10g/dl) or a hematocrit of less than 0.30 (30%). However, greater recognition of the risks of transfusion has alerted physicians to question and modify these criteria. The most important criteria for red blood cell transfusion is clinical judgement. Healthy patients with hemoglobin values of 100g/liter (10g/dl) or greater rarely require perioperative transfusion; those with hemoglobin values of less than 70g/liter (7g/dl) frequently require red blood cell transfusion. Some patients with chronic anemia, such as those with chronic renal failure, tolerate hemoglobin values of less than 70g/liter (7g/dl) (Consensus Conference, JAMA 260, 2700-2703, Nov. 11, 1988).

Alternatives to Red Blood Cell Transfusion: Alternatives to red blood cell transfusion are given in the next Table (Consensus Conference, JAMA 260, 2700-2703, Nov. 11, 1988):

Alternatives to Red Blood Cell Transfusion
Autologous Red Blood Cell Transfusion
Intraoperative Blood Salvage
Modification of usual Criteria for Red Blood Cell Transfusion, eg, Hemoglobin, 100g/liter (10g/dl); Hematocrit, 0.30 (30%).
Under Development: Modified Hemoglobin Solutions and improved Perfluorochemical Emulsions.
Drugs: Desmopressin; deliberately induced Hypotension; Erythropoietin therapy.

BONES (OSTEOMYELITIS)

Pathogens: The bacterial pathogens that are most likely to cause osteomyelitis are given in the next Table:(Handbook of Antimicrobial Therapy, The Medical Letter, 1990; Ingram, C. et al., Med. Clin. N. Am. 72, 723-738, May 1988; Nelson, J.D., Inf. Dis. Clin. N. Am. 4, 513-523, Sept. 1990):

Pathogens Causing Osteomyelitis
Staphylococcus aureus
Streptococci (Group A and Group B predominate)
Enterobacteriaceae
P. aeruginosa
Salmonella
Mycobacterium tuberculosis
Anaerobic streptococci (chronic)
Bacteroides (chronic)
Staphylococcus (coagulase negative)(more frequent in children)
Haemophilus influenzae (type b)(Children)
Streptococcus pneumoniae (Children)

The most common pathogens causing osteomyelitis in adults and older children are S. Aureus, Streptococci (predominantly Group A and Group B), and Pseudomonas aeruginosa; in younger children (<5 years and particularly <2 years), these organisms are common, but Haemophilus influenzae, Streptococcus pneumoniae, and coagulase-negative staphylococci are also frequent pathogens (Nelson, J.D., Inf. Dis. Clin. N. Am. 4, 513-523, Sept. 1990).

The types, cause(s) and site(s) of involve- ment of osteomyelitis are given in the next Table (Ingram, C. et al., Med. Clin. N. Am. 72, 723-738, May 1988):

Types, Cause and Site(s) of Involvement of Osteomyelitis

Types	Usual Cause(s)	Usual Site(s)
Contiguous septic focus	Trauma; surgical	Extremities
Vascular insufficiency	Diabetes; vasculitis; peripheral vascular disease.	Feet, ankles
Hematogeneous dissemination		Vertebrae, lower extremity
Prosthesis Infection	Compression plates; screws pins and wires	

Treatment of Osteomyelitis: Antibiotics used in the treatment of osteomyelitis are given in the next Table (Ingram, C. et al., Med. Clin. N. Am. 72, 723-738, 1988; Gentry, L.O., Inf. Dis. Clin. N. Am. 4, 485-499, Sept. 1990):

Organisms	Treatment
Anaerobic infections; also used in patients allergic to penicillins or cephalosporins	Clindamycin
P. aeruginosa	Aminoglycosides Ceftazidime
S. aureus	Nafcillin Cefazolin Ceftriaxone Clindamycin

Initial therapy is intravenous; choice of agent depends on identification of the organism or empiric therapy for most likely organisms. Inpatient IV therapy is often followed by outpatient IV or oral therapy. The serum bacteriocidal test may be useful to assess the adequacy of antibiotic dosages. Oral ciprofloxacin has shown some promise as monotherapy for osteomyelitis and provides broad coverage including S. Aureus and P. aeruginosa (Review: Gentry, L.O., Inf. Dis. Clin. N. Am. 4, 485-499, Sept. 1990).

Outcome of therapy depends on type, chronicity, cause, and pathogen. Hematogenously spread osteomyelitis (usually caused by S. aureus) has the best prognosis (88% cure) whereas vascular insufficiency has a poor prognosis (28% cure). Osteomyelitis associated with a contiguous septic focus or a prosthesis have an intermediate prognosis (58% and 52% cure). Acute infections are more easily cured than chronic infections, no matter what the type or cause. Since cause dictates the type of spread, causes associated with vascular insufficiency such as diabetes, vasculitis, or peripheral vascular disease have the worst prognosis. Pathogenic organism influences outcome, with S. aureus having the best prognosis (60% cure), with poorer prognosis associated with P. aeruginosa (46% cure) or Enterobacteriaceae (30% cure) (Ingram, C. et al., Med. Clin. N. Am. 72, 723-738, May 1988).

BRETYLIUM
(Bretylol)

USES: Bretylium is used as an **antiarrhythmic agent**; uses are given in the next Table:

Uses of Bretylium
Ventricular Fibrillation: Prophylaxis and Treatment
Ventricular Tachycardia: Acute treatment of Life-Threatening Tachycardia Unresponsive to Conventional Therapy, e.g., Lidocaine, Procainamide and Direct-Current Cardioversion

Bretylium is a **second choice drug** for three reasons: **delayed onset of action**, commonly causes **hypotension** and may increase **ventricular irritability**.

DOSAGE FORMS: Injection: 50mg/ml; In Dextrose: 1, 2, 4, 8mg/ml

DOSAGE: Bretylium tosylate is administered IM or IV. For the treatment of immediately life-threatening ventricular arrhythmias, the drug is administered undiluted by rapid IV injection over approximately 1 minute. Otherwise, in life threatening ventricular arrhythmias, the drug may be given IM or by intermittent or continuous IV infusion. No more than 5ml should be given by IM into one site.

For intermittent or continuous IV infusions, 500mg of bretylium tosylate is diluted to at least 50ml with 5% dextrose or 0.9% sodium chloride injection. For intermittent IV infusion, the dilute solution is given over a period of at least 8 minutes to minimize nausea and vomiting. Dosage of bretylium tosylate in treatment of ventricular arrhythmias is given in the next Table:

Dosage of Bretylium Tosylate in Treatment of Ventricular Arrhythmias

Condition	Age	Route	Dosage
Immediately Life-Threatening Ventricular Fibrillation such as Hemodynamically Unstable Ventricular Tachycardia Unresponsive to Conventional Anti-arrhythmic Drugs	Adult or Child	Rapid IV Injection (1 minute)	5mg/kg, undiluted (as a 5% Solution). Continue other cardiopulmonary resuscitation measures. If ventricular fibrillation persists, give 10mg/kg and repeat as necessary.
Other Ventricular	Adult	IM or IV	Initially: 5-10mg/kg; repeat in 1-2 hours if arrhythmias persist. Maintenance: 5-10mg/kg, IM every 6-8 h. or by intermittent IV infusion every 6 h. Dosage should be gradually reduced and discontinued in 3-5 days.

MONITOR: Electrocardiogram(ECG) and blood pressure(BP) continuously.

ADVERSE EFFECTS: Hypotension, dizziness, vertigo, anginal attacks, nausea, vomiting, transitory hypertension. **Antidote for Hypotension: Dopamine.**

BUMETANIDE
(Bumex)

USES: Bumetanide is a sulfonamide type **loop diuretic** with pharmacologic effects similar to those of furosemide; uses are given in the next Table:

Uses	Condition
Edema	Congestive heart failure (CHF) Impaired renal function Nephrotic syndrome Hepatic cirrhosis Acute pulmonary edema (IV administration)

DOSAGE FORMS: Tabs:0.5,1,2mg; Solution for IV: 0.25mg/ml in 2ml containers.

DOSAGE: Bumetanide is not recommended for children under 18 years. Bumetanide is usually administered orally. Dosage is given in the next Table:

Dosage of Bumetanide

Condition	Route	Dosage
Edema	Oral	Initially 0.5-2mg daily in the morning. If response inadequate, repeat doses at 4-to 5-hour intervals. Max. 10mg daily. Maintenance Dosage: Alternate days; or 3 or 4 consecutive days alternating with drug-free periods of 1 or 2 days. Higher doses may be necessary in patients with renal failure.
Acute Pulmonary Edema	IV	0.5 to 1mg. The dose may be repeated if necessary after 20 minutes.
Pediatrics	Oral or IV	0.015-0.1mg/kg/day.

PHARMACOKINETICS: Oral: 95% absorbed; Protein Bound: 95%; Volume of Distribution: 12-35 liters. Half-Life: 1-1.5 hours but prolonged in patients with renal failure.

ADVERSE EFFECTS: The most frequent adverse effects are hypokalemia, dehydration, hypotension and hypochloremic metabolic alkalosis. Other adverse effects include azotemia, hyperuricemia, and rarely, impaired glucose tolerance, nausea, vomiting, abdominal pain, rashes and ototoxicity. In patients with renal failure, large doses may cause myalgia.

CONTRAINDICATIONS: Anuria, hepatic coma, severe electrolyte depletion, lactation.

PRECAUTIONS: Hepatic cirrhosis, sulfonamide allergy, progressive renal disease, gout, diabetes, elderly, pregnancy.

MONITOR: Serum potassium often and other electrolytes, e.g. Na^+,Cl^-,CO_2 content, magnesium, blood glucose, uric acid, BUN and creatinine, occasionally.

BUSPIRONE
(BuSpar)

USES: Buspirone is used in the treatment of generalized anxiety disorder (GAD), but is chemically unrelated to the benzodiazepines.

The benzodiazepines, are most often used to treat anxiety; they possess characteristics that are not necessarily desirable, i.e., sedative, muscle-relaxant. motor-impairment, anticonvulsant, discriminative stimulus. or physical dependence properties (Taylor, D.P. et al., Pharmacol. Biochem. Behav. 23, 687-694, 1985). Buspirone does not have these side-effects.

Mechanism of Action: Buspirone has a high affinity for 5-hydroxytryptamine 1A receptors (Fozard, J.R., Trends Pharmacol. Sci 8, 501-506 1987; Taylor, D.P., FASEB J. 2, 2445-2452, 1988; Eison, A.S. and Temple, D.L., Am. J. Med. 80, (suppl 3B), 1-9, March 31, 1986).

DOSAGE FORMS: Tabs: 5 and 10mg.

DOSAGE: Initial dosage is 5mg, three times daily. The dosage may be adjusted every 2-3 days up to 60mg daily. For most patients, 15-30mg daily in divided doses is optimal.

ADVERSE EFFECTS: The most common adverse effects are dizziness (9%), nausea, headache (7%) nervousness (4%), lightheadedness (4%), excitability (2%), diarrhea (3%), paresthesia (2%) (Newton, R.E. Am. J. Med. 80, [suppl 3B], 17-21, 1986).

The most common adverse effects that have caused discontinuation of treatment are listed in the next Table:

Adverse Effects-Discontinuation of Treatment

System	Percent Discontinued	Features
Central Nervous System	3.4(%)	Dizziness, insomnia, nervousness, drowsiness, lightheadness.
Gastrointesinal System	1.2(%)	Nausea
Miscellaneous Disturbances	1.1(%)	Headache, fatigue

PHARMACOKINETICS: Absorption: Rapid and almost complete; Protein-binding: 95%; Half-Life: 2.1 hours; Metabolism: Liver.

BUTALBITAL, ASPIRIN, CAFFEINE
(Fiorinal)

USES: Fiorinal is used to relieve **muscle-contraction (tension) headache** and may be helpful as an analgesic in **migraine headache.**

DOSAGE FORMS: Tabs or caps: Butalbital 50mg; aspirin 325mg; caffeine 40mg, with or without codeine phosphate 30mg.

DOSAGE: 1-2 every 4 hours; max. 6 daily.

ADVERSE EFFECTS: Drowiness, dizziness, gastric upset, prolonged bleeding time, respiratory depression, salicylism with overdose.

CONTRAINDICATIONS: Severe bleeding or coagulation disorders, peptic ulcer, varicella or influenza in teenagers, pregnancy (last trimester), porphyria.

PRECAUTIONS: Asthma, impaired hepatic or renal function, gastritis, pregnancy, lactation, drug abusers.

INTERACTIONS: Potentiation with alcohol, CNS depressant, anticoagulants, hypoglycemics, NSAIDs.

BUTOCONAZOLE
(Femstat)

USES: Butoconazole is used to treat **vulvovaginal candidiasis.** Comparison of the cure rate for the treatment of vulvovaginal candidiasis of butoconazole and other drugs is given in the next Table:

Cure Rate for Vulvovaginal Candidiasis

Drug	Daily Dosage	Days of Therapy	Cure Rate	Reference
Butoconazole	5 gms	3	83%	Bradbeer, C.S. et al.,
Miconazole	10 gms	7	84%	Genitourin. Med. 61, 270, 1985.
Butoconazole	5 gms	3	95%	Droegemueller, W. et al.,
Clotrimazole	200 mg	3	91%	Obstet. Gynecol. 64, 530, 1984.

As shown in these studies, butoconazole is as least as effective as miconazole or clotrimazole in the treatment of vulvovaginal candidiasis.

Mechanism of Action: Butoconazole acts like other imidazole derivatives in that it alters cellular membranes, resulting in increased membrane permeability, secondary metabolic effects, and growth inhibition. The fungistatic activity of the drug may result from interference with ergosterol synthesis.

DOSAGE FORMS: Vaginal cream, 2%.

DOSAGE: One applicatorful (approximately 5g), 2% cream (100mg of the drug), intravaginally once daily at bedtime for 3 consecutive days.

During the second or third trimester of pregnancy, use one applicatorful once daily at bedtime for 6 consecutive days.

ADVERSE EFFECTS: Local burning or itching.

PRECAUTIONS: Do not use during first trimester of pregnancy.

BUTORPHANOL TARTRATE
(Stadol)

USES: **Butorphanol tartrate** is a **partial opiate agonist** used in patients with moderate to severe pain. Uses of butorphanol tartrate are given in the following Table:

Uses of Butorphanol Tartrate
Obstetrical Analgesia During Labor
Preoperative Sedation and Analgesia
Treatment of Moderate to Severe Pain in Acute and Chronic Medical Conditions, eg, Cancer, Surgery

When butorphanol is used during labor and delivery, respiratory depression may occur in the neonate.

DOSAGE FORMS: Parenteral: 1, 2mg/ml.

DOSAGE: Butorphanol tartrate is administered IM or IV. Dosage is given in the next Table:

Dosage of Butorphanol Tartrate

Condition	Route	Dosage
Usual	IM	2mg (range: 1-4mg) every 3-4 hours as needed.
	IV	1mg (range: 0.5-2mg) every 3-4 hours as needed.

ADVERSE EFFECTS: The most serious adverse effect is respiratory depression. Naloxone may be used to reverse respiratory depression. Sedation occurs in 40% of patients. Other CNS effects: headache, dizziness, lethargy, confusion, agitation, euphoria; GI effects: vomiting, constipation, abdominal cramps; Cardiovascular effects: bradycardia, hypotension; Other effects include urticaria, pruritis, miosis, blurred vision.

CALCITRIOL

[1,25-Dihydroxy-Cholecalciferol(1,25-DHCC), Rocaltrol]

USES: The usual uses of calcitriol are given in the next Table:

Usual Uses of Calcitriol
Chronic Renal Failure
Hypoparathyroidism and Pseudohypoparathyroidism
Vitamin D Dependent Rickets
Familial Hypophosphatemia (Vitamin D-Resistant Rickets)
Hypocalcemia in Premature Infants

Calcitriol is used to prevent or treat rickets or osteomalacia and to manage hypocalcemia associated with hypoparathyroidism or pseudohypoparathyroidism. Calcitriol may be useful for treatment of osteoporosis in postmenopausal women; synthetic calcitriol given for 2 years to a small group (50) of women with nontraumatic vertebral fractures demonstrated increased bone density and total body calcium with no adverse effects on renal function (Gallagher, J.C. and Goldgar, D., Ann. Intern. Med. 113, 649-655, 1990).

Mechanism of Action: Calcitriol, the potent physiologically active form of vitamin D, is synthesized, in-vivo, as illustrated in the next Figure:

Synthesis of Biologically Active Vitamin D

7-Dehydrocholesterol —Skin, U.V.Light→ **Cholecalciferol(CC) (Vit.D_3)** —Liver, +25-OH→ **25-OH-CC** —Kidney, +1-OH; PTH→ **Calcitriol ($1,25\text{-}OH_2CC$)**

Vitamin D_3 (cholecalciferol) is obtained in the diet or is synthesized in the skin from 7-dehydrocholesterol; vitamin D_3 is converted to 25-OH vitamin D in the liver and finally converted to $1,25\text{-}(OH)_2$ vitamin D (calcitriol) in the kidney. $1,25\text{-}(OH)_2$ vitamin D has 100 times the activity of 25(OH)vitamin D. The causes of 1,25-dihydroxyvitamin D deficiency are listed in the next Table:

Causes of 1,25-Dihydroxyvitamin D Deficiency

Cause	Mechanism
Lack of Sunlight	Failure to Convert 7-Dehydrocholesterol to D_3 (Cholecalciferol)
Poor Diet	Lack of D_2, (Ergocalciferol) in Diet
Malabsorption	Failure to Absorb Fat Soluble Vitamins and Loss of $25\text{-}(OH)D_3$ because of its Enterohepatic Circulation
Chronic Renal Failure	Reduced 1-Hydroxylation in Kidney, Elevated Serum Phosphate, Secondary Hyperparathyroidism, Acidosis
Anticonvulsant Therapy	Induction of Hepatic Microsomal Enzymes and Subsequent Inactivation of $25\text{-}(OH)D_3$
Vitamin D Dependent Rickets	Type I: Congenital (Autosomal Dominant) Lack or Decrease of Renal 1-Hydroxylase Activity
Others (Liver Disease Hyperthyroidism, Diabetes)	Reduced Vitamin D Metabolites

25-Hydroxyvitamin-D is increased in 25-OH-D deficient patients after even brief exposure to ultraviolet radiation (Adams, J.S., N. Engl. J. Med. 306, 722-725, 1982).

DOSAGE FORMS: Caps: 0.25, 0.50 microgram; Parenteral: 1.0, 2.0 micrograms/ml

DOSAGE: Calcitriol is administered orally, usually once daily. Dosage depends on degree of patient's hypocalcemia; maintain serum calcium concentrations, 9-11mg/dl.

The initial treatment of severe hypocalcemia is immediate IV administration of a calcium salt such as calcium gluconate or calcium chloride; then vitamin D analogs are used to maintain normocalcemia.

Dosage of Calcitriol		
Condition	Age	Dosage
Chronic Renal Failure, Patients undergoing Hemodialysis	Adults	Initially, 0.25 microgram daily or every other day or less frequently as necessary. If adequate clinical or biochemical responses are not obtained (increased serum calcium, decreased serum alkaline phosphatase), then dosage may be increased by 0.25 microgram daily at 4-to 8-week intervals. Maintenance:0.5-1.0 microgram daily
	Children	0.25-2 microgram daily
Renal Failure without Hemodialysis	Children	0.01-0.05 microgram/kg daily
Hypoparathyroidism and Pseudohypoparathyroidism	Adults, Children, >12 mos.	Initial: 0.25 microgram daily. If adequate clinical or biochemical responses are not obtained (increased serum calcium, decreased serum alkaline phosphatase), then increase dosage at 2-to 4-week intervals. Maintenance: 0.5-2.0 microgram daily
Hypoparathyroidism	1-5 yrs	0.25-0.75 microgram daily
	Pediatric	0.04-0.08 microgram/kg
Vitamin D-Dependent Rickets	Children	1 microgram daily
	Adults	1.0-17 microgram daily
Familial Hypophosphatemia (Vit. D-Resistant Rickets)		2.1 microgram daily; oral phosphate may be administered concomitantly
Hypocalcemia in Premature Infants	Infants	1 microgram daily for 5 days.
Hypocalcemic Tetany in Premature Infants	Infants	IV calcitriol, 0.05 microgram/kg daily for 5-12 days

MONITOR: Monitor serum calcium and serum alkaline phosphatase concentrations at least twice weekly, initially, and after dosage changes; or at least weekly for first 12 weeks of therapy and monthly after stabilization of dosage.
ADVERSE EFFECTS: Avoid concomitant use of Mg^{++} containing antacids; discontinue if hypercalcemia occurs.

CALCIUM CHLORIDE

(27% Calcium)

USES: Calcium chloride is the calcium salt of choice for symptomatic hypocalcemia. Calcium salts should not be used in cardiac resuscitation except for treatment of suspected or confirmed hypocalcemia, hyperkalemia, or calcium channel blocker overdose.

DOSAGE FORMS: Sol'n:100mg/ml(10%)(1.36mEq Ca^{++}/ml);13.6mEq Ca^{++}/gm salt; 73mg salt/mEq Ca^{++}). Dilute to 2% solution for oral administration.

DOSAGE: Calcium chloride is used IV or orally. It is not administered subcutaneously or IM. Dosage is given in the next table:

Dosage of Calcium Chloride

Condition	Age	Route	Dosage
Hypocalcemia	Adults	IV	0.2-1.0gm CaCl (2-10ml)
Hyperkalemia	Children	IV	20mg/kg CaCl (0.2ml/kg)
Ca^{++} Channel Blocker overdose			
Maintenance for hypocalcemia:	Adults	Oral	4-8gm/day in 4 divided doses
	Children	Oral	200-300mg/kg/day in 4 div. doses
		IV	70mg/kg/day

ADVERSE EFFECTS: When given by IV, irritation of the vein may occur. Treat local infiltration with hyaluronidase. Calcium chloride acts synergistically with digoxin and other cardiac glycosides; thus, IV administration of calcium should be avoided in patients receiving cardiac glycosides. If necessary, calcium should be given slowly in small amounts in patients receiving cardiac glycosides.

Calcium complexes tetracycline antibiotics rendering them inactive.

Calcium chloride is acidifying and generally should not be used when acidosis coincides with hypocalcemia, eg, renal failure.

Rapid infusion may cause bradycardia; should be given by slow IV infusion over 10 minutes.

CALCIUM GLUCONATE

(9% Calcium)

USES: Calcium gluconate is used to treat hypocalcemia; release of Ca^{++} is dependent on hepatic metabolism.

DOSAGE FORMS: Oral: 500(45mgCa^{++}), 650(58.5mgCa^{++}), 1g(90mgCa^{++})Tabs; Parenteral: 100mg/ml(10%)(9mg Ca^{++}/ml)

DOSAGE: Calcium gluconate is used orally or IV. Dosage must be individualized. Acute therapy for hypocalcemia or hyperkalemia warrants CaCl. The usual adult dosage for treatment of hypocalcemia is 1-2g of elemental calcium per day. Neonatal hypocalcemia is treated with 15-55mg/kg of elemental Ca^{++} per day (200-600mg/kg/day calcium gluconate).

ADVERSE EFFECTS: See Calcium Chloride.

CAPTOPRIL
(Capoten)

USES: Uses of captopril are given in the next Table:

Uses of Captopril
Hypertension
Congestive Heart Failure(CHF)

Hypertension: Captopril is used in the management of mild to severe hypertension. Treatment of hypertension with captopril is given in the next table (The 1988 Report of the Joint National Committee on Detection, Evaluation, and Treatment of High Blood Pressure, Arch. Intern Med. 148, 1023-1038, 1988):

Treatment of Hypertension with Captopril

Step 1: Nonpharmacologic Approaches (see Hypertension)

↓

Step 2: Captopril (Usual Minimum, 25-50 mg/day; Usual Maximum, 300 mg/day)
Observe up to 6 months; if captopril ineffective then,

↓

Step 3: Add a second drug of a different class
or Increase the dosage of captopril
or Substitute another drug

↓

Step 4: Add a third drug of a different class
or Substitute a second drug

↓

Step 5: Consider further evaluation and/or referral
or Add a third or fourth drug

"Step-Down": For patients with mild hypertension, after 1 year of control, consider decreasing or withdrawing captopril and other hypotensive drugs.

Congestive Heart Failure: Captopril is used in conjunction with cardiac glycosides and diuretics in the management of congestive heart failure resistant to or inadequately controlled by cardiac glycosides and diuretics.

Mechanism of Action: Captopril is an angiotensin-converting enzyme(ACE) inhibitor; ACE catalyses the reaction as illustrated in the next Figure:

Angiotensin-Converting Enzyme(ACE)

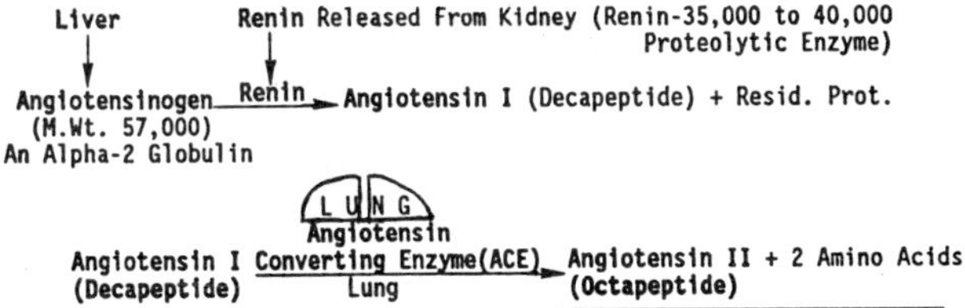

Captopril blocks the synthesis of angiotensin II; angiotensin II is a potent vasoconstrictor and stimulates the release of aldosterone from the adrenal cortex.

DOSAGE FORMS: Tabs: 12.5, 25, 50, 100mg

CAPTOPRIL (Cont.)

DOSAGE: Captopril is administered orally; the drug should be taken 1 hour before or 2 hours after meals. Dosage of captopril is given in the next Table:

Dosage of Captopril

Condition	Dosage
Hypertension	Except in patients with severe hypertension, discontinue other antihypertensive therapy one week prior to initiation of captopril to minimize the possibility of severe hypotension. 12.5mg, 3 times daily or 25mg, 2-3 times daily. If blood pressure not adequately controlled after 1-2 weeks, then 50mg, 2 or 3 times daily.If blood pressure not adequately controlled at a dosage of 50mg, 3 times daily, then give a thiazide at low dose, eg, 25mg, hydrochlorothiazide, daily; increase thiazide at 1-2 weeks intervals
Severe Hypertension (Malignant or Accelerated)	May be necessary to continue other anti-hypertensive drugs. 25mg, 2-3 times daily; dosage may be increased every 24 hours or less under continuous supervision until optimum blood pressure is attained or 450mg daily is given
Cong. Heart Fail.	6.25-12.5mg, 3 times daily or 25mg, 3 times daily

Dosage in Renal Failure: Initial dose should be reduced, that is, less than 75mg daily; increase dosage slowly at 1-2-week intervals. After the desired therapeutic effect is obtained, dosage should be decreased slowly to the minimum effective dose.

Dosage in Pediatrics: Experience is limited; Neonates: 0.1-0.4mg/kg/day, children: 0.5-1.0mg/kg/day divided every 8 hrs has been used. Max. dose 6mg/kg/day.

ADVERSE EFFECTS: Some adverse effects are given in the next Table:

Adverse Effects of Captopril
Neutropenia and Agranulocytosis
Angioedema
Proteinuria
Rash (Most Common)
Decrease in Taste Acuity
Hypotension
Tachycardia, Chest Pain, Palpitations
Hyperkalemia
Cough

Serious adverse effects are associated with captopril, eg, neutropenia and agranulocytosis. Neutropenia has occurred within 3-12 weeks after beginning treatment. The risk of captopril-induced neutropenia appears to depend principally on the degree of renal impairment and the presence of collagen vascular disease. Neutropenia occurs in 0.2% of patients with serum creatinine greater than 1.6mg/dl and in 3.7% of patients with collagen vascular disease and renal impairment. Other risk factors for neutropenia include patients with congestive heart failure(CHF) and impaired renal impairment and receiving procainamide concomitantly.

Angioedema may ocur with ACE inhibitors (0.1% of patients); patients should be aware of the signs and symptoms of this condition.

Proteinuria (urinary protein >1g/day) occurs in about 0.7% of patients and nephrotic syndrome occurs in about one-fifth of these patients. About 90% of patients who have developed proteinuria had evidence of prior renal disease and/or received relatively high dosages of the drug (greater than 150mg daily). Proteinuria usually develops by the 8th month of treatment.

The most common adverse effect of captopril is rash, occurring in 4-7% of patients depending on renal function and dosage. It generally occurs during the first 4 weeks of therapy. The rash is usually mild and disappears within a few days after dosage reduction, oral antihistamines and/or discontinuance of the drug.

Hyperkalemia can develop, particularly in patients with renal insufficiency.

DRUG INTERACTIONS: Nonsteroidal anti-inflammatory drugs may reduce the blood pressure reponse to captopril. Nonsteroidal anti-inflammatory drugs, including aspirin, may magnify potassium-retaining effects of captopril. Digoxin levels may increase 15-30% when captopril is added. Lithium levels may be increased.

CONTRAINDICATIONS: Can cause reversible, acute, renal failure in patients with bilateral renal arterial stenosis or unilateral stenosis in a solitary kidney.

CARBAMAZEPINE

(Tegretol)

USES: Carbamazepine is used as both an **anticonvulsant** and for the relief of pain associated wtih **trigeminal neuralgia** (tic douloureux); uses are given in the next Table:

Uses of Carbamazepine
Anticonvulsant
Complex Partial (Psychomotor or Temporal)
Tonic-Clonic (Grand Mal) Seizures
Mixed Seizure Patterns
Pain Associated with Trigeminal Neuralgia

Carbamazepine is used in the prophylactic management of partial seizures with complex symptomatology (psychomotor or temporal lobe seizures), generalized tonic-clonic (grand mal) seizures, and mixed seizure patterns. It has no effect on absence seizures (petit mal) or myoclonic seizures.

Carbamazepine is used in the symptomatic treatment of pain associated with true trigeminal neuralgia (tic douloureux).

DOSAGE FORMS: Tabs: 100mg chewable; 200mg; susp: 100mg/5ml.

DOSAGE: Carbamazepine is given by mouth and is slowly absorbed from the G.I. tract; it reaches a peak in the serum in 2 to 24 hours; about 3/4 of the drug is bound to albumin. Carbamazepine is metabolized (99%) by the liver. The clearance and half-life decrease with time so that it is advisable to initiate therapy gradually over two to four weeks; dose schedule and time to obtain blood specimens are as follows:

Dose Schedule and Blood Specimens

Age	Dose	Blood Specimens
Adults	Initially: 400mg/day in 2-4 divided doses Increase by 200mg/day every other day Maintenance: 600-1200 mg/day in 3 or 4 doses	Blood specimen obtained during weeks 3 or 4, several days after starting maintenance dose. Optimally, obtain blood specimen at start, middle and end (trough) of a dosing period; otherwise, obtain specimen at end of dosing period.
Children	Week 1: 5mg/kg/day (3 or 4 dose/day) Week 2: 10mg/kg/day (3 or 4 dose/day) Week 3: (Maint. Dose) 15-30mg/kg/day (3 or 4 dose/day)	Blood specimen obtained during weeks 3 or 4, several days after starting maintenance dose; optimally, obtain blood specimen at start, middle and end (trough) of a dosing period; otherwise, obtain specimen at end of dosing period.

Usual maximum adult dose is 1.2g daily, however, 1.6-2.4g daily is sometimes necessary.

There is variability in carbamazepine absorption and the trough concentration may not represent the lowest drug level during the dosing interval; therefore, multiple determinations may be necessary in some patients.

The time to peak concentration is about 3 hours after an oral dose when patients are on chronic therapy.

DRUG INTERACTIONS: The rate of clearance of carbamazepine in the presence of phenobarbital and phenytoin is increased. Clearance is decreased by erythromycin, calcium channel blockers, cimetidine, isoniazid and others. Carbamazepine accelerates the breakdown of estrogens necessitating higher estrogen doses in oral contraceptives. Metabolism of corticosteroids, theophylline, warfarin and haloperidol is increased (Review: "Carbamazepine Update" Lancet, 595-597, Sept. 9, 1989).

REFERENCE RANGE: Therapeutic: 2-10mcg/ml; Toxic: >12mcg/ml. Time to Obtain Serum Specimens (Steady State): 2-4 weeks (see dosage for initiation of therapy below); Half-life: chronic dosing, adults and children, 5 to 27 hours.

ADVERSE EFFECTS: Obtain pretreatment CBC. Minor hematologic changes (eg, decreased leukocyte counts) are not uncommon and do not necessarily require discontinuation of therapy unless there is evidence of infection ("Carbamazepine Update" Lancet, 595-597, Sept. 9, 1989). Aplastic anemia and agranulocytosis has been reported to occur in patients on carbamazepine; therefore, routine blood counts should be performed at 2-4 months intervals. Monitor hepatic toxicity (periodic liver function tests).

Side effects include rash, neuritis, drowsiness, dizziness, headache, tinnitus, diplopia, urinary retention and nausea. Mild asymptomatic hyponatremia is not uncommon; severe hyponatremia occurs rarely.

CARBENICILLIN

(Geopen, Geocillin)

USES: The only primary clinical indication for carbenicillin is suspected or proven systemic P. aeruginosa infection.

Carbenicillin is an extended-spectrum penicillin with a spectrum of activity similar to that of ticarcillin; activities of carbenicillin are given in the next Table (Parry, M.F., Med. Clin. No. Am. 71, 1093-1112, 1987):

Activities of Carbenicillin

	Gram-positive cocci			Gram-negative bacilli						Anaerobes	
	S. aureus	Streptococci	Strep. entero.	H. influenzae	P. mirabilis	E. coli	Klebsiella	Other Enterics	Pseudomonas a.	B. fragilis	Res. Anaerobes
Carbenicillin	■	4	■	4*	4	2	■	2	2	2	4

4=best activity; 3=good activity; 2=some activity; ■=little or no activity; Res.= Resident; *Beta-lactamase negative.

Note that carbenicillin has both anaerobic plus aerobic activity. Despite carbenicillin's broad spectrum of antibacterial activity, resistant bacteria are common and resistance may develop during therapy; thus, carbenicillin should not be used alone for empiric therapy of suspected infections.

Carbenicillin is an "old" drug and has been largely displaced by the newer, more effective antibiotics.

DOSAGE FORMS: Carbenicillin is commercially available for parenteral use as carbenicillin disodium; carbenicillin indanyl sodium is used for oral administration. Parenteral: 1, 2, 5, 10, 30g; Tabs: 382mg.

DOSAGE: Carbenicillin disodium is administered by slow IV injection or by deep IM injection. Carbenicillin is generally given IM only for the treatment of uncomplicated urinary tract infections. Dosage is given in the next Table:

Dosage of Carbenicillin Disodium

Condition	Age	Route	Dosage
Uncomplicated Urinary Tract Infections	Adults	IV or IM	1-2g every 6 hours.
	>1 month	IV or IM	50-200mg/kg daily, IM or IV in divided doses every 4-6 hours
Complicated Urinary Tract Infections	Adults	IV	200mg/kg daily in divided doses every 4 hours
Septicemia, Respiratory Tract Infections, Skin: Pseudomonas aeruginosa or Anerobes	Adults or >1 month	IV	400-500mg/kg (not exceeding 40g) daily IV in divided doses every 4 hours
Systemic Infections, Proteus, or E. Coli	Adults or >1 month	IV	250-400mg/kg daily IV in divided doses every 4 hours (max. 40g)
Systemic Infections in Neonates, Pseudomonas, Proteus, E. coli, H. Influenzae, S. Pneumoniae or Anaerobes	<2kg	15 min. IV Infusion	Loading dose of 100mg/kg followed by 75mg/kg every 8 hours (225mg/kg daily) during first week of life; dosage may be increased to 100mg/kg every 6 hours (400mg/kg daily) when neonate is older than 7 days of age.

Dosage of Carbenicillin Disodium

Condition	Age	Route	Dosage
	>2kg	15 min. IV Infusion	Loading dose of 100mg/kg followed by 75mg/kg every 6 hours (300mg/kg daily) during first 3 days of life; dosage may be increased to 100mg/kg every 6 hours (400mg/kg daily) when infant is older than 3 days.
Meningitis, H. Influenzae or S. Pneumonia	Adults or >1 month	IV	400-600mg/kg (maximum 40g) daily IV in divided doses every 4 hours.
Febrile Granulocytopenic Patients in Conjunction with other Drugs	Adults	IV	70-100mg/kg, IV, every 4 hours

Oral carbenicillin indanyl sodium has occasionally been used for treatment of acute or chronic urinary tract infection or acute or chronic prostatitis.

Renal and Hepatic Impairment: Modification of the usual dosage is unnecessary in patients with creatinine clearances greater than 10ml/minutes. Peritoneal Dialysis Patients: 2g IV every 6-12 hours. A maximum of 2g daily for adults with both renal and hepatic impairment.

ADVERSE EFFECTS: May cause anaphylaxis and platelet destruction. Unpredictable interaction with gentamicin. Give through separate IV tubing. May lead to urinary K^+ loss. Adjust dose with renal failure. Bleeding complications due to abnormal platelet aggregation and prolonged prothrombin time or bleeding time occurs rarely. Injection of carbenicillin is associated with a significant sodium load. (1gm carbenicillin = 4.7mMol Na)

CARISOPRODOL

(Soma, Rela, Soprodol, Soridol)

USES: Carisoprodol is a centrally acting skeletal muscle relaxant used to treat acute musculoskeletal pain; benefit may be due to sedative effects.

DOSAGE FORMS: Tabs: 350mg.

DOSAGE: Carisoprodol is administered orally, usual adult dosage is 350mg 4 times daily.

PHARMACOKINETICS: Onset: 30 minutes; Duration: 4-6 hours; Half-Life: 8 hours; Metabolism: Liver. Metabolized to meprobamate.

ADVERSE EFFECTS: The most frequent adverse effects are sedation and dizziness. Other adverse effects include nausea, vomiting, tachycardia, postural hypotension, and sensitivity reactions. Withdrawal symptoms may occur.

CEFACLOR - 2nd Gen. Ceph.
(Ceclor)

USES: Cefaclor is an orally administered second generation cephalosporin. Activities of cefaclor are given in the next Table (Fried, J.S. and Hinthorn, D.R., Disease-a-Month 31, No. 7, July 1985):

Activities of Cefaclor

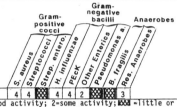

	Gram-positive cocci			Gram-negative bacilli				Anaerobes	
	S. aureus	Streptococci	Strep. entero.	H. influenzae	PEcK	Other Enterics	Pseudomonas a.	B. fragilis	Res. Anaerobes
Cefaclor (Ceclor)	4	4	▩	4	4	2	▩	▩	3

4=best activity; 3=good activity; 2=some activity; ▩ =little or no activity.
PEcK (Mnemonic)= P. mirabilis, E. coli, Klebsiella; Res.= Resident

Cefaclor has antibacterial activity similar to that of oral first generation cephalosporins except that it generally is more active against gram-negative bacilli.

Cefaclor is seldom the drug of choice for the treatment of any pathogen. It is used primarily in the treatment of acute otitis media and acute sinusitis caused by strains of H. influenzae or Moraxella (Branhamella) catarrhalis that are resistant to amoxicillin, the usual drug of choice.

Cefaclor usually is preferred in patients who are allergic to sulfonamides.It is an alternative to erythromycin/sulfisoxazole, trimethoprim/sulfamethoxazole and amoxicillin/potassium clavulanate for infections caused by bacterial strains resistant to these antibiotics.

DOSAGE FORMS: Caps: 250, 500mg; Susp.: 125mg/5ml, 187mg/5ml, 250mg/5ml, 375mg/5ml.

DOSAGE: Cefaclor is administered orally; dosage is given in the next Table:

Dosage of Cefaclor

Condition	Age	Dosage
Usual	Adults	750mg daily, 250mg every eight hours.
Severe Infections	Adults	1.5g daily, 500mg every eight hours; max. 4g daily.
Usual	Children and Infants >1 month	20-40mg/kg daily in equally divided doses every eight hours.
Otitis Media and Severe Infections	Children and Infants >1 month	40mg/kg daily in equally divided doses every eight hours; max. is 1g.

In patients with impaired renal failure, cefaclor usually can be administered in the usual dosage. For patients on hemodialysis, a supplemental dose should be administered after each dialysis session.

PHARMACOKINETICS: Peak following Absorption: 30-60 minutes; food delays absorption and decreases peak but the total amount of drug absorbed is not effected; Half-Life: 0.5-1 hours; 2.3-2.8 hours in anuria. Protein Bound: 25%; Apparent Volume of Distribution: 0.24-0.36 liter/kg. Therapeutic levels of the drug are not achieved in cerebrospinal fluid (CSF). Excretion: Urine, 60-85% unchanged. Excretion is delayed by probenecid.

ADVERSE EFFECTS: Gastrointestinal disturbances and hypersensitivity reations are most common. Prior to initiation of therapy, inquiry should be made concerning previous hypersensitivity reactions to cephalosporins, penicillins and other drugs. Adverse effects include pseudomembranous colitis, superinfection, diarrhea, G.I. rash, blood dyscrasias, hepatoxicity, CNS stimulation. Discontinue cefaclor if colitis occurs.

CEFADROXIL -1st Gen. Ceph.
(Duricef, Ultracef)

USES: Cefadroxil is a first generation cephalosporin; it is administered orally. Cefadroxil (Duricef, Ultracef), is the choice for oral use as compared to the other first generation oral cephalosporins, cephalexin or cephradine, because it has a longer serum half-life enabling twice daily dosing (500mg twice daily) rather than every six hours as for other oral first generation cephalosporins; in addition, cefadroxil is cheaper than these other oral cephalosporins. Furthermore, all of these oral cephalosporins have similar clinical effectiveness at similar doses. Activities of cefadroxil are given in the next Table (Goldberg, D.M. Med. Clin. No. Am. 71, 1113-1133, Nov. 1987; Fried, J.S. and Hinthorn, D.R., Disease-a-Month 31, No. 7, July 1985):

Activities of Cefadroxil

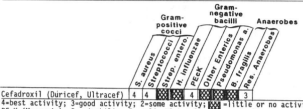

	Gram-positive cocci: S. aureus	Streptococci	Strep. entero.	Gram-negative bacilli: H. influenzae	PEcK	Other Enterics	Pseudomonas a.	Anaerobes: B. fragilis	Res. Anaerobes
Cefadroxil (Duricef, Ultracef)	4	4	▩	▩	4	▩	▩	▩	3

4=best activity; 3=good activity; 2=some activity; ▩ =little or no activity.
PEcK (Mnemonic)= P. mirabilis, E. coli, Klebsiella; Res.= Resident

Conditions commonly treated with cefadroxil are given in the next Table (Goldberg, D.M., Med. Clin. No. Am. 71, 1113-1133, 1987):

Conditions Commonly Treated with Cefadroxil

Most skin and soft tissue infections (Staph. and Strep. activity)
- Do not use for sacral decubitus and diabetic lower extremity infections which require better anaerobic coverage.

Community-acquired urinary tract infections (P. mirabilis, E. coli and K. pneumoniae activity).

Uncomplicated cholecystitis (P. mirabilis, E. coli and K. pneumoniae activity).

Pneumonia when H. influenzae and Klebsiella are not a concern. If Klebsiella, use newer cephalosporins.

DOSAGE FORMS: Caps:500mg; Susp:125mg/5ml, 250mg/5ml, 500mg/5ml; Tabs:1g.

DOSAGE: Cefadroxil is administered orally.Dosage is given in the next Table:

Dosage of Cefadroxil

Condition	Age	Dosage
Uncomplicated Urinary Tract Infections	Adults	1-2g daily as a single dose or in 2 equally divided doses.
Other Urinary Tract Infections	Adults	1g twice daily.
Skin and Skin Structures	Adults	1g daily as a single dose or in 2 equally divided doses.
Group A Beta-Hemolytic Streptococcal Pharyngitis and Tonsillitis	Adults	500mg twice daily for at least 10 days.
Usual	Pediatric	15mg/kg twice daily.
Dosage in Renal Impairment	Adults	Initial Dose:1g followed by 500mg maintenance doses at the following intervals

Creatinine Clearance ($ml/min/1.73m^2$)	Dosage Interval
25-50	every 12 hours
10-25	every 24 hours
0-10	every 36 hours

PHARMACOKINETICS: Absorption:Almost complete; Peak: 1-2 hours; Protein Bound: 15-20%; Half-Life: 1.4 hours; prolonged in renal failure; Excretion: Urine.

ADVERSE EFFECTS: Gastrointestinal disturbances, such as diarrhea, and hypersensitivity reactions, such as skin rash, are most common. See cefazolin.

CEFAZOLIN -1st Gen. Ceph.
(Ancef, Kefzol)

USES: Cefazolin is a parenteral first generation cephalosporin. Cefazolin is one of the most widely used first-generation cephalosporin because its longer half-life (2 hrs. versus 1 hr. or less) and superior tissue levels as compared to other first generation cephalosporin.

Activities of cefazolin are given in the next Table (Goldberg, D.M., Med. Clin. No. An. 71, 1113-113, 1987; Fried, J.S. and Hinthorn, D.R. Disease-A-Month 31, July 1985; Adams, H.G. Personal Comm.):

Activities of Cefazolin

	Gram-positive cocci			Gram-negative bacilli				Anaerobes	
	S. aureus	Streptococci	Strep. entero.	H. influenzae	PEcK	Other Enterics	Pseudomonas a.	B. fragilis	Res. Anaerobes
Cefazolin (Ancef, Kefzol)	4	4	▩	▩	4	▩	▩	▩	3

4=best activity; 3=good activity; 2=some activity; ▩=little or no activity.
PEcK (Mnemonic)= P. mirabilis, E. coli, Klebsiella; Res.= Resident

Cefazolin is usually active against gram-positive cocci including penicillinase-producing and nonpenicillinase-producing Staphylococcus aureus and S. epidermidis; group A beta-hemolytic streptococci (Streptococcus pyogenes); Streptococcus pneumoniae; and group B streptococci (S. agalactiae).

Uses of cefazolin are given in the next Table (Goldberg, D.M., Med. Clin. No. Am. 71, 1113-1133, 1987):

Uses of Cefazolin

Uses	Comments
Skin and Soft Tissue Infections except sacral decubitus and diabetic lower extremity infections.	Excellent activity against staphylococci and streptococci. However, sacral decubitus and diabetic lower extremity infections require anaerobic coverage.
Urinary Tract Infections, Community-Acquired and Uncomplicated Cholecystitis	Active against P. mirabilis, E. coli and K. pneumoniae.
Pneumonia	Do not use if H. influenzae or Klebsiella are present; newer cephalosporins are preferable.
Surgical Prophylaxis (DiPiro, J.T. et al., JAMA 252, 3277-3279, 1984).	See **SURGICAL PROPHYLAXIS.** Cefazolin is an antibiotic of choice for most types of surgical prophylaxis, including chest, abdominal, and orthopedic surgery. Colerectal requires better anaerobic coverage, eg, cefoxitin.

Cefazolin does not penetrate into the central nervous system (CNS) and is never used for infections involving the CNS. Cephalothin may be preferable for treatment of staphylococcal endocarditis.

CEFAZOLIN -1st Gen. Ceph. (Cont.)
DOSAGE FORMS: Parenteral: 250mg, 500mg, 1g.
DOSAGE: Cefazolin sodium is administered by IV injection or by deep IM injection. Dosage of cefazolin is identical for IM or IV administration and is given in the next Table:

Dosage (IM or IV) of Cefazolin Sodium

Condition	Age	Dosage
Usual	Adults	250mg every 8 h. to 1.5g every 6 h. In severe, life-threatening infections, up to 12g daily may be required.
	Child	25-100mg/kg/day in 3 or 4 divided doses
	Neonate <7d or >7d, <2kg	40mg/kg/day in 2 divided doses
	Neonate >7d, >2kg	60mg/kg/day in 3 divided doses
Perioperative Prophylaxis in Contaminated or Potentially Contaminated Surgery	Adults	1g 30-60 minutes prior to surgery and 500mg to 1g every 6-8 h. for 24 h. postoperatively. In lengthy operations (>1 h.), additional doses may be given. If necessary, prophylaxis may be continued for 3-5 days postoperatively.

Dosage in renal failure is given in the next Table:

Dosage of Cefazolin in Renal Failure

Clear. (ml/min)	Serum Creat. (mg/dl)	Age	Dosage
>54	<1.6	Adults	Full doses
35-54	1.6-3.0	Adults	Full doses at intervals of 8 hours
11-34	3.1-4.5	Adults	One-half usual dose every 12 hours
<11	>4.5	Adults	One-half usual dose every 18-24 hours
40-70		Children	60% of usual daily dose divided equally and administered every 12 hours
20-40		Children	25% of usual daily dose divided equally and administered every 12 hours
5-20		Children	10% of usual dose every 24 hours

ADVERSE EFFECTS: Like other cephalosporins, major side effects are rare. Adverse effects that do occur are allergic or toxic.

Allergic Reactions: The risk of allergy in a patient allergic to penicillin is 4-15%. Anaphylaxis is rare; allergic reactions to cephalosporins are usually skin rashes, drug fever, eosinophilia, or rarely serum sickness. Granulocytopenia, thrombocytopenia, or aplastic anemia are usually found only after prolonged or high-dose therapy. About 1-3% of patients develop a positive Coombs' test without clinical hemolysis.

Toxic Reactions: Toxic reactions include pseudomembranous colitis, diarrhea, G.I. upset and blood.

PHARMACOKINETICS: Half-life: 2 hours; Excretion: Unchanged by kidney; Tissue Distribution: High tissue levels but does not penetrate into CNS.

CEFIXIME
(Suprax)

USES: Cefixime is an **oral third generation cephalosporin**; it is distinct in that it is the only oral third generation cephalosporin and it can be dosed once or twice daily due to its long half-life. Activities of cefixime are given in the next Table:

Activites of Cefixime

	Gram-positive cocci			Gram-negative bacilli				Anaerobes	
	S. aureus	Streptococci	Strep. entero.	H. influenzae	PEcK	Other Enterics	Pseudomonas a.	B. fragilis	Res. Anaerobes
Cefixime (Suprax)	2	3	▨	4	4	4	▨	▨	2

4=best activity; 3=good activity; 2=some activity; ▨ =little or no activity.
PEcK (Mnemonic)= P. mirabilis, E. coli, Klebsiella; Res.= Resident

Cefixime is a relatively new drug and clinical efficacy has not been fully elucidated. The antimicrobial spectrum is similar to other third generation cephalosporins. Cefixime is particularly effective treatment for the following organisms: S. pneumoniae, S. pyogenes, H. influenzae (beta-lactamase positive and negative), Moraxella (Branhamella) catarrhalis, E. coli, and P. mirabilis. Indications for the use of cefixime are given in the following Table:

Uses of Cefixime

Uncomplicated Urinary Tract Infections - caused by E. coli and P. mirabilis
Otitis Media
Pharyngitis and Tonsilitis - caused by S. pyogenes
Acute Bronchitis or Acute Exacerbations of Chronic Bronchitis - caused by S. pneumoniae or H. influenzae

DOSAGE FORMS: Tabs: 200, 400mg; Oral Susp.: 100mg/5ml.

DOSAGE: Cefixime is administered orally; dosage is given in the following Table:

Dosage of Cefixime

Age	Dosage
Children	8mg/kg/day in 1-2 doses.
Adults	400mg daily in 1-2 doses.

Dosage in Renal Impairment: No adjustment is necessary if creatinine clearance (CrCl) is >60ml/min. Patients with CrCl of 21-60 or on hemodialysis should receive 75% of the standard dose. Patients with CrCl <20 or on continuous ambulatory peritoneal dialysis should receive 50% of the standard dose.

PHARMACOKINETICS: Half-Life: 3-4 hrs, up to 9 hrs in normal subjects; Absorption: 40-50%; Peak: 2-6 hrs; suspension produces levels 25-50% higher than equivalent dose in tablet form; Excretion: Urine (50%), Bile; Protein binding: 65%; Metabolism: None.

ADVERSE EFFECTS: Like other cephalosporins, major side effects are uncommon. Adverse effects that do occur are as follows: Hypersensitivity reactions (urticaria, skin rashes); transient transaminase elevations; headaches; GI symptoms: diarrhea (16%), nausea (7%), abdominal pain (3%). Overall, less than 4% of patients have to discontinue the drug due to adverse effects during trials.

CEFOPERAZONE -3rd Gen. Ceph.
(Cefobid)

USES: Cefoperazone is a parenteral third generation cephalosporin; activities of cefoperazone are given in the next Table (Fried, J.S. and Hinthorn, D.R., Disease-a-Month 31, July, 1985; Adams, H.G., Personal Comm.):

Activities of Cefoperazone

	Gram-positive cocci			Gram-negative bacilli				Anaerobes	
	S. aureus	Streptococci	Strep. entero.	H. influenzae	PEcK	Other Enterics	Pseudomonas a.	B. fragilis	Res. Anaerobes
Cefoperazone (Cefobid)	2	2	▩	4	4	4	3	▩	2

4=best activity; 3=good activity; 2=some activity; ▩ =little or no activity.
PEcK (Mnemonic)= P. mirabilis, E. coli, Klebsiella; Res.= Resident

Cefoperazone is very effective against gram-negative rods including virtually 100% of the usual hospital-acquired strains of E. coli and Proteus and is active against Klebsiella Serratia, Citrobacter and Providencia.

Cefoperazone has no role in surgical prophylaxis. The drug is not used in the treatment of abscesses; B. fragilis is the major pathogen responsible for abscess formation and is most effectively treated with cefoxitin, a second generation cephalosporin.

Some infections that may be treated with cefoperazone, include gram-negative osteomyelitis and septic arthritis; gram-negative rods causing endocarditis; hospital-acquired urinary tract infections; E. coli and Klebsiella pneumonia; H. influenzae pneumonia that is ampicillin resistant; community but not hospital acquired sepsis.

Structure:Cefoperazone has a methylthiotetrazole group substituted at position 3 of the dihydrothiazine rign; this substitution is associated with hypoprothrombinemia and a disulfiram a ("antabuse")-like effect. (see Adverse Effects)

DOSAGE FORMS: Parenteral: 1g, 2g

DOSAGE: Cefoperazone is administered by IV infusion or by deep IM injection; dosage is identical for IM or IV administration and is given in the next Table:

Dosage of Cefoperazone

Condition	Age	Dosage
Usual Adult	Adults	2-4g daily in equally divided doses every 12 h.
Severe, Life-Threatening Infections or Infections by Less Susceptible Organisms	Adults	6-12g daily in 2,3, or 4 equally divided doses
Usual Pediatric	Children	IV to Neonates and Children: 25-100mg/kg every 12 h.

Duration of Therapy: Therapy should generally be continued for at least 48-72 hours after the patient becomes afebrile or evidence of eradication of the infection is obtained.

Dosage in Hepatic and Renal Impairment: Dosage in hepatic and/or renal failure is given in the next Table:

Dosage of Cefoperazone in Hepatic and/or Renal Failure

Condition	Dosage
Hepatic Disease and/or Biliary Obstruction	Do not exceed 4g daily
Impaired Renal Function	Usual Dosage
Both Hepatic and Substantial Renal Impairment	1-2g daily
Hemodialysis Patients	Dosage at end of dialysis period

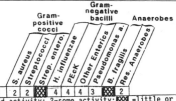

CEFOPERAZONE -3rd Gen. Ceph.
ADVERSE EFFECTS: Like other cephalosporins, major side effects are rare. Adverse effects that do occur are allergic or toxic.

Allergic Reactions: The risk of allergy in a patient allergic to penicillin is 4-15%. Anaphylaxis is rare; allergic reactions to cephalosporins are usually skin rashes, drug fever, eosinophilia, or rarely serum sickness. Granulocytopenia, thrombocytopenia, or aplastic anemia are usually found only after prolonged or high-dose therapy. About 1-3% of patients develop a positive Coombs' test without clinical hemolysis.

Toxic Reactions: Toxic reactions include nephrotoxicity, platelet aggregation defect, prolonged prothrombin time, and disulfiram reactions.

CEFOTAXIME -3rd Gen. Ceph.
(Claforan)
USES: Cefotaxime is a parenteral third generation cephalosporin; activities of cefotaxime are given in the next Table (Goldberg, D.M., Med. Clin. No. Am. 71, 1113-1133, 1987; Fried, J.S. and hinthorn, D.R., Disease-A-Month 31, July, 1985; Adams, H.G., Personal Comm.):

Activities of Cefotaxime

	Gram-positive cocci			Gram-negative bacilli				Anaerobes	
	S. aureus	Streptococci	Strep. entero.	H. influenzae	PEcK	Other Enterics	Pseudomonas a.	B. fragilis	Res. Anaerobes
Cefotaxime (Claforan)	3	3	▩	4	4	4	▩	▩	3

4=best activity; 3=good activity; 2=some activity; ▩ =little or no activity.
PEcK (Mnemonic)= P. mirabilis, E. coli, Klebsiella; Res.= Resident

Cefotaxime is very effective against gram-negative rods including E. coli, Proteus mirabilis, Klebsiella, Serratia, Proteus vularis, Providencia Morganella, Enterobacter, Citrobacter and Yersinia enterocolitica and is recommended for serious infections due to these organisms.

Cefotaxime is indicated for infections caused by relatively resistant gram-negative bacteria which usually occur in hospitalized patients. Conditions that are commonly treated with cefotaxime are given in the next Table (Goldberg, D.M., Med. Clin. No. Am. 71, 1113-1133, 1987):

Conditions Commony Treated with Cefotaxime

- Nosocomial Pneumonias
- Postoperative Wound Infections
- Catheter-Related Urinary Infections
- Community-Acquired Pneumonia when Klebsiella or H. Influenza is a possibility.
- Intra-abdominal and Pelvic Infections (add an anaerobic drug, eg, metronidazole or clindamycin)
- Empiric therapy for community acquired bacteremia, pneumonia and meningitis in infants and children

Cefotaxime is also used in the treatment of Neisseria meningitidis (meningococcus) or Strep. Pneumoniae as well as H. Influenzae which makes this drug useful for empiric therapy for bacteremia, pneumonia, or meningitis in infants and children.

CEFOTAXIME (Cont.)

DOSAGE FORMS: Injection: 500mg, 1.0 and 2.0 gram vials.

DOSAGE: Cefotaxime sodium is administered by IV or deep IM injection.

For direct intermittent IV injection, 10ml of sterile water for injection is added to a vial labeled as containing 1 or 2g of cefotaxime to provide a solution containing 95 or 180mg of cefotaxine per ml. Inject over a 3-5-minute period or slowly into the tubing of a freely-flowing compatible IV solution.

Dosage of cefotaxime is given in the next Table:

Dosage of Cefotaxime

Condition	Age	Dosage
Usual	Premature or Full-Term Neonates <1 week	50mg/kg every 12 hours
	1-4 weeks	50mg/kg every 8 hours
	1 month-12 yrs. <50 kg	50-200mg/kg daily in 4-6 equally divided doses
Uncomplicated Infections	>50kg or Adults	1g every 12 hours
Moderate to Severe Infect.	Adults	1-2g every 6-8 hours
Severe Life-Threatening Infections	Adults	2g every 4 hours; max. is 12g daily
Gonorrhea, Uncomplicated Penicillinase-Producing (PPNG)	Adults	1g IM, single dose
Gonorrhea, Disseminated	Adults	500mg IV, 4 times daily for at least 7 days
Gonococcal Ophthalmia caused by PPNG	Adults	500mg IV, 4 times daily for 5 days
Gonococcal Infections Neonate(PPNG)	Neonates	25-50mg/kg every 12 hours for 7-10 days
Perioperative Prophylaxis in Contaminated or Potentially Contaminated Surgery	Adults	1g IM or IV, 30-90 min. prior to surgery; consider preoperative bowel preparation using mechanical cleansing and a nonabsorbable anti-infective, eg, neomycin
Caesarean Section	Adults	1g IV as soon as umbilical cord is clamped followed by 1g IM or IV, 6 and 12 hours after first dose

Duration of Therapy: Usually, therapy should be continued for at least 48-72 hours after the patient becomes afebrile or evidence of eradication of infection is obtained. Chronic urinary tract infections(UTI) may require several weeks of therapy.

Dosage in Renal Impairment: Give usual dosage in patients with creatinine clearances of 20ml/min or greater per $1.73m^2$. If creatinine clearances are less than 20ml/min per $1.73m^2$, use half the usual dose at usual time interval. In patients undergoing hemodialysis, give 0.5-2g as single daily doses and supplemental dose after each dialysis period.

ADVERSE EFFECTS: Like other cephalosporins, major side effects are rare. Adverse effects that do occur are allergic or toxic.

Allergic Reactions: The risk of allergy in a patient allergic to penicillin is 4-15%. Anaphylaxis is rare; allergic reactions to cephalosporins are usually skin rashes, drug fever, eosinophilia, or rarely serum sickness. Granulocytopenia, thrombocytopenia, or aplastic anemia are usually found only after prolonged or high-dose therapy. About 1-3% of patients develop a positive Coombs' test without clinical hemolysis.

Toxic Reactions: Toxic reactions include pseudomembranous colitis, diarrhea, G.I. upset and blood dyscrasias.

CEFOTETAN-3rd Gen. Ceph.
(Cefotan)

USES: Cefotetan is a **parenteral** third generation cephalosporin , also classified as a cephamycin antibiotic. Activities of cefotetan are given in the next Table (Goldberg, D.M., Med. Clin. No. Am. 71, 1113-1133, 1987; Fried, J.S. and Hinthorn, D.R., Disease-a-Month 31, 1985; Adams, H.G., Personal Comm.):

	Gram-positive cocci			Gram-negative bacilli				Anaerobes	
	S. aureus	Streptococci	Strep. entero.	H. influenzae	PEcK	Other Enterics	Pseudomonas a.	B. fragilis	Res. Anaerobes
Cefotetan (Cefotan)	2	2	▩	1	4	2	▩	3	3

4=best activity; 3=good activity; 2=some activity; ▩=little or no activity.
PEcK (Mnemonic)= P. mirabilis, E. coli, Klebsiella; Res.= Resident

The main indication for the use of cefotetan is for treatment of severe infections due to Bacteroides fragilis (Wilkowske, C.J. and Hermans, P.E., Mayo Clin. Proc. 62, 789-798, 1987).

Cefotetan (like cefoxitin) is uniquely valuable as a single drug therapy for community-acquired infections caused by mixed aerobic and anaerobic bacteria as given in the next Table (Goldberg, D.M., Med. Clin. No. Am. 71, 1113-1133, 1987):

Cefotetan for Community-Acquired Mixed Aerobic and Anaerobic Bacteria

Tissue Involved	Examples
Intra-Abdominal Infections	Diverticulitis and perforated viscus.
Pelvic Infections	Endometritis and pelvic inflammatory disease (PID).
Lungs	Aspiration pneumonias involving aerobic gram-negative bacteria and anaerobes.
Soft-Tissue Infections, Chronic	Particularly diabetic lower extremity infections and sacral decubiti infected by anaerobes.

Cefotetan may be as effective as gentamicin and clindamycin for many of these conditions (Ward, A. and Richards, D.M., Drugs 30, 382-426, 1985).

Structure of Cefotetan: Cefotetan has the methylthiotetrazole group but has not been associated with hypoprothrombinemia as occurs with cefoperazone, cefamandole or moxalactam (Ward, A. and Richards, D.M., Drugs 30, 382-426, 1985).

DOSAGE FORMS: Powder: 1 and 2g (sodium 5.5mEq/g)

DOSAGE: Cefotetan is administered intramuscularly into a large muscle mass or intravenously by direct injection or by intermittent or continuous infusion. Dosage is given in the next Table:

Dosage of Cefotetan

Condition	Age	Route	Dosage
Mild to Severe Infections	Adults	IM or IV	500mg every 12 hours or 1 to 2g every 24 hours or 1 to 2g every 12 hours or 2g every 12 hours.
Life-Threatening Infections	Adults	IV	3g every 12 hours (max. 6g)

Pediatric Dosage: Limited clinical data is available, but 40-80mg/kg/day divided every 12 hours has been used.

Renal Impairment: Dosage of cefotetan in adults with renal failure is given in the next Table:

Dosage of Cefotetan in Adults with Renal Failure

Creatinine Clearance	Dosage
>30ml/min	Dosage modification unnecessary
10-30ml/min	Usual dose every 24 hours
<10ml/min	Usual dose every 48 hours

CEFOTETAN (Cont.)

ADVERSE EFFECTS: Like other cepalosporins, major side effects are rare. Adverse effects are given in the next Table:

Adverse Effects of Cefotetan	
System	Effect
Systemic	Hypersensitivity reactions (rash, pruritis, fever)
Gastrointestinal	Diarrhea, nausea, vomiting
Local Reactions	Phlebitis, local pain
Hematologic	Eosinophilia, leukopenia
Hepatic	Elevated SGOT, SGPT, alkaline phosphatase

PHARMACOKINETICS: Bioavailability: IM, 100%; Protein-Binding: 88%; Metabolism: Not metabolized; Half-Life : Adults: 3 to 4.4 hours; Children: 1.85 to 3.5 hours; Newborns with Urinary Tract Infections: 5.4 hours.

CEFOXITIN - 2nd Gen. Ceph.
(Mefoxin)

USES: Cefoxitin is a parenteral second generation cephalosporin also classified as a cephamycin antibiotic. Cefoxitin is one of the most widely used antibiotics because of its spectrum of activity includes both aerobic and anaerobic bacteria. Activities of cefoxitin are given in the next Table (Goldberg, D.M., Med. Clin. No. Am. 71, 1113-1133, 1987; Fried, J.S. and Hinthorn, D.R., Disease-A-Month 31, 32-34, July 1985; Adams, H.G., Personal Comm.):

Activities of Cefoxitin

	Gram-positive cocci			Gram-negative bacilli				Anaerobes	
	S. aureus	Streptococci	Strep. entero.	H. influenzae	PEcK	Other Enterics	Pseudomonas a.	B. fragilis	Res. Anaerobes
Cefoxitin (Mefoxin)	2	2	▩	1	4	2	▩	3	3

4=best activity; 3=good activity; 2=some activity; ▩=little or no activity.
PEcK (Mnemonic)= P. mirabilis, E. coli, Klebsiella; Res.= Resident

Cefoxitin resembles the second generation cephalosporins by having less gram-positive activity and increased gram-negative potency. However, cefoxitin is less active than the other second-generation cephalosporins against H. influenzae and E. aerogenes. Unlike other second-generation cephalosporins, cefoxitin is active against Serratia species. Cefoxitin is highly resistant to destruction by beta-lactamases and is the most potent cephalosporin of any generation against B. fragilis (Fried, J.S. and Hinthorn, D.R., Disease-A-Month 31, 32-34, July 1985).

Cefoxitin is uniquely valuable as single agent therapy for community-acquired infections caused by mixed aerobic and anaerobic bacteria as given in the next Table (Goldberg, D.M., Med. Clin. No. Am. 71, 1113-1133, 1987):

Cefoxitin for Community-Acquired Mixed Aerobic and Anaerobic Bacteria	
Tissue Involved	Examples
Intra-Abdominal Infections	Diverticulitis and perforated viscus.
Pelvic Infections	Endometritis and pelvic inflammatory disease(PID)
Lungs	Aspiration pneumonias involving aerobic gram-negative bacteria and anaerobes.
Soft-Tissue Infections, Chronic	Particularly diabetic lower extremity infections and sacral decubiti infected by anaerobes.

Cefoxitin compares favorable to gentamicin and clindamycin for many of these conditions (Drusano, G.L. et al., Surg. Gynecol. Obstet. 154, 715-720, 1982; Hofstetter, S.R., J. Trauma 24, 307-310, 1984).

DOSAGE FORMS: Parenteral: 1,2g vials. Parenteral for IV Infusion: 1g in 5% Dextrose; 2g in 5% Dextrose.

DOSAGE: Cefoxitin sodium is administered by IV injection or infusion or by deep IM injection. For direct IV injection, 1g of cefoxitin is dissolved in 10ml or 2g in 10 or 20ml of sterile water for injection. Inject directly in vein over a 3-to 5-minute period or slowly into the tubing of a compatible IV infusion fluid. Use of butterfly or scalp vein needles rather than polyethylene catheters may decrease the incidence of thrombophlebitis.

CEFOXITIN (Cont.)

Dosage of cefoxitin sodium is identical for IV or IM administration. Dosage is given in the next Table:

Dosage of Cefoxitin

Condition	Age	Dosage
Usual	Adults	1-2g every 6-8 h; up to 12g daily may be required
Usual	>3 Mos.	80-160mg/kg daily in 4-6 equally divided doses
Perioperative Prophylaxis	Adults	2g, 30-60 minutes prior to surgery and 2g every 6 h. for 24 hours
	>3 Mos.	30-40mg/kg dose given 30-60 minutes prior to surgery and 30-40mg/kg doses every 6 h. for 24 hours
Cesarean Section	Adults	2g IV as soon as umbilical cord is clamped followed by 2g IM or IV 4 h. and 8 h. after first dose. Subsequent 2g doses may be given every 6 h. for no more than 24 h.
Uncomplicated Gonorrhea Penicillinase or Nonpenicillinase	Adults	2g IM with 1g oral probenecid given at same time or up to 30 minutes before cefoxitin.
Disseminated Gonorrhea	Adults	1g IV, 4 times daily for at least 7 days.
Gonococcal Ophthalmia caused by Penicillinase-producing N. Gonorrhoeae(PPNG)	Adults	1g IV, 4 times daily for 5 days.
Acute Pelvic Inflammatory Disease(PID) (Hospitalized Patients)	Adults	2g IV, 4 times daily combined with 100mg of doxycycline, IV twice daily for at least 4 days and for at least 2 days after defervescence; doxycycline therapy should be continued after patient discharged at oral dosage of 100mg twice daily to complete 10-14 days of therapy.
Acute Pelvic Inflammatory Disease(PID) (Non-Hospitalized Patients)	Adults	2g IM plus 1g oral probenecid followed by an oral doxycycline dosage of 100mg twice daily for 10-14 days.
Transurethral Prostatectomy	Adults	1g IV, 30-60 minutes prior to surgery, followed by 1 g every 8 hours for up to 5 days. Prophylaxis should usually be discontinued within 24 h. after surgery; in prosthetic arthroplasty, continue for 72 h.

In infections by group A beta-hemolytic streptococci, continue therapy for at least 10 days.

Dosage in Renal Impairment: Give loading dose of 1-2g in adults and the maintenance dosage as given in the next Table:

Maintenance Dosage of Cefoxitin in Renal Impairment

Creatinine Clearance(ml/min)	Dosage
30-50	1-2g every 8-12 hours
10-29	1-2g every 12-24 hours
5-9	500mg to 1g every 12-24 hours
<5	500mg to 1g every 24-48 hours

ADVERSE EFFECTS: Like other cephalosporins, major side effects are rare. Adverse effects that do occur are allergic or toxic.

Allergic Reactions: The risk of allergy in a patient allergic to penicillin is 4-15%. Anaphylaxis is rare; allergic reactions to cephalosporins are usually skin rashes, drug fever, eosinophilia, or rarely serum sickness. Granulocytopenia, thrombocytopenia, or aplastic anemia are usually found only after prolonged or high-dose therapy. About 1-3% of patients develop a positive Coombs' test without clinical hemolysis.

Toxic Reactions: Toxic reactions include nephrotoxicity, prolonged prothrombin time, platelet aggregation defect, and disulfiram reactions.

CEFTAZIDIME -3rd Gen. Ceph.
(Fortaz, Tazicef, Tazidime)

USES: Ceftazidime is a parenteral third generation cephalosporin. It is more effective in vitro on a weight basis against Pseudomonas than other currently available third generation cephalosporins. Activities of ceftazidime are given in the next Table (Goldberg, D.M., Med. Clin. No. Am. 71, 1113-1133, 1987; Adams, H.G., Personal Comm.):

Activities of Ceftazidime

	Gram-positive cocci			Gram-negative bacilli				Anaerobes	
	S. aureus	Streptococci	Strep. entero.	H. influenzae	PEcK	Other Enterics	Pseudomonas a.	B. fragilis	Res. Anaerobes
Ceftazidime(Fortaz)	▩	2	▩	4	4	4	4	▩	2

4=best activity; 3=good activity; 2=some activity; ▩ =little or no activity.
PEcK (Mnemonic)= P. mirabilis, E. coli, Klebsiella; Res.= Resident

Ceftazidime should be reserved for patients with known or suspected Pseudomonas infections.

DOSAGE FORMS: Inj.: 500mg, 1, 2g. IV Infusion: 1, 2g.

DOSAGE: Ceftazidime is administered by IV injection or infusion or by deep IM injection. Dosage is given in the next Table:

Dosage of Ceftazidime

Age	Dosage
Adults	1.5-6gm/day; dosing interval, 8-12 hours, max. 6gm.
Children	90-150mg/kg/day; dosing interval 8-12 hours
Newborn (to 1 Week)	60mg/kg/day; dosing interval, every 12 hours
Newborn (1-4 Weeks)	60-100mg/kg/day; dosing interval, every 8-12 hours.

Therapy should continue for at least 48 hours after apparent eradication of the organisms.

Dosage in Renal Failure: Dosage of ceftazidime is given in the next Table (The Medical Letter, Handbook of Antimicrobial Therapy, The Medical Letter, Inc., New Rochelle, N.Y., 1986):

Maintenance Dosage of Ceftazidime in Renal Impairment

Creatinine Clearance (ml/min)	Dosage
31-50	1g every 12 hours
16-30	1g every 24 hours
6-15	500mg every 24 hours
<5	500mg every 48 hours

PHARMACOKINETICS: Distribution: Widespread including CNS; Distribution Half-Life: 0.1-0.6 hours; Elimination Half-Life: 1.4-2 hours; Metabolism: Ceftazidime is not metabolized and is excreted unchanged principally in the urine.

ADVERSE EFFECTS: Major side effects are rare. Adverse effects that do occur are allergic or toxic.

Allergic Reactions: The risk of allergy in a patient allergic to penicillin is 4-15%. Anaphylaxis is rare; allergic reactions to cephalosporins are usually skin rashes, drug fever, eosinophilia, or rarely serum sickness. Granulocytopenia, thrombocytopenia, or aplastic anemia are usually found only after prolonged or high-dose therapy. About 5% of patients develop a positive Coombs' test without clinical hemolysis.

Toxic Reactions: Toxic reactions include nephrotoxicity and hepatotoxicity.

CEFTRIAXONE -3rd Gen. Ceph.
(Rocephin)

USES: Ceftriaxone is a parenteral third generation cephalosporin; it is distinct in that it has a much longer half-life and dosing interval is long as compared to the other 3rd generation cephalosporins Activities of ceftriaxone are given in the next Table (Goldberg, D.M., Med. Clin. No. Am. 71, 1113-1133, 1987; Fried, J.S. and Hinthorn, D.R., Disease-a-Month 31, 1985; Adams, H.G., Personal Comm.):

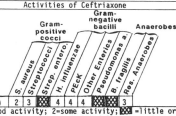

Activities of Ceftriaxone

	Gram-positive cocci			Gram-negative bacilli				Anaerobes	
	S. aureus	Streptococci	Strep. entero.	H. influenzae	PEcK	Other Enterics	Pseudomonas a.	B. fragilis	Res. Anaerobes
Ceftriaxone (Rocephin)	2	3	▩	4	4	4	▩	▩	3

4=best activity; 3=good activity; 2=some activity; ▩ =little or no activity.
PEcK (Mnemonic)= P. mirabilis, E. coli, Klebsiella; Res.= Resident

Drug of Choice: Ceftriaxone is a drug of first choice or alternate drug in the conditions listed in the next Table; (The Medical Letter, Handbook of Antimicrobial Therapy, The Medical Letter, Inc., N.Y. 1990):

Conditions in which Ceftriaxone is a Drug of First Choice or Alternative Drug

Drug of Choice	Alternative Drug
Neisseria gonorrhoeae	Neisseria meningitidis(meningococcus)
Enterobacter	Proteus mirabilis
Escherichia coli	Moraxella (Branhamella) catarrhalis
Proteus, Indole-Positive including Providencia rettgeri, Morganella morganii and Proteus vulgaris	Borrelia burgdorferi (causes Lyme Disease)[Ceftriaxone or Pen G are drugs of choice for Lyme Carditis or Meningitis (Rahn, D.W. and Malawista, S.E., Ann. Intern. Med. 114, 472-481, 1991)].
Providencia stuartii	
Salmonella	
Serratia	
Haemophilus ducreyi (causes chancroid)	
Klebsiella pneumoniae	
Haemophilus influenzae	

Neisseria Gonorrhoeae: Ceftriaxone (250mg IM) is as effective as 4.8 million units of procaine penicillin with probenicid or 2g of spectinomycin in the therapy of uncomplicated urethritis, proctitus, cervicitis, and pharyngitis caused by Neisseria gonorrhoeae (Rajan, V.S. et al., Br. J. Vener. Dis. 58, 314-316, 1982). Ceftriaxone has replaced penicillin for empiric therapy due to the emergence of penicillinase-producing gonorrhoeae. Cephalosporins are not active against chlamydiae; use tetracycline for coexisting chlamydial infections.

Gram-Negative Bacilli: Ceftriaxone is very effective against gram-negative rods. Conditions that are commonly treated with ceftriaxone are given in the next Table (Goldberg, D.M., Med. Clin. No. Am. 71, 1113-1133, 1987):

Conditions Commonly Treated with Ceftriaxone
Nosocomial Pneumonias
Postoperative Wound Infections
Catheter-Related Urinary Infections
Community-Acquired Pneumonia when Klebsiella or H. Influenza is a possibility.
Intra-abdominal and Pelvic Infections (add an anaerobic drug, eg, metronidazole or clindamycin)
Empiric therapy for community acquired bacteremia, pneumonia and meningitis in infants and children.

CEFTRIAXONE (Cont.)

DOSAGE FORMS: Parenteral: 250 and 500mg; 1 and 2g.

DOSAGE: Ceftriaxone is administered by intramuscular injection deep into a large muscle mass or intravenously by intermittent infusion. Dosage is identical for IM or IV administration; dosage is given in the next Table:

Dosage of Ceftriaxone

Condition	Age	Dosage
Usual	Adults	1-4g given once daily or in equally divided doses every 12 hrs.
Usual	Children	50-100mg/kg daily in equally divided doses every 12 hours.
Perioperative Prophylaxis	Adults	1g 0.5-2 hrs. prior to surgery
Gonorrhea, Uncomplicated	Adults	250mg IM plus Doxycycline
Gonorrhea, Disseminated	Adults	1g IV, once daily for 7 days
Gonococcal Ophthalmia	Adults	1g IM once
Acute, Sexually Transmitted Epididymo-Orchitis	Adults	250mg IM followed by oral tetracycline or erythromycin
Acute Pelvic Inflammatory Disease(PID) (not hospitalized)	Adults	250mg IM followed by oral doxycycline, 100mg twice daily for 10-14 days
Meningitis	Children	100mg/kg daily, divided doses, every 12 hrs.; a 75mg/kg loading dose may be given
Gonorrhea, Uncomplicated, Vulvovaginitis, Urethritis, Proctitis, Pharyngitis	Children, <45kg	125mg IM, single dose.
Acute Pelvic Inflammatory Disease(PID)	Children	100mg/kg daily IV in combination with IV erythromycin, sulfisoxazole, or tetracycline (in children 8 yrs. or older). Duration: minimum 4 days and 2 days after marked improvement. Thereafter, erythromycin, sulfisoxide, tetracycline, or doxycycline orally for at least 14 days

Duration: 4-14 days

Dosage in Renal or Hepatic Impairment: Adjustment of dosage is usually unnecessary.

PHARMACOKINETICS: Half-Life: 6-9 hrs.; Protein-Binding: 83%-96%; Volume of Distribution: 0.12-0.14liter/kg; Metabolism: not metabolized; Excretion: 60% in urine; 40% is excreted into the bile.

ADVERSE EFFECTS: Like other cephalosporins, major side effects are uncommon. Adverse effects that do occur are as follows: Hypersensitivity reactions (rash), diarrhea(3%-6%), hypoprothrombinemia (rare), other hematologic effects (eosinophilia, thrombocytosis, leukopenia), hepatic and renal toxicity.

Gallbladder sludge has been reported.

CEFUROXIME AXETIL - 2nd Gen. Ceph.
(Ceftin)

USES: **Cefuroxime axetil** is an oral form of **cefuroxime**, a **second-generation** parenteral **cephalosporin.** It is an ester of cefuroxime; after absorption from the gastrointestinal tract, cefuroxime axetil is hydrolyzed by carboxy esterases to release the active parent compound, cefuroxime. Activities of cefuroxime axetil are given in the next Table (Goldberg, D.M., Med. Clin. No. Am. 71,1113-1132, 1987; Adams, H.G. Personal Comm.):

Activities of Cefuroxime Axetil

	Gram-positive cocci: S. aureus	Gram-positive cocci: Streptococci	Gram-positive cocci: Strep. entero.	Gram-negative bacilli: H. influenzae	Gram-negative bacilli: PEcK	Gram-negative bacilli: Other Enterics	Gram-negative bacilli: Pseudomonas a.	Anaerobes: B. fragilis	Anaerobes: Res. Anaerobes
Cefuroxime (Zinacef)	3	3	▩	4	4	2	▩	2	3

4=best activity; 3=good activity; 2=some activity; ▩=little or no activity.
PEcK (Mnemonic)= P. mirabilis, E. coli, Klebsiella; Res.= Resident

Cefuroxime axetil is also active against the gram-negative cocci, Neisseria gonorrhoeae (gonococcus) and Moraxella (Branhamella) catarrhalis. Methicillin-resistant staphlococci are resistant to cefuroxime axetil. The chief advantage of cefuroxime axetil over the first-generation cephalosporins is that it is active against H. influenzae and N. gonorrhoeae without sacrificing gram positive activity (Goldberg, D.M., Med. Clin. No. Am. 71, 1113-1133, 1987).

Cefuroxime axetil is active against some other enterics: Salmonella, Shigella and Providencia. It has little activity against Serratia marcescens or indole positive Proteus. Listeria monocytogenes, Campylobacter jejuni and Acinetobacter are resistant to cefuroxime axetil.

DOSAGE FORMS: Tabs: 125, 250, 500mg.

DOSAGE: Cefuroxime axetil is administered orally. Dosage is given in the next Table:

Dosage of Cefuroxime Axetil

Condition	Age	Dosage
Usual	Adults & Child >12 yrs.	250mg, twice daily; dosage can be increased to 500mg, twice daily, for more severe infections.
Usual	Up to age 12	125-250mg, twice daily.
Otitis Media	>2 yrs.	250mg, twice daily.
	<2 yrs.	125mg, twice daily.

ADVERSE EFFECTS: Adverse effects are as follows; gastrointestinal diarrhea, nausea, and vomiting. Some patients stopped taking this drug because of G.I. effects. There is a high incidence of vomiting in young children; this may be due to the bitter taste of crushed tablets. Pseudomembranous colitis has been reported.

Other adverse effects include rash, headache, and vaginitis. Reversible laboratory abnormalities have included transient elevations of hepatic enzyme activity and a direct coombs test.

PHARMACOKINETICS: Bioavailability: 36% when fasting; 52% with food. Absorption is increased when taken with food. Excretion: Kidneys by glomerular filtration and tubular secretion; 95% of absorbed dose recoverable in urine within 24 hrs Concurrent use of probenecid (Benemid) increases serum concentrations of cefuroxime.

CEFUROXIME SODIUM -2nd Gen. Ceph.
(Zinacef, Kefurox)

USES: Cefuroxime is a second generation cephalosporin. Activities of cefuroxime are given in the next Table (Goldberg, D.M., Med. Clin. No. Am. 71,1113-1132, 1987; Adams, H.G. Personal Comm.):

Activities of Cefuroxime

	Gram-positive cocci			Gram-negative bacilli				Anaerobes	
	S. aureus	Streptococci	Strep. entero.	H. influenzae	PEcK	Other Enterics	Pseudomonas a.	B. fragilis	Res. Anaerobes
Cefuroxime (Zinacef)	3	3	▩	4	4	2	▩	2	3

4=best activity; 3=good activity; 2=some activity; ▩=little or no activity.
PEcK (Mnemonic)= P. mirabilis, E. coli, Klebsiella; Res.= Resident

Cefuroxime is also active against the gram-negative cocci, Neisseria gonorrhoeae (gonococcus) and Moraxella (Branhamella) catarrhalis. Methicillin-resistant staphlococci are resistant to cefuroxime. The chief advantage of cefuroxime over the first-generation cephalosporins is that it is active against H. influenzae and N. gonorrhoeae without sacrificing gram positive activity (Goldberg, D.M., Med. Clin. No. Am. 71, 1113-1133, 1987).

Cefuroxime is active against some other enterics: Salmonella, Shigella and Providencia. It has little activity against Serratia marcescens or indole-positive Proteus. Listeria monocytogenes, Campylobacter jejuni and Acinetobacter are resistant to cefuroxime.

Uses of cefuroxime are given in the next Table (Goldberg, D.M., Med. Clin. No. Am. 71, 1113-1133, 1987):

Uses of Cefuroxime

Use(s)	Comments
Community-Acquired Pneumonitis	Active against S. aureus and H. influenzae; do not use alone for Klebsiella pneumonia.
Community-Acquired Sepsis	May be used in childhood sepsis (except when Listeria monocytogenes is the causative bacteria). The 3rd gen. ceph. are preferred in the treatment of meningitis. Since CSF sterilization may be delayed in some patients treated with cefuroxime (Lebel, M.H. et al., J. Pediatr. 114, 1049-1054, 1989).

DOSAGE FORMS: Parenteral: 750mg and 1.5g (sodium 2.4mEq/g).

DOSAGE: Cefuroxime sodium is administered intramuscularly into a large muscle mass or intravenously by direct injection or by intermittent or continuous infusion. Dosage is given in the next Table:

Dosage of Cefuroxime Sodium

Condition	Age	Dosage
Uncomplicated Urinary Tract Infection; Skin and Skin Structure Infections; Disseminated Gonococcal Infections; Uncomplicated Pneumonia	Adults	750mg every eight hours.
Severe or Complicated Infections (eg, Bone, Joint Infections)	Adults	1.5g every eight hours.
Life-Threatening Infections (eg, sepsis)	Adults	1.5g every six hours, max. 9gm/day.
	Infants and Children over 3 months	200-240mg/kg daily in equally divided doses every 6-8 hours. The higher dose is given in more serious infections.
Mild to Mod Infections	Infants and Children over 3 months	50 to 100mg/kg daily in equally divided doses every 6-8 hours.

CEFUROXIME SODIUM (Cont.)
Renal Failure: Dosage of cefuroxime sodium in adults with renal failure is given in the next Table:

Dosage of Cefuroxime Sodium in Adults with Renal Failure

Creatinine Clearance	Dosage
>20ml/min	Dosage modification unnecessary
10-20ml/min	750mg every 12 hours
<10ml/min	750mg every 24 hours

In children with impaired renal failure, the frequency of administration is modified as in adults. In patients undergoing hemodialysis, a supplemental dose of cefuroxime should be given after each dialysis period.

ADVERSE EFFECTS: Like other cephalosporins, major side effects are rare. Adverse effects that do occur are allergic or toxic.

Allergic Reactions: The risk of allergy in a patient allergic to penicillin is 4-15%. Anaphylaxis is rare; allergic reactions to cephalosporins are usually skin rashes, drug fever, eosinophilia, or rarely serum sickness. Granulocytopenia, thrombocytopenia, or aplastic anemia are usually found only after prolonged or high-dose therapy. About 1-3% of patients develop a positive Coombs' test without clinical hemolysis.

PHARMACOKINETICS: Peak: IM, 45min; IV, 15min.; Protein-Binding: 33%; Excretion: Urine, 90% by glomerular filtration and renal tubular secretion and is delayed by probenecid. Half-Life: 1.3 to 1.7 hours; prolonged in renal impairment; the half-life in infants less than one week is 3.5 to 5.5 hours.

CEPHALEXIN 1st Gen. Ceph.
(Keflex)

USES: Cephalexin is a first generation cephalosporin; it is administered orally. Activities of cephalexin are given in the next Table (Fried, J.S. and Hinthorn, D.R., Disease-a-Month 31, July, 1985; Goldberg, D.M., Med. Clin. No. Am. 71, 1113-1133, 1987):

Activities of Cephalexin

	Gram-positive cocci: S. aureus	Gram-positive cocci: Streptococci	Gram-positive cocci: Strep. entero.	Gram-negative bacilli: H. influenzae	Gram-negative bacilli: PEcK	Gram-negative bacilli: Other Enterics	Gram-negative bacilli: Pseudomonas a.	Anaerobes: B. fragilis	Anaerobes: Res. Anaerobes
Cephalexin (Keflex)	4	4	▩	▩	4	▩	▩	▩	3

4=best activity; 3=good activity; 2=some activity; ▩ =little or no activity.
PEcK (Mnemonic)= P. mirabilis, E. coli, Klebsiella; Res.= Resident

It is more advantageous to use cefadroxil (Duricef, Ultracef) as a oral 1st generation cephalosporin rather than cephalexin (Keflex) or cephradine (Anspor, Velosef) because cefadroxil has a longer serum half-life enabling twice daily dosing rather than every 6 hours; in addition, cefadroxil is cheaper than other oral cephalosporins.

Conditions commonly treated with cephalexin are given in the next Table (Goldberg, D.M., Med. Clin. No. Am. 71, 1113-1133, 1987):

Conditions Commonly Treated with Cephalexin

Most skin and soft tissue infections (Staph. and Strep. activity)
Do not use for sacral decubitus and diabetic lower extremity infections which require better anaerobic coverage.
Community-acquired urinary tract infections (P. mirabilis, E. coli and K. pneumoniae activity).
Uncomplicated cholecystitis (P. mirabilis, E. coli and K. pneumoniae activity).
Pneumonia when H. influenzae and Klebsiella are not a concern. If Klebsiella, use newer cephalosporins.

DOSAGE FORMS: Caps: 250, 500mg; Susp: 125mg/5ml, 250mg/5ml, 100mg/ml; Tabs: 250, 500mg.

DOSAGE: Cephalexin is administered orally. Dosage is given in the next Table:

Dosage of Cephalexin

Condition	Age	Dosage
Usual	Adults	250mg every 6 hrs.
	Child.	25-50mg/kg daily in equally divided doses every 6 hours.
Skin and Skin Structures	Adults	500mg every 12 hours
Severe Infections	Adults	1 to 4g in equally divided doses every 6 hours.
	Child.	50-100mg/kg daily in equally divided every 6 hours
Dosage in Renal Impairment		If creatinine clearance is 10-50 ml/min increase dosing interval to 8 to 12 hrs If creatinine clearance is <10ml/min, increase dosing interval to 24 to 48 hrs

PHARMACOKINETICS: Absorption: Almost complete (adults); 50% (neonates); Peak: Within one hr. (<6 months), 2 hr. (9-12 months); <1 hr. (older children). Percent Protein Bound: 5-15%; Half-Life: 0.5-1.0hr.; 20-40 hr. (anuria); Excretion: Urine, 85-95% unchanged.

ADVERSE EFFECTS: Same as cefazolin

CEPHALOSPORINS

Classification: Cephalosporins are divided into three "generations" on the basis of activity against groups of gram-negative bacterial species.

Activities of cephalosporins are given in the next Table (Thompson, R.L., Mayo Clin. Proc. 62, 821-834, 1987; Adams, H.G., Personal Comm.):

Activities of Cephalosporins

Generation	Antibiotic (Trade Names)	Gram-positive cocci: S. aureus	Streptococci	Strep. entero.	Gram-negative bacilli: H. influenzae	PEcK	Other Enterics	Pseudomonas a.	Anaerobes: B. fragilis	Res. Anaerobes
First	Cefazolin (Ancef, Kefzol)	4	4	▩	▩	4	▩	▩	▩	3
Second	Cefuroxime (Zinacef)	3	3	▩	4	4	2	▩	2	3
	Cefoxitin (Mefoxin)	2	2	▩	1	4	2	▩	3	3
	Cefotetan (Cefotan)	2	2	▩	1	4	2	▩	3	3
Third	Cefotaxime (Claforan)	3	3	▩	4	4	4	▩	▩	3
	Ceftriaxone (Rocephin)	2	3	▩	4	4	4	▩	▩	3
	Cefoperazone (Cefobid)	2	2	▩	4	4	4	3	▩	2
	Ceftazidime (Fortaz)	▩	2	▩	4	4	4	4	▩	2

4=best activity; 3=good activity; 2=some activity; ▩=little or no activity.
PEcK (Mnemonic)= P. mirabilis, E. coli, Klebsiella; Res.= Resident

The activities of the cephalosporins against specific bacteria are given in the next Table (Goldberg, D.M., Med. Clin. N. Am. 71, 1113-1133, 1987):

Activities of Cephalosporins

Bacteria	Comments
Staphylococci	Best antistaph. activity: 1st gen. ceph. and cefuroxime (2nd gen. ceph). Methicillin-resistant staphylococci are resistant to all ceph.
Streptococci	All ceph. have excellent activity against strep. excluding enterococci which are resistant.
Haemophilus Influenzae	All 3rd gen. ceph. and cefuroxime (2nd gen. ceph). have excellent activity against H. influenza isolates resistant to ampicillin because of beta-lactamase production H. influenzae is resistant to 1st-gen. ceph.
Neisseria Gonorrhoeae	3rd-gen. ceph. and the 2nd gen. ceph. have excellent activity against N. gonorrhoeae including penicillinase-producing strains and chromosomally-mediated penicillin resisting strains.
Proteus mirabilis, Escherichia coli, Klebsiella	2nd and 3rd gen. ceph. have excellent activity against these bacteria.
Other Gram-Negative Bacteria	3rd gen. ceph. have good activity against these gram-negative bacteria: Enterobacter, Citrobacter, Serr., Providencia, Morganella, Proteus vulgaris.
Pseudomonas a.	Ceftazidime, a 3rd gen. ceph., is uniquely active.
B. fragilis	Relatively high conc. of the 2nd gen. ceph., cefoxitin and cefotetan inhibits B. fragilis; ceftizoxime (3rd gen. ceph.) shows mod. activity. B. fragilis generally is resistant to other cephalosporins.
Res. Anaerobes	Highly susceptible to the 2nd gen. ceph., cefoxitin and cefotetan; moderately susceptible to most other ceph. except for ceftazidime a 3rd gen. ceph.

CEPHALOSPORINS (Cont.)

As activity against enteric gram-negative bacilli increases from 1st through 3rd generation, more cephalosporins in each generation have reduced effectiveness against gram-positive cocci. The first and second generation cephalosporins are not effective against P. aeruginosa; third generation cephalosporins are variably effective. None of the cephalosporins are active against enterococci Streptococcus faecuim, S. faecalis and S. durans. The generic and brand names of the cephalosporins are given in the next Table:

Cephalosporins

First Generation		Second Generation		Third Generation	
Generic Name	Brand Name	Generic Name	Brand Name	Generic Name	Brand Name
Cefazolin	Ancef, Kefzol	Cefoxitin	Mefoxin	Cefoperazone	Cefobid
Cephalothin	Keflin, Seffin	Cefamandole	Mandole	Ceftriaxone	Rocephin
Cephalexin	Keflex	Cefaclor	Ceclor	Ceftazidime	Fortaz
Cephapirin	Cefadyl	Cefuroxime	Zinacef	Cefotaxime	Claforan
Cephradine	Anspor, Velosef	Cefuroxime Axetil	Ceftin	Moxalactam	Moxam
Cefadroxil	Duricef, Ultracef	Cefonicid	Monocid	Ceftizoxime	Cefizox
		Ceforanide	Precef	Cefixime	Suprax
		Cefotetan	Cefotan		

When prescribing cephalosporins, whether in a hospital or outpatient setting, give both the generic and brand names to avoid misinterpretation of the generic name.

Oral Cephalosporins: Cephalosporins that are absorbed orally are listed in the next Table:

Oral Cephalosporins

Generic Name	Brand Name	Generation
Cephalexin	Keflex	1st
Cephradine	Anspor, Velosef	1st
Cefadroxil	Duricef, Ultracef	1st
Cefaclor	Ceclor	2nd
Cefuroxime Axetil	Ceftin	2nd
Cefixime	Suprax	3rd

Activity for these oral cephalosporins is given in the next Table (Jones, R.N., The Antimicrobic Newsletter 5, No. 1, 1-7, Jan. 1988):

Activity for Oral Cephalosporins

Bacteria	First Generation: Cephalexin, Cephradine, Cefadroxil	Second Generation: Cefaclor	Second Generation: Cefuroxime Axetil
Gram-Positive Cocci			
S. Aureus	++	++	+++
S. Pneumoniae	+++	+++	+++
Enteric Gram-Neg. Bacilli			
P. Mirabilis	+	+++	+++
E. Coli	++	+++	-(+++)
Klebsiella species	+++	+++	+(+++)
M. Morganii	-	-	-
P. Vulgaris	-	-	-
P. Rettgeri	-	-	+(++)
P. Stuartii	-	-	+
Serratia species	-	-	-
Other Gram Neg. Bacilli			
H. Influenzae	++	++/+++	+++
Gram Neg. Cocci			
Moraxella/Gonococci	+++	+++	+++

CEPHALOSPORINS (Cont.)

Three cephalosporins, cephalexin, cephradine and cefadroxil have essentially identical activity against the three most important enteric pathogens, E. coli, Klebsiella species, and P. mirabilis, the gram-negative cocci, eg, Moraxella/gonococci, and fastidious strains.

Structure of Cephalosporins: The basic structure of the cephalosporins is given in the next Figure:

Basic Structure of Cephalosporins

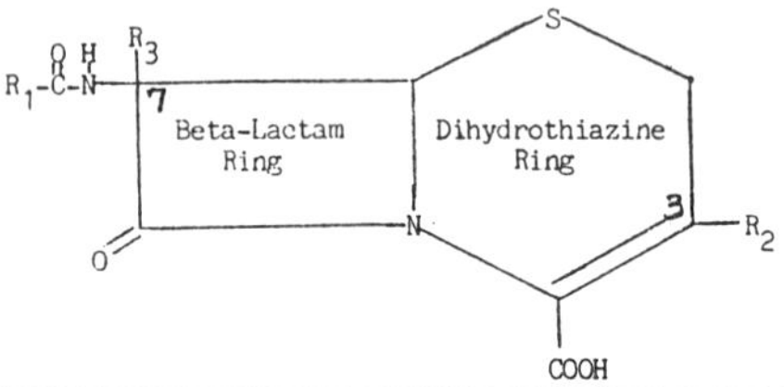

Cephalosporins are composed of a four-membered beta-lactam ring fused to a 6-membered dihydrothiazine ring. In contrast to the penicillin nucleus, the cephalosporin nucleus is more resistant to beta-lactamases and is more active against beta-lactamase-producing bacteria, eg, Staph. aureus and E. coli. The different cephalosporins are synthesized by modification of the molecule at R_1, R_2 and R_3.

Substitutions at position 3 of the dihydrothiazine ring have little effect on antibacterial activity but effects the half-life and toxicity as given in the next Table (Goldberg, D.M., Med. Clin. N. Am. 71, 1113-1133, Nov. 1987):

Substitution at Position 3 of Dihydrothiazine Ring

Substitution	Effect	Cephalosporin(s)
Triazine	Half-Life prolonged, 8 hrs.	Ceftriaxone
Methylthiotetrazole	Hypoprothrombinemia	Cefoperazone, Cefamandole, Moxalactam
	Disulfiram ("antabuse")-like effect due to inhibition of aldehyde dehydrogenase when alcohol is ingested.	Same as above

Cefotetan has the methylthiotetrazole group but has not been associated with hypoprothrombinemia (Ward, A., Richards, D.M., Drugs 30, 382-426, 1985).

Prophylactic vitamin K may be desirable when using cefoperazone, cefamandole or moxalactam; vitamin K reverses the hypoprothrombinemia. Vitamin K (adults, 10mg per week) is recommended for all patients receiving moxalactam.

Mechanism of Action of the Cephalosporins: Like other beta-lactam antibiotics, cephalosporins are bactericidal because they inhibit enzymes, known as penicillin binding proteins(PBP's) that catalyze important steps in the formation of the bacterial cell wall.

Mechanism of Bacterial Resistance to Beta-Lactam Antibiotics: The most important mechanism of bacterial resistance to the beta-lactam antibiotics is bacterial production of beta-lactamases, enzymes that hydrolyze the cyclic amide bond of the beta-lactam ring and render it inactive; the action of beta-lactamase on cephalosporins is illustrated in the next Figure:

Action of Beta-Lactamase on Cephalosporins

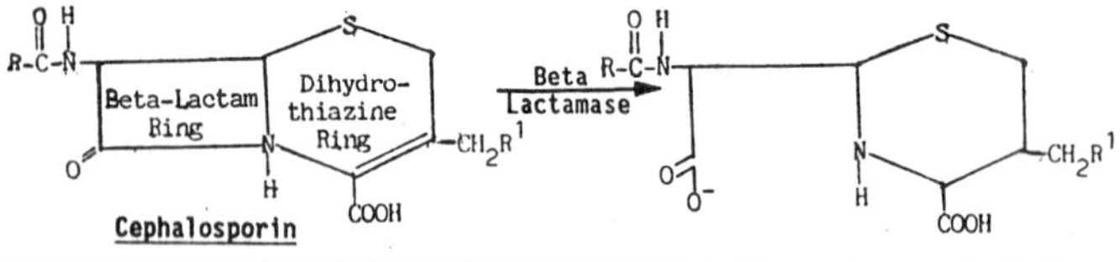

CEPHALOSPORINS (Cont.)

PHARMACOKINETICS: Half-Life: The serum half-life of most of the cephalosporins is 0.6-2 hrs. except for cefonicid (4 hrs.), cefotetan (4 hrs.) and ceftriaxone (8 hrs.) Excretion: The usual route of excretion for most cephalosporins is the urinary tract. Cephalosporins are eliminated unchanged except for cephalothin (1st gen.) and cefotaxime (3rd gen.) These latter cephalosporins are desacetylated; the desacetyl derivative of cefotaxime has antimicrobial activity and has a longer half-life than the parent compound (Quinitiliani, R. et al., Diagn. Microbiol. Infect. Dis. 2, 63S-70S, 1984). Ceftriaxone (3rd gen.) and cefoperazone (3rd gen.) are eliminated mainly by the biliary system which may account for their longer half-lives (8hrs. and 2 hrs. respectively). Conc. in Body Fluids: The first-generation and most of the second-generation cephalosporins do not penetrate the central nervous system (CNS); cefuroxime (2nd gen.) and 3rd gen. cephalosporins all yield significant levels in the CSF when the meninges are inflamed. (Trang, J.M. et al., Antimicrob. Agents Chemother. 28, 791-795 1985). Cefuroxime is not recommended for treatment of CNS infections.

First Generation Cephalosporins: The modes of administration of first generation cephalosporins are given in the next Table:

First Generation Cephalosporins

Generic Name	Brand Name	Oral	Parenteral
Cephalothin	Keflin, Seffin		X
Cephalexin	Keflex	X	
Cefazolin	Ancef, Kefzol		X
Cephapirin	Cefadyl		X
Cephradine	Anspor, Velosef	X	X
Cefadroxil	Duricef, Ultracef	X	

Cefadroxil (Duricef, Ultracef), is the choice for oral use as compared to cephalexin or cephradine, because it has a longer serum half-life enabling twice daily dosing (500mg twice daily) rather than every six hours as for other oral first generation cephalosporins; in addition, cefadroxil is cheaper than these other oral cephalosporins. Furthermore, these drugs have similar clinical effectiveness at similar doses.

With respect to parenteral use, cephalothin, cephapirin, and cephradine are interchangeable; cefazolin has two major advantages over the others: a substantially longer half-life and a much higher serum concentration.

The antibacterial activity of first generation cephalosporins is given in the next Table:

Antibacterial Activity of First Generation Cephalosporins

Gram-Positive Cocci	Gram-Negative Bacilli
Staph. aureus	P. mirabilis
Streptococci (not enterococci)	E. coli
	Klebsiella

The bacterial spectrum is the same for all drugs in this group; the first generation cephalosporins have been used as alternatives to the use of penicillins in patients allergic to penicillins; however, such patients may also have allergic reactions to cephalosporins.

The clinical uses of first generation cephalosporins reflect their antibacterial activity and are given in the next Table (Goldberg, D.M., Med. Clin. North Am. 71, 1113-1133, Nov. 1987):

Clinical Uses of First Generation Cephalosporins

- Surgical prophylaxis; cefazolin (see Section on Antibiotics for Surgical Procedures; Kaiser, A.B., N. Engl. J. Med 315, 1129-1138, Oct. 30, 1986).
- Most skin and soft tissue infections (Staph. and Strep activity). Do not use for sacral decubitus and diabetic lower extremity infections which require better anaerobic coverage.
- Community-acquired urinary tract infections (P. mirabilis, E. coli, and K. pneumoniae activity).
- Uncomplicated cholecystitis (P. mirabilis, E. coli and K. pneumoniae activity).
- Pneumonia when H. influenzae and Klebsiella are not a concern. If Klebsiella, use newer cephalosporins.
- Staphylococcal Endocarditis: Cefazolin or cephalothin.

CEPHALOSPORINS (Cont.)

The first-generation cephalosporins should never be used for infections involving or potentially involving the central nervous system because they fail to achieve therapeutic levels.

Second Generation Cephalosporins: Second generation cephalosporins and their characteristics are given in the next Table:

Second Generation Cephalosporins

Generic Name	Brand Name	Oral	Parenteral	Comments
Cefamandole	Mandol		X	Enhanced activity against H. Influenzae;associated with prothrombin deficiency and occasional bleeding.
Cefoxitin	Mefoxin		X	B. Fragilis
Cefaclor	Ceclor	X		
Cefuroxime	Zinacef		X	Enhanced activity against H. Influenzae
Cefuroxime Axetil	Ceftin	X		
Cefonicid	Monocid		X	Very Long Half-Life
Ceforanide	Precef		X	Very Long Half-Life
Cefotetan	Cefotan		X	B. Fragilis Very Long Half-Life

In comparison with first-generation cephalosporins, the second-generation cephalosporins are generally less active against staphylococci and streptococci and may be more active against certain gram-negative bacilli and anaerobes.

The chief advantage of cefuroxime over the first-generation cephalosporins is that it is active against H. influenzae and N. gonorrhoeae without sacrificing gram positive activity to any significant degree.

The antibacterial activity of second generation cephalosporins (cefuroxime) is given in the next Table:

Antibacterial Activity of Second Generation Cephalosporins (Cefuroxime)

Gram-Positive Cocci	Enteric Gram-Negative Bacilli	Other Gram-Negative Bacilli
Staph. aureus	P. mirabilis	H. influenzae
Streptococci (not enterococci)	E. coli	
	Klebsiella	

The clinical uses of some second generation cephalosporins are given in the next Table:

Clinical Uses of Some Second Generation Cephalosporins

Cephalosporins	Uses
Cefuroxime	Community-Acquired Sepsis and Pneumonitis
Cefuroxime plus Erythromycin	Severe Pneumonia
Cefonicid, Ceforanide, Cefotetan	Outpatient I.V. Treatment, once or twice daily
Cefaclor	Oral treatment of otitis media

The main indications for second-generation cephalosporins are given in the next Table (Wilkowske, C.J. and Hermans, P.E. Mayo Clin. Proc. 62, 789-798, 1987):

Main Indications for Second-Generation Cephalosporins

Cephalosporin	Main Indication
Cefoxitin	Severe infections due to Bacteroides fragilis-for example, pelvic inflammatory disease
Cefuroxime	Severe infections due to streptococci (not enterococci), Enterbacteriaceae (not Serratia), and Haemophilus influenzae. May be used in childhood sepsis(except when Listeria monocytogenes is causative agent) & pneumonia
Cefotetan	Severe infections due to B. fragilis

CEPHALOSPORINS (Cont.)

Third Generation Cephalosporins: Third generation cephalosporins and their half-life are given in the next Table:

Third Generation Cephalosporins

Generic Name	Brand Name	Half Life(hrs.)
Cefotaxime	Claforan	1
Moxalactam	Moxam	2.1
Cefoperazone	Cefobid	2.0
Ceftizoxime	Cefizox	1.6
Ceftriaxone	Rocephin	7.5
Ceftazidime	Fortaz	1.8

Ceftriaxone has a much longer half-life as compared to the other third-generation cephalosporins. The third generation cephalosporins are administered by intravenous or intramuscular injection.

The third generation cephalosporins may be divided into two groups-those with important activity against Pseudomonas aeruginosa and those without such activity; these are given in the next Table:

Activity of Third-Generation Cephalosporins Against Pseudomonas Aeruginosa

Active	Inactive
Cefoperazone	Cefotaxime
Ceftazidime	Ceftizoxime
Cefsulodin	Ceftriaxone
	Moxalactam

Cefotaxime is the third-generation cephalosporin with which there has been the most experience.

Activity of Third-Generation Cephalosporins: Recommendations by consultants of the Medical Letter for use of third-generation cephalosporins as first choice or alternative antimicrobial therapy are given in the next Table (The Medical Letter 30, 33-40, Mar. 25, 1988):

Third-Generation Cephalosporins as First or Alternative Choice Antimicrobial Therapy

Bacterial Pathogen	Cephalosporin
GRAM-NEGATIVE COCCI	
Moraxella (Branhamella) catarrhalis	Alternative
Neisseria gonorrhoeae (gonococcus)	Ceftriaxone as first choice
Neisseria meningitidis (meningococcus)	Alternative
ENTERIC GRAM-NEGATIVE BACILLI	
Enterobacter	First Choice
E. coli	First Choice or Alternative
K. pneumoniae	First Choice
Proteus mirabilis	Alternative
Proteus, indole-positive (including Providencia, rettgeri, Morganella morganii and Proteus vulgaris)	First Choice
Providencia stuartii	First Choice
Salmonella	First Choice
Serratia	First Choice
Yersinia enterocolitica	Alternative
OTHER GRAM-NEGATIVE BACILLI	
Haemophilus ducreyi (chancroid)	First Choice
Haemophilus influenzae	First Choice
Pasteurella multocida	
Urinary tract infection	Alternative
other infections	Alternative
Pseudomonas maltophilia	Aminoglycoside with Ceftazidime
Pseudomonas cepacia	Alternative
SPIROCHETES	
Borrelia burgdorferi (Lyme disease)	Alternative; may be first choice in Lyme carditis or meningitis (see **CEFTRIAXONE**)

CHLORAL HYDRATE
(Noctec, Aquachloral)

USES: Uses of chloral hydrate are given in the next Table:

Uses of Chloral Hydrate

Hypnotic in Treatment of **Insomnia** only for Short-Term Use, that is, up to Two Weeks
- EEG: Induce Sleep Prior to EEG Evaluation

Sedative:
- Preoperatively: Allay Anxiety and Produce Sedation and/or Sleep
- Postoperatively: Adjunct to Opiates and Analgesics in Control of Pain
- Alcohol Withdrawal
- Withdrawal of other Drugs, eg, Opiates or Barbiturates

Chloral hydrate is a halogenated aliphatic alcohol, rapidly reduced to trichloroethanol which is responsible for CNS depression.

Chloral hydrate loses its hypnotic efficacy by the second week of use (Kales, A. et al., J.Clin. Pharmacol. 17, 207-213, 1977). Unlike barbiturates, chloral hydrate causes no significant enzyme induction, and there is no significant effect on REM sleep or difficulty with REM rebound for most patients (Greenblatt,D.J. & Miller,R.R., Am.J.Hosp. Pharm. 31, 990-995,1974).

DOSAGE FORMS: Caps: 250, 500mg; Syrup: 250, 500mg/5ml; Supp: 325, 500, 650mg

DOSAGE: Chloral hydrate is administered orally or rectally. When chloral hydrate is administered orally, capsules should be taken with a full glass of water or liquid; eg, fruit juice, ginger ale. Dosage is given in the next Table:

Dosage of Chloral Hydrate

Condition	Age	Route	Dosage
Hypnotic	Adults	Oral or Supp.	500mg to 1g, 15-30 min. before retiring
	Children	Oral or Supp.	50-75mg/kg; max. 1g
Preoperative	Adults	Oral or Supp.	500mg to 1g, 30 min. before surgery
Sedative	Adults	Oral or Supp.	250mg, 3 times daily after meals
	Children	Oral or Supp.	5-15mg/kg, 3 times daily with a max. dosage of 500mg 3 times a day.
Alcohol Withdrawal	Adults	Oral or Supp.	500mg to 1g, 6 hour intervals, if needed.
EEG Premedication	Children	Oral or Supp.	20-25mg/kg

Single doses or daily dosage for adults should not exceed 2g.

PHARMACOKINETICS: Onset, 30-60 min.; half-life (trichloroethanol), 8 hours.

ADVERSE EFFECTS: Occasionally, gastric irritation and nausea occur; rarely, excitement, delirium, disorientation, erythematous and urticarial allergic reactions occur.

CONTRAINDICATIONS: Marked hepatic and renal impairment.

PRECAUTIONS: Pregnancy, gastritis, severe cardiac disease.

CHLORAMPHENICOL
(Chloromycetin)

USES: Chloramphenicol is used only for the treatment of serious infections; activities of chloramphenicol are given in the next Table (Francke, E.L. and Neu, H.C., Med. Clin. No. Am. 71, 1155-1168, 1987; Adams, H.G., Personal Comm.):

Activities of Chloramphenicol

	Gram-positive cocci			Gram-negative bacilli						Anaerobes		
	S. aureus	Streptococci	Strep. entero.	H. influenzae	P. mirabilis	E. coli	Klebsiella	Other Enterics	Pseudomonas a.	B. fragilis	Res. Anaerobes	Rickettsia
Chloramphenicol	3	4	XXX	4	4	3	3	3	XXX	4	4	3

4=best activity; 3=good activity; 2=some activity; XXX =little or no activity.
Res.= Resident

CHLORAMPHENICOL (Cont.)

Other organisms that are sensitive to chloramphenicol are chlamydia and mycoplasma.

The indications for the use of chloramphenicol are as follows: **anaerobic infections,** especially with **Bacteroides fragilis; typhoid fever; Haemophilus influenzae meningitis; pneumococcal and meningococcal meningitis** in patients allergic to penicillin; **brain abscess;** and **rickettsial infections.**

Chloramphenicol is the **drug of choice** for the treatment of severe cases of **typhoid fever. Haemophilus Infections:** Chloramphenicol may be used in conjunction with ampicillin for the initial treatment of meningitis, osteomyelitis, septic arthritis, cellulitis, epiglottitis, septicemia, or other serious infections caused by **H. influenzae** although third generation cephalosporins are more commonly used. **Rickettsial Infections:** Tetracyclines are the drugs of choice for the treatment of **Rocky Mountain spotted fever** and other **rickettsial infections;** however, chloramphenicol is the drug of choice when tetracyclines cannot be used. **In children younger than 8 years, tetracycline may color the teeth.**

DOSAGE FORMS: Caps: 250mg; Susp.: 150mg/5ml; Parenteral: 1g (100mg/ml); Otic. Sol'n: 0.5%; Ophthal. Sol'n: 0.16, 0.25, 0.5%; Ophthal. Ointment: 1%; Topical Cream: 1%

DOSAGE: Chloramphenicol and chloramphenicol palmitate are administered orally; chloramphenicol sodium succinate is administered IV. When taken orally, drug should be taken with a full glass of water on an empty stomach(1 h before or 2 h after meals) for best absorption. Dosage is given in the next Table:

Dosage of Chloramphenicol

Age	Route	Dosage
Neonate <7 days or >7 days <2kg	Orally or IV	25mg/kg/day in one dose
Neonate >7d, >2kg	Orally or IV	50mg/kg/day in 2 divided doses
Children, Adults		
Meningitis	Orally or IV	75-100mg/kg/day in 4 divided doses
Other Infections	Orally or IV	50-75mg/kg/day in 4 divided doses

PHARMACOKINETICS: Therapeutic: 10-20mcg/ml; Toxic: >25mcg/ml.
Half-Life: Adults and Children: 1.5-5 hours; Premature Infants (one to two days old): 24-48 hours; Premature Infants (13 to 23 days old): 8-15 hours.

ADVERSE EFFECTS: Bone Marrow Depression: Bone-marrow depression is dose-related. Plasma levels >25mcg/ml is frequently associated with reversible bone marrow depression with decreased reticulocytes, decreased hemoglobin, decreased thrombocytes, decreased WBC's and increased serum iron. Anemia most often follows parenteral therapy, large doses, long duration of therapy or impaired drug elimination. Patients do not respond to iron or vitamin B_{12} therapy while receiving chloramphenicol. Complete recovery usually occurs within 1-2 weeks after drug discontinuation.

Gray Baby Syndrome: Fatal cardiovascular-respiratory collapse (gray baby syndrome) may develop in neonates given excessive doses and having plasma levels above 50-100mcg/ml. Large overdoses may induce a gray baby like syndrome in children and adults (Slaughter, R.L. et al., Clin. Pharmacol. Ther. 28, 69-77, 1980).

Chloramphenicol is converted to chloramphenicol-glucuronide by glucuronyl transferase in the liver and then excreted rapidly (80 to 90 percent of the dose) in the urine by the kidney. In the neonate, conversion of chloramphenicol to the glucuronide is slow because the activity of the enzyme, glucuronyl transferase, is low; thus, chloramphenicol may accumulate. Chloramphenicol levels must be monitored, particularly in neonates and infants.

Aplastic Anemia: Aplastic anemia is rare, non-dose related, and fatal and can occur long after a short course of oral or parenteral therapy (Meissner, H.C. and Smith, A.L., Pediatrics 64, 348-356, 1979).

MONITOR: Complete blood count should be obtained every two days to recognize reticulocytopenia, leukopenia, thrombocytopenia and anemia.

DRUG INTERACTIONS: Chloramphenicol may increase the effects of many drugs that undergo hepatic metabolism (eg, phenytoin and oral hypoglycemic agents). Effects of anticoagulants may be increased. Phenobarbital may increase chloramphenicol metabolism.

CHLORDIAZEPOXIDE
(Librium)

USES: Chlordiazepoxide is a benzodiazepine; uses are given in the next Table:

Uses of Chlordiazepoxide
Anxiety
Preanesthetic Medication
Alcohol Withdrawal

Chloridiazepoxide is used in the management of situational anxiety and generalized anxiety disorder; it is used to ameliorate the symptoms of alcohol withdrawal and as a preanesthetic medication.

DOSAGE FORMS: Caps: 5, 10 and 25mg; Tabs: 5, 10 and 25mg; Chlordiazepoxide hydrochloride for IV: Powder 100mg in 5ml containers.

DOSAGE: Dosage of chlordiazepoxide is given in the next Table:

Dosage of Chlordiazepoxide

Condition	Age	Route	Dosage
Anxiety	Adults	Oral	15 to 40mg daily divided into three or four doses.
	Elderly or Debilitated	Oral	5mg, two to four times daily.
	Children >6 years	Oral	5mg, two to four times daily or 0.5mg/kg daily in divided doses.
Severe Withdrawal Symptoms in Acute Alcoholism **Acute Severe Anxiety**	Adults	IV	50 to 100mg given cautiously over at least one minute;repeat if necessary in two to four hours. The dose may be reduced to 25 to 50mg three or four times daily if necessary. The total daily dose generally should not exceed 300mg, but doses as high as 800mg have been used. Change to oral administration as soon as possible. Reduce dose by one-half in elderly or debilitated patients.

ADVERSE REACTIONS: The smallest dose that produces the desired effect should be used. Large doses have caused hypotension and syncope; usual oral doses may exacerbate ventilatory failure in patients with chronic lung disease. Adverse effects that occur rarely are increased or decreased libido, agranulocytosis, jaundice, and a lupus erythematosus-like syndrome; other effects include excitement, depression, confusion and hallucinations.

Long-term use may produce psychological and physical dependence.

Alcohol and other central nervous system depressants may exacerbate adverse effects.

CHLOROTHIAZIDE
(Diuril)

USES: Chlorothiazide is a thiazide diuretic; uses are given in the next Table:

Uses of Chlorothiazide
Hypertension: Thiazide Diuretics are often Drugs of First Choice
Edema:
Right Heart Failure: Thiazide Diuretics are often Drugs of First Choice
Left Heart Failure: Thiazide Diuretics are often Drugs of First Choice
Cirrhotic Edema and Ascites: Thiazide Diuretics are usually Drugs of Second Choice; Spironolactone is Diuretic of First Choice.
Nephrogenic Diabetes Insipidus: Thiazide Diuretics are often Drugs of First Choice.
Hypercalciuria: Thiazide Diuretics are Drugs of First Choice

Thiazide diuretics are not used as diuretics of first or second choice in patients with pulmonary edema, acute renal failure, chronic renal failure, nephrotic syndrome, drug poisoning, or hypercalcemia.

Hypertension: Treatment of hypertension with chlorothiazide is given in the next Table (The 1988 Report of the Joint National Committee on Detection, Evaluation, and Treatment of High Blood Pressure, Arch. Intern Med. 148, 1023-1038, 1988):

Treatment of Hypertension with Chlorothiazide

Step 1: Nonpharmacologic Approaches (see **HYPERTENSION**)
↓
Step 2: Chlorothiazide(Usual Minimum, 125-250mg/day; Usual Maximum, 500mg/day
↓ Observe up to 6 months; if chlorothiazide ineffective then,
Step 3: Add a second drug of a different class
or Increase the dosage of chlorothiazide
or Substitute another drug
↓
Step 4: Add a third drug of a different class **or** Substitute a second drug
↓
Step 5: Consider evaluation and/or referral **or** Add a third or fourth drug

"Step-Down": With mild hypertension, after 1 year of control, consider decreasing or withdrawing chlorothiazide and other hypotensive drugs.

Mechanism of Action: Chlorothiazides, like other thiazides, act mainly on the early segments of the distal tubule where they inhibit the absorption of NaCl from the tubular lumen. Excretion of Cl^-, Na^+ and water is increased. The increased Na^+ load in the distal tubule stimulates Na^+ exchange with K^+ and H^+, increasing their excretion; hypokalemia and a metabolic alkalosis may develop.

Thiazides reduce blood pressure mainly by lowering the body sodium stores. Initially, the blood pressure falls because of a decrease in blood volume, venous return and cardiac output. Gradually, the cardiac output returns to normal but the hypotensive effect remains because the peripheral resistance has in the meantime decreased for unknown reasons.

DOSAGE FORMS: Tabs: 250, 500mg; Susp.: 250mg/5ml; Parenteral: 500mg

DOSAGE: Chlorothiazide is administered orally; chlorothiazide sodium is administered IV, usually by infusion. The IV route should only be used when the patient cannot take the drug orally or in emergency situations. Dosage is given in the next Table:

Oral Dosage of Chlorothiazide

Condition	Age	Dosage
Hypertension	Adults	Initial: 125-250mg daily, single dose or two divided doses, orally. Maintenance: Determined by b.p.; Stepped Approach: 250mg, max. 500mg orally
Edema	Adults	500mg to 2g daily in 1 or 2 doses; after several days or when nonedematous state attained, reduce dosage. **or** alternate days or 3-5 days weekly
Toxemia of Pregnacy	Adults	1g daily; max. 2g daily
Pediatric	<6 mos.	20-30mg/kg daily in two divided doses
	6 mos.-12 yrs.	20mg/kg daily in two divided doses

CHLOROTHIAZIDE (Cont.)

PHARMACOKINETICS: Duration of diuretic action, oral, 6-12 h; not metabolized but excreted unchanged in urine.

ADVERSE EFFECTS: Potassium depletion occurs in most patients; it is usually not severe or progressive and rarely causes symptoms. Potassium supplement, such as potassium chloride, may be necessary in patients whose serum potassium is less than 3mmol/liter, or those on digitalis glycosides, older patients, those with cirrhosis or those taking other potassium-wasting drugs.

Hypochloremic alkalosis may occur with hypokalemia, especially in patients with other losses of potassium and chloride, eg, vomiting, diarrhea, and gastric suction. Hyponatremia may occur.

Volume depletion, hypotension and weakness may occur with high doses and salt restriction.

Hyperuricemia occurs in many patients but is usually asymptomatic except in patients with a history or predisposition of gout or chronic renal failure.

Hyperglycemia (especially in diabetics on oral hypoglycemic agents), hypercalcemia, hypercholesterolemia, and hypertriglyceridemia may occur.

Sexual dysfunction may occur and can be emotionally disturbing.

Weakness, cramps, drowsiness, lethargy may be signs of electrolyte disturbances.

CONTRAINDICATIONS: Allergy to other sulfonamide derivatives, anuria, pregnancy unless accompanied by severe edema.

PRECAUTIONS: May be ineffective in renal failure; hypokalemia increases digitalis toxicity; may precipitate acute gout. Use with caution in patients with diabetes and in patients with liver disease.

DRUG INTERACTIONS: Increases digitalis; decreases effect of oral hypoglycemics; can raise lithium blood levels by enhancing proximal tubular reabsorption of lithium. ACE inhibitors blunt hypokalemia induced by thiazide diuretics.

MONITOR: Serum potassium weekly to monthly initially; every 3-6 months when stable. Monitor other electrolytes, including magnesium periodically.

CHLORPHENIRAMINE

(Chlorpro, Chlor-Trimetron, etc.)

USES: Chlorpheniramine is an antihistamine used to treat rhinitis and allergic reactions to blood or plasma.

DOSAGE FORMS: Oral: 2,4mg; extended release: 6,8,12mg; solution: 1, 2mg/5ml; Parenteral: 10mg/ml (IV) or 100mg/ml (IM or SQ).

DOSAGE:

Oral Dosage of Chlorpheniramine

Age	Dosage
Adults Children > 12 yrs	4mg every 4-6 hrs or 8-12mg extended release twice a day
6-12 yrs	2mg every 4-6 hrs or 8mg extended release once a day
2-6 yrs	1mg every 4-6 hrs
Pediatric, by weight	0.35mg/kg daily in 4 divided doses

ADVERSE EFFECTS, CONTRAINDICATIONS, DRUG INTERACTIONS: see **ANTIHISTAMINES**.

CHLORPROMAZINE
(Thorazine)

USES: Chlorpromazine is a derivative of phenothiazine; uses are given in the next Table:

Uses of Chlorpromazine
Psychotic Disorders and Excessive Anxiety, Tension and Agitation
Restlessness and Apprehension before Surgery
Nausea and Vomiting
Intractable Hiccups
Adjunctive Treatment of Tetanus
Acute Intermittent Porphyria

Chlorpromazine was the first phenothiazine used in schizophrenia but is now obsolete for prolonged treatment. It has more serious adverse effects than the newer drugs.

Psychotic Disorders: Chlorpromazine is used primarily to treat schizophrenia and acute active psychoses and to control the manifestations of mania; it is used less commonly in schizoaffective disorders and paranoia.

Other Uses: Other uses of chlorpromazine include treatment of intractable hiccups, nausea, vomiting and as a premedication to reduce restlessness and apprehension before surgery.

Chlorpromazine binds strongly to and blocks dopaminergic receptors of the forebrain and basal ganglia.

DOSAGE FORMS: Tabs: 10, 25, 50, 100, 200mg; Caps (Extended Release): 30, 75, 150, 200, 300mg; Sol'n.(Oral): 10mg/5ml; Oral Conc.: 30, 100mg/ml; Supp.: 25, 100mg; Injection: 25mg/ml (1 and 2 ml vials)

DOSAGE: Chloropromazine hydrochloride is administered orally, by deep and slow IM or direct IV injection. Direct IV injection is intended for use only during surgery to control nausea and vomiting, as an adjunctive treatment of tetanus and in controlled settings for chemotherapy patients or in the ICU. IM administration may cause severe hypotension and should only be used when oral therapy is not feasible.

When taken orally, dilute with fruit juice, milk, carbonated drink, coffee, tea or water. Chlorpromazine is administered rectally. The drug should not be used in children under 6 months. Dosage is given in the next Table:

Dosage of Chlorpromazine

Condition	Age	Route	Dosage
Psychotic Disorders & Excessive Anxiety, Tension, & Agitation	Adults	Oral	30-75mg daily in 2-4 divided doses; if necessary, increase dosage twice weekly by 20-50mg; maintain optimal dosage for 2 weeks & gradually reduce dosage to minimal effective level; 200-800mg daily may be required for maintenance.
Prompt Relief of Anxiety, Tension & Agitation (Outpatients)	Adults	IM	25mg; repeat in one hour as needed. After symptoms controlled, replace with oral therapy, 25-50mg, 3 times daily.
Psychotic Disorders (Hospitalized Patients)	Adults	IM	25mg; 25-50mg in one hour. Gradually increase over several days to a max. of 400mg every 4-6 hours until symptoms controlled. Patients become quiet & cooperative in 24-48 hours. Continue with 500mg daily. Up to 2g daily may be required.
Psychotic Disorders & Behavioral Problems	>6 mos.	Oral	0.5mg/kg every 4-6 hours.
		Rectal	1mg/kg every 6-8 hours.
		IM	0.5mg/kg every 6-8 hours
Nausea and Vomiting	Adults	Oral	10-25mg every 4-6 h, as necessary
		Rectal	50-100mg every 6-8 h.
		IM	25mg; if hypotension does not occur, additional IM doses of 25-50mg may be given every 3-4 h. Oral therapy should replace IM
	>6 mos.	Oral	0.5mg/kg every 4-6 h.
		Rectal	1mg/kg every 4-8 h
		IM	0.5mg/kg every 6-8 h.(Max. in child. >5 and <22.7kg is 40mg daily); Max. in child. 5-12 yrs. & 22.7-45.5kg is 75mg daily

CHLORPROMAZINE (Cont.)

Dosage of Chlorpromazine			
Condition	Age	Route	Dosage
Restlessness & Apprehension Before Surgery	Adults	Oral	25-50mg, 2-3 h. before surgery
		IM	12.5-25mg, 1-2 h. before surgery
	>6 mos.	Oral	0.5mg/kg, 2-3 h. before surgery
		IM	0.5mg/kg, 1-2 h. before surgery
Nausea & Vomiting During Surgery	Adults	IM	12.5mg; may repeat in 30 minutes if hypotension does not occur.
		IV	2mg at 2 min., max. 25mg
	>6 mos.	IM	0.275mg/kg; repeat in 30 min. if necessary & if hypotension does not occur.
		IV	1mg at 2 min. intervals, maximum 0.275mg/kg, repeat as necessary
Following Surgery	Adults	Oral	10-25mg every 4-6 h., as necessary
		IM	12.5-25mg;repeat in 1 h., as needed.
	>6 mos.	Oral	0.5mg/kg; repeat every 4-6 h., as needed.
		IM	0.5mg/kg; repeat in 1 h., as needed.

PHARMACOKINETICS: Oral bioavailability, 20-40%; orally, time to peak plasma conc. is 2-4 h. IM: Onset, 20-30 min., Peak, 2-3 h.; Plasma Binding, 95-98%. Half-Life: 23-37 h. Metabolized in liver and kidneys.

ADVERSE EFFECTS: The relative frequency of side effects is as follows: sedation, high; anti-cholinergic effects, also called antimuscarinic or atropinic, (dryness of the mouth, orthostatic hypotension, blurred vision, urinary retention and constipation) moderate. These reactions tend to diminish after the first week of continual therapy. Extrapyramidal effects (dystonia - often bizarre and abrupt; akathisia - characterized by feeling of restlessness; and Parkinsonism - rigidity, bradykinesia, shuffling gait, postural abnormalities) moderate.

Hypotension may occur, especially with IV or IM administration.

Chlorpromazine may produce agranulocytosis and cholestatic jaundice but both are rare.

Allergic skin reactions are uncommon but mild photosensitivity occurs relatively often and the patient should be informed.

Patients should be examined periodically for conjunctival melanosis, pigmentary opacities in the cornea and lens and glaucoma. Menstrual irregularities, galactorrhea, gynecomastia, and impotence have been reported occasionally.

DRUG INTERACTIONS: Chlorpromazine may enhance the action of other central nervous system depressants such as antianxiety agents, hypnotics, analgesics, and alcohol. It interferes with the neuronal uptate of guanethidine. Combined with lithium, may cause encephalopathic syndrome rarely. Increased seizure risk with metrizamide. Decreases metabolism of phenytoin.

MONITOR: Monitor blood pressure because of high incidence of hypotension.

CHLORPROPAMIDE

(Diabinase, Glucamide)

USES: Chlorpropamide is a "first" generation **sulfonylurea** compound which is used to lower glucose levels in patients with **non-insulin dependent diabetes mellitus** (NIDDM; Type II diabetes mellitus). Chlorpropamide is only used following dietary management; dietary management is continued during therapy.

Mechanism of Action: Sulfonylureas act by stimulating the release of insulin from pancreatic islets by increasing the sensitivity of the beta cells to glucose, which stimulates insulin secretion. Sulfonylureas may suppress the secretion of glucagon and the production of hepatic glucose and potentiate insulin-stimulated glucose transport in adipose tissue and across skeletal muscle membrane.

DOSAGE FORMS: Tabs:100, 250mg

DOSAGE: Chlorpropamide is usually given once daily with breakfast. Dosage is given in the next Table:

Dosage of Chlorpropamide

Age	Dosage
Elderly	Initially, 100-125mg daily;
Middle-Aged	Initially up to 250mg daily

After 5-7 days, the blood glucose levels reach a plateau and the dose is increased or decreased by 50-125mg at weekly intervals.

Maintenance Dose: Usual range, 100-500mg daily. Patients who do not respond adequately to 500mg daily usually will not respond to larger doses.

PHARMACOKINETICS: Metabolism: Liver to an active metabolite; Half-Life: 36 hours (range, 25-60 hours) Duration of Action: 24-72 hours.

ADVERSE EFFECTS: Untoward effects occur more frequently with chlorpropamide than with other sulfonylureas probably secondary to the accumulation of the active metabolite. Rarely, life-threatening hypoglycemia and water retention with hyponatremia (especially in patients with congestive heart failure or hepatic cirrhosis) have occurred (similar to SIADH).

PRECAUTIONS: Chemically related to sulfonamides. Chlorpropamide should not be administration to patients with renal impairment because the duration of action of the drug is greatly prolonged. Disulfiram (Antabuse)-like reaction may occur with alcohol consumption.

MONITOR: Blood glucose is monitored every one to two weeks until the dosage of chlorpropamide is established and monthly thereafter; therapy is continued if the response is satisfactory.

CHLORTHALIDONE
(Hygroton, Biogroton)

USES: Chlorthalidone is structurally and pharmacologically similar to **thiazide diuretics**; uses are given in the next Table:

Uses of Chlorthalidone
Edema
Hypertension

Hypertension: Treatment of hypertension with chlorthalidone as a step 2 drug is given in the next Table (The 1988 Report of the Joint National Committee on Detection, Evaluation, and Treatment of High Blood Pressure, Arch. Intern.Med. 148, 1023-1038, 1988):

Treatment of Hypertension with Chlorthalidone

Step 1: Nonpharmacologic Approaches (see **HYPERTENSION**)

↓

Step 2: Chlorthalidone (Usual Minimum, 12.5-25mg/day; Usual Maximum,50mg/day)
Observe up to 6 months; if chlorthalidone ineffective then,

↓

Step 3: Add a second drug of a different class
or Increase the dosage of chlorthalidone
or Substitute another drug

↓

Step 4: Add a third drug of a different class
or Substitute a second drug

↓

Step 5: Consider further evaluation and/or referral
or Add a third or fourth drug

"Step-Down": For patients with mild hypertension, after 1 year of control, consider decreasing or withdrawing chlorthalidone and other hypotensive drugs.

Chlorthalidone was used to treat 4800 elderly patients with isolated systolic hypertension. In this study, patients were treated with chlorthalidone 12.5mg daily; dose was increased to 25mg daily, then atenolol 25mg/day then 50mg/day was added if patients did not respond adequately to the initial therapy. The study was double-blind and placebo controlled. Antihypertensive therapy resulted in a 36% reduction in the incidence of stroke and a 32% reduction in the incidence of major cardiovascular events. Death rate from all causes was reduced by 13% (Systolic Hypertension in the Elderly [SHEP] Cooperative Research Group, JAMA 265, 3255-3264, 1991).

Mechanism of Action: Chlorthalidone acts like thiazide diuretics on the cortical diluting segment of the nephron.

DOSAGE FORMS: Tabs: 25, 50 and 100mg.

DOSAGE: Chlorthalidone is administered orally; the dosage of chlorthalidone is given in the next Table:

Dosage of Chlorthalidone

Condition	Dosage
Edema	Adults: 50 to 100mg daily in a single dose after breakfast fast or 100mg every other day or 3 times per week; some patients may require 200mg daily. Children: 2mg/kg 3 times weekly; maintenance dose adjusted individually.
Hypertension	Adults: initially, 25mg daily; may be increased to 50mg daily. Children: 1-2mg/kg daily.

PHARMACOKINETICS: Binding 90%, principally to or in red blood cells; Half-Life: 54 hours.

ADVERSE EFFECTS: Potassium depletion, orthostatic hypotension, hyperglycemia, hyperuricemia, hypercholesterolemia, hypertriglyceridemia, sexual dysfunction, weakness. GI upset, dizziness, rash, urticaria.

DRUG INTERACTIONS: May increase digitalis, lithium, diazoxide toxicity.

PRECAUTIONS: May be ineffective in renal failure; hypokalemia increases digitalis toxicity; may precipitate acute gout.

CHLORZOXAZONE

(Paraflex, Parafon Forte)

USES: Chlorzoxazone is a CNS depressant which is used to treat the pain of local muscle spasm; it is not effective in spastic or dyskinetic movement disorders. The skeletal muscle relaxant effects are minimal and are probably related to its sedative effect.

DOSAGE FORMS: Tabs: 250, 500mg.

DOSAGE: Dosage is given in the next Table:

Dosage of Chlorzoxazone

Age	Dosage
Adults	250 to 750 mg, three or four times daily.
Children	20mg/kg daily in 3 or 4 divided doses.

PHARMOCOKINETICS: Peak: 3-4 hours; Metabolism: Liver; conjugated with glucuronic acid; Half-Life: 1.1 hours.

ADVERSE EFFECTS: Drowsiness (15%); headache, gastrointestinal irritation, and rarely gastrointestinal bleeding, hypersensitivity reactions, hepatic dysfunction.

CHOLESTEROL-LOWERING DRUGS

Drugs used in the treatment of hypercholesterolemia are given in the next Table (Medical Letter 30, 85-88, Sept. 9, 1988):

Drugs Used in the Treatment of Hypercholesterolemia

Drugs	Reduces Coronary Artery Risk	Long-Term Safety	LDL-Chol. Lowering
Bile Acid Sequestrants: Cholestyramine and Cholestipol	Yes	Yes	15-30%
Niacin (Nicotinic Acid)	Yes	Yes	15-30%
Lovastatin (Mevacor) (HMG CoA Reductase Inhibitor)	Not proven	Not Established	25-45%

The effect of antilipemic drugs on lipoproteins is given in the next Table (Dunn, F.L., Clinical Monograph, Roche Biomedical Lab, 1988):

Effect of Antilipemic Drugs on Lipoproteins

Drug	Low Density Lipoprotein(LDL)	Very Low Density Lipoprotein(VLDL)	High Density Lipoprotein(HDL)
Bile Acid Sequestrants	↓	↑	+/-
Nicotinic Acid	↓	↓	↑
Lovastatin	↓↓	↓	↑

Bile Acid Sequestrants: The bile acid sequestrants, cholestyramine (Questran) and colestipol (Colestid) have been shown to reduce coronary artery risk, to lower LDL-cholesterol and are not associated with systemic toxicity. They can be used in the treatment of children and women considering pregnancy. The most frequent side effects of bile acid sequestrants are gastrointestinal.

In a large study, cholestyramine lowered serum cholesterol 8.5%, LDL-cholesterol 12.6% and the incidence of coronary heart disease from 8.6% in the placebo-treated patients to 7.0% in the cholestyramine group (JAMA 251, 351, 365, 1984). In another study, cholestyramine inhibited the progression of coronary artery stenosis (Brensike, J.F. et al., Circulation 69, 313, 1984).

The choice of drug, cholestyramine or colestipol, depends on individual patient preference with respect to taste and palatability.

The bile acid sequestrants are contraindicated as single-drug therapy in patients with marked hypertriglyceridemia [triglyceride >500mg/dl (>5.7mmol/liter)] or patients with severe constipation.

Niacin (Nicotinic Acid): Niacin, a water soluble B vitamin, has been shown to lower LDL-cholesterol, to lower triglycerides and to reduce coronary artery risk (Canner, P.L. et al., J. Am. Coll. Cardiol. 8, 1245, 1986); niacin raises HDL-cholesterol levels.

Niacin is preferred for patients with concurrent hypertriglyceridemia (triglyceride >250mg/dl), because it lowers LDL-cholesterol without exacerbating the hypertriglyceridemia.

Combined niacin with cholestipol inhibits atherosclerosis in native coronary arteries and surgical coronary artery grafts (Blankenhorn, D.H. et. al., JAMA 257, 3233, 1987).

Flushing may be a prominent side effect in some patients.

Lovastatin (Mevacor): Lovastatin is a specific competitive inhibitor of the rate-limiting enzyme (HMG CoA reductase) in cholesterol biosynthesis. It is effective in reduction of LDL-cholesterol (JAMA 260, 359, July 15, 1988). However, long term safety studies are not available.

The effects of lovastatin, niacin and colestipol are additive (Malloy, M.J. et al., Ann. Intern. Med. 107, 616, 1987).

CHOLESTEROL-LOWERING DRUGS (Cont.)

OTHER DRUGS: Other drugs that are used to treat hyperlipidemias are given in the next Table:

Other Drugs to Treat Hyperlipidemias

Drug	Comment
Gemfibrozil (Lopid)	FDA approved for lowering serum triglyceride to reduce the risk of pancreatitis.
Clofibrate (Atromid-S)	FDA approved for lowering serum triglyceride to reduce the risk of pancreatitis. Clofibrate is used less frequently than gemfibrozil because of reports of long-term toxicity (WHO Clofibrate Trial, Br. Heart J. 40, 1069-1118, 1978).
Probucol (Lorelco)	Probucol reduces LDL-cholesterol (10-15%) but also reduces HDL-cholesterol up to 25%. The role of probucol in the treatment of patients with elevated LDL-cholesterol is uncertain because of concerns about the reduction of HDL-cholesterol (Durrington, P.N. and Miller, J.P. Atherosclersis 55, 187, 1985).
Dextrothyroxine (Choloxin)	Not recommended; causes moderate hyperthyroidism.
Neomycin	Not recommended for general use; neomycin, as an aminoglycoside, may cause ototoxicity and nephrotoxicity.

COMBINED DRUG THERAPY FOR HYPERLIPIDEMIA: If the response to a single drug is inadequate, combination drug therapy is considered as given in the next Table:

Combined Drug Therapy for Hyperlipidemia

Condition	Recommendation
Increased LDL-Cholesterol	Bile acid sequestrant plus niacin or lovastatin.
Increased LDL-Cholesterol plus Increased Triglycerides	Niacin plus lovastatin usual drugs of choice. Bile acid sequestrant plus gemfibrozil.

CHOLESTEROL-LOWERING DRUGS (Cont.)

PROTOCOL FOR TREATMENT OF ELEVATED LDL-CHOLESTEROL: A protocol for the treatment of patients with elevated LDL-cholesterol is given in the next Figure:

Treatment of Elevated LDL-Cholesterol

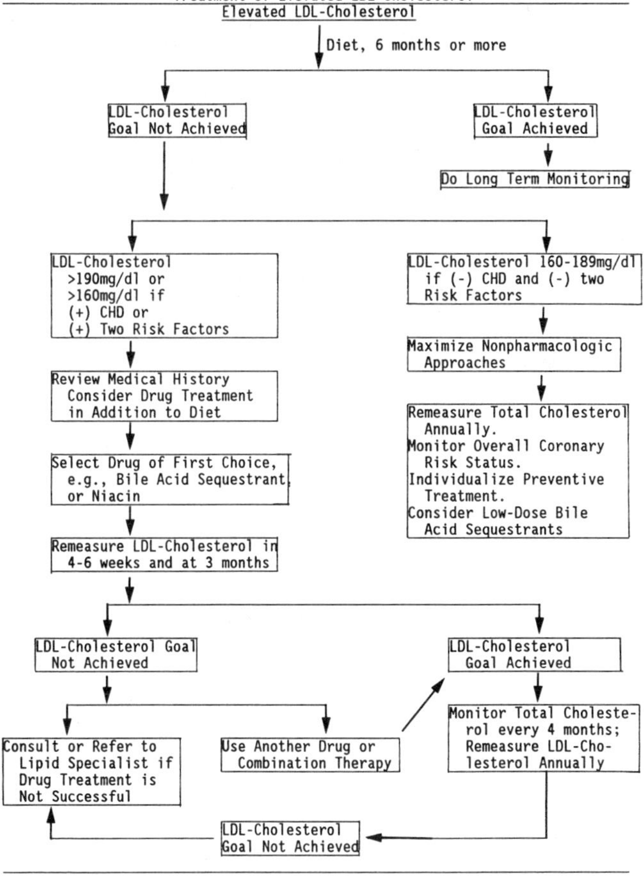

CHOLESTYRAMINE

(Questran, Cholybar)

USES: Cholestyramine is used primarily to lower serum cholesterol; uses are given in the next Table:

Uses of Cholestyramine
Decrease Elevated Cholesterol and LDL Concentration
Relief of Pruritis Associated with Cholestasis
Diarrhea associated with excess fecal bile acids

Decrease of Elevated Cholesterol: Cholestyramine is used in patients with type II hyperlipoproteinemia to lower serum cholesterol and low density lipoprotein(LDL) which carries cholesterol. Decreases in LDL-cholesterol of 10-15% may be obtained with the initial starting dosage schedule of 4g of cholestyramine taken twice daily; on average, there is a reduction of 15-30% in the concentration of LDL-cholesterol with 16-24g daily of cholestyramine.

Relief of Pruritis Associated with Cholestasis: Cholestyramine resin provides symptomatic relief of pruritis associated with partial obstructive jaundice and primary biliary cirrhosis. The pruritis in cholestasis is due to increase in bile salts in the circulation.

Mechanism of Action: Cholestyramine is an anion exchange resin which binds bile acids in the intestine to form an insoluble complex that is excreted in the feces; this interrupts the enterohepatic circulation of bile acids and leads to an increased hepatic synthesis of bile acids from cholesterol as illustrated in the next Figure (Brown, M.S. and Goldstein, J.L., Science 232, 34-47, April 4, 1986):

Effect of Cholestyramine Binding to Bile Acids on Cholesterol Metabolism

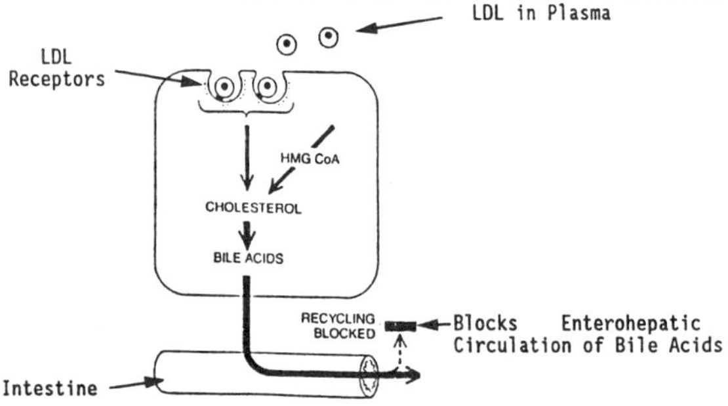

Depletion of the hepatic pool of cholesterol results in an increase in LDL receptor activity in the liver; this stimulates removal of LDL from plasma and lowers the concentration of LDL-cholesterol. Bile acid sequestration may increase hepatic VLDL production and this increases the plasma concentration of triglycerides.

DOSAGE FORMS: 4g of dried cholestyramine resin per 9g of powder or per chewable bar.

DOSAGE: Cholestyramine resin is administered orally. The dose should be mixed with 60-180ml of water, milk, fruit juice or other noncarbonated beverage. Dosage is given in the next Table:

Dosage of Cholestyramine

Condition	Age	Dosage
Hypercholesterolemia	Adults	Initial: 4g, 2 times daily within an hour of major meals. Maintenance: 16-24g/day in 2 divided doses.
	Children	80mg/kg, three times a day.
Pruritis of Cholestasis	Adults	4g, 3-4 times a day.

CHOLESTYRAMINE (Cont.)

PHARMACOKINETICS: Cholestyramine is not absorbed from the G.I. tract. It takes 1-3 weeks for lipid lowering effect to occur; lipids return to pretreatment levels 2-4 weeks after the drug is discontinued.

ADVERSE EFFECTS: Cholestyramine is not absorbed from the gastrointestinal tract and systemic toxicity is minimal. However, gastrointestinal side effects are frequent. Constipation is the most frequent adverse effect, occurring especially in the elderly. Other adverse effects that occur occasionally include nausea, vomiting, flatulence, diarrhea, steatorrhea at high doses, abdominal distension and cramps.

Cholestyramine resin contains chloride as its anion exchanger. This chloride may be absorbed instead of bicarbonate and lead to hyperchloremic metabolic acidosis especially in children; this effect may be partially offset by reducing chloride intake.

Cholestyramine occasionally interferes with the absorption of fat soluble vitamins A,D,E and K. Prolonged use of cholestyramine may be associated with an increased bleeding tendency as a result of hypoprothrombinemia secondary to vitamin K deficiency.

Increased urinary calcium excretion may occur, leading potentially to osteoporosis.

There may be a moderate increase in plasma triglycerides in some patients.

An occasional mild and usually transient increase in alkaline phosphatase and transaminases may occur.

Folate deficiency may occur during long-term treatment and patients, especially children, should receive 5mg of folic acid daily, if necessary.

DRUG INTERACTIONS: Cholestyramine can decrease the absorption of other anionic drugs if these are taken concurrently. It is advisable to take other medications at least 1 hour before or 4 hours after taking cholestyramine. Cholestyramine can interfere with the absorption of digoxin, warfarin, thyroxine, thiazide diuretics, beta blockers and other drugs.

There may be decreased absorption of the fat soluble vitamins (A,D,E and K) and folic acid especially in patients treated with prolonged high doses of cholestyramine, primarily in patients with severe liver or small bowel disease; routine vitamin supplementation is not needed or recommended in adult patients.

CONTRAINDICATIONS: Cholestyramine can increase triglyceride levels and should not be used as single-drug therapy in patients with marked hypertriglyceridemia [triglyceride >500mg/dl (>5.7mmol/liter.)]

It is also contraindicated in patients with severe constipation.

MONITOR: Monitor total cholesterol and LDL-cholesterol just prior to starting therapy, in 4-6 weeks, and at 3 months. If LDL-cholesterol goal is achieved, monitor total cholesterol at 4 month intervals, and LDL-cholesterol annually. Electrolytes should be determined at two month intervals, especially in children. Prothrombin time (PT) should be determined at 3 month intervals.

CIMETIDINE
(Tagamet)

USES: Uses of cimetidine are given in the next Table:

Uses of Cimetidine
Active Duodenal Ulcers
Prophylaxis of Recurrent Duodenal Ulcers
Active Gastric Ulcers
Pathologic Hypersecretory Conditions, e.g., Zollinger-Ellison Syndrome, Systemic Mastocytosis and Multiple Endocrine Adenomas

Cimetidine and antacids may be administered concomitantly but not simultaneously since antacids interfere with absorption of cimetidine. Antacids are used for the relief of pain.

Cimetidine is used in pathologic hypersecretory conditions, eg, Zollinger-Ellison syndrome, systemic mastocytosis and multiple endocrine adenomas. Cimetidine reduces diarrhea, anorexia and pain and promotes healing of intractable ulcers in patients with these conditions.

Mechanism of Action: Cimetidine competitively inhibits the action of histamine on H_2 receptors of parietal cells, thus reduces acid secretion by parietal cells of the stomach; it acts like the other H_2 receptor antagonists,ie., ranitidine (Zantac),famotidine(Pepcid) and nizatidine (Axid).

DOSAGE FORMS: Tabs: 200, 300, 400, 800mg; Syrup: 300mg/5ml; Inject: 150mg/ml

DOSAGE: Cimetidine and cimetidine hydrochloride are administered orally. Cimetidine hydrochloride may be given by IM or slow IV injection or by slow IV infusion. Dosage is given in the next Table:

Dosage of Cimetidine

Condition	Age	Route	Dosage
Acute Duodenal Ulcer, Gastric Ulcer or Hypersecretory Conditions	Adults	Oral, IM or slow IV	300mg, every 6 h., max. 2.4g/day Treat duodenal ulcer for 4-6 weeks Doses larger than 300mg may be necessary for hypersecretory states
Prophylaxis of Recurrent Duodenal Ulcer	Adults	Oral	300 or 400g at bedtime
	Newborn	Oral, IM or slow IV	10-20mg/kg/day in 4 divided doses
	Child.	Oral, IM or slow IV	20-40mg/kg/day in 4 divided doses

Renal Impairment: 300mg every 12 h. at creatinine clearance <30ml/min.

PHARMACOKINETICS: Onset, 0.5-1 h.; Peak: 1-2 hours; Duration, 4-6 h.; Oral Absorption: 70-80%; Metabolized: Liver. Excretion: 75% in urine. Half-Life: 2 h.; liver disease, 2.9 h.; renal failure, 4-5 h.; liver and renal disease, 6.7 h.

ADVERSE EFFECTS: Fever, rashes, hypersensitivity reactions. Mental alterations, eg, hallucinations, confusion, delirium and encephalopathy, occur especially with IV use in the elderly, renal or hepatic impaired patients. Rarely, leukopenia, thrombocytopenia and oligospermia may occur. Gynecomastia and impotence after 2-4 months of therapy. Rarely, bradycardia, hypotension, and cardiac arrhythmias.

MONITOR: CBC, serum creatinine and liver enzymes should be monitored at two week intervals.

DRUG INTERACTIONS: Numerous drug interactions exist, some of the major ones are listed. Antacids and metoclopramide reduces bioavailability of cimetidine by 20% to 30%; these reactions may not be clinically significant; however, these drugs should not be used within an hour of the use of cimetidine. Cimetidine increases the half-life of warfarin and similar anticoagulants, theophylline, phenobarbital, phenytoin, carbamazepine, propranolol, diazepam, chlordiazepoxide and probably prazepam and chlorazepate; this occurs because cimetidine inhibits drug metabolizing enzymes in the liver.

Cimetidine increases the serum concentration of lidocaine and nifedipine

CIPROFLOXACIN
(Cipro)

USES: Ciprofloxacin is the second oral fluoroquinolone to be marketed in the United States; norfloxacin (Noroxin) which is marketed only for treatment of urinary tract infections was the first fluoroquinolone. The older quinolones are nalidixic acid (Negram), cinoxacin (Cinobac) and oxolinic acid. Activities of ciprofloxacin are given in the next Table (Neu, H.C., Med. Clin. No. Am. 72, 623-636, 1988; Adams, H.G., Personal Comm.):

Activities of Ciprofloxacin

	Gram-positive cocci			Gram-negative bacilli				Gram-negative cocci	Anaerobes	
	S. aureus	Streptococci	Strep. entero.	H. influenzae	PEcK	Other Enterics	Pseudomonas a.	Neisseria	B. fragilis	Res. Anaerobes
Ciprofloxacin	+	±	+	+	+	+	+	+		

PEcK (Mnemonic)= P. mirabilis, E. coli, Klebsiella; Res.= Resident

Ciprofloxacin is active against the gram-negative cocci: Moraxella (Branhamella) catarrhalis; Neisseria gonorrhea (gonococcus) and Neisseria meningitides (meningococcus).

Oral ciprofloxacin offers an alternative to parenteral therapy for serious infections, such as **urinary tract infections, bacterial gastroenteritis, gonococcal infections, osteomyelitis,** and **respiratory infections** in patients with **cystic fibrosis.** It should not be used to treat anaerobic infections, and a penicillin or a cephalosporin is preferred for known or suspected pneumococcal or streptococcal infections (The Medical Letter 30, 11-13, Jan. 29, 1988; Walker, R.C. and Wright, A.J., Mayo Clin. Proc. 62, 1007-1012, 1987).

Infectious Diarrhea: Pathogens that have a high degree of susceptibility are those associated with enteric (intestinal) disease, eg, Salmonella species, Shigella species, Yersinia enterocolitica, Campylobacter species, Vibrio species, Aeromonas species. It is not active against Clostridium difficile.

Other Infections: Ciprofloxacin readily penetrates into various organs and tissues. It has been used to treat infections of the **upper and lower respiratory tract, skin, soft tissue, bone (osteomyelitis)** (Arcieri, G. et al., Am. J. Med. 82, Suppl. 4A, 381, 1987). Ciprofloxacin has decreased the incidence of gram-negative infections in patients with neutropenia (Dekker, A.W. et al., Ann. Intern. Med. 106, 7, 1987).

Mechanism of Action: Fluoroquinolones apparently act to block DNA gyrase (topoisomerase II) (Wolfson, J.S. and Hooper, D.C., Antimicrob. Agents Chemother. 28, 581, 1985). DNA gyrase is responsible for proper coiling of DNA, for DNA replication, transcription of certain genes, and aspects of DNA repair and recombination.

DOSAGE FORMS: 250, 500 and 750mg.

DOSAGE: Ciprofloxacin is not recommended for children or during pregnancy. It is given orally. Dosage is given in the next Table:

Dosage of Ciprofloxacin

Condition	Oral Dosage
"Usual" Condition	500-750mg every 12 hours
Uncomplicated Urinary Tract Infection	250-500mg every 12 hours
Infectious Diarrhea	500mg every 12 hours
Creatinine Clearance <30ml/min	250-500mg every 18 hours

No dosage alterations are recommended in the elderly or in patients with hepatic dysfunction.

Continue treatment for 2 days after symptoms improve.

CIPROFLOXACIN (Cont.)

PHARMACOKINETICS: Oral Bioavailability: 60-80%; Peak Serum Concentration: 1-2 hours; food increases time to peak concentration; Protein-Binding: 40%; Volume of Distribution: 3 liter/kg. Tissue Penetration: Excellent but penetration into the brain is poor (10% of serum concentration); Metabolism: 50-60% metabolized in the liver to at least four metabolites, three of which have some antimicrobial activity; Excretion: primarily eliminated by kidneys and some eliminated in feces. Elimination Half-Life: 3-4 hours.

ADVERSE EFFECTS: The incidence of adverse effects is 15%; 4% of patients discontinued drug. Adverse effects are given in the next Table:

Adverse Effects of Ciprofloxacin

System	Effects
Gastrointestinal Tract	Incidence, 5%; nausea, vomiting, diarrhea.
Central Nervous System	Incidence, 3%; dizziness, restlessness, tremor and headache. Seizures occur rarely.
Metabolic	Incidence, 2%; transient elevation of SGOT (AST) and SGPT (ALT), urea and creatinine.
Other	Incidence, 1.5%; rash, pruritis.
Cartilage Deterioration	Fluoroquinolones are not recommended for use in children or in pregnancy because of reports of cartilage deterioration in animals.

CONTRAINDICATIONS: Children or during pregnancy because of reports of cartilage deterioration in animals.

DRUG INTERACTIONS: Drug interactions are given in the next Table:

Drug Interactions of Ciprofloxacin

Drug	Effect
Aluminum and Magnesium Hydroxide (Maalox)	Ten fold reduction in serum peak ciprofloxacin concentration.
Theophylline	Elevation in serum theophylline due to reduced theophylline clearance by 30-60% possibly due to inhibition of hepatic metabolism.

Sucralfate, iron, calcium and bismuth also interfere with ciprofloxacin absorption.

CISPLATIN
(Platinol)

USES: Cisplatin is one of the most effective drugs against testicular tumors and is used, most often in combination regimens, to treat tumors listed in the next Table:

Uses of Cisplatin in Treatment of Tumors
Testicular Tumors
Ovarian Tumors
Bladder Carcinomas
Cervical Carcinomas
Head and Neck Squamous Cell Carcinomas
Osteogenic Sarcomas
Small Cell (Oat Cell) Carcinomas of the Lung
Esophageal and Gastric Carcinomas
Adrenocortical Carcinoma
Medulloblastoma
Neuroblastoma
Prostate Carcinomas

Testicular Carcinomas: Combination therapy, cisplatin, bleomycin, and vinblastine, is particularly effective against disseminated seminomatous and nonseminomatous testicular cancer; long-term survival and probable cures occur in about 70% of patients.

Mechanism of Action: Cisplatin is a platinum-containing antitumor agent. Cisplatin binds to DNA and inhibits DNA synthesis; protein and RNA synthesis are also inhibited.

DOSAGE FORMS: Injection: 10 and 50mg

DOSAGE: Cisplatin is administered by IV.

The most frequent and serious toxicity produced by cisplatin is impaired renal function. To reduce nephrotoxicity, pretreatment hydration with 1 to 2 liters of IV fluids is recommended.

Mannitol with or without furosemide is often administered concomitantly with cisplatin to ensure adequated diuresis. Dosage of cisplatin is given in the next Table (consult specific protocols prior to initiating therapy):

Dosage of Cisplatin

Condition	Route	Dosage
Treatment of Testicular Cancer	IV	Single Agent: 120mg/m^2 once every 3-4 weeks
		Combination Therapy: When combined with vinblastine and bleomycin, 20mg/m^2 daily for five days (days 1 to 5), administered every three weeks for four courses.

Before proceeding to repeat dosage, monitor parameters as listed in the next Table:

Parameters to Monitor Before Repeat Dosage of Cisplatin

Parameter	Comment
Serum Creatinine	Do not repeat dosage until level is <1.5mg/dl
BUN	Do not repeat dosage until level is <25mg/dl
Platelet Count	Do not repeat dosage until level is >100,000/microliter
Leukocyte Count	Do not repeat dosage until level is >4,000/microliter
Auditory Acuity	Maintain within normal limits

PHARMACOKINETICS: Half-Life: Biphasic: 25-48 min.; 58-73 hrs.; Protein-Binding: 90% Excretion; Urinary: 60% with mannitol; 40% without.

ADVERSE EFFECTS: Adverse effects of cisplatin are listed in the next Table:

Adverse Effects of Cisplatin

Effect	Comment
Impaired Renal Function	Most common adverse effect; noted during second week of therapy after initial dose; dose related and cumulative.
Electrolyte abnormalities	Most common effects are hypomagnesemia, hypocalcemia, and hypokalemia.
Myelosuppression	25%-30% of patients; nadirs in platelets and leukocyte counts 18-23 days (range, 7.5-45 days) recovery by day 39 (range, 13 to 62)
Nausea and Vomiting	Almost all patients; begins within 1-4 hrs. after treatment; last up to 24 hrs.
Ototoxicity	Up to 30%;
CNS	Peripheral neuropathies, generally sensory.

MONITOR: Serum creatinine, BUN, platelet count, leukocyte count, auditory acuity.

CLEMASTINE
(Tavist, Tavist-1)

USES: Clemastine is an ethanolamine derivative **antihistamine;** it is most often used to provide symptomatic relief of nasal allergies. It is also used for symptomatic treatment of dermatologic conditions.

DOSAGE FORMS: Tabs: 1.34mg; 2.68mg. Oral Solution: 0.67ml/5ml.

DOSAGE: Clemastine is administered orally.Dosage is given in the next Table:

Dosage of Clemastine

Age	Dosage
Adults and Children >11 years	1.34mg twice daily or 2.68mg one to three times daily; give 2.68mg for dermatologic conditions
Children 6-11 years	0.67mg twice daily, max dose 4.0mg per day.

PHARMACOKINETICS: Peak: 2-4 hrs. Max. Therapeutic Effect: 5-7 hrs.

ADVERSE EFFECTS: Sedation; anticholinergic symptoms such as dry mouth; and gastrointestinal symptoms such as nausea, constipation and abdominal pain. See **ANTIHISTAMINES** section.

CLIDINIUM BROMIDE AND CHLORDIAZEPOXIDE
(Librax)

USES: **Clidinium bromide** is an **anticholinergic antispasmodic** and **chlordiazepoxide** is an **antianxiety** agent; uses of Librax are given in the next Table:

Uses of Librax
Adjunct in the Treatment of Peptic Ulcer Disease
Irritable Bowel Syndrome

DOSAGE FORMS: Each capsule contains chlordiazepoxide hydrochloride 5mg and clidinium bromide 2.5mg.

DOSAGE: Librax is given orally. Dosage for adults is as follows: 1-2 caps, three or four times daily, max. 8 caps daily. For elderly or debilitated, initially 1 cap twice daily and then gradually increase dosage.

ADVERSE EFFECTS: The adverse effects of the clidinium bromide as an anticholinergic antispasmodic, competitively antagonizing the effect of acetylcholine at parasympathetic postganglionic muscarinic receptors are as follows: dilated pupils, blurred vision, dry mouth, constipation, difficulty urinating, and tachycardia. Adverse effects associated with chlordiazepoxide include drowsiness, hypotension and syncope, jaundice, paradoxical excitement and agranulocytosis.

CONTRAINDICATIONS: Pregnancy, glaucoma, GI or urinary tract obstruction, paralytic ileus or intestinal atony.

CLINDAMYCIN
(Cleocin)

USES: **Clindamycin** is widely used in the treatment of **anaerobic** infections and when both **S. aureus** and **anaerobes** occur together. Activities of clindamycin are given in the next Table (Klainer, A.S., Med. Clin. No. Am. 71, 1169-1175, 1987; Adams, H.G., Personal Comm.):

Activities of Clindamycin

	Gram-positive cocci			Gram-negative bacilli				Anaerobes	
	S. aureus	Streptococci	Strep. entero.	H. influenzae	PEcK	Other Enterics	Pseudomonas a.	B. fragilis	Res. Anaerobes
Clindamycin	3	4	▨	▨	▨	▨	▨	4	4

4=best activity; 3=good activity; 2=some activity; ▨=little or no activity; PEcK (Mnemonic)= P. mirabilis, E. coli, Klebsiella; Res.= Resident

Clindamycin is also active against the anaerobe, Clostridium.

Clindamycin is considered to be the **drug of choice** in the treatment of infections caused by **B. fragilis**. In the treatment of mixed **aerobic-anaerobic** bacterial infections, clindamycin has been used in conjunction with an aminoglycoside. The CDC suggests using clindamycin in combination with gentamcin as one possible regimen for the treatment of **acute pelvic inflammatory disease (PID)** in hospitalized patients.

Clindamycin is used in the treatment of serious infections by susceptible organisms involving tissues listed in the next Table:

Infections Treated with Clindamycin

Respiratory Tract Infections (Empyema, Pneumonia, Lung Abcess)
Serious Skin and Soft Tissue Infections
Septicemia
Intra-Abdominal Infections
Infections of the Female Pelvis and Genital Tract (Pelvic Inflammatory Disease (PID)): Endometritis, Nongonococcal Tubo-Ovarian Abscess, Pelvic Cellulitis, Postsurgical Vaginal Cuff Infections
Acne Vulgaris (Failure to respond to Oral Tetracycline, Erythromycin, or Co-Trimoxazole)
Osteomyelitis

Structure: Clindamycin is a semisynthetic derivative of **lincomycin.**

DOSAGE FORMS: Caps: 75, 150, 300mg; Oral Soln: 75mg/5ml; Parenteral (Inject): 150mg/ml

DOSAGE: Clindamycin hydrochloride and clindamycin palmitate hydrochloride are administered orally. Clindamycin phosphate is administered IM or by IV infusion. Dosage is given in the next Table:

Dosage of Clindamycin

Age	Route	Dosage
Adults	Oral	150-450mg every 6 hours
Children	Oral	10-25mg/kg daily in 3 or 4 equally divided doses
Adults	IM or IV	600mg-2.7g daily in 2-4 equally divided doses (max. 600mg for single IM dose; max. 1.2g IV infusion in 1-hour period; max. IV 4.8g. daily. Suggested Rate of Infusion: 10mg/min for 30 min. followed by 0.75mg/min.
Children >1 month	IM or IV	15-40mg/kg daily in 3 or 4 divided doses
Neonates <1 month	IM or IV	>2kg >7d: 5mg/kg every 6 h.; >2kg <7d or <2kg >7d: 5mg/kg every 8 h.; <2kg <7d: 5mg/kg every 12 h.

Acne Vulgaris: Clindamycin phosphate is applied topically to the skin (1%). A thin film is applied to cleaned affected area twice daily. Months or years of therapy may be necessary.

CLINDAMYCIN (Cont.)
PHARMACOKINETICS: Half-Life: 1.5-4 hour (av, 2.5 hour); unchanged or slightly increased in severe renal or liver disease. Peak: Oral dose, 1 hr., IM, 1-2hr. Protein Bound: 80-94%. Metabolism: Liver.
ADVERSE EFFECTS: Oral Route: Anorexia, nausea, vomiting, cramps, and diarrhea occur frequently. Clindamycin has neuromuscular blocking properties which may enhance effects of other neuromuscular blocking agents.

Pseudomembranous colitis (PMC) may occur following oral and rarely parenteral injection; PMC is secondary to overgrowth of toxin-producing Clostridium difficile. PMC may resolve by discontinuing clindamycin immediately; if diarrhea persists, treat with vancomycin.
MONITOR Bowel frequency; PMC usually manifests by severe diarrhea and abdominal cramps.

CLONAZEPAM
(Klonopin; formerly Clonopin)
USES: Clonazepam is a **benzodiazepine-derivative anticonvulsant;** uses are given in the next Table:

Uses of Clonazepam
Myoclonic Seizures
Akinetic Seizures
Partial Complex Seizures
Absence (Petit Mal) Seizures in Patients who do not Respond to Succinimides

Clonazepam is used to treat myoclonic, atonic and absence seizures that may be resistant to treatment with other anticonvulsants. It is generally less effective for absence seizures than ethosuximide or valproate.

A decreased response may occur after several months or years of clonazepam therapy.
DOSAGE FORMS: Tabs: 0.5, 1.0 and 2.0mg; Route: Orally
DOSAGE: Clonazepam is administered orally; daily dosage is usually given in 3 equally divided doses. Dosage is given in the next Table:

Dosage of Clonazepam

Age	Dosage
Infants and Children up to 10 years or 30kg	Initial: 0.01-0.05mg/kg/day divided every 8 hours Increments: Not >0.25-0.5mg every 3 days, up to max. maintenance dose of 0.1-0.2mg/kg/day divided every 8h
Adults	Initial: 1.5mg/day three times daily Increments: 0.5-1mg every third day Maximum dose: 20mg/day

PHARMACOKINETICS: Half-Life: 19-60 h. (av. 36); Time to Steady State: 4-12 days. Plasma Protein Bound: 45-85%
ADVERSE EFFECTS: CNS depression, drowsiness and ataxia common. May cause behavioral changes, and other CNS symptoms; increased bronchial secretions. GI, CV, GU and hematopoietic toxicity may occur.
CONTRAINDICATIONS: Significant liver disease; acute narrow angle glaucoma. Use with caution in renal impairment.
PRECAUTIONS: Pregnancy. May increase frequency of generalized seizures in patients with mixed seizure disorders. Abrupt withdrawal of drug in patients with epilepsy may precipitate status epilepticus.

CLONIDINE
(Catapres)

USES: Clonidine is used in the management of hypertension. Treatment of hypertension with clonidine is given in the next table (The 1988 Report of the Joint National Committee on Detection, Evaluation, and Treatment of High Blood Pressure, Arch. Intern Med. 148, 1023-1038, 1988):

Treatment of Hypertension with Clonidine

Step 1: Nonpharmacologic Approaches (see **HYPERTENSION**)
↓
Step 2: **Diuretic** or **Beta-Blocker** or **Calcium Antagonist** or **ACE Inhibitor**
Observe up to 6 months; if treatment ineffective then,
↓
Step 3: Add a second drug of a different class, usually one of the group of four listed above.
or Increase dosage of the first drug
or Substitute for one of the drugs in Step 2, usually another drug in Step 2.
↓
Step 4: Add a third drug of a different class, such as **clonidine**
or Substitute a second drug, eg, **clonidine**
↓
Step 5: Consider further evaluation and/or referral
or Add a third or fourth drug

"Step-Down": For patients with mild hypertension, after 1 year of control, consider decreasing or withdrawing clonidine and other hypotensive drugs.

Clonidine is generally reserved for patients who fail to respond to therapy with a step 1 drug (diuretics or beta-adrenergic blocking agents).

Clonidine may be used to treat hypertensive urgencies. It is used as an aid in the diagnosis of pheochromocytoma.

Clonidine (transdermal) has been used to ameliorate withdrawal symptoms associated with smoking cessation (Ornish, S.A. et al., Arch. Intern. Med. 148, 2027-2031, 1988).

Mechanism of Action: Clonidine lowers blood pressure by inhibiting sympathetic outflow from the brain following stimulation of the alpha-2 receptors in the vasomotor center of the medulla. Its hypotensive effect is associated with a fall in total peripheral resistance.

DOSAGE FORMS: Topical System: 0.1mg/day, 0.2mg/day, 0.3mg/day. Each transdermal patch delivers dose for 1 week. Tabs: 0.1, 0.2, 0.3mg.

DOSAGE: Clonidine is administered transdermally or orally; dosage is given in the next Table:

Dosage of Clonidine

Route	Dosage
Oral	Initially: 0.1mg once daily at bedtime for several weeks followed by 0.1mg twice daily. Dosage may be increased gradually by 0.1 or 0.2mg. Maintenance: 0.2 to 0.8mg in divided amounts. Usual max., 1.2mg daily. Max.: 2.4mg daily. If the patient complains of drowsiness, two-thirds of the total dose may be given at bedtime.
Transdermal	Initially: 0.1mg patch weekly applied to intact, hairless area of upper arm or anterior torso. Taper withdrawal of other antihypertensives that are to be discontinued. Increase after 1-2 weeks if necessary; max. 0.6mg daily. Rotate application sites.

Abrupt discontinuation of clonidine may result in a rapid increase in blood pressure; plan withdrawal over at least one week. Pediatric dosage of 0.005-0.01mg/kg daily in 2-3 divided doses has been suggested, but there is minimal pediatric experience.

PHARMACOKINETICS: Clonidine is readily absorbed after oral administration; bioavailability is 75%. Onset: 1 hour; Duration: 6-8 hours; Max. Effect: 3-4 hours. Volume of distribution is 2.1 liter/kg; Half-Life: 8.5 hours. Metabolism: Hepatic metabolism, 50%; 50% is eliminated unchanged in the urine; clearance is 3.1 ml/min/kg .

ADVERSE EFFECTS: The most common side effects of clonidine are drowsiness, dryness of the mouth, and constipation. Other adverse effects include weakness, sedation, pruritis, myalgia, urticaria, nausea, insomnia, arrhythmias, agitation, orthostatic hypotension, impotence. May cause depression.

CLONIDINE (Cont.)

PRECAUTIONS: Severe coronary insufficiency; recent myocardial infarction; cerebrovascular disease; renal failure. If local reaction occurs during patch use, oral substitution may cause generalized rash. Pregnancy (Cat.C).

Rebound hypertension may occur with abrupt discontinuance, particularly with prior administration of high doses or with continuation of concomitant beta-blocker therapy.

INTERACTIONS: Clonidine may be additive with, or may potentiate the action of other CNS depressants such as opiates, other analgesics, barbiturates or other sedatives, anesthetics or alcohol.

Tricyclic antidepressants, i.e., imipramine, desipramine, inhibit the hypotensive effect of clonidine.

CLORAZEPATE

(Tranxene, Cloraze Caps)

USES: Clorazepate is a benzodiazepine; uses are given in the next Table:

Uses of Clorazepate
Anxiety Disorders or Short Term Relief of Symptoms of Anxiety
Management of Agitation associated with Acute Alcohol Withdrawal
Adjunct in the Management of Partial Seizures

Clorazepate is metabolized to active metabolites.

DOSAGE FORMS: Caps and Tabs: 3.75, 7.5, and 15mg; Tabs: 11.25 and 22.5mg.

DOSAGE: The dosage of clorazepate is given in the next Table:

Dosage of Clorazepate

Condition	Dosage
Anxiety	30mg daily in divided doses; or a single daily dose at bedtime not to exceed 15mg; dosage range, 15 to 60mg in two to four divided doses.
Acute Alcohol Withdrawal	Initially, 30mg; day 1, 30-60mg; day 2, 45-90mg; day 3, 22.5-45mg; day 4, 15-30mg. Thereafter, gradually reduce daily dosage to 7.5-15mg and discontinue when the patients condition in stable
Partial Seizures	Adults and children >12: 7.5mg 3 times daily; dosage should be increased by no more than 7.5mg per week and should not exceed 90mg daily. Ages 9-12 Years: Initial dosage of 3.75 to 7.5mg twice daily; dosage should be increased by no more than 3.75mg weekly, max. 60mg daily.

Clorazepate is not recommended for children <9 years old.

PHARMACOKINETICS: Clorazepate is converted to desmethyldiazepam in the stomach and is absorbed rapidly in the intestine; steady-state concentrations of desmethyldiazepam are reached in 1-2 weeks.

ADVERSE EFFECTS: Frequent: drowsiness, ataxia; Occasional: confusion, amnesia, paradoxical excitement, dizziness, withdrawal symptoms including convulsions on abrupt discontinuation, rebound insomnia or excitment, blurred vision, depression; Rare: hypotension, blood dyscrasias, jaundice, allergic reactions, paradoxical rage reactions.

CLOTRIMAZOLE

(Lotrimin, Mycelex, Gyne-Lotrimin as vaginal cream)

USES: Clotrimazole is an **antifungal agent (Candida,** confirm by KOH microscopic mounts and/or culture); uses are given in the next Table:

Uses of Clotrimazole
Vulvovaginal Candidiasis (Moniliasis) and Trichomoniasis
Skin: Cutaneous Candidiasis (Moniliasis)
Dermatophytoses: Tinea pedis, Tinea Cruris and Tinea Corporis caused by T. Rubrum, T. Mentagrophyties, E. Floccosum or M. Canis; Tinea Vesicolor
Oropharyngeal Candidiasis

Vagina: Clotrimazole is used intravaginally for the treatment of vulvovaginal candidiasis (moniliasis) which has been confirmed by potassium hydroxide microscopic mounts and/or culture. Cure rates are similar to those achieved with nystatin vaginal tablets.

Clotrimazole has been used intravaginally in the treatment of trichomonal vaginitis; the drug is less effective than oral therapy with metronidazole. However, metronidazole is contraindicated during the first trimester of pregnancy and should be avoided during pregnancy, the CDC currently states that a 7-day regimen using 100-g vaginal tablets of clotrimazole daily can be used for the treatment of trichomoniasis in pregnant women.

Skin: Clotrimazole, like ciclopirox olamine, econazole nitrate, or miconazole, is active against bothCandida and dermatophytes.

Oropharynx: Clotrimazole is used in the form of a lozenge for the topical treatment of oropharyngeal candidiasis.

DOSAGE FORMS: Cream: 1% (15, 30g); Sol'n: 1% (10, 30ml); Vag. Cream: 1%; (45g with applicator); Vag. Tabs: 100mg, 500mg; Lozenges (10mg) for oral topical use.

DOSAGE: Clotrimazole is administered intravaginally as a cream or tablets; to the skin as a cream, lotion or solution; or as an oral lozenge for treatment of candidiasis of the oropharynx. Dosage is given in the next Table:

Dosage of Clotrimazole

Condition	Form of Drug	Dosage
Vulvovaginal Candidiasis	Tablet	100mg, intravaginally once daily (bedtime) for 7 consecutive days; can be used during pregnancy **or** 2 tablets, 100mg each, once daily (bedtime) for 3 consecutive days **or** 500mg vaginal tablet, single-dose (less effective)
	Cream	One applicatorful (approx. 5g), once daily(bedtime)for 7-14 consecutive days; can be used during pregnancy
Skin, Candidiasis or Dermatophytes	1% Cream or 1% Lotion or 1% Sol'n.	Apply sparingly and gently, morning and evening; expect improvement in one week and, in extreme, at 4 weeks. Up to 8 weeks may be necessary for tinea pedis.
Oropharynx	Lozenges	Dissolve slowly in the mouth over approx. 15-30 min. Use one 10mg lozenge 5 times daily for 14 consecutive days.

ADVERSE EFFECTS: Vaginal Tablets: Mild burning, vulval irritation, vaginal soreness during intercourse and dyspareunia. Topical: May cause erythema, blistering or urticaria.

CLOTRIMAZOLE, BETAMETHASONE
(Lotrisone)

USES: Clotrimazole is an antifungal agent; betamethasone is a glucocorticoid. Uses of Lotrisone are given in the next Table:

Uses of Lotrisone
Tinea Pedis, Tinea Cruris and Tinea Corporis caused by T. rubrum, T. mentagrophtes, E. floccosum and M. cunis.

Clinical studies indicate that clotrimazole is as effective as other topical imidazole derivates, eg, econazole and ketoconazole.

Clotrimazole exerts its antifungal effect by binding to phospholipid in the fungal cell membrane and thus altering cell membrane permeability.

The combination, clotrimazole and betamethasone in Lotrisone decreased the onset of therapeutic effects as opposed to the use of clotrimazole alone.

DOSAGE FORMS: Lotrisone is a cream containing clotrimazole, 10%, and betamethasone, 0.05% in 15g and 45g containers.

DOSAGE: Apply sparingly and massage in twice daily. Max. two weeks use for tinea cruris or tinea corporis; four weeks for tinea pedis.

ADVERSE EFFECTS: Erythema, stinging, blistering, peeling of skin, epidermal and dermal atrophy, local irritation, folliculitis, hypertrichosis and dermatitis.

Prolonged use of Lotrisone may cause suppression of the hypothalamic-pituitary-adrenal axis because of the glucocorticoid effects of betamethasone.

CLOXACILLIN
(Tegopen, Cloxapen)

USES: Cloxacillin is a penicillinase-resistant penicillin and is generally used only in the treatment of infections caused by, or suspected of being caused by, penicillinase-producing staphylococci. Cloxacillin should not be used orally for the initial treatment of severe, life-threatening infections, including endocarditis or meningitis, but may be used as follow-up therapy after parenteral penicillinase-resistant penicillin therapy.

DOSAGE FORMS: Caps: 250, 500mg; Sol'n: 125mg/5ml; Route: Orally

DOSAGE: Cloxacillin sodium is administered orally. The drug should be administered with a glass of water, at least 1 hour before or 2 hours after meals. Dosage is given in the next Table:

Dosage of Cloxacillin

Age	Dosage
>20 kg	50-100mg/kg daily in 4 divided doses; 2-4 times higher doses may be used in severe infections
>20 kg & Adults	1-2g/day divided every 6h; max. dose: 4g/day

PHARMACOKINETICS: Half-Life: 30 min.; 50 min. with severe renal impairment. 50% absorbed orally; peak at 1 hour; 75% of absorbed drug is excreted unchanged in urine.

ADVERSE EFFECTS: Hypersensitivity reactions: rash, fever, eosinophilia, pruritis and serum sickness-like reactions with fever, chills and myalgia. Anaphylaxis occurs rarely. Hematologic effects: eosinophilia, hemolytic anemia, transient neutropenia, leukopenia, thrombocytopenia. G.I. effects: nausea, vomiting, epigastric distress, loose stools, diarrhea and flatulence. Renal effects: acute interstitial nephritis; Hepatic effects: hepatitis or intrahepatic cholestasis.

PRECAUTIONS: Use with caution or not at all in patients with a history of penicillin or cephalosporin hypersensitivity.

CODEINE

USES: Codeine is 3-methoxy morphine and shares the general pharmacologic properties of morphine. Uses of codeine are given in the next Table:

Uses of Codeine
Mild Analgesic: Relief of Mild to Moderate Pain
Antitussive: Suppresses Cough Reflex

Codeine is a mild analgesic used in the relief of mild to moderate pain which is not relieved by a non-opiate analgesic. Codeine and acetaminophen, in combination, probably produce additive analgesic effects.

Codeine causes suppression of the cough reflex by direct effect on the cough center in the medulla of the brain; it is used, alone or in combination with other antitussives or expectorants, in the symptomatic relief of nonproductive cough.

DOSAGE FORMS: Tab: 15, 30, 60mg; Oral Sol'n: 15mg/5ml; Inj.: 15, 30, 60mg/ml. Formulated as phosphate or sulfate salt.

DOSAGE: Codeine Sulfate: Orally; Codeine Phosphate: Orally, Subcutaneously or IM. Dosage is given in the next Table:

Dosage of Codeine

Condition	Age	Route	Dosage
Analgesic	Adults	Oral, SubQ, IM	15-60mg every 4 hours, as needed
	Children	Oral, SubQ, IM	0.5-1.0mg/kg/dose every 4-6 h.
Antitussive	Adults & >11 yrs.	Oral	15-30mg every 4-6 h.; max. 120mg daily
	6-11 yrs.	Oral	5-10mg every 4-6h.; max. 60mg daily
	2-5 yrs.	Oral	1mg/kg/day divided every 4-6h.; max. 30mg daily

PHARMACOKINETICS: Onset, 15-30 min., Duration: 4-6 h.; Protein Bound: 7%; Metabolized in liver to narcodeine and morphine.

ADVERSE EFFECTS: Sedation, dizziness, nausea, vomiting, constipation and respiratory depression are most frequently observed. May be habit forming.

CODEINE, BUTALBITAL, ASPIRIN, CAFFEINE
(Fiorinal/Codeine)

USES: Fiorinal/codeine is used to treat mild to moderate pain associated with muscle contraction (tension) headache and may be helpful as an analgesic in migraine headache.

DOSAGE FORMS: Dosage forms of Fiorinal/codeine are given in the next Table:

Dosage Forms of Fiorinal/Codeine

Drug	Codeine Phosphate	Butalbital	Aspirin	Caffeine
Fiorinal/Codeine #1,Caps	7.5mg	50mg	325mg	40mg
Fiorinal/Codeine #2,Caps	15.0mg	50mg	325mg	40mg
Fiorinal/Codeine #3,Caps	30.0mg	50mg	325mg	40mg

DOSAGE: 1-2 caps, 3-4 times daily as needed; max. 6 caps daily.

CONTRAINDICATIONS: Severe bleeding or coagulation disorders, peptic ulcer, pregnancy (last trimester), porphyria

PRECAUTIONS: Asthma, gastritis, head injury, increased intracranial pressure, acute abdominal conditions, impaired renal, hepatic, thyroid, or adrenocortical function, prostatic hypertrophy or urethral stricture, elderly or debilitated.

ADVERSE EFFECTS: Drowsiness, dizziness, allergic reactions, gastric upset, nausea, vomiting, constipation, urinary retention, prolonged bleeding time, respiratory depression, salicylism with overdose, abuse potential.

INTERACTIONS: Alcohol, CNS depressants, anticoagulants, hypoglycemics, tricyclic antidepressants, MAOs, anticholinergics.

COLESTIPOL

(Colestid)

USES: **Colestipol** is used primarily to **lower serum cholesterol;** uses are given in the next Table:

Uses of Colestipol
Decrease Elevated Cholesterol and LDL Concentration
Relief of Pruritis Associated with Cholestasis

Decrease of Elevated Cholesterol: Colestipol is used in patients with type II hyperlipoproteinemia to lower serum cholesterol and low density lipoprotein(LDL) which carries cholesterol. Decreases in LDL-cholesterol of 10-15% may be obtained with the initial starting dosage schedule of 5g of colestipol taken twice daily; on average, there is a reduction of 15-30% in the concentration of LDL-cholesterol with 15-25g daily of colestipol.

Relief of Pruritis Associated with Cholestasis: Colestipol resin provides symptomatic relief of pruritis associated with partial obstructive jaundice and primary biliary cirrhosis. The pruritis in cholestasis is due to increase in bile salts in the circulation.

Mechanism of Action: Colestipol is an anion exchange resin which binds with bile acids in the intestine to form an insoluble complex that is excreted in the feces; this interrupts the enterohepatic circulation of bile acids and leads to an increased hepatic synthesis of bile acids from cholesterol as illustrated in the next Figure (Brown, M.S. and Goldstein, J.L., Science 232, 34-47, April 4, 1986):

Effect of Colestipol Binding to Bile Acids on Cholesterol Metabolism

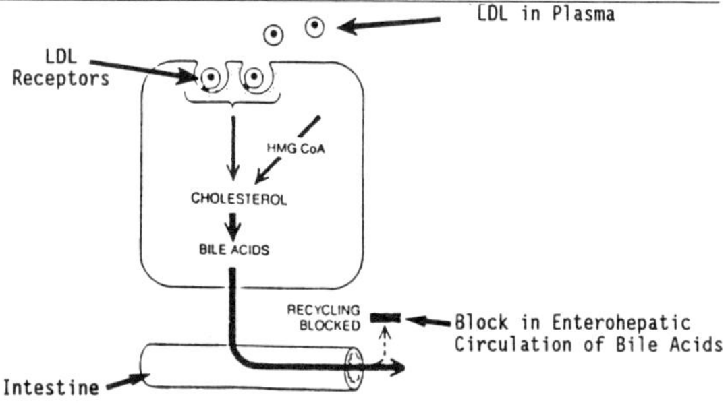

Depletion of the hepatic pool of cholesterol results in an increase in LDL receptor activity in the liver; this stimulates removal of LDL from plasma and lowers the concentration of LDL-cholesterol. Bile acid sequestration may increase hepatic VLDL production and thus increase the plasma concentration of triglycerides.

DOSAGE FORMS: 5 gram packet or scoop; granules.

DOSAGE: Colestipol dosage is given in the next Table:

Dosage or Colestipol

Age	Dosage
Adults	Initially, 5g twice daily; Max. dose: 30g daily in 2-4 divided doses
Children	125-500mg/kg daily in 2-4 divided doses. Experience is limited.

PHARMACOKINETICS: Colestipol is not absorbed from the G.I. tract. It takes 1-3 weeks for lipid lowering effect to occur; lipids return to pretreatment levels 2-4 weeks after the drug is discontinued.

ADVERSE EFFECTS: Colestipol is not absorbed from the gastrointestinal tract and systemic toxicity is minimal. However, gastrointestinal side effects are frequent. Constipation is the most frequent adverse effect, occurring especially in the elderly. Other adverse effects that occur occasionally include nausea, vomiting, flatulence, diarrhea, steatorrhea at high doses, abdominal distension and cramps.

COLESTIPOL (Cont.)

Colestipol resin contains chloride as its anion exchanger. This chloride may be absorbed instead of bicarbonate and lead to hyperchloremic metabolic acidosis especially in children; this effect may be partially offset by reducing chloride intake.

Colestipol occasionally interferes with the absorption of fat soluble vitamins, A,D,E and K. Prolonged use of colestipol may be associated with an increased bleeding tendency as a result of hypoprothrombinemia secondary to vitamin K deficiency.

Increased urinary calcium excretion may occur, leading potentially to osteoporosis.

There may be a moderate increase in plasma triglycerides in some patients.

An occasional mild and usually transient increase in alkaline phosphatase and transaminases may occur.

Folate deficiency may occur during long-term treatments and patients, especially children, should receive 5mg of folic acid daily, if necessary.

DRUG INTERACTIONS: Colestipol can decrease the absorption of other anionic drugs if these are taken concurrently. It is advisable to take other medications at least 1 hour before or 4 hours after taking colestipol. Colestipol can interfere with the absorption of digoxin, warfarin, thyroxine, thiazide diuretics, beta blockers and other drugs.

There may be decreased absorption of the fat soluble vitamins (A,D,E and K) and folic acid especially in patients treated with prolonged high doses of colestipol, primarily in patients with severe liver or small bowel disease; routine vitamin supplementation is not needed or recommended in adult patients.

CONTRAINDICATIONS: Colestipol can increase triglyceride levels and should not be used as single-drug therapy in patients with marked hypertriglyceridemia [triglyceride >500mg/dl (>5.7mmol/liter)].

It is also contraindicated in patients with severe constipation.

MONITOR: Monitor total cholesterol and LDL-cholesterol just prior to starting therapy, in 4-6 weeks, and at 3 months. If LDL-cholesterol goal is achieved, monitor total cholesterol at 4 month intervals and LDL-cholesterol annually. Electrolytes should be determined at two month intervals, especially in children. Prothrombin time(PT) should be determined at 3 month intervals.

CONTRACEPTIVES, ORAL

USES: Oral contraceptives contain estrogen and progestin or progestin alone. Oral contraceptives prevent pregnancy by inhibition of ovulation, endometrial changes hostile to egg implantation and cervical mucus changes.

Oral contraceptives inhibit ovulation through negative feed-back to the hypothalamus as illustrated in the next Figure:

Plasma FSH and LH Concentration in Normal Cycle and Following Oral Contraceptives

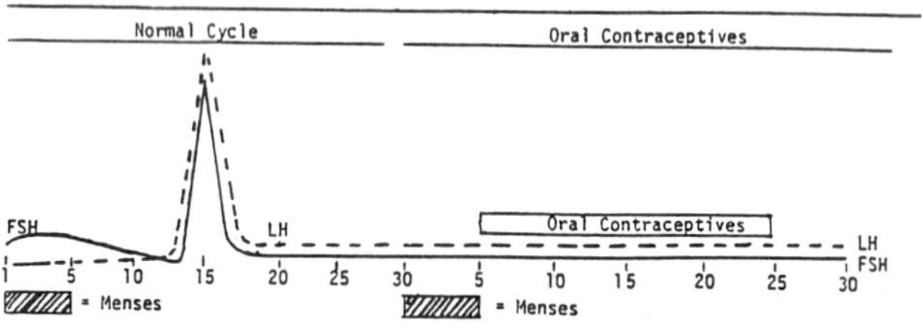

The estrogen acts mainly by suppressing secretion of follicle-stimulating hormone(FSH), resulting in prevention of follicular development and preventing the subsequent rise of plasma estradiol concentration which is thought to be the stimulus for release of luteinizing hormone (LH). Progestin acts mainly by inhibiting the preovulatory rise of LH.

Oral contraceptives causes thickening of the cervical mucus (except high estrogen concentration preparations); this thickening makes it difficult for the sperm to penetrate and travel into the uterus. In addition, the alteration in the uterus is unfavorable for nidation. Furthermore, tubal transport of the ova may be affected.

When progestin-only is used, inhibition of ovulation is not prominent; thick cervical mucus that is relatively impenetrable by sperm is produced. Tubular transport time may be increased and the endometrium may involute.

Ovulation usually resumes within 3 menstrual cycles after oral contraceptives have been discontinued; however, anovulation and amenorrhea may persist for 6 months or longer. After the drug is discontinued, recovery in sequence, is as follows: first, pituitary; second, ovary; third, uterus.

Administration of combination oral contraceptives may be started 2-4 weeks after full-term pregnancy.

DOSAGE FORMS AND DOSAGE: Oral contraceptives are mixtures of a synthetic estrogen (ethinyl estradiol or mestranol) and a progestin (norethindrone, norethindrone acetate, ethynodiol diacetate, norethynodrel, norgestrel, or levonorgestrel). Some preparations contain a progestin alone.

Combinations products may be classified according to estrogen content as shown in the next Table:

Classification of Oral Contraceptives According to Estrogen Content

Classification	Estrogen Content(mcg)
"Low Dose"	<50
"Regular"	50 or more
"Biphasic"	Two dosage regimens in a cycle
"Triphasic"	Three dosage regimens in a cycle

Combination oral contraceptives are started on the fifth day after onset of menses and are continued for a total of 21 days (days 5 through 24), followed by seven days without medication during which withdrawal bleeding occurs. Preparations are usually available in one or two forms. In one preparation, there are 21 tablets and the patient takes one tablet daily for 21 days followed by 7 tablet-free days. In another preparation, there are 28 tablets and the patient takes one oral contraception daily for 21 days followed by 7 inert tablets or 7 iron tablets.

CONTRACEPTIVES ORAL (Cont.)

Commercially available oral contraceptive preparations are given in the next Table (Medical Letter 30, 106, Nov. 18, 1988):

Oral Contraceptives

Type	Drug	Manufacturer	Estrogen (micrograms)	Progestin (mg)	No. of Tablets
COMBINED					
Ethinyl estradiol/ norethindrone	Loestrin 1/20	Parke-Davis	20	1*	21
	Loestrin(Fe)1/20	Parke-Davis	20	1*	28
	Loestrin 1.5/30	Parke-Davis	30	1.5*	21
	Loestrin(Fe)1.5/30	Parke-Davis	30	1.5*	28
	Brevicon	Syntex	35	0.5	21 or 28
*as norethindrone acetate	Modicon	Ortho	35	0.5	21 or 28
	Norinyl 1+35	Syntex	35	1	21 or 28
	Ortho-Novum 1/35	Ortho	35	1	21 or 28
	Ovcon-35	Mead Johnson	35	0.4	21 or 28
	Norlestrin 1/50	Parke-Davis	50	1*	21 or 28
	Norlestrin(Fe)1/50	Parke-Davis	50	1*	28
	Norlestrin2.5/50	Parke-Davis	50	2.5*	21
	Norlestrin(Fe)2.5/50	Parke-Davis	50	2.5*	28
	Ovcon-50	Mead Johnson	50	1	21 or 28
Ethinyl estradiol/ levonorgestrel	Levlen	Berlex	30	0.15	21 or 28
	Nordette	Wyeth	30	0.15	21 or 28
Ethinyl estradiol/ norgestrel	**Lo/Ovral**	Wyeth	30	0.3	21 or 28
	Ovral	Wyeth	50	0.5	21 or 28
Ethinyl estradiol/ ethynodiol diacetate	Demulen 1/35	Searle	35	1	21 or 28
	Demulen 1/50	Searle	50	1	21 or 28
Mestranol/ norethindrone	Norinyl 1+50	Syntex	50	1	21 or 28
	Ortho-Novum 1/50	Ortho	50	1	21 or 28
	Genora 1/50	Rugby	50	1	21 or 28
	Nelova 1/50	Warner Chilcott	50	1	21 or 28
	Norethin 1/50	Searle	50	1	21 or 28
Mestranol/ norethynodrel	Enovid 5mg	Searle	75	5	21
	Enovid 10mg	Searle	150	9.85	
BIPHASIC					
Ethinyl estradiol/ norethindrone	Ortho-Novum 10/11	Ortho	(10tabs)35 (11tabs)35	0.5 1	21 or 28
TRIPHASIC					
Ethinyl estradiol/ norethindrone	**Ortho-Novum 7/7/7**	Ortho	(7tabs)35 (7tabs)35 (7tabs)35	0.5 0.75 1	21 or 28
	Tri-Norinyl	Syntex	(7tabs)35 (9tabs)35 (5tabs)35	0.5 1 0.5	21 or 28
Ethinyl estradiol/ levonorgestrel	Tri-Levlen	Berlex	(6tabs)30 (5tabs)40 (10tabs)30	0.05 0.075 0.125	21 or 28
	Triphasil-21	Wyeth	(6tabs)30 (5tabs)40 (10tabs)30	0.05 0.075 0.125	21 or 28
PROGESTIN-ONLY					
Norethindrone	Micronor	Ortho	-	0.35	28
	Nor-Q.D.	Syntex	-	0.35	42
Norgestrel	Ovrette	Wyeth	-	0.075	28

The products in bold are those that are most commonly prescribed.

CONTRACEPTIVES ORAL (Cont.)

The oral contraceptive preparations that are most frequently used based on estrogen content are given in the next Table:

Most Frequently Used Oral Contraceptives

Estrogen Content	Product
Less than 50mcg Estrogen	Ortho-Novum 1/35-21 or 28; Lo/Ovral-21 or 28.
Less than 50mcg Estrogen, Triphasic	Ortho-Novum 7/7/7-21 or 28
50mcg Extrogen	Ortho-Novum 1/50-21 or 28; Ovral

Preparations containing 35mcg of estrogen or less and a low dose of a progestin are preferred to minimize the risk of cardiovascular adverse effects. The pharmaceutical firms (Ortho, Searle and Syntex) phased out during 1988-1990 sale of pills with more than 50micrograms of estrogen because of the higher incidence of thromboembolism in the high estrogen preparations.

FAILURE RATE: The percent accidental pregnancy during first year of use is given in the next Table (Trussell, J. and Kost, K., Stud. Fam. Plann. 18, 237, 1987; Sivin, I. and Schmidt, F., Contraception 36, 55, 1987):

Percent Accidental Pregnancy

Oral Contraceptive	Failure Rate: Optimal	Failure Rate: Typical
Combined (Estrogen plus Progestin)	0.1	3
Progestin only	0.5	2

PROGESTIN-ONLY: Oral contraceptives containing only a progestin have a higher failure rate than combination contraceptives and my cause irregular bleeding.

The principal indication for progestin-only contraceptives is for nursing mothers who want to use an oral contraceptive; estrogens are contra-indicated during nursing because they decrease lactation.

SUMMARY: A summary of uses of oral contraceptives in different conditions is given in the next Table:

Uses of Oral Contraceptives

Use	Dosage
Contraception	One tablet daily beginning on fifth day after onset of menses and continued for 21 days; stop for 7 days or take 7 inert tablets and restart the next cycle. Onset of contraception after one week.
Contraception Postpartum	Start 2-4 weeks postpartum
Contraception Post-abortion	Start immediately if gestation terminated at 12 weeks or less; Start in one week if gestation terminated at 13-28 weeks.
Dysfunctional Uterine Bleeding (Anovulatory Cycles)	Any combination contraceptive; one tablet 4 times daily for 5-7 days for acute bleeding; then 1 tablet daily cyclically as for contraception to prevent further bleeding. Dysfunctional uterine bleeding should decrease within 12 to 24 hours.
Dysmenorrhea or Endometriosis	Use minimal estrogen, maximal progestin combination, such as Ovral, Demulen, Norlestrin 2.5mg. One tablet cyclically as for contraception for 3-9 months to induce a pseudopregnant state.
Emergency Postcoital Contraception	Two tablets of Ovral taken as soon as possible after coitus, and two more tablets taken 12 hrs. later but within 72 hours after coitus. See Table below.

PATIENT INSTRUCTIONS FOR CONTRACEPTION: If one dose is missed, take it as soon as it is remembered or take two tablets the next day. If two doses are missed, take two tablets daily for the next two days. If more than two doses are missed and bleeding occurs, consider as a normal period and restart cycle; also use an alternative form of contraception for the remainder of the cycle. Report if no menses occur for two months.

MEDROXYPROGESTERONE ACETATE: Parenteral medroxyprogesterone acetate is used in many countries other than the United States for contraception; it has a failure rate less than that of any other method of contraception. Dosage is 150mg of medroxyprogesterone acetate, IM, every 3 months.

CONTRACEPTIVES, ORAL (Cont.)

Medroxyprogesterone acetate (Depo-Provera), a synthetic progestin, is approved by the FDA in the United States for treatment of endometrial and renal cancer and in Canada for treatment of endometriosis and breast cancer.

POSTCOITAL "MORNING AFTER" CONTRACEPTIVE REGIMENS: Postcoital contraceptive regimens are given in the next Table (Drug Evaluations, 6th ed., Am. Med. Assoc., Chicago, Ill., 1986, pg. 730):

Postcoital Contraceptive Regimens

Estrogen	Dosage
Ethinyl Estradiol and Norgestrel(available as Ovral)	100mcg ethinyl estradiol and 1mg norgestrel (two Ovral tablets)taken twice 12 hours apart.
Ethinyl Estradiol	2.5mg twice daily for five days.
Conjugated Estrogens	10mg three times daily for five days.
Estrone	5mg three times daily for five days.
Diethylstilbestrol	25mg twice daily for five days.

PATIENT INSTRUCTIONS FOR ACUTE ANOVULATORY BLEEDING: Expect heavy and severely cramping flow 2-4 days after stopping pills with normal periods thereafter.

PHARMACOKINETICS: Onset of Contraception: After one week of starting regimen. Dysfunctional Uterine Bleeding: Within 12-24 hours of starting regimen; Half-Life: Ethinyl estradiol: 6-20 hours; Norgestrel: 11-45 hours; Norethindrone, 5-14 hours; Norethindrone, 5-14 hours. Metabolism: Ethinyl estradiol is metabolized by the liver; 20% is excreted in the urine as the glucuronide and 50% is excreted in the bile. For the metabolism of norgestrel, 30% is excreted unchanged in the urine and 70% is metabolized by the liver.

"ABORTION PILL": An "abortion pill" (trade name, Mifepristone) has been introduced in France; this compound blocks the action of progesterone and induces abortion. It is effective in 80% of patients when used alone and in 95% when used with prostaglandin. It cannot be taken later than 49 days after pregnancy starts because French legislation authorizes abortion until the 12th week of pregnancy.

A major side effect is prolonged bleeding. The drug is teratogenic in several animal species and one woman who had taken it at an early stage of pregnancy is reported to have given birth to a child with multiple deformities.

This drug may be useful in treating some forms of cancer.

There has been no attempt to obtain FDA approval of this drug in the United States.

CONTRACEPTIVES, ORAL (Cont.)

ADVERSE EFFECTS: Adverse effects of oral contraceptives are given in the next Table:

Adverse effects of Oral Contraceptives

Adverse Effect	Comment
Myocardial Infarction	Risk 2.8 times; especially in females>35 years, smokers and presence of other risk factors such as increased cholesterol (increased low density lipoprotein), and increased blood pressure; risk may persist after discontinuation in long term users. May be related to increased estrogen/progestin ratio.
Thromboembolism and Thrombophlebitis with possible Pulmonary Embolism	Risk 4-11 times; especially females >35 years, smokers and duration of use >5 years. Risk decreased with estrogen <50mcg. Estrogens decrease antithrombin III and increase coagulation factors and platelet factors.
Stroke and Transient Ischemic Attacks	Risk of thrombolic stroke, 10 times; risk of hemorrhagic stroke, 2 times. The usual cause of fatal stroke is subarachnoid hemorrhage.
Hypertension	Risk 3-6 times. The increase in blood pressure is usually reversible within 1-6 months after cessation of therapy. The mechanism of hypertension probably involves the renin-angiotensin system; the concentration of angiotensin the substrate for renin, is increased and the negative feedback control of renin is impaired; elevated levels of angiotensin and aldosterone results.
Gallstones	Risk 2 times especially in older women;estrogens increase cholesterol excretion in bile.
Cholestatic Jaundice	Increased risk in women who developed jaundice during pregnancy or women with a genetic predisposition.
Hepatic Tumors	Risk greater with duration of use. Tumor may be highly vascular and rupture of tumor and hemorrhage may occur.
Endometrial and Ovarian Cancer	Oral contraceptive use protects against endometrial and ovarian cancer (CDC, JAMA 257, 796, 1986; N. Engl. J. Med. 316, 650, 1987; WHO Collaborative Study, Int. J. Epidemiol. 17, 263, 1988).
Postpill Amenorrhea	Prevalence 0.2-2.6%. Unrelated to duration or dose.
Metabolic	Abnormal glucose tolerance in predisposed individuals.

CONTRAINDICATIONS: Known or suspected pregnancy; presence or history of thrombophlebitis or thromboembolic disorders; cerebral or coronary artery disease; impaired liver function; heavy smoking in women 35 years or older; undiagnosed abnormal genital bleeding; estrogen-dependent tumors such as breast carcinoma and endometrial carcinoma: patients with hyperlipidemia.

PRECAUTIONS: Use with caution in patients with hypercholesterolemia, diabetes, severe varicosities, in adolescents in whom regular menses are not established and in conditions which may be aggravated by fluid retention, such as hypertension, cardiac or renal dysfunction.

ABNORMAL LABORATORY VALUES: Oral contraceptives cause elevation of laboratory as follows: blood glucose, iron and iron binding capacity, coagulation factors, total T-4, cortisol.

DRUG INTERACTIONS: The following drugs decrease the effectiveness of oral contraceptives in preventing pregnancy: rifampin, barbiturates, anticonvulsants, griseofulvin. These drugs taken concurrently can increase the metabolism of contraceptive hormones.

The bioavailability of imipramine and theophylline may be increased.

CORTISONE ACETATE
(Cortone)

USES: Cortisone acetate or hydrocortisone is usually the corticosteroid of choice for replacement therapy in patients with adrenocortical insuffiency; these drugs have both glucocorticoid and mineralcorticoid properties. Concomittant administration of a more potent mineralocorticoid such as desoxy-corticosterone or fludrocortisone may be required in some patients.

Cortisone acetate is not used for anti-inflammatory or immunosuppressive conditions; synthetic glucocorticoids which have mineral mineralocorticoids activity are preferred.

DOSAGE FORMS: Tabs:5, 10, 25mg; Parenteral: 50mg/ml; Route: Oral or IM

DOSAGE: Cortisone acetate is administered orally or IM; IM therapy is used in patients who are unable to take the drug orally. Following long-term therapy, cortisone should be withdrawn gradually. Dosage is given in the next Table:

Dosage of Cortisone Acetate

Condition	Age	Route	Dosage
Physiologic Replacement	Adults	Oral	25-30mg daily in 4 divided doses
		IM	0.25-0.35mg/kg/day
	Children	Oral	0.5-0.75mg/kg/day in 3 divided doses
		IM	0.25-0.35mg/kg/day

Stressful situations require 2-4 times physiologic replacement dose.

PHARMACOKINETICS: Half-Life: 0.5 hrs.

ADVERSE EFFECTS: Common side effects following prolonged use include: hypokalemic alkalosis, hyperglycemia and glycosuria, increased susceptibility to infection, exacerbation of peptic ulcers, myopathy, psychoses, osteoporosis, vertebral compression fractures, Cushing's habitus, acne, hirsutism, cataracts, hypertension.

Acute withdrawal is associated with hypotension, hypoglycemia, shock, fever, myalgia, arthralgia and malaise.

MONITOR: Electrolytes at 2-3 month intervals.

CROMOLYN SODIUM

(Intal, Nasalcrom, Opticrom)

USES: Uses of cromolyn sodium are given in the next Table:

Uses of Cromolyn
Asthma
Prevention of Exercise-Induced Bronchospasm
Allergic Rhinitis
Allergic Conjunctivitis
Systemic Mastocytosis

Cromolyn sodium is used prophylactically for the treatment of asthma, allergic rhinitis and prevention and treatment of allergic conjunctivitis.

Asthma: Cromolyn sodium is not a bronchodilator and has no anti-inflammatory or antihistaminic effect. It prevents the release of chemical mediators that cause the signs and symptoms of an acute asthmatic attack; it can only be used prophylactically. In patients who respond, it takes at least 3-5 days and often up to one month to become effective. It is effective in the prevention of nonimmune responses such as cold air-induced, hyperventilation-induced and exercise-induced airway obstruction. It is used to prevent antigen-induced asthma, eg, extrinsic allergic asthma (severe perennial asthma). It is helpful in permitting gradual steroid reduction by 25-80% or even withdrawal in selected patients. Routine daily administration is necessary.

Allergic Rhinitis: Cromolyn sodium is an effective medication in the treatment of allergic rhinitis and reduces the need for antihistaminics (Chandra, R.K., et al., Ann. Allergy 49, 131, 1983).

Allergic Conjunctivitis: Allergic conjunctivitis may be associated with hay fever, a particular time of year (vernal or seasonal keratoconjunctivitis), atopic dermatitis or eczema (atopic keratoconjunctivitis), or with contact lenses or plastic ocular prostheses (giant papillary conjunctivitis). Cromolyn sodium apears to be safe and may relieve or prevent some symptoms in some types of allergic conjunctivitis and associated keratitis; it may take several days to a week or more for symptoms to improve (Medical Letter 27, 7-8, Jan. 18, 1985).

It has not been determined whether cromolyn sodium is as effective as topical corticosteroids; however, prolonged ophthalmic use of steroids can cause glaucoma, cataracts, and other serious complications.

Mechanism of Action: Cromolyn sodium blocks degranulation of mast cells, preventing release of histamine and other substances stored in its granules that cause hypersensitivity reactions. The most likely mechanism for this action is the prevention of entry of calcium ions into the mast cells by interference with the calcium gate mechanism. It is not effective in counteracting the effects of mediators once they are released. It has no direct vasoconstrictor, antihistaminic or anti-inflammatory activity.

Cromolyn acts on cells of the lung mucosa, nasal mucosa and eyes. Cromolyn prevents release of the mediators of type I allergic reactions, including histamine and slow-reacting substance of anaphylaxis (SRS-A) from sensitized mast cells after the antigen-antibody reaction has occurred. Cromolyn does not inhibit the binding of IgE to mast cells nor the interaction between cell-bound IgE and the specific antigen; however, cromolyn suppresses the release of substances, histamine, SRS-A that occurs following this reaction. Cromolyn also inhibits type III (late allergic, Arthus) reactions. Cromolyn has no bronchodilator, antihistaminic or anti-inflammatory activity.

DOSAGE FORMS: Cromolyn sodium is available as a dry powder aerosol or as a 1% solution for treatment of asthma (Intal), as a liquid nasal spray for allergic rhinitis (Nasalcrom), and as a 4% ophthalmic solution for prevention and treatment of allergic conjunctivitis (Opticrom). Oral Inhalation: Powder for inhalation (contained in capsules) 20mg (Intal); Solution for nebulization, 20mg/2ml, (Intal nebulizer solution). Aerosol for inhalation: 800micrograms/metered spray. Nasal Solution: 5.2mg/metered spray (40mg/ml) (Nasalcrom). Ophthalmic Solution: 4% (Opticrom). Capsules (oral administration) (Gastrocrom): 100mg.

CROMOLYN SODIUM (Cont.)
DOSAGE: Cromolyn sodium must be taken daily. It is not absorbed orally and is only effective by inhalation or by application to the eye. Oral Inhalation: Cromolyn sodium powder is administered by inhalation from capsules containing the powder using a special oral inhaler (Spinhaler).

Cromolyn sodium oral solution is administered by nebulization using a power-operated nebulizer and face mask. Cromolyn sodium inhaler delivers 800micrograms/metered spray.

Nasal Inhalation: Cromolyn sodium nasal solution is administered by nasal inhalation using a special nasal inhaler (Nasalmatic). The nasal inhaler delivers 5.2mg of cromolyn sodium per metered spray; the commercially available preparation delivers about 100 metered sprays.

Dosage of cromolyn sodium to be give in the next Table:

Dosage of Cromolyn Sodium

Condition	Age	Route	Dosage
Asthma	Adults and Children 2 years and older	Oral Inhal. Sol'n	20mg inhaled four times daily at regular intervals; when stabilized, reduce to 3 times daily.
	5 years or older and adults	Powder for Oral Inhal.	20mg inhaled 4 times daily at regular intervals;when stabilized, reduce to 3 times daily.
		Metered dose Inhaler	1.6mg (2 inhalations) 4 times daily; reduce to 3 times daily when stable.
Exercise-Induced Bronchospasm	Adults & Child, 2 yrs. or older	Oral Inhal. Sol'n	20mg inhaled not longer than 1 hour before anticipated exercise.
	5 yrs. or Older and Adults	Powder for Oral Inhal.	20mg inhaled not longer than 1 hour before anticipated exercise.
		Metered dose Inhaler	1.6mg (2 inhalations) not longer than 1 hour before anticipated exercise.
Allergic Rhinitis (Prevention and Treatment)	Adults and Child.>5 yrs.	Nasal Inhaler	Nasal inhaler delivers 5.2 mg of cromolyn sodium per metered spray. One spray in each nostril 3 or 6 times daily. For seasonal rhinitis, continue therapy until pollen season is over. Symptomatic relief,2-4 wks.
Allergic Ocular Disorders	Adults and Child. >3 years	Ocular Drops	One or two drops in each eye 4-6 times daily.
Systematic Mastocytosis	Adults	Oral	100-200mg, 4 times daily

PHARMACOKINETICS: Onset: 1 min. Duration: 5 hr. Half-Life: 80-90 min. after inhalation. Fate: About 1% of inhaled dose is absorbed orally; about 8% is absorbed from lung; most is cleared by mucociliary mechanisms and appears in feces.
ADVERSE EFFECTS: Cromolyn sodium is the only asthma drug that is virtually free of serious side effects; only 2% of patients experienced side effects, most being transient skin eruptions (Settipane, G.A., et al., JAMA 241, 811, 1979). Bronchospasm and pharyngeal irritation, coughing and sneezing occur occasionally; use of a bronchodilator aerosol just prior to cromolyn may prevent bronchospasm. Other adverse effects include rash, urticaria, dizziness, nausea, vomiting and hoarseness.
CONTRAINDICATIONS: Acute wheezing. Not recommended in patients with renal or hepatic dysfunction.

CROTAMITON
(Eurax)

USES: **Crotamiton** is used for the topical treatment of the **parasitic mite**, Sarcoptes scabiei, the causative agent of scabies.
DOSAGE FORMS: Cream (10%): 60g; Lotion (10%): 60ml; Route: Topical
DOSAGE: One treatment (2 applications) with crotamiton is usually highly effective in eradicating scabies.

Massage into skin from neck down, with particular attention to skin folds and creases. Clothing and bed sheets should be changed on the morning following the first application. Repeat in 24h. Bath 48 hours after last application.
ADVERSE EFFECTS: Mildly irritating. Do not apply to raw or weeping skin. Avoid application near eyes or mouth.

CYCLOBENZAPRINE
(Flexeril)

USES: Cyclobenzaprine is used as an adjunct to rest, physical therapy, and other appropriate therapy in the short-term treatment of painful local muscle spasm.

It is structurally and pharmacologically related to the tricyclic antidepressants.
DOSAGE FORMS: Tabs, 10mg
DOSAGE: Adults: 10-20mg three times daily (maximum 60mg daily); limit treatment to 3 weeks.
PHARMACOKINETICS: Absorption: rapid; Metabolism: G.I. tract or liver; Onset: one hour; Duration of Action: 12-24 hours. Protein-Binding: 93%; Excretion: kidney as glucuronide conjugates.
ADVERSE EFFECTS: The most common side effects are drowsiness (39%), dryness of the mouth (27%), and dizziness (11%). These effects reflect the anticholinergic and sedative actions of cyclobenzaprine as an tricyclic antidepressant. Other adverse effects that occur occasionally are as follows: tachycardia, weakness, dyspepsia, paresthesia, blurred vision, unpleasant taste, nausea and insomnia. Adverse effects that occur rarely are as follows: sweating, myalgia, dyspnea, abdominal pain, constipation, coated tongue, tremors, dysarthria, euphoria, nervousness, disorientation, confusion, headache, urinary retention, decreased bladder tonus, ataxia and allergic reactions.
PRECAUTIONS: Urinary retention, glaucoma, pregnancy (Cat. B), lactation.
CONTRAINDICATIONS: Acute recovery phase of myocardial infarction, patients with arrhythmias, heart block, conduction disturbances, or congestive heart failure.
DRUG INTERACTIONS: Cyclobenzaprine may interact with monoamine oxidase inhibitors when given concomitantly or within 14 days after their discontinuation. It may enhance effects of alcohol, other central nervous system depressants and drugs with anticholinergic actions.

The antihypertensive action of guanethidine and related drugs may be antagonized.

CYCLOPHOSPHAMIDE
(Cytoxan, Neosar)

USES: Cyclophosphamide, an antineoplastic agent, is the most widely used alkylating agent; indications are given in the next Table:

Uses of Cyclophosphamide
Cancer: Hodgkin's Disease and Malignant Lymphomas, Multiple Myeloma, Leukemias, Mycosis Fungoides, Neuroblastoma, Ovarian Carcinoma, Retinoblastoma, Breast Carcinoma, Choriocarcinoma, Lung Cancer, Rhabdomyosarcoma and others.
Rheumatoid Arthritis
Nephrotic Syndrome in Children
Wegener's Granulomatosis
Following Bone Marrow, Kidney, Heart, Liver Transplant

DOSAGE FORMS: Inj: 100, 200, 500mg; 1g, 2g; Tabs: 25,50mg

DOSAGE: Cyclophosphamide is administered orally or by IV injection. Dosage is given in the next Table (check specific treatment protocols):

Dosage of Cyclophosphamide

Age	Dosage
Adults	Patients with no hematologic deficiences Loading Dose: 40-50mg/kg (1.5-1.8g/m^2), IV, in divided doses over 2-5 days; if induction therapy is administered orally, 1-5mg/kg/day. Maintenance Dose: 1-5mg/kg/day orally; or 10-15mg/kg(350-550mg/m^2) IV every 7-10 days; or 3-5 mg/kg (110-185 mg/m^2) IV twice weekly.
Children	Loading Dose: 2-8mg/kg or 60-250mg/m^2/day orally or IV. Maintenance Dose: 2-5mg/kg orally or 50-150mg/m^2 orally, administered twice weekly.

PHARMACOKINETICS: Oral: max. conc. 1 hour; Distribution: throughout the body; Protein Binding: 0-10%; Serum Half-Life: 4.0-6.5 hours. Metabolism: liver; Excretion: urine.

ADVERSE EFFECTS: Hematologic effects: leukopenia, thrombocytopenia, hypoprothrombinemia, and anemia. Leukopenia nadirs occur at 8-15 days following a single dose and recovery usually occurs within 17-28 days. Thrombocytopenia nadirs occur at 10-15 days. Anemia may occur after large doses or prolonged therapy. Hypoprothrombinemia occurs rarely.

GI Effects: Anorexia, nausea, and vomiting occur commonly, especially at high doses; these effects may respond to treatment with antiemetics. Occasionally, diarrhea, hemorrhagic colitis, mucosal irritation, and oral ulceration have occurred. Rarely, aphthous stomatitis (oral cavity lesions: small whitish lesions surrounded by a red border which ulcerate before healing) and enterocolitis occur. Hepatotoxicity has been reported.

Genitourinary Effects: Sterile hemorrhagic cystitis is observed in up to 20% or patients, especially children. Nephrotoxicity and tubular necrosis have been reported.

Dermatologic Effects: About 33% of patients develop alopecia, generally beginning 3 weeks after initiation of therapy; the condition is reversible. Skin pigmentation and fingernail ridging, growth retardation and pigmentation may occur.

Pulmonary Effects: Fatal interstitial pulmonary fibrosis may develop in patients who receive high doses over prolonged periods; discontinuance of the drug and administration of steroids do not necessarily reverse this condition.

Metabolic Effects: Hyperuricemia may occur, especially in those patients with non-Hodgkin's lymphoma or leukemia. Hyperuricemia is minimized by adequate hydration, alkalinization of the urine and/or administration of allopurinol.

Other metabolic effects that may be observed are hyperkalemia, hyponatremia secondary to inappropriate antidiuretic hormone syndrome(SIADH) may occur.

Cardiac Effects: Diffuse hemorrhagic myocardial necrosis and pericarditis have been reported.

Other Adverse Effects: Other adverse effects include headache, dizziness, and myxedema. Following IV administration, faintness, facial flushing, diaphoresis and oropharyngeal sensation have occurred.

PARAMETERS MONITOR: Prior to induction therapy, white cells should be greater than 3,500/cu mm and platelets greater than 120,000/cu mm. With chronic dosing, WBC's and platelets should be assayed at least monthly.

CYCLOSPORINE
(Sandimmune)

USES: Cyclosporine is widely used as an immunosuppressant,with the ability to prolong graft survival by inhibiting delay hypersensitivity without bone marrow suppression.It is used for the prevention of rejection in human kidney, liver, heart, heart-lung, and bone marrow transplantation. Cyclosporine is preferable to azathioprine in preventing renal transplant rejection (Multi-centre Transplant Study Group, N.Engl. J. Med. 309, 809-815, 1983).

Cyclosporine is a cyclic non-polar polypeptide consisting of 11 amino acids and is of fungal origin.

Cyclosporine selectively inhibits T-helper cell function and number. The drug depletes medullary thymocytes and splenic T-lymphocytes. There is a relative sparing of T-suppressor cells.

Cyclosporine reversibly inhibits the macrophage T-lymphocyte activation and impairs the production of interleukin-2, a growth factor essential for T-cell proliferation and differentiation into cytotoxic T-cells. The drug does not inhibit mature, proliferating T-cells.

Cyclosporine suppresses primary and, to a lesser degree, secondary antibody responses to T-cell-dependent antigens. The inhibition of antibody production to T-cell-dependent antigens is a consequence of impaired T-helper cell function, which is required for B-cell growth and differentiation (Review: Kahan, B.D., N. Engl. J. Med. 321, 1725-1738, 1989).

DOSAGE FORMS: Caps: 25, 100mg; Oral solution: 100mg/ml; Parenteral concentrate: 50mg/ml.

DOSAGE: Cyclosporine is administered orally or by IV infusion. The gastrointestinal absorption of cyclosporine is erratic; therefore, cyclosporine blood concentrations should be monitored frequently and the dosage adjusted accordingly. Cyclosporine is routinely administered with adrenal corticosteroids.

To increase the palatability of the oral solution, a measured dose of cyclosporine is diluted at room temperature with milk, chocolate milk, or orange juice and then stirred well and administered immediately. Do not store oral solution in the refrigerator; use glass containers only. Usual dosage or`adults and children is given in the next Table:

Usual Dosage for Adults and Children of Cyclosporine

Route	Dosage
Oral	Initial (4-12 hours before transplantation): 15mg/kg Postoperatively:15mg/kg daily as a single dose for 1-2 weeks and then tapered by 5% per week (over about 6-8 weeks) to a maintenance dosage of 5-10 mg/kg daily.
IV Infusion	IV infusion is used in patients unable to take the drug orally. Initial IV dosage: 5-6mg/kg as a single dose 4-12 hours before transplatation. Postoperatively: 5-6mg/kg once daily until the patient is able to tolerate oral administration of the drug.

MONITOR: Cyclosporine is monitored by radioimmunoassary (RIA) or by high performance liquid chromatography (HPLC).

The trough concentration determined just prior to the next dose (24 hours after the previous dose) should be 250-800ng/ml (blood) or 100-250ng/ml (plasma) to minimize adverse effects and graft rejection. The level should be determined 3 times weekly during the early posttransplantation period and then periodically.

PHARMACOKINETICS: Absorption: Absorption from the gastrointestinal tract is variable. Peak blood and plasma concentrations occur in approximately 3.5 hrs. The maximum concentration is about 1ng/ml/mg of dose and 1.4 to 2.7ng/ml/mg of dose for blood. Administration of cyclosporine with food increases peak and trough concentrations. Distribution: Most of cyclosporine is distributed outside the blood volume. The distribution is concentration-dependent in blood: 33%-47% in plasma; 4%-9% in leukocytes; 5%-12% in granulocytes; 40%-60% in erythrocytes. Protein Binding: Approximately 90% of cyclosporine is bound to lipoprotein; binding to lipoprotein might be expected considering the non - polar characteristics of cyclosporine. Metabolism: Cyclosporine is extensively metabolized with only 0.1% excreted unchanged in the urine. There is no major metabolic pathway. Half-Life: The elimination half-life is 10 to 27 hours. Elimination: Cyclosporine is excreted primarily in the bile; only 6% is excreted in the urine.

CYCLOSPORINE (Cont.)
ADVERSE EFFECTS: The principal adverse effects of cyclosporine are given in the next Table:

Adverse Effects of Cyclosporine
Renal Dysfunction (25% to 40% of patients)
Neurotoxicity
Hepatotoxicity
Hypertension
Thromboembolism

Nephrotoxicity: The main adverse effect of cyclosporine is nephrotoxicity. Cyclosporine-induced nephrotoxicity is associated with serum creatinine concentrations that rise rapidly or slowly over several weeks. Clues to graft rejection are fever, graft tenderness or enlargement.
Neurotoxicity: Neurotoxicity includes hallucinations, generalized epileptic seizures, convulsions, limb paresthesias and tremor. Seizures may be due to renal magnesium wasting and is resolved by magnesium replacement.
Hepatotoxicity: Hepatotoxicity occurs in about 5% of patients. A reduction in cyclosporine dosage rapidly reverses the hepatoxicity effects.
Hypertension: Hypertension occurs in about 25% of patients.
DRUG INTERACTIONS: Numerous drug interactions, some of the more important of which are listed here. Cyclosporine is very nephrotoxic; other nephrotoxic drugs may potentiate this effect (eg, aminoglycosides, amphotericin B, acyclovir). Drugs that increase the plasma concentration of cyclosporine include ketoconazole, erythromycin, corticosteroids, and diltiazem; mechanism is probably inhibition of hepatic microsomal enzymes. Drugs that decrease the plasma concentration of cyclosporine include phenobarbital, phenytoin, and rifampin, probably by increasing hepatic metabolism. Therapeutic drug monitoring is critical to the management of patients receiving cyclosporine, especially with concomittant administration of other drugs.

CYPROHEPTADINE
(Periactin)
USES: Cyproheptadine is a potent antihistaminic; in allergic conditions, it shares the actions and uses of other antihistamines. It is considered by some clinicians as the drug of choice for treatment of cold urticaria.
OTHER USES: Cyproheptadine is effective in some patients for the treatment of Cushing's syndrome secondary to pituitary disorders; the beneficial effects are generally believed to result from the drugs antiserotonergic activity.
DOSAGE FORMS: Tabs: 4mg; Syrup: 2mg/5ml; Route: Orally
DOSAGE: Cyproheptadine hydrochloride is administered orally; dosage is given in the next Table:

Dosage of Cyproheptadine

Age	Dosage
Adults	4mg, 3-4 times daily; max. 0.5mg/kg daily
7-14 years	4mg, 2-3 times daily; max. 16mg daily
2-6 years	2mg, 2-3 times daily; max. 12mg daily
Pediatric (by wt)	0.25-0.5mg/kg daily in 2-3 divided doses

PHARMACOKINETICS: About 70% excreted in urine as conjugate of glucuronic acid; remainder excreted in feces.
ADVERSE EFFECTS: Drowsiness, dry mouth, dizziness and irritability with intermittent therapy; however, most patients develop tolerance to these side effects during continuous therapy as dose is increased slowly. Stimulates appetite and weight gain. See **ANTIHISTAMINES.**
CONTRAINDICATIONS: Concurrent use of MAO inhibitors, asthma, lactation, glaucoma, gastrointestinal or urinary tract obstruction.

DANTROLENE
(Dantrium)

USES: Dantrolene is a hydantoin derivative. It causes **skeletal muscle relaxation** through a direct effect on skeletal muscle. Uses are given in the next Table:

Uses of Dantrolene
Spasticity from Upper Motor Neuron Disorders, e.g., **Cerebral Palsy, Spinal Cord Injury, Stroke Syndrome** **Multiple Sclerosis**
Malignant Hyperthermia
Neuroleptic Malignant Syndrome (NMS)

Dantrolene is used in the management of spasticity resulting from upper motor neuron disorders such as cerebral palsy, spinal cord injury, stroke syndrome and multiple sclerosis.

Oral dantrolene is also used for the prophylaxis of malignant hyperthermia crisis in individuals thought to be at risk; IV dantrolene is used in the management of malignant hyperthermia crisis.

DOSAGE FORMS: Caps: 25, 50, 100mg; IV: 0.33mg/ml in 60ml vials with 3gm mannitol.

DOSAGE: Dantrolene sodium is administered orally for the management of spasticity, for preoperative prophylaxis of malignant hyperthermia crisis in patients at risk, and to prevent recurrence of the manifestations of malignant hyperthermia following initial IV therapy. Dosage is given in the next Table:

Dosage of Dantrolene

Condition	Age	Route	Dosage
Chronic Spasticity	Adults	Oral	Dosage increased at 4-7 day intervals. Initial: 25mg daily; then give 25mg 2-4 times a day & increase by 25mg increments up to 100mg 4 times a day as needed. Some patients require 400mg daily
	Child.	Oral	Dosage increased at 4-7 day intervals. Initial:0.5mg/kg twice a day; then give 0.5mg/kg three or four times daily and increase by 0.5mg/kg up to 3mg/kg 2, 3 or 4 times daily - do not exceed 100mg four times daily.
Prevention of Malignant Hyperthermia Crisis		Oral	4-8mg/kg daily in 3 or 4 divided doses for 1-2 days prior to surgery with last dose 3-4 h. prior to surgery or 2.5mg/kg IV over 1 h. beginning 1.25 h. prior to surgery.
Malignant Hyperthermia Crisis	Adults Child.	IV	Initial: 1mg/kg. If needed, repeat; max. 10mg/kg. To prevent recurrence, oral dantrolene, 4-8mg/kg daily in 4 divided doses for up to 3 days.

PHARMACOKINETICS: Half-Life: 7-9 hours. Metabolism: Liver

ADVERSE EFFECTS: Hepatitis, muscle weakness; GI Effects: diarrhea, anorexia, vomiting, gastric irritation, constipation. These symptoms usually respond to reduction of dosage. Neurologic Effects: speech disturbance, headache, visual disturbances, insomnia, depression.

MONITOR: AST(SGOT), ALT(SGPT), Alkaline Phosphatase and total serum bilirubin prior to therapy and repeated periodically or with symptoms of hepatitis.

DRUG INTERACTIONS: Concomittant use of calcium channel blockers may lead to marked hyperkalemia.

DEFEROXAMINE
(Desferal)

USES: Deferoxamine is used in the treatment of **acute iron intoxication** and **chronic iron overload** from multiple transfusions or iron storage diseases.
Mechanism of Action: Deferoxamine chelates ferric ions.
DOSAGE FORMS: Injection: 500mg
DOSAGE: Deferoxamine mesylate may be administered by IM injection, by slow or continuous IV infusion or by subcutaneous infusion via a portable controlled-infusion device. For the treatment of acute iron intoxication, IM or IV administration is preferred and should be used for all patients who are not in shock. Dosage is given in the next Table:

Dosage of Deferoxamine

Condition	Age	Route	Dosage
Acute Iron Intoxication	Adults	IM or Slow IV	One gram followed by 500mg at 4 h. intervals for 2 doses. If needed, 500mg every 4-12 h.
	Children	IM or Slow IV	or 20mg/kg or 600mg/m^2 followed by 10mg/kg or 300mg/m^2 at 4 h. intervals for 2 doses. If needed, 10mg/kg or 300mg/m^2 every 4-12 h.
		Continuous IV	Rate should not exceed 15mg/kg/hr. Max. 6g daily.
Chronic Iron Overload (eg, Thalassemia or sickle cell hypertransfusion)	Adults and Children	IM	0.5-1 gram daily. In addition, give 2g by slow IV infusion with, but separate from each unit of blood transfused.
		Subcut.	20-40mg/kg up to 1-2 grams daily over 8-12 hours.

ADVERSE EFFECTS: Relatively non-toxic in acute iron intoxication. Long-Term Therapy: Allergic-type reactions, abdominal discomfort, diarrhea, ocular toxicity (blurred vision, cataracts, color blindness, night blindness, etc), ototoxicity (tinnitus, hearing deficits, deafness), and may predispose to infection due to Yersinia enterocolitica and mucormycosis. Rapid IV infusion may be associated with skin flushing, erythema, urticaria, hypotension, and shock - possibly due to histamine release.

DEPRESSION

Neurotransmitter Hypothesis of Depression: Neurotransmitters are synthesized and released by neurons to communicate with other neural cells; neurotransmitters include **norepinephrine**, **acetylcholine**, **gamma-aminobutyric acid (GABA)** and **serotonin**. There is evidence that norepinephrine is involved in the pathogenesis of depression. The mechanism of regulation by norepinephrine of neurotransmission is illustrated in the next Figure (Siever, L.J. and Davis, K.L., Am. J. Psychiatry 142, 1017-1031, 1985):

Regulation by Norepinephrine of Neurotransmission

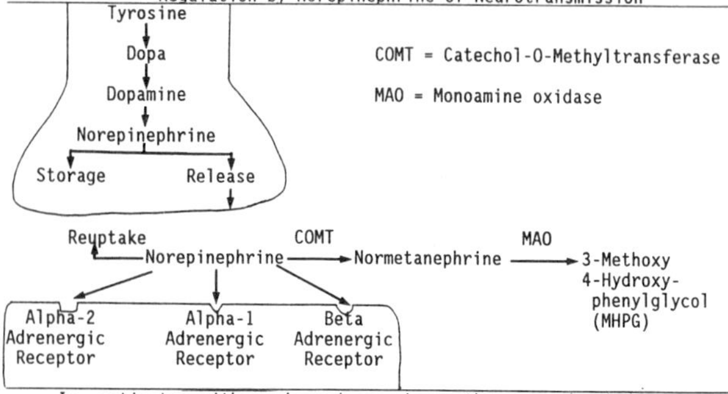

In patients with major depression, the **norepinephrine** system is **activated;** there are normal or increased levels of CSF norepinephrine, increased plasma norepinephrine, and increased CSF and urinary MHPG. Furthermore, successful responses to antidepressants are associated with decrease in CSF and plasma MHPG in patients with major depression and the involvement of norepinephrine and other neurotransmitters in depression is discussed in a review (Gold, P.N. etal.,N Engl. J. Med. 319, 348-353, Aug. 11, 1988).

The different categories of depression and drug therapy are given in the next Table:

Drug Therapy for Depressive Disorders

Depressive Disorders	Treatment
Bipolar	
Depression	Lithium alone or with an heterocyclic antidepressant.
Mania	Lithium (85% of patients respond); carbamazepine as an alternative drug.
Mixed	Lithium alone or lithium plus antidepressant.
Major Depression	Heterocyclic antidepressants are drugs of choice for acute treatment and prophylaxis. Monamine oxidase inhibitors are useful when psychomotor agitation or anxiety is a presenting symptom agitation or anxiety is a presenting symptom (Davidson, J., Drug Ther. 13, 197-202, 1983) or when heterocyclic antidepressants have failed.
Cyclothymic	Lithium is used in hypomania.
Dysthymic	Heterocyclic antidepressants or monoamine oxidase inhibitor in selected patients
Atypical with panic attacks and hysteroid dysphoria	Monoamine oxidase ingibitors

Biopolar Disorder: Diagnosis is based on the duration of episodes (depression for at least two weeks, mania for at least one week) and their severity .

Major Depression (Unipolar Depression): Diagnosis is based on dysphoric mood (emotional state marked by anxiety, depression and restlessness) or loss of interest or pleasure in usual activities plus classic signs and symptoms of depression; present nearly every day for at least two weeks.

Cyclothmic Disorder: Cyclothymic disorder is a chronic illness (at least two year's duration) with recurring episodes of hypomania and depression that are not of sufficient duration and severity for a diagnosis of bipolar disorder.

DEPRESSION (Cont.)

Dysthmic Disorder: Dysthymic disorder is characterized by duration of at least two years in adults and one year in children; some signs and symptoms resembling those of major depression but less severe and shorter duration; often, coexisting personality disorder.

Atypical Depression: Atypical depression is a residual category for depressive symptoms that are not classifiable as bipolar, major, cyclothmic or dysthymic.

DRUG THERAPY: Drugs used in therapy of the major depressive disorders are lithuim, heterocyclic antidepressants, monoamine oxidase inhibitors and psychomotor stimulants. Four to eight weeks are required for the patient to become nearly symptom-free. Then, the daily dose is reduced to lessen adverse effects.

Lithium Lithium decreases the intensity and frequency of successive episodes in manic-depression.

Heterocyclic Antidepressants: The pharmacology of heterocyclic antidepressants is given in the next Table (Richelson, E., J. Clin. Psychiatry 43: 11 (Sec. 2), 4-11, 1982; Rudorfer, M. and Potter, W., Drugs 37, 713-738, 1989; Peckar, Paul, J., Personal Communication, 1988):

Pharmacology of Heterocyclic Antidepressants

ANTI-DEPRESSANT	Potency; Blockage of Serotonin Uptake	Potency; Blockage of Norepinephrine (NE)Uptake	Adverse Effects; Blockage of Receptors to Histamine (H_1)	Adverse Effects; Blockage of Receptors to Muscurinic Acetylcholine	Adverse Effects; Blockage of Receptors to Alpha-1 Adrenergic
Fluoxe-*** tine(Prozac)	3+ to 4+	0 to 1+	Min.	Min.	Min.
Amitrip.* (Elavil)	2+ to 4+	1+ to 2+	Max.	Max.	Max.
Imipramine* (Tofranil)	1+ to 4+	1+ to 2+	Intermed. to Min.	Intermed.	Min.
Trazodone*** (Desyrel)	1+ to 3+	1+	Min.	Min.	Max. to Intermed.
Nortrip.* (Pamelor)	1+ to 3+	2+	Intermed. to Min.	Intermed. to Min.	Intermed. to Min.
Protrip.* (Vivactil)	3+	3+	Min.	Max.	Min.
Desipramine* (Norpramin)	0 to 3+	4+	Min.	Min.	Min.
Doxepin* (Sinequan)	3+	1+	Max.	Intermed.	Max.
Amoxapine** (Asendin)	0 to 2+	2+ to 3+	Intermed. to Min.	Min.	Intermed.
Trimipramine* (Surmontil)	1+	1+	Max.	Intermed.	Max.
Maprotiline** (Ludiomil)	0 to 1+	2+	Intermed.	Min.	Min.

*Tricyclics; **Tetracyclics; ***Other Meterocyclics.

The tricyclics that are usually preferred are those associated with a low incidence of adverse effects, eg, **desipramine** and **nortriptyline;** slow induction of the tricyclics can diminish side effects.

Because tricyclics can cause significant cardiac conduction changes, a baseline ECG should be obtained. All tricyclic dosages should be tapered slowly once depression is under control, especially when anticholinergic side-effects are significant.

Fluoxetine Fluoxetine is a new antidepressant which is putatively a "pure" serotonin uptake blocker; it has a long half-life so that once-a-day (20mg) is effective in most patients. Furthermore, fluoxetine does not promote weight gain.

Fluoxetine seems to help about half of those patients unresponsive to tricyclic antidepressants and MAO inhibitors.

Fluoxetine and trazodone, both with serotoninergic effects, are similarly effective in depressed patients (Debus, J. etal.,J. Clin. Psychiatry 49, 422-426, Nov. 1988)

DEPRESSION (Cont.)
Adverse Effects of Antidepressants: Adverse effects of antidepressants are medicated through blockage of serotonin, norepinephrine, histamine (H_1), muscarinic acetylcholine, and alpha-1 adrenergic receptors; the clinical manifestations of blockage of these receptors are given in the next Table (Richelson, E., J. Clin. Psychiatry 43: 11 [Sec, 2], 4-11, 1982):

Adverse Effects of Antidepressants

Property	Possible Clinical Consequence
Blockade of serotonin uptake at nerve endings.	Postural hypotension.
Blockade of norepinephrine uptake at nerve endings.	Blockade of the antihypertensive effects of guanethidine(Ismelin and Esimil), Clonidine (Catapres), and alpha-methyldopa(Aldomet). Augementation of pressor effects of sympathomimetic amines.
Blockade of histamine H_1 receptors.	Potentiation of central depressant drugs. Sedation, drowsiness, weight gain, hypotension.
Blockade of muscarinic acetylcholine receptors.	Blurred vision, dry mouth, sinus tachycardia, constipation, urinary retention, memory dysfunction.
Blockade of alpha-1-adrenergic receptors.	Potentiation of the antihypertensive effect of prazosin(Minipress). Postural hypotension, dizziness, reflex tachycardia.

Monoamine Oxidase (MAO) Inhibitors: The monoamine oxidase inhibitors are useful in major depression, particularly when psychomotor agitation or anxiety is a presenting symptom. **Monoamine oxidase** inhibitors include isocarboxazid, naialamide, phenelzine and tranylcypromine. These substances increase concentrations of serotonin and norepinephrine in the brain and are used to treat more severe cases of depression or as second line therapy.

Patients taking MAO inhibitors must avoid tyramine-rich and dopamine containing foods. Tyramine and MAO inhibitors can lead to hypertensive emergency.

Clinical response to MAO inhibitors often takes five to eight weeks.

Psychomotor Stimulants: Psychomotor stimulants, such as methylphenidate, act by cholinergic reinforcement. Combination forms of perphenazine and amitriptyline (Etrafon, Schering; Triavil, Merck) are used for treatment of patients with neuroses or psychoses characterized by both anxiety and depression. Antidepressant and antianxiety effect is also claimed for thioridazine.

Side effects of psychomotor stimulants include nervousness, restlessness, insomnia, and cardiovascular and gastrointestinal disorders.

DESIPRAMINE
(Norpramin, Pertofrane)

USES: Desipramine is a **tricyclic antidepressant,** a metabolite of imipramine, which is used to treat **depression.**

DOSAGE FORMS: Norpramin Tabs: 10, 25, 50, 75, 100, and 150mg; Pertofrane Caps: 25 and 50mg.

DOSAGE: Desipramine is administered orally. The dosage must be individualized and the minimum effective dose should be used. The patient must be clinically monitored closely at all stages of treatment. Dosage is given in the next Table:

Dosage of Desipramine

Age	Dosage
Adults (Hospitalized)	Initially, 75mg daily in divided doses; increase gradually to 200mg daily. If necessary, after two weeks, the dosage may be increased gradually to 300mg daily
Adults (Outpatients)	Initially, 25mg twice daily for three days, 50mg twice daily for three days and 75mg twice daily for the next ten days. If insomnia is prominent, it may be desirable to give the major portion of the daily dose at bedtime. If little benefit is obtained by the third week, the dose may be increased by 50mg daily every week. (max 300mg daily). Maintenance: Use the lowest dose that will maintenance remission.
Elderly Patients and Adolescents	Initially, 25 to 50mg daily, increased to 100mg daily in divided doses.

ADVERSE EFFECTS: The most frequent adverse effects are **anticholinergic effects (dry mouth, mydriasis, cycloplegia, urinary retention, decreased GI motility, tachycardia and delirium in high doses),** hypotension, drowsiness, weight gain.

Occasional Adverse Effects: Mania, psychosis, tremors, first-degree heart block, tachycardia and other arrhythmias, rash, sweating, confusion, insomnia, sexual disturbances.

Rare Adverse Effects: Hepatic toxicity, tinnitus, bone marrow depression including agranulocytosis, seizures, peripheral neuropathy, severe cardiovascular effects in patients with cardiac disease, photosensitivity, dysarthria, stuttering, withdrawal symptoms; death has been reported to have occurred.

PHARMACOKINETICS: Well absorbed; Time to Peak: 80 minutes; Protein Binding: 90%; Metabolized to Active Metabolites; Half-Life: 8 hours; half-life of active metabolite: 30 hours.

DRUG INTERACTIONS: Hyperpyrexic crisis, convulsions and death with monoamine oxidase inhibitors, potentiates alcohol, sympathomimetics, benzodiazepines and other CNS depressants. Paralytic ileus with anticholinergics, blocks guanethidine.

DESMOPRESSIN ACETATE
(DDAVP)

USES: Desmopressin is a synthetic polypeptide structurally related to **arginine vasopressin (antidiuretic hormone).** Uses are given in the next Table:

Uses of Desmopressin Acetate
Diabetes Insipidus
Bleeding in Hemophilia A and Type I von Willebrand's Disease
Primary Nocturnal Enuresis

Diabetes Insipidus: Desmopressin is used intranasally or parenterally to prevent or control polyuria, polydipsia and dehydration in patients with diabetes insipidus secondary to deficiency of posterior pituitary vasopressin (antidiuretic hormone) and to manage temporary diabetes insipidus associated with trauma or surgery in the pituitary region.

Hemophilia A and Type I von Willebrand's Disease: Desmopressin is used parenterally for the management of spontaneous or trauma-induced bleeding episodes in patients with hemophilia A whose plasma factor VIII activity is greater than 5%. The drug is also used parenterally to maintain hemostasis during surgical procedures and postoperatively in these hemophiliacs. The drug is not indicated for patients with hemophilia A whose factor VIII activity is 5% or less or for patients with hemophilia B or those with factor VIII antibodies. Desmopressin causes a dose-dependent increase in plasma factor VIII (antihemophilic factor), plasminogen activator, and, to a smaller degree, factor VIII-related antigen and ristocetin cofactor activities.

A nasal spray preparation of desmopressin is being tested for treatment of bleeding episodes and prophylactically for minor surgical procedures in patients with hemophilia A and von Willebrand disease; preliminary results are encouraging (Rose, E.H. and Aledort, L.M., Ann. Intern. Med. 114, 563-568, April, 1991).

DOSAGE FORMS: Nasal Solution: 0.1mg/ml (in 2.5ml vial with applicator)
Parenteral Inject.: 4mcg/ml

DOSAGE: Desmopressin acetate is administered intranasally, subcutaneously or direct IV for the management of diabetes insipidus or by slow IV infusion for the management of hemophilia A or von Willebrand's Disease. Dosage is given in the next Table:

Dosage of Desmopressin

Condition	Age	Route	Dosage
Diabetes Insipidus	Adults	Intranasally	2.5-10mcg (0.025-0.1ml of 0.01% sol'n). Titrate dose to achieve control of excessive thirst and urination. Max. adult dose: 0.4ml/day
	>3 months to 12 yrs.	Intranasally	2.5-5mcg (0.025-0.05ml of 0.01% sol'n). Titrate dose and frequency to thirst and urination. Range: 0.05ml-0.3ml/day
Bleeding Hemophilia A and Type I von Willebrand's Disease	Adults and Children 3 months and older	Slow IV Infusion	0.3mcg/kg; if administered preoperatively, inject 30 min. prior to procedure.
Enuresis	Children 6 yrs. and older	Intranasally	20mcg at bedtime (range: 10-40mcg)

PHARMACOKINETICS: Desmopressin is destroyed in GI tract. Following intranasal administration, antidiuretic effects occur within 1 hour, peak in 1-5 hours, and persists for 8-20 hours. Following IV infusion of desmopressin, factor VIII activity occurs within 15-30 minutes, peaks between 90 min. and 3 hrs.

ADVERSE EFFECTS: Infrequent and mild.

MONITOR: Intake and output, thirst, electrolytes.

DESOXYCORTICOSTERONE

(DOCA, Percorten)

USES: **Desoxycorticosterone** is a **mineralocorticoid** secreted by the adrenal glands; it has practically no glucocorticoid activity. Uses are given in the next Table:

Uses of Desoxycorticosterone
Mineralocorticoid Replacement Therapy:
Adrenocortical Insufficiency
Salt-Losing Forms of Congenital Adrenogenital Syndrome, eg,
21-Hydroxylase Deficiency, after Electrolyte Balance has been Restored.

Desoxycorticosterone is used only for parenteral mineralocorticoid replacement therapy in patients with adrenocortical insufficiency or salt-losing forms of congenital adrenogenital syndrome after electrolyte balance has been restored. Drug is contraindicated in all conditions except those which require a high degree of mineralocorticoid activity. The treatment of adrenocortical insufficiency or salt-losing forms of congenital adrenogenital syndrome is as follows:

Treatment of Adrenocortical Insufficiency or Salt-Losing Forms of Congenital Adrenogenital Syndrome

Initially	If Mineralocorticoid Required, Add
Hydrocortisone or Cortisone plus Liberal Salt Intake	Desoxycorticosterone (IM) or Fludrocortisone (oral)

DOSAGE FORMS: Injection: IM: 5mg/ml (in oil); Pellets: 125mg

DOSAGE: First, desoxycorticosterone acetate injection is used. Then, desoxycorticosterone acetate sterile pellets are used only after dosage requirements have been established using desoxycorticosterone acetate injection.

Desoxycorticosterone acetate injection is administered IM into the upper outer quadrant of the buttocks. Use a 19 gauge needle to withdraw the drug into the syringe and a 23 gauge needle for injection. Dosage is given in the next Table:

Dosage of Desoxycorticosterone

Condition	Age	Route	Dosage
Adrenocortical Insuff.	Adults	IM	DOC Acetate Injection: 1-5mg daily. Max. 10mg Daily
	Children	IM	DOC Acetate: 1.5-2mg/m^2 daily
Congenital Adreno-genital Syndrome	Adults	IM	DOC Acetate Injection: 2-6mg daily for first 3-4 days. Then, adjust dosage.
	Children	IM	DOC Acetate Injection:1.5-2mg/m^2 daily. Then, adjust dosage
Adrenocortical Insuff. or Congenital Adrenogenital Syndrome (Maintenance Therapy)		Implant of Pellets	DOC Acetate Pellets implanted below skin over scapula. This is done only after DOC acetate injection has been given for at least 2-3 mos. One 125mg pellet for each 0.5mg DOC acetate administered IM daily, e.g.,5mg IM daily=10 pellets

ADVERSE EFFECTS: If the dose or intake of dietary sodium is excessive, adverse effects result from sodium and water retention and potassium loss (hypertension, edema, hypokalemia, congestive heart failure).

DEXAMETHASONE
(Decadron, Dexone, Hexadrol)

USES: Dexamethasone is a potent, long-acting synthetic **glucocorticoid** having only minimal mineralocorticoid activity. It is used principally to treat inflammatory or allergic conditions. Uses are given in the next Table:

Uses of Dexamethasone
Screening Test for Cushing's Syndrome
Cerebral Edema (some situations)
Septic Shock (controversial)
Allergic Conditions
Inflammatory Diseases
Bronchial Asthma and Bronchospasm (oral inhalation)
Bacterial Meningitis in Children
Croup
Prevent Hyaline Membrane Disease in Premature Infants
Cancer Therapy-Induced Nausea and Vomiting

Dexamethasone is inadequate alone for the treatment of adrenocortical insufficiency because it has only minimal mineralocorticoid activity.

Screening Test for Cushing's Syndrome: The dexamethasone suppression test for the diagnosis of Cushing's syndrome is as follows: Dexamethasone, 1mg, is taken orally by the patient between 11:00 P.M. and midnight; a fasting blood cortisol is obtained the next morning at 8:00 A.M. in green (heparin) top tube, separate plasma, or red top tube, separate serum. Store and ship frozen. Suppression by dexamethasone in normal individuals of blood cortisol is less than 5mcg/dl. A value of blood cortisol greater than 5mcg/dl is compatible with Cushing's syndrome.

Cerebral Edema: Dexamethasone is commonly used to treat vasogenic cerebral edema.

DOSAGE FORMS: Oral: Tabs: 0.25, 0.5, 0.75, 1, 1.5, 2, 4, 6mg; Elixir: 0.1mg/ml; Solution: 0.1, 1mg/ml; Parenteral: 4, 8, 10, 16, 20, 24mg/ml; Oral inhalation: 100mcg per spray.

DOSAGE: The forms of dexamethasone and the routes of administration are given in the next Table:

Forms and Routes of Administration of Dexamethasone

Form	Routes
Dexamethasone	Oral
Dexamethasone Acetate	IM, Intra-Articular, Intralesional Soft-Tissue
Dexamethasone Sodium Phosphate	Oral Inhalation, Intra-Articular, Intrasynovial, Intralesional, Soft-Tissue, IM, IV Injection, IV Infusion

Dosage is given in the next Table:

Dosage of Dexamethasone

Condition	Age	Route	Dosage
Screening Test for Cushing's	Adults	Oral	1mg at midnight
Usual Dose Range	Adults	Oral	0.75-9mg daily in 2-4 divided doses.
Usual Dose Range	Children	Oral	0.024-0.34mg/kg or 0.66-10mg/m^2 in 4 divided doses.
Usual Dose Range	Adults	IM	Initial:8-16mg; additional doses at 1-3 week intervals as needed.
		Intra-lesional	0.8-1.6mg per injection site.
		Intra-Articular or Soft Tissue	4-16mg; repeat at 1-3 weeks as needed.

DEXAMETHASONE (Cont.)

Dosage of Dexamethasone

Condition	Age	Route	Dosage
Shock, Life Threatening	Adults Children	IV	1-6mg/kg or 40mg repeated every 2-6 h. as needed. **or** 20mg IV initially followed by continuous IV infusion of 3mg/kg per 24 h. High-dose therapy should not be continued beyond 48-72 hrs. Use is controversial. No proven benefit.
Cerebral Edema	Adults	IV or IM then Oral	10mg IV followed by 4mg IV every 6h. until edema subsides. Dosage reduced after 2-4 days and gradually discontinued over 5-7 days. Use oral dose (1-3mg, 3 times daily) to replace IM when possible.
	Children	IV or IM	Initially, 0.5-1.5mg/kg IV or IM followed by 0.2-0.5mg/kg/day IV or IM divided every 6 h. for 5 days, then taper.
Allergic Conditions (Acute Self-Limited or Acute Exacerbation of chronic)	Adults	IM or IV	4-8mg IM or IV on first day, 3mg orally in 2 divided doses on second and third days; 1.5mg orally in 2 divided doses on the fourth day; and a single oral daily dose of 0.75mg on the fifth and sixth days.
Inflammatory Diseases	Adults		Large Joints, eg, knee: 2-4mg Smaller Joints: 0.8-1mg Bursae: 2-3mg Tendon Sheath: 0.4-1mg Soft-Tissue: 2-6mg Injections may be repeated from once every 3-5 days for bursae to once every 2-3 weeks for joints.
Bronchial Asthma & Bronchospasm	Adult	Oral Inhal.	300mcg (3 inhalations) 3-4 times daily.
	Children	Oral Inhal.	200mcg (2 inhalations) 3-4 times daily.
Bacterial Meningitis	Children	IV	0.6mg/kg/day divided 4 times daily for 4 days (see **MENINGITIS**)
Croup	Children	Oral, IM or IV	0.5-0.6mg/kg/dose for 1-4 IM or IV doses, every 6 hours.
Prevent Hyaline Membrane Disease	Adult	IM	4mg IM 3 times daily for 2 days prior to delivery.
Cancer Therapy Nausea and Vomiting	Adult	IV and Oral	Mild Vomiting: 10mg IV over 3-5 minutes 30 min before chemotherapy followed by oral administration of 8mg, 6, 12 and 18 hours after chemotherapy. Moderate Vomiting: 10 to 20mg IV, 30 min before chemotherapy followed by oral administration of 8mg, 6, 12, and 18 hours after chemotherapy. Severe Vomiting: 20mg IV, plus metoclopramide 1 to 3mg/kg and diphenhydramine 50mg given concomitantly, 30 min before chemotherapy.

DEXAMETHASONE (Cont.)
ADVERSE EFFECTS: Adverse effects are associated with long term use of dexamethasone and other steroids are given in the next Table:

Adverse Effects of Dexamethasone

Condition	Comment
Adrenocortical Insufficiency	Long-term therapy may cause decreased secretion of endogenous corticosteroids by suppressing pituitary release of ACTH; this effect may be minimized by alternate-day therapy. Acute adrenal insufficiency may occur if dexamethasone is withdrawn abruptly or the patient is subject to stress. Adrenal suppression may persist for up to 12 months.
Musculoskeletal Effects	Muscle weakness, muscle wasting, muscle pain, delayed wound healing, osteoporosis.
Increased Susceptibility to Infection	Oral inhalation therapy is associated with fungi, candida albicans or Aspergillus niger infections of the mouth, pharynx and occasionally the larynx. The occurrence of these fungal infections is dose dependent.
Ocular Effects	Subcapsular cataracts, especially in children; exophthalmos, increased intraocular pressure which may result in glaucoma.
Endocrine Effects	Prolonged dexamethasone therapy may result in hypercorticism (Cushingoid state) and amenorrhea or menstrual difficulties.
GI Effects	Nausea, vomiting, anorexia or increased appetite, diarrhea or constipation, abdominal distension, pancreatitis, gastric irritation, and ulcerative esophagitis, development and delayed healing of ulcers (<2%).
Nervous System Effects	Headache, vertigo, insomnia, seizures
Dermatologic Effects	Skin atrophy, thinning and acne, increased sweating, hirsutism, easy bruising.
Cardiovascular Effects	Bradycardia in preterm infants with bronchopulmonary dysplasia (Puntis, J.W.L. et al., Lancet 2, 1372, Dec. 10, 1988). Hypertension.

DEXTROAMPHETAMINE
(Dexedrine)

USES: Dextroamphetamine is the dextrorotatory isomer of amphetamine; uses are given in the next Table:

Uses of Dextroamphetamine
Narcolepsy (Brief Attacks of Deep Sleep)
Attention Deficit Disorder with Hyperactivity (Hyperkinetic Syndrome of Childhood, Minimal Brain Dysfunction) in Children
Obesity

Dextroamphetamine sulfate is used in the treatment of narcolepsy and as an adjunct to other remedial measures in the treatment of attention deficit disorder with hyperactivity (hyperkinetic syndrome of childhood, minimal brain dysfunction) in children. Dextroamphetamine (as a resin complex) and dextroamphetamine sulfate are used to reduce appetite in obese patients.

DOSAGE FORMS: Tabs: 5, 10mg; Elixir: 5mg/5ml; Sustained-Release Caps: 5, 10, 15mg

DOSAGE: Dextroamphetamine (as a resin complex) and dextroamphetamine sulfate are administered orally. Amphetamine causes insomnia; therefore, the last dose is given at least 6 hours before retiring. Dosage is given in the next Table:

Dosage of Amphetamine

Condition	Age	Dosage
Narcolepsy	6-12 years	5mg daily; incr. daily dose by 5mg at weekly intervals until optimum response is attained
	>12 years	10mg daily; increase daily dose by 10mg at weekly intervals until optimum response is attained. 60mg daily may be required.
Attention Deficit Disorder	6 years and older	5mg once or twice daily; increase daily dose by 5mg at weekly intervals until optimum response is attained.
	3-5 years	2.5mg daily; increase daily dose by 2.5mg at weekly intervals until optimum response is attained.
Obesity	12 years and older	5-30mg daily given 30-60 minutes before meals in divided doses of 5-10mg. or extended-release capsules, 10-15mg daily as a single dose in the morning.

In narcolepsy, interrupt therapy occasionally to determine need for continued therapy. Tolerance may develop.

ADVERSE EFFECTS: Nervousness, insomnia, irritability, talkativeness, increased libido, dizziness, headaches, increased motor activity, chilliness, pallor or flushing, blurred vision, mydriasis and hyperexcitability.

Hypertension or hypotension, tachycardia, palpitation or cardiac arrhythmias may occur in some patients.

This drug has significant abuse potential; alternative therapies should be considered whenever possible.

DIARRHEA; PATHOGENS, TREATMENT

Pathogens:

Clinical features of acute infectious diarrheas are given in the next Table;(Kluge, R.M., E.R. Reports 4, Nos.12 & 13, 71-80, June 13 and 27,1983):

Acute Infectious Diarrheas

Agent	Usual Age	Fever	Vomiting	Incubation Period	Stool Bloody	Stool Leukocytes
S. Aureus, Toxigenic(T)	Any	No	Yes	1-6 Hr	No	No
B. Cereus, Diarrhea(T)	Any	No	Yes	8-16 Hr	No	No
B. Cereus, Emetic(T)	Any	No	Yes	1-3 Hr	No	No
E. Coli, Toxigenic(T)	Any	No	Yes	1-2 Days	No	No
C. Perfringens(T)	Any	No	No	8-24 Hr	No	No
Shigella(I)	<5 Yrs	Yes	No	1-3 Days	Yes	Yes
Salmonella, Non-Typhoid(I)	<5 Yrs	Yes	No	1-2 Days	+/-	Yes
C. Fetus Jejuni(I)	Child	Yes	Yes	3-5 Days	Yes	Yes
E. Coli, Invasive(I)	Any	Yes	Yes	8-24 Hr	Yes	Yes
Y. Enterocolitica(I)	5-20 Yrs	Yes	No	1-2 Days	No	Yes
V. Parahaemolyticus(I)	Any	Yes	Yes	1-4 Days	+/-	Yes
C. Difficile(T,I)	Any	Yes	No	4-10 Days	Yes	Yes
Rotavirus(E)	6 Mos.-2 Yrs	Yes	Yes	2-4 Days	No	No
Norwalk-Like Agents(E)	School/ Adults	Yes	Yes	1-2 Days	No	No
G. Lamblia(E)	Any	No	No	3 Days-3 Wks	No	No
E. Histolytica(I)	Any	Yes	No	3 Days-3 Wks	Yes	No
Cryptosporidium(E)	1-4 Yrs 30-39 Yrs	No	No	-	No	No

T=Toxin-Producing Bacteria; E=Enterocyte Injury; I=Mucosal Invasion

Rotaviral and Norwalk-like viral diarrhea are seen in the winter months; most bacterial diarrhea predominates during the summer or fall; however, Y. enterocolitica is isolated more frequently during the winter months.

Bacterial agents usually cause diarrhea by (1) Toxin-producing bacteria or (2) Damage to the intestinal mucosa cells (enterocyte injury) or (3) Mucosal invasion.

(1) Toxin-Producing Bacteria: Certain bacteria attach to the small bowel mucosa and produce exotoxins; these toxins interact with adenylate cyclase of the mucosal cells to augment secretion, decrease active reabsorption or both. The large volume of this luminal fluid exceeds the capacity of the colon; a large volume, non-inflammatory, watery stool is produced. There is no evidence of bowel wall inflammation. Patients have abdominal cramps and are afebrile. Examples: S. aureus (toxin produced in meats, poultry or dairy products and then ingested); B. cereus (heat-stable toxin produced in boiled or fried rice); E. coli, toxigenic; C. Perfringens (bacteria ingested in meat or poultry; toxin produced in gut lumen).

(2) Enterocyte Injury (Damage to Intestinal Mucosal Cells): Enterocytes are affected (infected by viruses, rotavirus or Norwalk-like viruses; binding, Cryptosporidium; enterocyte injury of upper small bowel, G. lamblia). There may be loss of brush border, villous flattening, loss of absorptive capacity, and stimulation of motility. An inflammatory infiltrate may be found in the submucosa. Clinically, there is a noninflammatory water loss diarrhea or malabsorptive stool in a nontoxic, variably febrile patient.

(3) Mucosal Invasion: Actively invasive pathogens (Shigella, Non-Typhoidal Salmonella, E. coli, Campylobacter) cause inflammation, mucus bleeding and irritation which produce the frequent, small volume stool with bloody mucus and abdominal cramps. The colon and occasionally the ileum are involved.

Age: The most common cause of diarrhea in infants is rotavirus, accounting for more than 50% of hospitalized cases in children. Enterotoxigenic E. coli is the second most common cause in infants.

Fever: Fever is associated with viral infection, the parasites, E. histolytica and invasive bacteria, e.g., salmonella, non-typhoid; shigella; C. fetus jejuni; E. coli, invasive; Y. enterocolitica; V. parahaemolyticas; C. difficile.

DIARRHEA; PATHOGENS, TREATMENT (Cont.)

Vomiting: Vomiting is associated with viral infections and some bacterial infections; it is not associated infection by the bacteria: C. perfringens; salmonella, non-typhoid; shigella; Y. enterocolitica, and C. difficile; and parasitic infections.

Incubation Period: The incubation period tends to be shorter for those bacteria that produce toxins, eg., S. aureus, B. cereus, C. perfringens as compared to those bacteria that are invasive.

Patients with diarrhea of more than 3-5 days likely do not have a viral or enterotoxigenic cause, unless they have an infection with C. difficile, which can persist for weeks.

Blood: Blood and mucus in the stool are more prevalent with the invasive bacteria, E. histolytica and cases of diarrhea due to C. difficile.

Clues to the etiology of infectious diarrhea are given in the next Table:

Infectious Diarrhea - Clues Associated with Specific Infectious Agents

Clue	Suspect Agent
Specific Food Item Incriminated	
Poultry or Eggs	Salmonella and C. Jejuni
Seafood	V. Parahaemolyticus
Raw Milk	Campylobacter(Most Common), Salmonella, E. Coli,Brucella,Listeria, or Yersinia
Fried Rice or Bean Sprouts	B. Cereus
Family Pets	Y. Enterocolitica or C. Jejuni
Homosexual Activity; Anal Sexual Intercourse	Gonococcal and Chlamydial Proctitis, Amoeba, Shigella, or Campylobacter

Treatment: Treatment of diarrhea is directed toward rehydration, if necessary, and appropriate antibiotics therapy; only supportive therapy is appropriate for patients with diarrhea due to viruses and toxins (except C. difficile).

a. Hydration: Calculations of maintenance and deficit water and electrolytes, eg., sodium and potassium requirements are given in the next Table:

Calculations of Daily Maintenance and Deficit Water and Electrolyte Requirements

	Maintenance		Deficit	Examples
	Wt. in Kg.	Water(Day)	(% Dehydra. x Body Wt. in kg.)	Wt. 10kg.; Dehydra.,10%
H_2O	0-10	100ml/kg	5% = 50ml/kg	Maint. = 1000ml
	11-20	1000ml/kg+50ml/kg	10% = 100ml/kg	Deficit= 1000ml
	>20	1500ml/kg+20ml/kg	15% = 150ml/kg	Total = 2000ml/24 hrs. Approx. 80ml/hr
Na^{+}	2-4mEq/kg/Day		Isotonic Dehyra. (Na^{+}=130-150mEq/l) 7-11mEq/kg	Wt. 10kg; Dehyda.,10% Maint. = 30mEq Deficit= 100mEq Total = 130mEq/24hrs
K^{+}	2-3mEq/kg/Day		Isotonic Dehyra. 3-6mEq/kg	Maint. = 20mEq Deficit= 40mEq Total = 60mEq/24 hrs.

Rehydration may be accomplished orally or IV, depending on the particular clinical situation. Severely ill patients will require IV therapy. A summary of the American Academy of Pediatrics (AAP) recommendations for oral therapy of enteritis are given in the following Table (AAP Committee on Nutrition, Pediatrics 75, 358-361, 1985):

AAP Recommendations for Oral Therapy of Enteritis
Oral rehydration may be used for mild, moderate, or severe dehydration.
Vomiting is not a contraindication.
Sodium concentration in glucose-electrolyte solutions should be 75-90mEq/L for rehydration, 40-60mEq/L for maintenance.
Carbohydrate to sodium ratio should not exceed 2:1.
Reintroduce feedings within 24 hrs: Infants, breast milk, diluted formula or milk; older infants and children, BRAT diet (see below).
Follow state of hydration closely.

DIARRHEA; PATHOGENS, TREATMENT (Cont.)

The sodium, potassium and carbohydrate composition of various oral solutions is given in the next Table (Link, D.A., E.R. Reports 3, 101-106, Sept. 20, 1986; Santosham, M. and Greenough, W.B., J. Pediatr. 118, S44-S51, April, 1991; Snyder, J.D., Pediatr. 87, 28-33, 1991):

Composition of Oral Solutions for Outpatient Therapy

Type	Na+(mEq/l)	K+(mEq/l)	CHO(mmol/L)
Rehydration Solutions			
WHO	90	20	111
Pedialyte	45	20	140
Rehydralyte	75	20	140
RiceLyte	50	25	?
Infalyte	50	20	111
Resol	50	20	111
Other Fluids			
Pepsi	7	4	700
Coke	1	13	700
Gingerale	4	1	?
Apple Juice	3	32	690
Human Milk	7	13	?
Gatorade	20	3	255
Boiled Skim Milk	Very High	Very High	?
Whole Cow's Milk	25	35	?
Chicken Broth	250	8.2	0

If the patient responds well to oral solutions, solids may be resumed with the BRAT diet: Bananas, Rice, Applesauce and Toast.

Criteria for Hospitalization in Pediatric Dehydration: Criteria for hospitalization in pediatric dehydration are given in the next Table; (Link, D.A., ER Reports 3, No. 18, 101-106, Sept. 20, 1982):

Criteria for Hospitalization in Pediatric Dehydration

Clinical Criteria
- (a) Dehydration of any Degree and Under Two Months of Age
- (b) Dehydration Over 5% of Body Weight
- (c) Inability to Tolerate Oral Fluids
- (d) Bloody Diarrhea

Laboratory Criteria
- (a) Severe Hyponatremia (<125mEq/liter)
- (b) Hypernatremia (>150mEq/liter)
- (c) Hypokalemia (<3.0mEq/liter)
- (d) Hyperkalemia (>6.0mEq/liter)
- (e) Marked Acidosis (pH < 7.20 or Bicarbonate < 15mEq/liter)
- (f) Azotemia; Elevated Creatinine

Other Criteria: Pathology of Renal, Endocrine, Non-infectious or Surgical Origin

The objectives in treatment of moderate and severe dehydration are given in the next Table:

Objectives in Treatment of Moderate and Severe Dehydration
- (1) Restoration or Maintenance of Circulation
- (2) Expansion of the Plasma Volume
- (3) Replacement of Lose Electrolytes
- (4) Correction of Acid-Base Imbalance

Patient in Shock: Initially, give 20ml/kg of Ringer's lactate or normal saline intravenously over 20 minutes or less. Evaluate patient's circulatory status and urinary output. If there is no response, repeat fluid load. If the child's circulation returns, adjust fluid administration to replace half the total fluid deficit over the first 8 hours, complete rehydration by 24 hrs. Rapid determination of blood glucose by reagent strip (eg, Dextrostix, Chemstrip).

DIARRHEA; PATHOGENS, TREATMENT (Cont.)

Therapeutic Agents for Acute Diarrhea: Therapeutic agents for acute diarrhea are given in the next Table; (Levine, M.L. and Pickering, L.K., Patient Care, pgs. 125-150, Feb. 15, 1985; Kluge, R.M., ER Reports 4, 75-80, June 27, 1983):

Therapeutic Agents for Acute Diarrhea

Infectious Agent	Drug	Pediatric Dosage (Adult Dosage)
BACTERIA		
Campylobacter	**Erythromycin**	40mg/kg/d po in 4 doses; 7-10 days(500mg, po, bid, 7-10 days)
Clostridium Difficile	**Vancomycin** (Vancocin)	Usually no drug therapy is needed. 40-50mg/kg/d in 4 doses for 10-14 days po with replacement fluids (0.5-2g/d, po, in 3-4 doses, 10-14 days)
Escherichia Coli (Entero-pathogenic	**Neomycin Sulfate Suspension (Mycifradin)**	50mg/kg/d po in 3-4 doses for 2-3 days. Adults 3g daily in 3-4 divided doses for 2-3 days.
	Ampicillin, Oral	100-200mg/kg/d, po, 4 doses, 5-7 days (500mg, po, qid, for pregnant women, 5-7 days)
	Trimethoprim and Sulfamethoxazole (Bactrim, Septra, generic)	8mg/kg/d Trimethoprim and 40mg/kg/d Sulfamethoxazole, po, bid, 5 days (160mg/d trimethoprim and 800mg/d sulfamethoxazole for 5 days)
Salmonella		Treatment not indicated for uncomplicated gastroenteritis caused by nontyphi species since disease course is not altered and antibiotics can prolong duration of salmonella excretion.
	Trimethoprim and Sulfamethoxazole (Bactrim, Septra, generic)	8mg/kg/d Trimethoprim and 40mg/kg/d Sulfamethoxazole, po, or IV in 2 doses 2 weeks (160mg/800mg, po, bid 5 days) (Contraindicated in infants less than 2 mos. of age); consider use if Shigella or Salmonella is Ampicillin resistant
	Ampicillin	100-200mg/kg/d IV, 4-6 doses, 10-14 d or 100-200mg/kg/d po in 4 doses, 10-14 d (1g, IV, q4-6h, 14 days).
	Chloramphenicol	Suspension (give only for sepsis and only when less potentially harmful agents are ineffective)(Chloromycetin Palmitate) Orally or Chloramphenicol Sodium Succinate (Chloromycetin Sodium Succinate) IV 75-100mg/kg/d in 4 doses, 7-10 days (1g, po, q8h, 7-10 days).
Shigella	**Trimethoprim and Sulfamethoxazole (Bactrim, Septra)**	8mg/kg/d Trimethoprim and 40mg/kg/d Sulfamethoxazole po or IV in 2 doses for 5 days (160mg/800mg, po, bid, 5 days)
	Ampicillin	75-100mg/kg/d IV or po in 4 doses, 5 days (1g, IV, q4-6h, 14 days)
Vibrio Cholerae	**Tetracycline**	Generally contraindicated in children less than 8 yrs. of age, but drug of choice for this disorder. 40mg/kg/d po, 4 doses, 3-5 days.
Vibrio Parahaemolyticus		None.
Yersinia Enterocolitica		None.
PARASITES		
Entamoeba Histolytica, Mild-to-Moderate Disease	**Metronidazole (Flagyl)**	35-50mg/kg/d, po, 3 doses, 10 days (750mg, po, 3 doses, 10 days)
	and Iodoquinol (Yodoxin)	30-40mg/kg/d, po, 3 doses, 20 days (650mg/dose, po, 3 doses, 20 days)
Severe Intestinal Disease	**Paromomycin (Humatin)**	25-35mg/kg/d, 3 doses, with meals, 7 days.
	Metronidazole (Flagyl)	35-50mg/kg/d, 3 doses, 10 days (750mg, po, 3 doses, 10 days)
	and Iodoquinol (Yodoxin)	30-40mg/kg/d, 3 doses, 20 days (650mg/dose, po, 3 doses, 20 days)

DIARRHEA; PATHOGENS, TREATMENT (Cont.)

Infectious Agent	Drug	Pediatric Dosage (Adult Dosage)
	Dehydroemetine (Obtain from CDC)	1.0-1.5mg/kg/d (Max. dosage, 90mg/d), IM in 2 doses for up to 5 days.
	and Iodoquinol (Yodoxin)	30-40mg/kg/d in 3 doses for 20 days (650mg/dose, po, 3 doses, 20 days) (Dosage and duration of administration should not be exceeded because of possibility of causing optic neuritis)
Giardia Lamblia	**Furazolidone (Furoxone)**	6mg/kg/d po in 4 doses for 7 days (100mg po 4 times daily for 7 days)
	Quinacrine HCl (Atabrine)	6mg/kg/d po in 3 doses after meals, 7 days (maximum dosage 300mg/day) (100mg, po tid, 7 days)
Strongyloides Sterocoralis	**Thiabendazole (Mintezol)**	50mg/kg/d po in 2 doses for 2 days (Maximum dosage, 3g/d)

DIAZEPAM
(Valium)

USES: Diazepam (Valium) is a **benzodiazepine;** the uses of diazepam are given in the next Table:

Uses of Diazepam

Usually, diazepam is used for the treatment of **anxiety**
Preoperative: Relieve anxiety, provide sedation, light anesthesia, and anterograde amnesia
Adjunct During Endoscopy: Relieve anxiety, provide sedation, light anesthesia and anterograde amnesia
Relief of Acute, Painful Musculoskeletal Conditions
Manage Skeletal Muscle Spasticity such as reflex spasm secondary to local pathology (eg, trauma, inflammation), spasticity caused by upper motor neuron disorders (eg, cerebral palsy, paraplegia), athetosis, stiff-man syndrome, or tetanus.
Anticonvulsant: **IV diazepam is drug of choice for termination of status epilepticus;** must be followed by long acting anticonvulsant.
Other uses of diazepam that are not currently approved by the FDA are as follows: reduce requirements for opiate analgesics, produce anterograde amnesia during labor and delivery, manage neonatal opiate withdrawal; acute alcohol withdrawal.

Mechanism of Action: The action of diazepam is thought to be mediated through facilitation of inhibitory gamma-aminobutyric acid (GABA) neurotransmission.

DOSAGE FORMS: Tabs:2,5,10mg; Oral sol'n: 5mg/5ml, 5mg/ml; Sustained Release:15mg; Amp:5mg/ml for injection

DOSAGE: Diazepam is administered orally or slow IV (rate not > 5mg/minute in adults and not >1mg/minute or over a 3 minute period in children). IM administration is possible, but absorption is slow and erratic. Dosage is given in the next Table:

Dosage of Diazepam

Condition	Age	Route	Dosage
Sedative/Muscle Relaxant	Child.	IV	0.04-0.2mg/kg/dose every 2-4 h.(max. dose: 0.6mg/kg within an 8 h. period).
		Orally	0.12-0.8mg/kg/day 3 to 4 times a day.
	Adults	IV	2-10mg/dose every 3-4 h. as necessary.
		Orally	2-10mg/dose every 6-8 h. as necessary.
Status Epilepticus	1 mo. to 5 yr.	IV every 15-30 min.	0.1-0.5mg/kg/dose.(Max. total dose:5mg)
	>5 yr.	IV every 15-30 min.	0.1-0.5mg/kg/dose (Max. total dose: 10mg)
	Adults	IV every 10-15 min.	5-10mg/dose. (Max. total dose: 30mg).

PHARMACOKINETICS: Half-Life: 20-50 hrs.; Peak (oral): 1-2 hrs.; Therapeutic Range: 100-150ng/ml; Toxic Range: 3,000-14,000ng/ml; Protein Bound: 85%-95%.

Diazepam acts rapidly when taken as a single dose; it is absorbed rapidly from the GI tract, and since it is soluble in lipids, it quickly reaches therapeutic concentrations (serum therapeutic range, 100-1500ng/dl) in the CNS. Diazepam is metabolized in the liver by oxidation and has active metabolites N-desmethyldiazepam and oxazepam. Half-Life at steady state for diazepam, 55 hours; half-life for N-desmethydiazepam, 40 hours. Half-life increases with age. Steady-State: Seven days. It may be more hazardous for the elderly and for patients with liver diseases.

DIAZEPAM (Cont.)

ADVERSE EFFECTS: The main risk with IV infusion of diazepam is respiratory arrest, particularly in infants, elderly, and with rapid infusion. Resuscitative equipment should be available when IV diazepam is used.

Daytime sedation and hangover are the most common initial untoward effects. Other common adverse effects include dizziness and ataxia which are dose related.

Untoward effects noted occasionally are headaches, blurred vision, diplopia, bradycardia, hypotension, amnesia, slurred speech, tremor, urinary incontinence, constipation, depression.

Death is rare in overdose when diazepam is taken alone; the actual cause of death is more likely attributable to the other drugs ingested (Finkle, B.S. et al., JAMA 242, 429-434, 1979; Jatlow, P. et al., Am. J. Clin. Path. 72, 571-577, 1979). Dose-dependent adverse CNS effects are common.

DRUG INTERACTIONS: When diazepam is used with a narcotic analgesic, the dosage of the narcotic should be reduced by at least one third. Cimetidine inhibits the metabolism of diazepam.

Rifampin may significantly decrease serum levels of diazepam.

DIAZOXIDE

(Hyperstat, Proglycem)

USES: **Diazoxide** is a **nondiuretic thiazide** that reduces total peripheral resistance by a direct action on arteriolar smooth muscle; it reduces blood pressure rapidly when given intravenously. Heart rate and cardiac output are increased. Diazoxide increases blood glucose by inhibiting insulin release and by other means. Uses are given in the next Table:

Uses of Diazoxide

Severe Hypertension: IV diazoxide is used for emergency lowering of blood pressure; it is of particular value in patients with malignant hypertension associated with renal impairment. Diazoxide is ineffective in hypertension caused by pheochromocytoma and contraindicated in hypertension associated with aortic coarctation or arteriovenous shunt.

Hypoglycemia: In infants and children, diazoxide is used orally in the management of hypoglycemia associated with leucine sensitivity, islet cell hyperplasia, nesidioblastosis, extrapancreatic malignancy, islet cell adenoma or adenomatosis.

PHARMACOKINETICS: Onset:1-2 min.(IV); 1 hr.(oral), Peak Effect:2-3 min.(IV); Duration: 4-12 hr.(IV); 8 hr. (oral). Protein Bound: 90%; Elimination: Renal excretion; Half-Life: 10-72 hrs.

DOSAGE FORMS: Amp.: 15mg/ml; (Proglycem) Caps: 50mg; Susp. 50mg/ml

DOSAGE: Diazoxide is administered orally for the treatment of hypoglycemia. Diazoxide is administered undiluted by rapid IV injection over a period of 30 seconds or less into a peripheral vein via an IV line. Dosage is given in the next Table:

Dosage of Diazoxide

Condition	Age	Route	Dosage
Hypertensive Crisis	Children & Adults	IV	1-3mg/kg up to 150mg; repeat 5-15 min. as necessary, then every 4-24 h.
Hypoglycemia (due to insulin producing tumors)	Newborns & Infants	Orally or IV	8-15mg/kg/day divided every 8-12 h.
	Children & Adults	Orally or IV	3-8mg/kg/day divided 8-12 h.

ADVERSE EFFECTS: Rarely occur when drug administered IV for short periods. Hypotension, nausea and vomiting, dizziness and weakness.

Hyperglycemia frequently occurs in patients receiving diazoxide IV in the management of hypertension.

CONTRAINDICATIONS: Allergy to thiazides; hypertension secondary to arteriovenous shunt or coarctation of the aorta.

MONITOR: Blood pressure continuously or every 5 minutes during emergency treatment of severe hypertension. Blood glucose and serum uric acid.

DICLOXACILLIN

(Dynapen, Dycill, Pathocil)

USES: **Dicloxacillin** is a semisynthetic penicillinase-resistant penicillin generally used only in the oral treatment of infections caused by, or suspected of being caused by, **penicillinase-resistant staphylococci.**

DOSAGE FORMS: Cap: 125, 250, 500mg; Susp: 62.5mg/5ml

DOSAGE: Dicloxacillin sodium is administered orally; it is taken at least 1 hour before or 2 hours after meals. Dosage is given in the next Table:

Dosage of Dicloxacillin

Condition	Age	Dosage
Mild-Moderate Infections	Adults & >40 kg	125-250mg every 6 hours.
	Children >1 month	25-50mg/kg daily in divided doses every 6 hours
Severe Infections & Follow-Up of Osteomyelitis	Adults & >40 kg	250-500mg every 6 hours. Max: 4gm daily
	Children >1 month	50-100mg/kg daily in divided doses every 6 hours. Max: 4gm daily.

Duration of Therapy:At least 14 days; however, for follow-up of osteomyelitis, 3-6 weeks is necessary, and compliance must be assured; serum bacteriocidal titers may be useful to assess adequacy of therapy.

PHARMACOKINETICS: Half-life: 45 min.; Protein Binding: 96%; Excretion: 70% unchanged in urine.

ADVERSE EFFECTS: Similar to other penicillins.

DICYCLOMINE
(Bentyl)
USES: Dicyclomine is an **anticholinergic, antispasmodic** which is used in the treatment of functional disturbances of GI motility such as **irritable bowel syndrome.**

Dicyclomine has been used alone and in combination with phenobarbital in the treatment of **infant colic** and **acute enterocolitis;** these uses are not labeling approved by the FDA. Adverse effects may outweigh potential benefits
DOSAGE FORMS: Caps: 10, 20mg Tabs: 20mg, Syrup:10mg/5ml; Sol'n for Injection: 10mg/ml.
DOSAGE Adults: Oral or IM: Initially, 10-20mg four times daily; increase to 40mg four times daily if tolerated. Discontinue if not effective within 2 weeks or daily doses of 80mg or above are not tolerated.

Children: This drug should be avoided. Fatal reactions have occurred in infants treated for colic.
PHARMACOKINETICS: Apparent volume of distribution is 3.65 liter/kg. Half-Life; Initial Phase: 1.8 hours; Terminal Phase: 9-10 hours.
ADVERSE EFFECTS: Fatal reactions have occurred in infants. Anticholinergic effects: blurred vision; dryness of mucous membranes; difficulty in swallowing; urinary retention; tachycardia; hypertension.

DIFLUNISAL
(Dolobid)
USES: Diflunisal is a fluoridated salicylic acid derivative that, like other **non-steroidal anti-inflammatory drugs** (NSAIDs), has analgesic, anti-inflammatory and antipyretic activities and inhibits prostaglandin synthesis. Uses of diflunisal are given in the next Table:

Uses of Diflunisal
Osteoarthritis
Rheumatoid Arthritis
Mild to Moderate Pain

DOSAGE FORMS: Tabs:250, 500mg
DOSAGE: Diflunisal is administered orally; dosage is given in the next Table:

Dosage of Diflunisal

Condition	Dosage
Osteoarthritis	500 to 1g daily in two divided doses. Dosage may be increased or decreased according to the patients response.
Rheumatoid Arthritis	One g daily in two divided doses.
Mild to Moderate Pain	Initially, 1g followed by 500mg every 8-12 hours.

PHARMACOKINETICS: Absorption:Well absorbed and may be taken with food; Peak: 2-3 hours; Half-Life: 10 hours; Protein Binding: 99%.
ADVERSE EFFECTS: The most frequent adverse reactions are nausea, dyspepsia, gastrointestinal pain, and diarrhea. Rash and headache are observed in 3% to 9% of patients. Other adverse effects include vomiting, constipation, flatulence, dizziness, tinnitus, fatigue, somnolence and insomnia.

The effect of diflunisal on platelet function and bleeding time is dose related but reversible. Other reactions that have been reported are acute interstitial nephritis, acute renal failure, peripheral edema, borderline elevation of liver function test, peptic ulceration, GI bleeding and cholestasis. As with other salicylates, use of this drug in children should be weighed against the risk of developing Reyes syndrome.

Falsely elevates salicylate levels performed by colorimetric technique.

DIGOXIN

(Lanoxin)

USES: Uses of digoxin are listed in the next Table:

Uses of Digoxin
Congestive Heart Failure
Atrial Fibrillation or Flutter (Digitalis is Drug of Choice)
Supraventricular Tachycardia

Congestive Heart Failure: Digitalis is most effective when cardiac failure is caused by ischemic, hypertensive, valvular or congenital heart disease or dilated cardiomyopathy. Digoxin may not be required in patients with heart failure and/or arrhythmias associated with hypertension, anemia, beriberi, thyrotoxicosis or valvular heart disease after treatment or correction of the underlying disease.

In cardiac failure, the direct positive inotropic action (increase in the strength of contraction of the heart) may increase cardiac output and thereby decrease venous pressure, reduce heart size, and slow compensatory reflex tachycardia. Digoxin decreases ventricular volume, and thus does not increase myocardial oxygen consumption in the failing heart. Renal hemodynamics are improved and diuresis is promoted, thus reducing blood volume and relieving edema.

Atrial Fibrillation or Flutter: In patients with atrial flutter, digoxin may convert atrial flutter to atrial fibrillation with a slow ventricular rate; subsequently, atrial fibrillation may convert spontaneously to normal sinus rhythm during digoxin therapy or when digoxin is withdrawn.

Mechanism of Action: The direct action of digoxin is believed to be mediated through inhibition of the (Na^+-K^+)-ATPase enzyme system - the sodium pump that provides the energy for active transport of sodium and potassium ions across the myocardial cell membrane. Digoxin combines reversibly with the (Na^+-K^+)-ATPase on the cell membrane; the binding of the intracellular ATP is prevented. Inactivation of the sodium pump increases intracellular sodium ions and decreases intracellular potassium ions. Inhibition of the sodium-potassium transport system is accompanied by increased cellular uptake of calcium ions.

Digitalis slows the heart rate by directly suppressing the conduction of electric impulses at the atrioventricular (AV) node. The cardiac output increases and peripheral circulation improves.

DOSAGE FORMS: Tabs: 0.125, 0.25, 0.5mg; Elixir: 0.05mg/ml; IV Solutions: 0.1mg/ml (pediatric); 0.25mg/ml; Digoxin Solutions in Capsules (Lanoxicaps): 0.05, 0.1 and 0.2mg. The oral bioavailability of digoxin in capsules is greater than that of the tablet formulations.

DOSAGE: In adults, maintenance dosage of digoxin is usually administered as a single daily dose; however, it may be necessary to give divided doses to some patients with recurrent supraventricular tachyarrhythmias. In infants and young children, divided daily doses are typically given, but preliminary data suggests that single daily dosing may be equivalent (Zalzstein, E. et al., J. Pediatr. 116, 137-139, 1990).

Digoxin has a low therapeutic index. Furthermore, there is variation in individual requirements and response. Dosage may be modified according to the cardiovascular status and renal function of the patient. Dosage should be based on lean or ideal body weight.

There is no substantial difference in bioavailability of digoxin tablets or elixir. When changing from oral (tablets or elixir) or IM to IV therapy, digoxin dosage should be reduced by about 20-25%. When changing from tablets, elixir or IM therapy to liquid-filled capsules, digoxin dosage should be reduced by about 20%. The liquid-filled capsules are 90-100% absorbed.

Digitalization is the process of establishing a safe and effective serum concentration of a digitalis glycoside in a patient. In adults, the average digitalizing dose is 0.75 to 1.5mg.

Rapid digitalization may be accomplished by the I.V. or by oral route. Rapid digitalization by IV may be necessary in patients with rapid supraventricular arrhythmias when early control of the ventricular rate is desirable.

ECG monitoring of cardiac function should be performed during initial digitalization of infants and children; monitoring should be done in adults when the drug is given IV, when it is given orally for prolonged periods, or when it is given to patients with increased risk of adverse reactions to digoxin, such as those with severe heart or renal disease.

DIGOXIN (Cont.)

In neonates, ECG signs of toxicity may include sinus bradycardia, SA arrest and prolongation of the PR interval.

All orders for digoxin should be recorded in micrograms, milligrams, and milliliters (ml). Dosage of digoxin is given in the next Table:

Dosage of Digoxin

Condition	Age	Route	Dosage
Slow Digitalization (example, reduced left ventricular ejection)	Adults	Oral	0.125 to 0.5mg daily (usually 0.25mg in the elderly). Digitalization is usually accomplished in 7 to 10 days. Check digoxin level at 2 weeks to assure that it is in 1.0 to 1.8ng/ml range. In another schedule, 0.5mg daily for 3 days followed by usual maintenance dose.
Maintenace Dose	Adults	Oral	0.125 to 0.5mg daily depending on renal function, body size, age, thyroid function, and gastrointestinal absorption. Unless the end point of therapy is control of the ventricular response in atrial fibrillation, measure the serum digoxin levels after 1 week.
Rapid Digitalization	Adults	Oral	Initially, 0.5 to 0.75mg followed by 0.25 to 0.5mg every 6-8 hours until full digitalization is achieved (usually 0.75-1.25mg). In another schedule, 1-1.25mg are administered in divided dosages over the first 24 hours; 0.5mg is given during the second 24 hours.
Rapid Digitalization (example: rapid supra-ventricular arrhythmias when early control of the ventricular rate is desirable)	Adults	IV	Initially, 0.25-0.5mg given slowly over 10-20min;to avoid an immediate hypertensive response. IV digoxin begins to have an effect after 1.5-3 hours. Additional 0.125mg doses may be administered every 4-8 hours (up to max 1.5mg total) or until the ventricular response is controlled.
Rapid Digitalization	Infants & Children	Oral	Digitalizing doses are given in the next Table: (see Digitalizing Doses of Digoxin below) Digitalizing doses are given as follows: Initially, give 50% of the total dose; then give 25% fractions orally at 6-8 hours. The daily oral maintenance dose for premature neonates is 20-30% of oral loading dose, the daily oral maintenance dose for full-term and children is 25% to 35% of the oral loading dose.

Digitalizing Doses of Digoxin

Age	Dosage(mg/kg)
Premature Infants	0.020-0.030
Full Term, Newborn	0.025-0.035
1 Month-Two Years	0.035-0.060
2 to 5 Years	0.030-0.040
5 to 10 Years	0.020-0.035
Over 10 Years	0.010-0.015 (or adult dose)

DIGOXIN (Cont.)
Table Cont.

Dosage of Digoxin			
Condition	Age	Route	Dosage
	Children	IV	Digitalizing doses are given in the next Table:

Digitalizing Doses of Digoxin	
Age	Dosage (mg/kg)
Premature Infants	0.015 to 0.025
Full-Term, Newborn	0.020 to 0.030
One mon. to Two yrs.	0.030 to 0.050
Two to Five yrs.	0.025 to 0.035
Five to Ten yrs.	0.015 to 0.030
Over 10 years	0.010 to 0.015 (or adult dose)

The digitalizing doses are given in divided amounts at 6-8 hour intervals.
The daily intravenous maintenance dose is 20% to 30% of the oral loading dose in premature infants and 25% to 30% of the oral loading dose in full-term infants and children.

Renal insufficiency requires dosage adjustment.

PHARMACOKINETICS: Bioavailability: Lanoxin tablets, 60% to 80%; Lanoxin elixir, 70% to 85%; Lanoxicaps, 90% to 100%. Apparent Volume of Distribution: 6 liter/kg; decreased in elderly patients and in those with impaired renal function. Protein-Binding: 20% to 25%. Half-Life: 1.5 days and proportional to glomerular filtration rate.

Digoxin crosses the placenta, and, at delivery, the serum concentration in the newborn is similar to that in the mother. Excretion: 50% to 75% of a dose is excreted unchanged in the urine via glomerular filtration and tubular secretion.

DRUG INTERACTIONS: Many drugs affect digoxin levels; interactions should be investigated prior to initiating any additional drug therapy in patients on digoxin. Quinidine increases digoxin level in average twofold. The effect begins in 24 hours and a new steady state is attained in 4 days. Quinidine increases digoxin levels by decreasing renal clearance and tissue binding of digoxin. Calcium channel blockers, especially verapamil, increase digoxin levels by up to 75%. Amiodarone increases digoxin levels by 100% or more. Erythromycin may also double digoxin levels.

Cholestyramine may bind digoxin in the gut. Kaolin and pectin reduces GI absorption.

Spironolactone reduces elimination of digoxin.

CONTRAINDICATIONS: Hypertrophic obstructive cardiomyopathy except for supraventricular arrhythmias; second or third degree heart block in the absence of mechanical pacing.

TOXICITY: The most effective therapeutic dose of digoxin is a large fraction of the toxic dose, meaning that the therapeutic index is very low with only a very narrow difference between therapeutic and toxic dosages.

Digoxin toxicity dropped from 14% to 6% after the assay of digoxin was introduced (Koch-Weser, J. Therapeutic Drug Monitoring 3, 3-16, 1981). The toxic reaction to digoxin has a reported 20% mortality (Smith, T.W., Am. J. Med. 58 470-476, 1975).

DIGOXIN (Cont.)

The features of chronic digitalis toxicity are given in the next Table (Anderson, G.J., Geriatrics, pgs. 57-65, June, 1980):

Features of Chronic Digitalis Toxicity

Precipitating or potentiating factors	
Hypokalemia	Impaired excretion
Hypercalcemia	Severe heart disease
Hypoxia	Hypomagnesemia
Overdose	Hypothyroidism
	Drug interactions:
	Quinidine
	Spironolactone
	Verapamil
Clinical signs and symptoms	
Anorexia	Abdominal pain
Nausea	Psychosis
Vomiting	Mesenteric venous occlusion
Diarrhea	Weight loss
Headache	Scotomas
Depression	Blue-yellow vision
Congestive heart failure	
Incidence of cardiac arrhythmias	
Ventricular arrhythmias	55-85%
Atrioventricular (AV) block	20-40%
Atrial arrhythmias	20-25%
Junctional arrhythmias	12-18%
Sinotrial arrhythmias	5-15%
AV dissociation	10-20%

The systems that are most commonly involved are the gastrointestinal tract and the central nervous system. ECG Manifestations of Digitalis Toxicity: Between 30% and 70% of patients with ECG manifestations of digitalis toxicity will not have any clinical signs or symptoms; ECG changes occur in 85% to 95% of patients with digitalis toxicity. The changes are listed in the previous Table. Ventricular arrhythmias are the most prevalent ECG finding and are observed in about 60% of patients.

Precipitating or Potentiating Factors:

Hypokalemia: Hypokalemia potentiates or precipitates digitalis toxicity because the potassium ion competitively inhibits the binding of cardiac glycosides to the cardiac membrane.

Hypercalcemia: An increase in calcium concentration potentiates digitalis toxicity and induces abnormal automaticity through its effects on membranes.

Quinidine Effect on Digoxin: The simultaneous administration of quinidine and digoxin results in increased digoxin blood level. Therefore, digoxin dose should be decreased by one-third to one-half when quindine is given.

THERAPEUTIC DRUG MONITORING: Specimen: Red top tube; remove serum and freeze if greater than 24 hours; Reject specimen if not clotted. Blood specimen must be drawn 6-8 hours after administration of the last dose.

Reference Range: Therapeutic range: 0.5-2ng/ml; Toxic: >2ng/ml; potentially, >1.5ng/ml; in patients whose plasma potassium concentrations are below normal, plasma digoxin concentrations between 1.3 and 2.0ng/ml may be associated with toxicity. Half-Life: 1.6 days (normal renal and hepatic function); 5.0 days (markedly reduced renal and hepatic function.)

The time to steady state is 1 or 2 weeks; the time to steady state may be prolonged with either renal or hepatic dysfunction. Therapeutic monitoring is done after steady state has been achieved.

Serum Digoxin in Uremia: Blood samples from uremic patients, who are not receiving digoxin, may give false values for digoxin; two-thirds of blood specimens were positive for digoxin when measured by immunoassay methods (Graves, S.W. et al., Ann. Intern. Med. 99, 604-608, 1983).

DIGOXIN (Cont.)

In another study, acute renal failure with uremia was found to be associated with a two-fold rise in serum digoxin concentration during a nine-day period after the last dose of the drug, when measured by immunoassy. The apparent increase in serum digoxin may have been caused by a decrease in the apparent volume of distribution of digoxin and its metabolites secondary to renal failure, or the occurrence of an endogenous digoxin-like substance or polar digoxin metabolites (Craver, J.L. et al., Ann. Intern. med. 98, 483-484, 1983). In uremia, it may be that substances are produced that have both immunological activity and physiological activity similar to digoxin (Editorial, The Lancet 2 pgs. 1463-1464, Dec. 24 and 31, 1983).

Therapy is usually begun with or without a loading dose and therapeutic serum levels are maintained on a long-term basis after plasma-tissue equilibrium. The time course of distribution and elimination of a single oral dose of digoxin is shown in the next Figure; (Fenster, P.E. and Ewy, G.A., Resident and Staff Physician, 2s-15s, Dec. 1981):

Time Course of Distribution and Elimination of
a Single Oral Dose of Digoxin

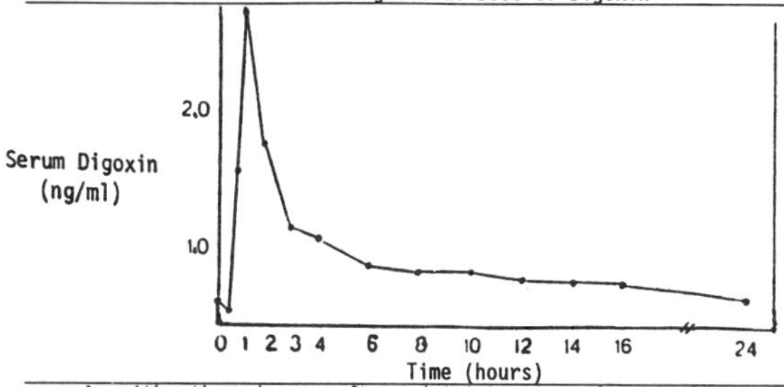

As with other drugs, after administration of a single dose, drug levels increase and then decline. The relatively high concentration of digoxin during the first six hours after oral dose reflects the relatively slow distribution of digoxin from the central compartment to the peripheral compartment. The serum level to determine peak activity should be obtained after the serum digoxin has had time to equilbrate with the tissues, that is, 8 to 24 hours after the oral dose.

TREATMENT: Absorption from the gastrointestinal tract should be prevented with either cholestyramine or colestipol. Restore body stores of potassium; mild intoxication can be corrected with oral potassium. The cardiac aspects of digoxin toxicity are treated with lidocaine or phenytoin. Severe digoxin toxicity may be treated with digoxin-specific Fab antibody fragments (Smith, T.W. et al., N. Engl. J. Med. 307, 1357-1362, 1982).

DIHYDROERGOTAMINE MESYLATE
(D.H.E. 45)

USES: Dihydroergotamine, given by IV or IM, is the drug of choice in physician's offices and hospital emergency rooms for the termination of acute migraine headaches, or cluster headaches. IV dihydroergotamine has terminated status migrainosus and repeated IV administration terminated the cycles of attacks (Raskin, N.H. and Raskin, K.E., Neurology 34, 245, 1984).

Mechanism of Action: Ergotamine causes peripheral **vasoconstriction,** especially in the dilated external carotid artery. It acts as a vasoconstrictor if the tonus of the blood vessel is low and as a vasodilator if the tonus is high.

The remarkably specific antimigraine action of ergotamine is thought to be related to its actions on vascular or neuronal serotonin receptors.

DOSAGE FORMS: D.H.E. 45 solution, 1mg/ml in 1ml containers.

DOSAGE: Dosage of dihydroergotamine mesylate for adults is given in the next Table:

Dosage of Dihydroergotamine

Route	Dosage
IM	One mg at the onset of an attack, repeated if necessary at hourly intervals to a total of 3mg. IM route is preferred.
IV	One mg repeated if necessary once after one hr. (max. 2mg).

DIHYDROERGOTAMINE MESYLATE (Cont.)

ADVERSE EFFECTS: The most frequent adverse effects are nausea, vomiting, epigastric discomfort, diarrhea, polydipsia, and drowsiness. Other more serious adverse effects may occur due to vasospasm and include paresthesias of the extremities, cramps and weakness of the legs, myalgia, precordial pain and rarely, gangrene. These effects can be reduced with vasocilator therapy. Rebound headaches can occur during chronic use, possibly leading to escalation of dosage by the patient.

There is a risk of provoking bronchospasm in asthmatic patients when ergotamine is administered by inhalation.

CONTRAINDICATIONS: Hypertension, cerebrovascular disease, coronary artery disease, angina pectoris, severe peripheral vascular disease, thyrotoxicosis, hepatic or renal impairment, sepsis, severe pruritis, malnutrition, pregnancy (category X).

PHARMACOKINETICS: Peak Plasma Conc.: 2 to 11 minutes; Metabolism: Liver. The low bioavailability is the result of significant degradation (97%) first-pass effect. Half-Life: 96 minutes; Excretion: Bile (90%); urine (3-4%).

DRUG INTERACTIONS: Erythromycin may increase toxicity.

DIHYDROTACHYSTEROL

(DHT, Hytakerol)

USES: **Dihydrotachysterol** is a **vitamin D analog,** activated by 25-hydroxylation in the liver;it does not require 1-hydroxylation in kidney. Dihydrotachysterol is used in the treatment of **hypocalcemia** associated with conditions listed in the next Table:

Uses of Dihydrotachysterol in Hypocalcemia
Renal Failure
Hypoparathyroidism
Pseudohypoparathyroidism
Familial Hypophosphatemia
Thyroidectomy-Induced Hypocalcemia
Osteoporosis

Dihydrotachysterol is used in the treatment of hypocalcemia associated with renal failure, hypoparathyroidism and pseudohypoparathyroidism, familial hypophosphatemia, thyroidectomy-induced hypocalcemia, osteoporosis.

DOSAGE FORMS: Caps: 0.125mg; Sol'n with alcohol: 0.2mg/ml; Sol'n in oil: 0.25mg/ml; Tabs: 0.125, 0.2, 0.4mg.

DOSAGE: Dihydrotachysterol is administered orally, usually once daily. Dosage is regulated to maintain serum calcium concentrations of 9-10mg/dl. Dosage is given in the next Table:

Dosage of Dihydrotachysterol

Condition	Age	Dosage
Renal Osteodystrophy	Children	0.1-0.5mg daily until healing occurs; then 0.25-0.6mg daily
	Adults	0.6-6mg daily until healing occurs; then 0.25-0.6mg daily
Hypoparathyroidism and Pseudohypoparathyroidism*	Neonates	0.05-0.1mg daily
	Infants and Young Children	0.1-0.5mg daily
	Older Children and Adults	0.5-1.0mg daily
Hypophosphatemic Vit. D Resistant Rickets		0.25-1.0mg daily
Nutritional Rickets		0.5mg daily

*Higher doses (usually, 4 times maintenance dose) may be necessary for several days initially.

One mg of dihydrotachysterol usually is equivalent to 3mg(120,000 units) of ergocalciferol.

MONITOR: Monitor serum calcium and serum phosphorus at least once weekly for first month and then monthly. Thereafter, maintain serum calcium in range 9-10mg/dl.

ADVERSE EFFECTS: Hypercalcemia with associated signs and symptoms.

DILTIAZEM
(Cardizem)

USES: **Diltiazem** is a **calcium-entry blocker** (calcium antagonist)used for its vasodilating properties; uses are given in the next Table:

Uses of Diltiazem
Prinzmetal Variant Angina
Chronic Stable Angina Pectoris
Hypertension

Prinzmetal Variant Angina (Vasospastic Angina): Diltiazem inhibits spontaneous coronary artery spasm resulting in increased myocardial oxygen.
Chronic Stable Angina Pectoris: Diltiazem has the following effects: dilation of systemic arteries resulting in decrease in total peripheral resistance; decrease in systemic b.p. (5-10mm Hg); decrease in afterload of the heart; small reflex increase in heart rate. The reduction in afterload and its resultant decrease in myocardial oxygen consumption is probably responsible for the effects of diltiazem in patients with angina.
Hypertension: Treatment of hypertension with diltiazem is given in the next Table (Report of the Joint National Committee on Detection, Evaluation, and Treatment of High Blood Pressure, Arch. Intern Med. 148, 1023 1988):

Treatment of Hypertension with Diltiazem

Step 1: Nonpharmacologic Approaches (see **HYPERTENSION**)
↓
Step 2: Diltiazem (Usual Minimum, 60 mg/day; Usual Maximum, 360 mg/day)
Observe up to 6 months; if diltiazem ineffective then,
↓
Step 3: Add a second drug of a different class
or Increase the dosage of diltiazem
or Substitute another drug
↓
Step 4: Add a third drug of a different class
or Substitute a second drug
↓
Step 5: Consider further evaluation and/or referral
or Add a third or fourth drug

"Step-Down": For patients with mild hypertension, after 1 year of control, consider decreasing or withdrawing diltiazem and other hypotensive drugs.
Mechanism of Action: Diltiazem inhibits calcium influx, thus inhibiting the contractile processes of cardiac and vascular smooth muscles; coronary arteries and systemic arteries dilate.
DOSAGE FORMS: Tabs: 30, 60, 90, 120mg; Caps(extended release): 60, 90, 120mg
DOSAGE: Diltiazem is administered orally before meals and at bedtime. Dosage is given in the next table:

Dosage of Diltiazem

Condition	Dosage
Prinzmetal Variant Angina or Chronic Stable Angina Pectoris	Initial: 30mg, 4 times daily; then, dosage is gradually increased at 1- to 2-day intervals until optimum control. Ave. 180-360mg/day.

PHARMACOKINETICS: Absorption: 80% rapid; Peak: 2-3 hrs.; Plasma Protein Binding: 80%; Half-Life:3-5 hrs.; Metabolism:Liver; Excretion:Urine and bile.
ADVERSE EFFECTS: The most common adverse effects are anorexia and nausea (3% of patients). Vomiting, diarrhea, constipation, indigestion occur in less than 1% of patients. Edema, arrhythmia, headache, rash and fatigue occur in 1-3% of patients. Diltiazem may cause liver dysfunction.

In contrast to nifedipine, diltiazem inhibits the cardiac conduction system, eg, reduces rate of sinoatrial(SA) node discharge or recovery time, reduces heart rate slightly. Adverse effects include bradycardia, asymptomatic asystole, congestive heart failure, 2° and 3° AV block occurs in less than 1% of patients.
DRUG INTERACTIONS: Diltiazem with quinidine may induce hypotension particularly in patients with idiopathic hypertrophic subaortic stenosis. Diltiazem may induce increases in plasma digoxin levels.
PRECAUTIONS: Use with caution in patients with congestive heart failure; contraindicated in patients with 2° or 3° heart block.

DIMENHYDRINATE

(Dramamine, etc)

USES: Dimenhydrinate is an ethanolamine derivative antihistamine that is especially useful in preventing and treating **vertigo** associated with **Meniere's disease and motion sickness**. It is also effective in treating **nausea and vomiting during pregnancy**.

Note that scopolamine, promethazine, meclizine or cyclizine may be more effective for the prevention and treatment of motion sickness.

DOSAGE FORMS: Tabs:50mg; Sol'n: 15mg/5ml; Amp.: 50mg/ml Injection.

DOSAGE: Dimenhydrinate may be administered orally, IM, or IV injection. For IV injection, each 50mg of dimenhydrinate must be diluted with 10ml of 0.9% sodium chloride injection and administered slowly over a period of 2 minutes. Dosage is given in the next Table:

Dosage of Dimenhydrinate

Condition	Age	Route	Dosage
Motion Sickness		Oral	Take 30 min. before exposure to motion
	Adults	Oral	50-100mg every 4 hr, as needed. Max: 400mg/day
	Children	Oral or IM	1.25mg/kg/dose every 6 hrs; Max: age 2-6 yrs, 75mg/day, age 6-12 yrs, 150mg/day
Meniere's Disease		Oral	25-50mg, 3 times daily for maintenance, or 50mg IM for acute attacks

PHARMACOKINETICS: Antiemetic Effects: Almost immediately after IV administration; within 15-30 minutes after oral administration and 20-30 minutes after IM administration. Duration of Action: 3-6 hours.

ADVERSE EFFECTS: Drowsiness or paradoxical CNS stimulation. Headache, blurred vision, tinnitus, dryness of mouth and respiratory passages, incoordination, palpitation, dizziness and hypotension.

DIMERCAPROL

(B.A.L., British Anti-Lewisite)

USES: **Dimercaprol** is a **chelating agent**; uses are given in the next Table:

Uses of Dimercaprol

Uses	Comments
Acute Arsenic Poisoning	**Treatment of Choice**
Acute Mercury Poisoning	**Treatment of Choice**
Acute Gold Poisoning	**Treatment of Choice**
Mercury-Induced Acrodynia	
Acute Lead Encephalopathy and/or Blood Lead Conc. >70mcg/dl	**Adjunct to Edetate Calcium Disodium**

Dimercaprol is the **antidote of choice** in the treatment of **acute arsenic** (except arsine), mercury, or gold poisoning. Mercury-induced acrodynia (pink disease) in infants and children responds to treatment with dimercaprol.

Dimercaprol is used as an adjunct to edetate calcium disodium and concomitant administration of the drugs is preferred in the management of acute lead encephalopathy and/or when blood lead concentration is greater than 100mcg/dl or in patients with symptomatic lead poisoning.

DOSAGE FORMS: Injection (in oil): 100mg/ml.

DOSAGE: Dimercaprol is administered only by deep IM injection; dosage is given in the next Table:

Dosage of Dimercaprol

Condition	Dosage
Arsenic or Gold Poisoning	
Severe	3mg/kg every 4 h. for first 2 days, 4 times daily on third day, then twice daily for 10 days or until recovery is complete.
Mild	2.5mg/kg, 4 times daily on first 2 days, twice daily on the third day, & once daily for 10 days.
Severe Gold Dermatitis	2.5mg/kg every 4 h. for 2 days; then twice daily for one week.
Gold-Induced Thrombocytopenia	100mg, twice daily for 15 days.
Acute Mercury Poisoning	5mg/kg followed by 2.5mg/kg once or twice daily for 10 days.
Acrodynia In Infants and Children	3mg/kg every 4 h. for 2 days; then every 6 h. for 1 day; then every 12 h. for 7-8 days.
Lead Poisoning:	
Lead Encephalopathy and/or Blood Lead >70mcg/dl	Initially: 4mg/kg or 80mg/m^2; then, 4mg/kg or 80mg/m^2 4 h. later and at 4 h. intervals for 5 days. Note edetate calcium disodium 250mg/m^2 is given simultaneously IM at separate sites or edetate calcium disodium may be given by continuous IV infusion (1.5g/m^2/day).

ADVERSE EFFECTS: Potentially nephrotoxic; urine must be kept alkaline during dimercaprol therapy to protect the kidneys. If acute renal failure develops during therapy, discontinue or use very cautiously.

Mild and transitory effects in about one-half of patients receiving IM dose of 5mg/kg. Antihistamines may prevent or relieve mild effects. If dose exceeds 5mg/kg, most patients experience vomiting, seizures, and stupor or coma which may begin within 30 minutes after injection and usually subsides in 1-6 hours. Hypertension and tachycardia are dose related. Fever occurs in 30% of children. May induce hemolysis in patients with G6PD deficiency. Sterile abscesses may occur, especially if not given deep IM.

CONTRAINDICATIONS: Acute hepatocellular injury, G6PD deficiency.

DIPHENHYDRAMINE
(Benadryl, etc.)

USES: Diphenhydramine is a **competitive antagonist** of **histamine** at the H-1 histamine receptor. Uses are given in the next Table:

Uses of Diphenhydramine

Usual Antihistamine Actions:
- **Nasal Allergies:** Seasonal allergic rhinitis; eg, hayfever and perennial (nonseasonal) allergic rhinitis.
- **Other Allergic Conditions:** Allergic dermatoses; allergic conjunctivitis caused by foods or inhaled allergens; allergic or hypersensitivity reactions to drugs; atopic dermatitis; contact dermatitis, pruritus ani or vulvae, & insect bites; dermatographism; mild transfusion reactions not caused by ABO incompatibility or pyrogens.
- **Adjunct Therapy** to epinephrine in treatment of **anaphylactic reactions** and laryngeal edema after acute manifestations controlled.

Other Uses:
- **Prevention of motion sickness**
- **Relief of cough** caused by minor throat and bronchial irritation
- Used in patients with mild insomnia
- Topically for temporary relief of itching: poison ivy, poison oak, sunburn, insect bites
- Parkinsonian Syndrome

It also has anticholinergic effects (dry mouth due to decreased salivary secretion, constipation due to decreased GI motility, blurring of vision, decreased sweating) and sedative effects.

DOSAGE FORMS: Caps: 25, 50mg; Tabs: 25, 50mg; Elixir/Sol'n: 12.5mg/5ml; Injection: 10, 50mg/ml; Topical: Cream, 1%; Lotion, 1%

DOSAGE: Diphenhydramine hydrochloride is usually administered orally. When oral therapy is not feasible, the drug may be given by deep IM, or preferably IV injection. Dosage is given in the next Table:

Dosage of Diphenhydramine

Condition	Age	Route	Dosage
Usual	Adults	Oral	25-50mg, 3-4 times daily, 4-6 h. intervals Max dosage: 300-400mg/day.
	Children	Oral IV, IM	5mg/kg daily in 3 or 4 doses up to adult dosage
Prevention of Motion Sickness	Adults	Oral	50mg, 30 min. before exposure; then, 50mg before meals and at bedtime.
Mild Insomnia	Adults	Oral	50mg, 20 min. before retiring.
Parkinsonian Syndrome	Adults	Oral	25mg, 3 times daily; then, gradually increased to 50mg, 4 times daily
Relief of Itching	Adults & Child. >2 yrs.	Topical	1% creams or lotions, 3-4 times daily for up to 7 days.

PHARMACOKINETICS: Onset: 15 min.; Peak: 1-4 h.; Duration: 4-6 h.; Half-Life: 3-9 h.; Protein Binding: 80%; Metabolism: Liver; Excretion: Urine

ADVERSE EFFECTS: CNS depression: sedation, drowsiness, dizziness, lassitude, disturbed coordination, muscle weakness, headache. GI Effects: Epigastric distress, anorexia, nausea, vomiting, diarrhea, constipation. Other Effects: Dry mouth, nose and throat; urinary retention; hypotension; thickening of bronchial secretions.

DRUG INTERACTION: Diphenhydramine may have additive CNS depressant effects with alcohol, sedatives, hypnotics, tranquilizers and narcotics.

CONTRAINDICATIONS: Prolonged acute asthma symptoms, i.e., status asthmaticus; narrow angle glaucoma, symptomatic prostatic hypertrophy, intestinal stasis and duodenal obstruction.

DIPHENOXYLATE WITH ATROPINE
(Lomotil, etc.)

USES: **Lomotil** is used to treat **diarrhea.** It is an opioid that slows GI motility; atropine is added in subtherapeutic amounts to decrease abuse potential.

Mechanism of Action: Diphenoxylate is an **opioid** which limits peristalsis by inhibiting mucosal receptors thus abolishing the local mucosal peristaltic reflex, and by stimulating segmental contraction. Lomotil decreases frequency of bowel movements and stool volume.

DOSAGE FORMS: Lomotil or generic: Each tablet or 5ml of liquid contains diphenoxylate hydrochloride 2.5mg and atropine sulfate 0.025mg.

DOSAGE: Dosage of Lomotil is given in the next Table:

Dosage of Lomotil

Age	Route	Dosage
Adults	Tablets or Liquid	5mg(two tablets) or 10ml three or four times daily.
8-12 years	Liquid	10mg (20ml) daily in five divided doses.
5-8 years	Liquid	8mg (16ml) daily in four divided doses.
2-5 years	Liquid	6mg (12ml) daily in three divided doses.
Children (by wt.)	Liquid	0.3-0.4mg/kg daily in divided doses.

Use with extreme caution in children; young children are particularly prone to toxicity, which may mask signs of dehydration, electrolyte imbalance or surgical abdomen.

ADVERSE EFFECTS: The incidence of adverse reactions is relatively low; these include abdominal distention, intestinal obstruction, dilation of the colon, rash, drowsiness, dizziness, mental depression, restlessness, nausea, headache and blurred vision.

Large doses (40 to 60mg) of diphenoxylate may produce a morphine-like euphoria. Toxic doses may cause respiratory depression and coma. Narcotic antagonists, e.g. naloxone (Narcan) or naltrexone (Trexan) may be used in treatment of poisoning.

PHARMACOKINETICS: Onset: 45-60 min.; Duration: 3-4 hours; Metabolism: Metabolized to an active metabolite, diphenoxylic acid. Half-Life: Diphenoxylate, 2.5 hours, diphenoxylic acid, 3-14 hours.

DIPYRIDAMOLE

(Persantine)

USES: Dipyridamole is a widely prescribed antithrombotic drug, used commonly in combination with aspirin; proposed uses of dipyridamole as a **platelet inhibitor** and coronary vasodilator are given in the next Table (FitzGerald, G.A., N. Engl. J. Med. 316, 1247-1257, 1987):

Proposed Uses of Dipyridamole
Secondary Prevention of Acute Myocardial Infarction.
Secondary Prevention of Transient Cerebral Ischemia and Stroke.
Preservation of Patency after Coronary-Artery Bypass.
Prevent:
Occlusion in Obliterative Arterial Disease of Lower Limbs.
Venous Thrombosis and Thromboembolism.
Thromboembolic Complications of Cardiac Valve Disease.

Secondary Prevention of Acute Myocardial Infarction: Treatment with aspirin plus dipyridamole reduces the incidence of nonfatal myocardial infarction by about one fifth in patients who have previously had a heart attack (Klimt, C.R. et al., J. Am. Coll. Cardiol. 7, 251-269, 1986). This is similar to the results obtained by using aspirin alone (Lancet 1, 1172-1173, 1980).

Secondary Prevention of Transient Cerebral Ischemia and Stroke: Dipyridamole adds nothing to the effiacy of aspirin in the secondary prevention of cerebral infarction (Bousser, M.G., Stroke 14, 5-14, 1983; Stroke 16, 406-415, 1985).

Preservation of Patency after Coronary-Artery Bypass: Dipyridamole is unlikely to contribute substantially to the efficacy of aspirin in maintaining the patency of saphenous vein aortocoronary-bypass grafts (Brown, B.G. et al., Circulation 72, 138-146, 1985).

Peripheral Vascular Disease: Combination therapy, eg., aspirin (330mg) plus dipyridamole (75mg), is significantly superior to placebo and to aspirin alone in preventing progression of peripheral vascular disease (Hess, H. et al., Lancet 1, 415-419, 1985).

Mechanism of Action: The proposed mechanisms of action of dipyridamole as an antithrombotic drug are given in the next Table (FitzGerald, G.A., N. Engl. J. Med 316, 1247-1257, May 14, 1987):

Proposed Mechanisms of Action of Dipyridamole
1. Inhibition of the phosphodiesterase enzyme in platelets resulting in an increase in intraplatelet cyclic AMP and the consequent potentiation of the platelet-inhibiting acts of prostacyclin.
2. Direct stimulation of the release of this eicosanoid by vascular endothelium.
3. Inhibition of cellular uptake and metabolism of adenosine, thereby increasing its concentration at the platelet-vascular interface.
4. Dipyridamole may augment the platelet-inhibiting action of aspirin through a pharmacokinetic interaction.

Prospective comparisons of aspirin plus dipyridamole (combination) with aspirin alone is given in the next Table (FitzGerald, G.A., N. Engl. J. Med. 316, 1247-1257, 1987):

Prospective Comparisons of Aspirin plus Dipyridamole in Combination with Aspirin Alone

Event	Daily Dose: Aspirin	Daily Dose: Dipyridamole	Combination vs. Aspirin Alone	Comment	Ref.
TIA, Stroke	1g	225mg	No difference	Both treatments superior to placebo	1
TIA, Stroke	325mg	75mg	No difference	No placebo group	2
Coronary-Graft Occlusion	975mg	225mg	No difference		3
Peripheral Vascular Disease	330mg	75mg	Combination superior	Both treatments superior to placebo.	4

1. Bousser, M.G. et al., Stroke 14, 5-14, 1983; 2. Stroke, 16, 406-415, 1985; 3. Brown, B.G. et al., Circulation 72, 138-146, 1985; 4. Hess, H. et al., Lancet 1, 415-419, 1985.

DOSAGE FORMS: Tabs: 25, 50, 75mg.

DOSAGE: Dosage of dipyridamole is given in the next Table:

Dosage of Dipyridamole

Condition	Dosage
Prevent Thromboembolism	75-100mg four times daily
Chronic Angina	50mg, 3 times daily given at least 1 hr before meals.

PHARMACOKINETICS: Dipyridamole is metabolized in liver.

ADVERSE EFFECTS: Headache, dizziness, GI intolerance, nausea, vomiting, diarrhea, peripheral vasodilation, flushing weakness, syncope and rash.

PRECAUTIONS: Use cautiously in patients with hypotension (vasodilator properties).

DISOPYRAMIDE
(Norpace)

USES: Disopyramide is a class I antiarrhythmic agent used to **prevent ventricular extrasystoles** and **ventricular tachycardia;** it may be less effective than quinidine in treatment of supraventricular tachyarrhythmias; uses are given in the next Table:

Uses of Disopyramide

Prophylactic Therapy to Maintain Normal Sinus Rhythm after Conversion of Atrial Fibrillation and/or Flutter by other methods
Prevent Recurrence:
- **Paroxysmal Atrial Fibrillation**
- **Paroxysmal Atrial Tachycardia**
- **Paroxysmal AV Junctional Rhythm**
- **Paroxysmal Ventricular Tachycardia**

Disopyramide is used, especially in patients refractory to quinidine or procainamide therapy or in patients in whom the side effects of other antiarrhythmic therapy are unacceptable.

Mechanism of Action: The mechanism of action of disopyramide is like that of quinidine and procainamide. Disopyramide has a direct action on the cell membrane; it depresses automaticity, especially in ectopic sites. It slows conduction and increases refractoriness of the atria, His-Purkinje system, accessory pathways and ventricles.

Disopyramide, like quinidine and procainamide, has anticholinergic properties which may modify the direct myocardial effects of the drug.

DOSAGE FORMS: Disopyramide is given orally; Caps:100,150mg regular and timed-release preparations. The timed-release preparations should not be used in patients with severe renal insufficiency, cardiomegaly or cardiac decompensation

Dosage of disopyramide is given in the next Table:

Dosage of Disopyramide

Condition	Preparation	Age	Dosage
Usual Dose; Normal Renal Function	Conventional	Adults >50kg	100-150mg every 6 hours.
Usual	Timed-Release	Adults	300mg every 12 hours; dosage should be reduced to 200mg every 12 hours in patients with small stature or moderate renal insufficiency.
Renal or Hepatic	Conventional	Adults	Maintenance dose of 100mg with or without a loading dose of 150mg at the following intervals: Clearance — Dosage Intervals(hr) 30-40(ml/min) — 8 15-30(ml/min) — 12 >15(ml/min) — 24
Usual	Conventional	<1yr	10-30mg/kg/day 4 divided doses
	Conventional	1 to 4yrs	10-20mg/kg/day 4 divided doses
	Conventional	4 to 12yrs	10-15mg/kg/day 4 divided doses
	Conventional	12 to 18yrs	6-15mg/kg/day 4 divided doses
Rapid Control, Normal Renal Function	Conventional	Adults	Loading Dose: 300mg; Maintenance Dose: 150mg every 6 hrs. If there is no therapeutic response and if no toxic effects occur within 6 hrs after the initial 300mg dose, 200mg doses may be given every 6 hrs. If there is no response in 48 hrs, the drug is discontinued and alternative therapy initiated or the patient should be hospitalized, closely evaluated, and continuously monitored while the dosage is increased to 250-300 every 6 hrs.

DISOPYRAMIDE (Cont.)

DOSAGE: Dosage is modified in the conditions listed in the next Table:

Modification of Dosage of Disopyramide

Condition	Effect	Modification of Dosage
Renal Failure	Half-Life Longer Serum Conc. Higher	Decrease by increasing dosing interval
Acute Myocardial Infarction	Half-Life Longer Volume of Distribution Higher	Decrease by decreasing maintenance dose
Congestive Heart Failure	Avoid disopyramide unless failure is caused by arrhythmias	
Hypokalemia		Higher Doses Are Necessary

PHARMACOKINETICS: Absorption: Rapid and complete; Onset: Within 1 hr; Duration: 6-12hrs; Excretion: 50% unchanged, 30% as metabolites in urine, 10% in feces. Range: Therapeutic: 2.0-5.0mcg/ml. Time to Obtain First Serum Specimen (Steady State): 36-48 hours. Peak: 2-3 hours. Sampling Time: Just before next dose. Half-Life: 4 to 10 hours. Toxicity: >7mcg/ml.

ADVERSE EFFECTS: Hypotension may occur and may be severe. Torsades de pointes and cardiac arrest occur rarely. Hypoglycemia has been reported. Anticholinergic effects (dry mouth, blurred vision, constipation, and urinary retention). Other reactions that may occur are nausea, vomiting, gastric pain and diarrhea; these reactions occur less often than with quinidine. Rarely, acute angle-closure glaucoma may be precipitated.

CONTRAINDICATIONS: Second or third degree AV block unless a ventricular pacemaker is in place; sinus node dysfunction; congestive heart failure.

GUIDELINES FOR THERAPY: Guidelines for therapy and serum specimen monitoring are given in the next Table:

Guidelines for Therapy and Monitoring

Therapy	Monitoring
Loading Dose: 300mg Maintenance Dose: 100-150mg every 6 hours	36-48 hours and at least 6 hours after last dose

DOBUTAMINE

(Dobutrex)

USES: **Dobutamine** is a **sympathomimetic drug** stimulating primarily **cardiac beta-1 adrenergic receptors;** dobutamine is used to increase cardiac output in the short-term treatment of patients with severe chronic cardiac failure caused by depressed contractility from organic heart disease or cardiac surgical procedures; dobutamine does not significantly increase heart rate. However, in patients with marked mechanical obstruction, such as severe valvular aortic stenosis, the drug may be ineffective and potentially harmful.

The relative beta-1 specificity is dose-dependent and at low doses, dobutamine has only a slight agonist effect on beta-2 and alpha-adrenergic receptors. However, specificity is lost at high doses.

DOSAGE FORMS: Injection: 250mg/20ml vials

DOSAGE: Continuous IV infusion: 2.5-20mcg/kg/min. To prepare for infusion:

6 x wt(kg) = mg of drug to add to 100ml IV fluids

Then:

IV infusion rate (ml/hr)(eg, 2.5ml/hr) = Dose (mcg/kg/min)(eg, 2.5mcg/kg/min)

Initially, the dosage is 2.5-5mcg/kg/min. Increase gradually in increments of 2.5-5mcg/kg/min. up to 20mcg/kg/min., titrating to desired response in each patient. Most patients can be maintained on 10mcg/kg/min. or less. Maximum recommended dose: 40mcg/kg/min.

PHARMACOKINETICS: Onset: 1-2 min.; Peak: Within 10 min.; Duration: <10 min.; Half-Life: 2 min.; Metabolism: Liver; Excretion: Urine

ADVERSE EFFECTS: Side effects of tachycardia, hypertension, arrhythmias (PVC's) may occasionally occur (especially at higher infusion rates). Correct hypovolemic state before use. Increases AV conduction, may precipitate ventricular ectopic activity.

CONTRAINDICATIONS: Contraindicated in idiopathic hypertrophic subaortic stenosis.

MONITOR: Heart rate, arterial blood pressure, urine output, pulmonary artery wedge pressure, cardiac index; ECG for ectopic activity and infusion rate of solution.

DOCUSATE
(Colace, etc.)
USES: Docusate is a stool softener. It is used in patients who have constipation secondary to hard stools and in patients who have painful anorectal conditions in which ease of defecation is desirable.
Mechanism of Action: Docusate, a salt of dioctylsulfosuccinate, is an **anionic surfactant (detergent)** that lowers the surface tension at the oil-water interface of the stool, allowing water and fat to penetrate the fecal material and, thus **softening the stool.**
DOSAGE FORMS: Caps: 50, 100, 240, 250, 300mg; Syrup: 16.7, 20mg/5ml; Tab: 50, 100mg; Solution: 10mg/ml, 50mg/ml; Rectal: 283mg/4ml.
DOSAGE: Docusate is administered orally or rectally. Take with a full glass of fluid; dosage is given in the next Table:

Dosage of Docusate

Age	Dosage
<3 yr.	10-40mg/day, 1-4 times a day
3-6 yrs.	20-60mg/day, 1-4 times a day
6-12 yrs.	40-120mg/day, 1-4 times a day
>12 yrs.	50-360mg/day, 1-4 times a day

PHARMACOKINETICS: Onset: 1-3 days after first dose with continuous use; Fate: May be partially absorbed in the duodenum and jejunum and secreted in bile.
CONTRAINDICATIONS: Intestinal obstruction and undiagnosed abdominal pain.
ADVERSE EFFECTS: Occasional abdominal pain.

DOPAMINE
(Intropin)
USES: Dopamine is the immediate **precursor of norepinephrine;** uses are given in the next Table:

Uses of Dopamine

Shock: Dopamine increases cardiac output(CO), blood pressure(BP), and **urine output.**
Chronic Refractory Congestive Heart Failure

Dopamine is indicated in shock caused by myocardial infarction, trauma, renal failure, and endotoxic septicemia.

The actions of dopamine are dose related as follows: low dose (0.5-2mg/kg/min.) acts on dopaminergic receptors; moderate dose (1-10mcg/kg/min.), beta-1 receptors; high dose (>10mcg/kg/min), alpha-adrenergic receptors and release of norepinephrine.

The in-vivo synthesis of dopamine is as follows:

Tyrosine ⟶ Phenylalanine ⟶ L-Dopa ⟶ Dopamine

DOSAGE FORMS: Injection: 40, 80, 160mg/ml
DOSAGE: Dopamine is administered by IV infusion using an infusion pump. Actions of dopamine at increasing dosages are given in the next Table:

Actions of Dopamine at Different Dosages

Low Dosage (0.5-2mcg/kg/min.) **(Dopaminergic Receptors)**	Moderate Dosage (1-10mcg/kg/min.) **(Beta-1 Receptors)**	High Dosage (>10mcg/kg/min.) **(Alpha-Adrenergic Receptors)**
Vasodilation of Arteries:	**Heart:**	**Vasoconstriction:**
Renal	Increased Heart Rate	Decreased Renal Blood Flow
Mesenteric	Increased Cardiac Contractility	
Coronary	Increased Cardiac Output(CO) with Increased Pulse Pressure	
Intracerebral with Increased Blood Flow	Increased Systolic B.P. however, with Peripheral Vasodilation, B.P. may remain unchanged	
Increased Renal Blood Flow — Increased Glomerular Filtration Rate(GFR)		

Dopamine infusion is usually begun at 1-5mcg/kg/min.; the infusion rate may be increased by 1-5mcg/kg/min. at 10-30 min. intervals. To prepare for infusion:

6 x wt(kg) = mg of drug to add to 100ml IV fluids

Then:
IV infusion rate (ml/hr)(eg, 2.5ml/hr) = Dose (mcg/kg/min)(eg, 2.5mcg/kg/min)

Max. dose recommended: 20-50mcg/kg/min.

DOPAMINE (Cont.)
PHARMACOKINETICS: Onset: 2-4 min.; Half-Life: 1-2 min.; Duration: <10 min.; Fate: 75% metabolized to homovanillic acid (HVA) and other metabolites; 25% metabolized to norepinephrine.
MONITOR: Vital signs and blood pressure continuously; correct hypovolemic states.
ADVERSE EFFECTS: Tachyarrhythmias; ectopic beats; hypotension at low infusion rates indicates rate should be increased; hypertension may occur at high infusion rates. Nausea, vomiting and angina pectoris may occur. Extravasation may cause tissue necrosis; if extravasation occurs, the area may be infiltrated with 5-10mg of phentolamine diluted in 10ml normal saline.
DRUG INTERACTIONS: Dopamine is metabolized by monoamine oxidase (MAO); the effects of dopamine are prolonged and intensified by monoamine oxidase inhibitors such as isocarboxazid, phenelzine and tranylcypromine. (These drugs are considered to be second-line drugs in the treatment of affective disorders). The dose should be reduced to one-tenth the usual amount in patients receiving monoamine oxidase inhibitors.

The cardiac effects of dopamine are antagonized by beta-adrenergic blockage agents such as propranolol and metoprolol, and the peripheral vasoconstriction caused by high doses of dopamine is antagonized by alpha-adrenergic blocking agents.

When general anesthetics are used, eg, halothane or cyclopropane anesthesia, ventricular arrhythmias and hypertension may occur.

IV phenytoin to patients receiving dopamine has resulted in hypotension and bradycardia.
CONTRAINDICATIONS: Pheochromocytoma; presence of uncorrected tachyarrhythmias or ventricular fibrillation.

DOXEPIN

(Adapin, Sinequan)

USES: Doxepin is a heterocyclic **antidepressant** used to treat depression and **anxiety**. Uses of doxepin in patients with depression are given in the next Table:

Uses of Doxepin in Depression
Major Depressive Episodes of Major Depression
Mixed Bipolar Disorder
Depressed Bipolar Disorder
Depressive Periods of Dysthymic Disorder
Atypical Depression

Doxepin is as effective as imipramine in the treatment of the first three conditions listed in the previous Table and also may be effective in the depressive periods of dysthymic disorder and atypical depression.

DOSAGE FORMS: Caps: 10, 25, 50, 75, 100, 150mg; Sol'n concentrate: 10mg/ml. Dilute just before administering with 4 oz of juice, water or milk.

DOSAGE: Doxepin is administered orally. Maximum antidepressant effects may not occur for 2-3 weeks; doxepin should not be withdrawn abruptly in patients who have received high dosages for prolonged periods. Dosage should be individualized; start with low dose and increase as tolerated until the desired clinical effect has been achieved. Dosage is given in the next Table:

Dosage of Doxepin

Condition	Dosage
Moderate Symptoms	25mg, three times a day; max. 150mg daily
Severe Symptoms	50mg, three times a day; max. 300 mg daily

Use lower doses in elderly and adolescents.

PHARMOCOKINETICS: Peak plasma concentrations occur within 2 hours. Mean half-life and range in hours 16.8 (8.2 to 24.5).

CONTRAINDICATIONS: Do not use during or within 14 days of monoamine oxidase inhibitors. Post myocardial infarction. Urinary retention. Glaucoma.

PRECAUTIONS: Cardiovascular disease, Epilepsy, Suicidal tendencies, Psychosis Diabetes, Abrupt cessation may produce withdrawal symptoms.

ADVERSE EFFECTS The most common adverse effects are due to their anticholinergic and alpha-adrenergic blocking activities: flushing, diaphoresis, dryness of the mouth, blurred vision, constipation, tachycardia and hypotension.

Central nervous system effects include sedation, fine tremor, speech blockage, anxiety and insomnia. Increased appetite with overeating may occur. Seizures may be observed in patients who have had a previous history of such disorders and those with a history of alcoholism.

Parkinsonism occurs occasionally especially on abrupt withdrawal of the drug.

DOXORUBICIN

(Adriamycin)

USES: Doxorubicin, an anthracycline, **antitumor antibiotic,** is produced from Streptomyces peucetius.

Doxorubicin is one of the most effective antineoplastic agents and is used, most often in combination regimens, to treat tumors listed in the next Table:

Uses of Doxorubicin in Treatment of Tumors
Leukemia: Acute Lymphocytic and Acute Myelogenous Leukemia
Hodgkin's Disease and Non-Hodgkin's Lymphoma
Sarcomas: Ewing's, Osteogenic, Rhabdomyosarcoma, Soft Tissue Sarcomas.
Neuroblastoma
Wilm's Tumor
Carcinomas: Breast, Lung, Stomach, Pancreas, Bladder, Prostate, Ovary, Endometrium, Cervix, Testes, Thyroid, Squamous Cell Carcinomas of Head and Neck, Hepatoma.

Mechanism of Action: Doxorubicin slips between neighboring base pairs of DNA; the intercalation process forces the base pairs apart and lengthens the double helical DNA so it cannot function as an effective template for RNA synthesis.

DOXORUBICIN (Cont.)
DOSAGE FORMS: Injection: 10, 20, 50, 100, 150mg
DOSAGE: Doxorubicin hydrochloride is administered by IV; extravasation of doxorubicin produces severe local tissue damage. The drug is administered slowly by direct intravenous administration into the side arm of a freely running intravenous line. Dosage is given in the next Table:

Dosage of Doxorubicin

Age	Dosage
Adults, Children	60-75mg/m^2 given as a single dose at 21-day intervals; the lower dose is given to patients with inadequate bone marrow secondary to old age, prior therapy, or marrow infiltration with malignant cells. or 20mg/m^2 once weekly. Cumulative Dose Limits: 550mg/m^2; 400mg/m^2 with prior chest irradiation.

No dosage adjustment necessary in renal impairment; reduce dosage with severe hepatic dysfunction.
PHARMACOKINETICS: Drug enters cells rapidly with subsequent concentration in the nucleus. Tissue concentrations are highest in lung, kidney, spleen, small intestine and liver; only a very small amount penetrates into the CNS.

Half-Life: The plasma decay curve is triphasic with half-lives of 12 min., 3.3 hrs., and 30 hrs. Metabolism: Liver; Elimination: After seven days, 40%-50% eliminated in bile, 50% as unchanged drug and 23% as active metabolite (adriamycinol). Only 5% to 10% is excreted in the urine.
ADVERSE EFFECTS: Toxicity effects the hematopoietic, cardiac, dermatologic and gastrointestinal systems as described in the next Table:

Toxicity of Doxorubicin

System	Effect
Hematopoietic	Bone Marrow Depression: Leukopenia is the usual dose-limiting toxicity; the lowest counts occur 10 to 15 days after the initial administration. Blood counts return to normal approximately 21 days after administration. Thrombocytopenia and anemia follow a similar pattern Monitor blood counts!
Cardiac	Acute Effects: Develop within a few minutes after a single IV dose and may persist for two weeks. ECG changes may include sinus tachycardia, flattening of T-wave, depressed S-T segment, voltage reduction and arrhythmias. These changes are usually transient and reversible. Delayed Effects: This effect is delayed, cumulative, dose-dependent cardiomyopathy occurring during or several weeks after completion of treatment. Doxorubin must be discontinued when congestive heart failure secondary to diffuse cardiomyopathy develops. The drug should not be given to patients with significantly impaired cardiac function. Children treated with cumulative doses of 228-550mg/m^2 often have impaired myocardial growth with increased left ventricular afterload and occasionally, decreased contractility (Lipshultz, S.E. et al., N. Engl. J. Med. 324, 808-815, March, 1991).
Dermatologic	Alopecia is observed in about 80% of patients, and regrowth of hair is usually complete two to five months after cessation of therapy.
Gastrointestinal	Nausea and vomiting are common; diarrhea occurs occasionally. Stomatitis and esophagitis may be severe.
Other	The urine may become red due to red colored doxorubicin.

MONITOR: Pretreatment and at least monthly complete blood count(CBC) including platelet count. Monitor general cardiac status; serial radionuclide scans of the heart in high risk patients.

DOXYCYCLINE
(Vibramycin, etc.)

USES: **Doxycycline** is a **tetracycline** antibiotic; uses in the treatment of infections are given in the next Table:

Uses of Doxycycline in Infections
Rickettsia
Chlamydia
Mycoplasma
Gonorrhea and Associated Infections
Brucellosis
Legionella Pneumophilia
Anti-Infective prophylaxis in Rape Victims
Traveler's Diarrhea
Suppression or Chemoprophylaxis of Malaria

DOSAGE FORMS: Caps: 50, 100mg; Tabs: 50, 100mg; Oral Susp: 25, 50mg/5ml; Parenteral: 100, 200mg

DOSAGE: Doxycycline calcium, doxycycline hyclate, and doxycycline monohydrate are administered orally; since doxycycline may cause esophageal irritation, it should be administered with fluids and should not be taken at bedtime.

Doxycycline hyclate may be administered by slow IV infusion; thrombophlebitis is a complication of IV therapy. Dosage is given in the next Table:

Dosage of Doxycycline

Condition	Age	Route	Dosage
Usual	Adults & Child. >8 yrs. Wt. >45kg	Oral IV	100mg every 12 h. on first day; then 100-200mg daily in 1-2 doses. If given IV, infuse over 1-4 hrs.
	Child. >8 yrs. Wt. <45kg	Oral IV	5mg/kg every 12 h. on first day; then 2.5-5mg/kg daily in 1-2 doses. If given IV, infuse over 1-4 hrs.
Rickettsial Infect. Rocky Mountain Spotted Fever; Endemic (Murine) Typhyus; Q Fever; Rickettsial pox	Adults & Child. >8 yrs. Wt. >45kg	Oral IV	100mg every 12 h. on first day; then 100-200mg daily in 1-2 doses. IV infusion over 1-4 hrs. Duration of Treatment:10-15 days or until patient is afebrile.
	Child. >8 yrs. Wt. <45kg	Oral IV	5mg/kg every 12 h. on first day; then 2.5-5mg/kg daily in 1-2 doses. IV infusion over 1-4 hrs. Duration of Treatment: 10-15 days or until patient is afebrile.
Louse-Borne (Epidemic) Typhus	Adults	Oral	100mg as single oral dose
Brill-Zinsser Dis Scrub Typhus	Child.	Oral	50mg as single oral dose
Chlamydia Trachomatis Uncomplicated Urethral Endocervical or Rectal	Adults	Oral	100mg twice daily for 7 days
Lymphogranuloma Venereum Serotype of Trachomatis	Adults	Oral	100mg twice daily for 3 wks.
Mycoplasma Urethritis	Adults	Oral	100mg,1 or 2 times daily for 1-3 wks
Gonorrhea (Patients Allergic to Penicillin Cephalosporin or Probenecid)	Adults	Oral	100mg twice daily for 7 days
Rape Victims	Adults	Oral	100mg twice daily for 7 days
Traveler's Diarrhea	Adults	Oral	100mg once daily for up to 2 wks. on beginning day of travel and continuing 2 days after returning home.

PHARMACOKINETICS: Half-Life: 15 h. adults.

CONTRAINDICATIONS: Do not give doxycycline to children under 8 years.

ADVERSE REACTIONS: IV is frequently associated with phlebitis. Nausea and diarrhea. Do not use in children because doxycycline binds to calcium in teeth and bones and may cause discoloration of teeth. Occasionally, phototoxic skin reactions may occur.

EDETATE CALCIUM DISODIUM
(Calcium EDTA)

USES: Edetate calcium disodium is a **chelating agent.** The calcium in calcium EDTA can be displaced by divalent and trivalent metals particularly lead. Parenterally administered calcium EDTA is the **chelating agent of choice** for the reduction of blood and depot **lead** in the treatment of acute and chronic **lead poisoning and lead encephalopathy**.

DOSAGE FORMS: Amp: 200mg/ml (5ml)

DOSAGE: Calcium EDTA may be administered by slow IV infusion or by IM injection. Daily doses by IV infusion are preferably administered over 12-24 hours. IM administration has been recommended as the preferred route of administration in children and in all patients with incipient or overt lead encephalopathy. Dosage is the same for either IV or IM administration. Dosage is given in the next Table:

Dosage of Edetate Calcium Disodium for Lead Poisoning
1-1.5gm/M^2/day or 50-75mg/kg/day, divided every 4-12 h. and given for 3-7 days depending on severity. Do not exceed 7 days duration of administration. Can add procaine (final conc. 0.5%) when giving IM. IM route preferred. Usual adult dose: 2-4gm/day.

CONTRAINDICATIONS: Anuria

ADVERSE EFFECTS: May cause renal tubular necrosis with hematuria, proteinuria, and uremia. May cause hypocalcemia, hypomagnesemia, and transient elevation of transaminases. Rapid IV infusion may cause sudden increase in intracranial pressure in patients with cerebral edema. May cause zinc deficiency by chelating zinc.

MONITOR: Urinalysis and renal function. Monitor ECG.

EDROPHONIUM

(Tensilon)

USES: Edrophonium, a parasympathomimetic, is usually the drug of choice for the differential diagnosis of myasthenia gravis and may be used to terminate A-V nodal reentrant tachycardia when vagal maneuvers fail.

Myasthenia Gravis: Myasthenia gravis is manifested, clinically, by weakness of skeletal muscle. Muscular contraction is mediated by release of acetylcholine from motor nerve terminals and its binding to receptor proteins on muscle; contraction is terminated by the enzyme acetylcholinesterase which catalyzes the hydrolysis of acetylcholine to choline plus acetate. Myasthenia gravis is an autoimmune disease in which antibodies to acetylcholine receptor proteins reduce the acetylcholine sensitivity of the receptor.

Acetylcholinesterase has a well-defined physiological role at the motor end-plate; it acts on acetylcholine, which is an important mediator of nerve conduction. The reaction catalyzed by acetylcholinesterase is as follows:

$$\text{Acetylcholine} + H_2O \xrightarrow{\text{Acetyl-Cholinesterase}} \text{Acetate} + \text{Choline}$$

Edrophonium attaches to acetylcholinesterase at the site of binding of acetylcholine and thus inhibits the hydrolysis of acetylcholine. Acetylcholine accumulates and its effects are prolonged and exaggerated at cholinergic synapses (parasympathomimetic effects). Edrophonium produces cholinergic responses of short duration including miosis, increased tonus of intestinal musculature, constriction of bronchi and ureters, bradycardia and stimulation of secretion by salivary and sweat glands, depressed conduction through A-V node and increase in tonus of skeletal musculature.

Patients with myasthenia gravis show a dramatic, transient increase in muscle strength in response to IV edrophonium chloride. After IV edrophonium administration, muscle strength increases in patients with myasthenia gravis within 1-3 minutes and lasts for 5-10 minutes.

Arrhythmias: Edrophonium may be used to terminate A-V nodal reentrant tachycardia when vagal maneuvers fail.

DOSAGE FORMS: Injection: 10mg/ml (1ml)

DOSAGE: Edrophonium chloride is usually administered IV. For the diagnosis of myasthenia gravis, all anticholinesterase medications should be discontinued for at least 8 hours before administering edrophonium. Placebo response should be determined; measure muscle strength before and after administration of atropine sulfate or sodium chloride injection. To counteract the untoward actions of edrophonium, both atropine in a syringe and resuscitation equipment must be available. Muscle strength of cranial musculature is usually measured. Dosage is given in the next Table:

Dosage of Edrophonium

Condition	Age	Dosage
Diagnosis of Myasthenia Gravis	Adults and Children >34kg	Draw 10mg of edrophonium into syringe. Inject 2mg over 15-30 seconds. If a cholinergic reaction occurs, the test should be discontinued and 0.4-0.5mg of atropine sulfate administered IV. If no response to edrophonium occurs, the remaining 8mg of the drug is given 45 seconds later; after 30 minutes, the test may be repeated if needed.
	Children <35kg	Draw 5mg of edrophonium into syringe. Inject 1mg over 15-30 seconds. If a cholinergic reaction occurs, the test should be discontinued and atropine 0.01-0.04mg/kg/dose is administered. If no response occurs within 45 seconds of the initial dose of edrophonium, 1mg is given every 30-45 seconds up to 5mg. Or give 0.04mg/kg as test dose. If no reaction in one minute, give 0.16mg/kg.
	Neonate	0.1mg single dose.
Cardiac Arrhythmias A-V Nodal Reentrant Tachycardia	Adults	An initial test dose of 1 to 2mg to elderly patients, those receiving digitalis and in those with a history of cardiac disease. 5mg; if ineffective, give 5-10mg.
	Children	0.1-0.2mg/kg IV, max: 2mg administered slowly.

PHARMACOKINETICS: Half-Life:110 min.; Onset:30-60 seconds; Duration:5-10 min.

ADVERSE EFFECTS: May precipitate cholinergic crisis,arrhythmias,bronchospasm.

ENALAPRIL
(Vasotec)

USES: Enalapril, like captopril is an **angiotensin-converting enzyme(ACE) inhibitor**; it reduces peripheral vascular resistance and venous tone. Uses of enalapril are given in the next Table:

Uses of Enalapril
Hypertension
Congestive Heart Failure

Hypertension: Enalapril is used in mild to severe essential hypertension and renovascular hypertension; it may be particularly useful in hypertensive patients with coexisting congestive heart failure. Treatment of hypertension with enalapril is given in the next Table (The 1988 Report of the Joint National Committee on Detection, Evaluation, and Treatment of High Blood Pressure, Arch. Intern. Med. 148, 1023-1038, 1988):

Treatment of Hypertension with Enalapril

Step 1: Nonpharmacologic Approaches (see **HYPERTENSION**)
↓
Step 2: Enalapril (Usual Minimum, 2.5-5.0 mg/day; Usual Maximum, 40mg/day)
Observe up to 6 months; if enalapril ineffective then,
↓
Step 3: Add a second drug of a different class
or Increase the dosage of enalapril
or Substitute another drug
↓
Step 4: Add a third drug of a different class
or Substitute a second drug
↓
Step 5: Consider further evaluation and/or referral
or Add a third or fourth drug

"Step-Down": For patients with mild hypertension, after 1 year of control, consider decreasing or withdrawing enalapril and other hypotensive drugs.

Congestive Heart Failure: Enalapril acts predominantly to reduce left ventricular volume and filling pressure and increase cardiac output. Heart rate may be reduced initially and blood pressure may be reduced markedly after the first few doses.

Molecular Form: Enalapril is a pro-drug, activated by the liver to enalaprilat, the active form.

DOSAGE FORMS: 2.5, 5, 10 and 20mg

DOSAGE: Enalapril is administered orally. The drug can be given before, during or after meals since food does not appear to substantially affect the rate or extent of absorption.

Dosage of enalapril is given in the next Table:

Dosage of Enalapril

Condition	Dosage
Hypertensive Patient on Diuretics	Discontinue diuretic for 2-3 days to minimize the possibility of hypotension. Initially, 2.5mg daily; monitor b.p. closely for two weeks. Maintenance: Titrate dose at 2-4 weeks intervals to the usual maintenance dose of 10-40mg daily as a single dose or in two divided doses daily.
Hypertensive Patient Creatinine Clearance, <30ml/min.	Initially, 2.5mg daily. If necessary, dosage may then be gradually increased to a max. dosage of 40mg daily.
Hypertensive Patient, Not Taking Diuretics and Creatinine Clearance >30ml/min.	Initially, 5mg daily. If necessary, titrate dose at 2-4 weeks intervals to the usual maintenance dose of 10 to 40mg daily as a single dose or in 2 divided doses daily.
Congestive Heart Failure with Normal Renal Function	Enalapril is administered in conjunction with cardiac glycoside and diuretic. Initially: 2.5mg once or twice daily. Dose may be increased gradually by titrating at 2-3 weeks intervals to a range of10-40mg daily as a single dose or in 2 divided doses daily.

PHARMACOKINETICS: Bioavailability: 40%; Metabolism: Liver to its active form, enalaprilat; Half-Life of Enalaprilat: 11 hours and increased in renal failure.

ENALAPRIL (Cont.)
ADVERSE EFFECTS: Severe, symptomatic hypotension may occur after the first dose; acute renal failure has been reported. Hirsutism, pruritis, rash, cough, and angioneurotic edema. Headache, dizziness, nausea and diarrhea may occur.
DRUG INTERACTIONS: Nonsteroidal anti-inflammatory drugs, including aspirin, may magnify potassium-retaining effects of enalapril. Increases lithium levels.
PRECAUTIONS: Can cause reversible, acute, renal failure in patients with bilateral renal arterial stenosis or unilateral stenosis in a solitary kidney; proteinuria may occur; hyperkalemia can develop, particularly in patients with insufficiency; rarely can induce neutropenia.

ENCAINIDE
(Enkaid)
USES: Encainide, a class IC antiarrhythmic drug (sodium-channel blockage), is used to treat supraventricular and ventricular arrhythmias (Woosley, R.L. et al., N. Engl. J. Med. 318, 1107-1115, 1988). It is approved by the FDA for only the treatment of ventricular arrhythmias, and should be used only in patients with life-threatening, refractory arrhythmias, where potential benefits are judged to outweigh the risks - see ADVERSE EFFECTS.
Mechanism of Action: Encainide, as a class IC antiarrhythmic drug, decreases the rate of rise of phase 0 of the action potential but has little effect on the duration or amplitude of the action potential. It depresses the fast sodium channel and decreases myocardial conduction velocity (Wehmeyer, A.E. and Thomas, R.L., Drug Intell. Clin. Pharm. 20, 9-13, 1986).
DOSAGE FORMS: Caps: 25, 35 and 50mg.
DOSAGE: Encainide is administered orally. The initial dosage is 25mg, three times daily. Changes can be made every 3 to 5 days as follows: 35mg, 3 times daily; 50mg, 3 times daily, 50mg, 4 times daily.
ADVERSE EFFECTS: Adverse effects of encainide occur in 30% of patients causing 10% to discontinue the drug; adverse effects are given in the next Table(Kreeger, R.W. and Hammill, S.C., Mayo Clin. Proc. 62, 1033-1050, 1987):

Adverse Effects of Encainide

Adverse Effects	Percent (%)
Cardiac toxicity	
Proarrhythmia	5-20% (increased to 20% in patients with reduced ejection fraction and history of ventricular tachycardia or fibrillation).
Congestive heart failure	<1%
Noncardiac toxicity	
Dizziness	26%
Blurred vision	19%
Nausea	4%
Tremor	4%
Headache	4%

PHARMACOKINETICS: G.I. Absorption: Completely absorbed; Protein Binding: 70%-80%; Metabolism: Metabolism occurs in the liver and depends on phenotypic mode of metabolism; 90% of the population are extensive metabolizers, whereas 10% are poor metabolizers. Encainide is metabolized to two active metabolites: O-demethyl encainide (ODE) and 3-methoxy-O-demethyl encainide (3-MODE).

The pharmacokinetics of encainide and its metabolites are given in the next Table (Wang, T. et al., J. Pharmacol. Exp. Ther. 228, 605-611, 1984; Woosley, R.L. et al., N. Engl. J. Med. 318, 1107-1115, 1988):

Pharmacokinetics of Encainide and its Metabolites

Feature	Extensive Metabolism	Poor Metabolism
Elimination Half-Life (Hr.)	0.5-4	8-22
Clearance (liters/min)	1.9	0.18
Plasma Protein Binding (%)	70	78
Plasma Conc. at Steady State(ng/ml)		
Encainide	18	200-1100
ODE	115	~12
MODE	94	Not detectable

ODE accumulates during long-term treatment and is primarily responsible for the effects of the drug in extensive metabolizers. Encainide is primarily responsible for the effects of the drug in poor metabolizers. Plasma Levels: Plasma levels of encainide are more than 20 times higher in poor metabolizers as compared to extensive metabolizers. Excretion: Urine.

ENCAINIDE (Cont.)

ADVERSE EFFECTS: Encainide can induce new life-threatening arrhythmias including sinus arrest, AV block and intraventricular conduction disturbances, particularly in patients with poor left ventricular function and sustained ventricular arrhythmias. Encainide can also aggravate congestive heart failure (Gottlief, S.S. et al., Ann. Inter. Med. 110, 505, 1989). Encainide (and flecainide) was associated with an increase in mortality and nonfatal cardiac arrest compared with controls in post-myocardial infarction patients treated for asymptomatic nonlife-threatening arrhythmias (Echt, D.S., et al., N. Engl. J. Med. 324, 781-788, March, 1991).

ENDOCARDITIS, PATHOGENS, TREATMENT

Pathogens: The pathogens that are most likely to cause endocarditis are given in the next Table (Handbook of Antimicrobial Therapy, The Medical Letter, 1990):

Pathogens Causing Endocarditis
1. Viridans group of Streptococcus
2. Enterococci
3. Streptococcus bovis
4. Staphylococcus aureus
5. Staphylococcus epidermidis
6. Candida albicans and other fungi
7. Gram-negative bacilli
8. Streptococcus pneumoniae
9. Streptococcus pyogenes (Group A)
10. Corynebacterium sp. (especially with prosthetic valves)
11. Haemophilus, Actinobacillus, or Cardiobacterium
Other:
Legionella species (Tompkins, L.S. et al., N. Engl. J. Med. 318, 530-535, 1988.
Q fever
Neisseria gonorrhoeae (Williams, C. and Corey, R., South. Med. J. 80, 1194-1195, 1987).

Over 80% of cases of endocarditis are caused by streptococci (Bain, R.J.I. et al., J. Antimicrob. Chemother. 20 (suppl. A), 17-24, 1987). Between 60-80% of patients with endocarditis have predisposing cardiac conditions, most usually damage associated with rheumatic heart disease.

Treatment: Empirical antimicrobial therapy is given in the next Table:

Empirical Antimicrobial Therapy of Endocarditis

Probable Cause	Drug Treatment
Streptococcal Endocarditis	Fully Sensitive to Penicillin: Benzylpenicillin plus low-dose gentamicin (60-80mg 12-hours) for 14 days followed by amoxicillin for a further 14 days. Reduced Sensitivity to Penicillin: Benzylpenicillin plus low-dose gentamicin (60-80mg 12-hours) for 28 days Penicillin Allergic Patients: Vancomycin plus gentamicin
Staphylococcal Endocarditis	Staphylococcus Aureus: Parenteral nafcillin or oxacillin plus low-dose gentamicin for 14 days followed by nafcillin or oxacillin by mouth for a further 14 days. Vancomycin is used in patients allergic to penicillin. Staphylococcus Epidermidis: Vancomycin for 21 days; consider giving rifampin in addition to vancomycin for prosthetic valve endocarditis caused by this organism.

ENDOCARDITIS, PROPHYLAXIS

Some conditions may predispose to endocarditis. These conditions include the following (Dajani, A.S., JAMA 264, 2919-2922, 1990):

Conditions Predisposing to Endocarditis
1. Congenital cardiac defects
2. Prosthetic cardiac valves
3. Rheumatic and other acquired valvular dysfunction
4. Idiopathic hypertrophic subaortic stenosis
5. Mitral valve prolapse with insufficiency
6. Previous history of bacterial endocarditis
7. Surgically constructed systemic-pulmonary shunts

Conditions for which the risk of endocarditis is small and antibiotic prophylaxis is not recommended include the following (Shulman, S.T. et al., Circulation 70, 1123A-1127A, 1984; Dajani, A.S., Pediatr. Inf. Dis. 4, 349-352, 1985; Dajani, A.S., et al., JAMA 264, 2919-2922, 1990):

Conditions with Minimal Risk of Endocarditis
1. Isolated secundum atrial septal defect
2. Secundum atrial septal defect repaired without a patch 6 months or more earlier
3. Patent ductus arteriosus ligated and divided 6 months or more earlier
4. Post coronary artery bypass graft surgery
5. Routine diagnostic cardiac catheterization and angiography

Procedures for which endocarditis prophylaxis is indicated include two major categories: dental and upper respiratory procedures, and gastrointestinal and genitourinary procedures (Shulman, S.T. et al., Circulation 70, 1123A-1127A, 1984; Dajani, A.S. et al., JAMA 264, 2919-2922, 1990):

Procedures Necessitating Endocarditis Prophylaxis
Dental and Upper Respiratory Procedures
Dental procedures likely to induce gingival bleeding
Tonsillectomy and/or adenoidectomy
Surgical procedures or biopsy of respiratory mucosa
Bronchoscopy
Genitourinary and Gastrointestinal Tract Surgery and Instrumentation
Cystoscopy
Prostatic Surgery
Urethral catheterization
Urinary tract surgery
Vaginal hysterectomy
Gallbladder surgery
Colonoscopy, colonic surgery
Esophageal dilatation, sclerotherapy of esophageal varices

Streptococcus viridans (following intra-oral procedures) and enterococci (following genitourinary or gastrointestinal procedures) are the most common causes of endocarditis in high risk individuals. Present guidelines for antimicrobial prophylaxis prior to procedures are based on recommendations of the American Heart Association as follows (Dajani, A.S., et al., JAMA 264, 2919-2922, 1990):

Endocarditis Prophylaxis for Dental and Upper Respiratory Procedures

Route	Adults	Children
Oral (Standard)	Amoxicillin 3g 1 hr prior and 1.5g 6 hrs later. Pen allergy: Erythromycin stearate 1g 2 hrs prior and 500mg 6 hrs later (EES: 800mg followed by 400mg 6 hrs later) or Clindamycin 300mg 1 hr prior and 150mg 6 hrs later.	Amoxicillin 50mg/kg 1 hr prior and 25mg/kg 6 hrs later. Pen allergy: Erythromycin stearate (or EES) 20mg/kg 2 hrs prior and 10mg/kg 6 hrs later or Clindamycin 10mg/kg 1 hr prior and 5mg/kg 6 hrs later.
Parenteral (Low Risk)	Ampicillin 2g IM or IV 30 min prior and 1g 6 hrs later (or amoxicillin 1.5g 6 hrs later). Pen allergy: Clindamycin 300mg 30 min prior and 150mg 6 hrs later.	Ampicillin 50mg/kg IM or IV 30 min prior and 25mg/kg 6 hrs later(or amoxicillin 25mg/kg 6 hrs later). Pen allergy: Clindamycin 10mg/kg 30 min prior and 5mg/kg 6 hrs later.

ENDOCARDITIS, PROPHYLAXIS (Cont.)

Endocarditis Prophylaxis for Dental and Upper Respiratory Procedures		
Parenteral (High risk)	Ampicillin 2g and Gentamicin 1.5mg/kg (Max. 80mg) IM or IV 30 min prior followed by repeat half doses 8 hrs later or amoxicillin 1.5g orally 6 hrs later. Pen allergy: Vancomycin 1g IV over 1 hr starting 1 hr prior to procedure, no follow-up dose.	Ampicillin 50mg/kg and Gentamicin 2mg/kg IM or IV 30 min prior followed by repeat half doses 8 hrs later or amoxicillin 25mg/kg orally 6 hrs later Pen allergy: Vancomycin 20mg/kg IV over 1 hr starting 1 hr prior to procedure; no follow-up dose.
Endocarditis Prophylaxis for GI and GU Procedures		
Route	Adults	Children
Oral (Low risk)	Amoxicillin 3g orally 1 hr prior followed by 1.5g 6 hrs later.	Amoxicillin 50mg/kg orally 1 hr prior followed by 25m/kg 6 hrs later.
Parenteral (Standard)	Ampicillin 2g and Gentamicin 1.5mg/kg (max. 80mg) IM or IV 30 min prior followed by repeat half doses 8 hrs later or amoxicillin 1.5g orally 6 hrs later. Pen allergy: Vancomycin 1g over 1 hr and Gentamicin 1.5mg/kg (max. 80mg) IV 1 hr prior followed by repeat half doses 8 hrs later.	Ampicillin 50mg/kg and Gentamicin 2mg/kg IM or IV 30 min prior followed by repeat half doses 8 hrs later or amoxicillin 25mg/kg 6 hrs later. Pen allergy: Vancomycin 20mg/kg over 1 hr and Gentamicin 2mg/kg IV 1 hr prior followed by repeat half doses 8 hrs later.

EPHEDRINE

USES: **Ephedrine** is a **sympathomimetic** drug; it stimulates alpha-, beta-1 and beta-2 receptors and releases norepinephrine from its storage sites. Uses of ephedrine are given in the next Table:

Uses of Ephedrine
Bronchospasm
Nasal Congestion
Hypotension and Shock

Bronchospasm: Ephedrine is used as a bronchodilator in the symptomatic treatment of mild bronchial asthma and reversible bronchospasm in association with chronic bronchitis, emphysema, and other obstructive pulmonary diseases. Other bronchodilators are more effective than ephedrine as a bronchodilator.

Nasal Congestion: Oral ephedrine is of little or no value in the treatment of nasal congestion. Solutions of 0.5-3%, applied topically, produces decongestion.

Hypotension and Shock: The effectiveness of parenteral ephedrine in the treatment of hypotension and shock is not proven.

DOSAGE FORMS: Syrup: 11mg/5ml or 20mg/5ml; Caps: 25, 50mg; Caps, Extended-Release: 15, 30, 60mg; Nasal drops: 0.5%, 1%; Nasal Jelly: 0.6%; Parenteral: 25, 50mg/ml.

EPHEDRINE (Cont.)
DOSAGE: As a nasal decongestant, ephedrine is applied intranasally. Ephedrine and its salts are administered orally, IM, subcutaneously, or IV. Dosage is given in the next Table:

Dosage of Ephedrine

Condition	Age	Route	Dosage
Bronchospasm	Adults	Oral	25-50mg every 3 or 4 h. as needed; every 8-12 h. with extended-release caps.
	Children	Oral	2-3mg/kg daily or 100mg/m^2 daily in 4-6 divided doses.
Orthostatic Hypotension	Adults	Oral	25mg ephedrine sulfate, 1-4 times daily.
	Children	Oral	3mg/kg daily ephedrine sulfate, 4-6 times.
Myasthenia Gravis		Oral	25mg, 3 or 4 times daily.
Enuresis	Adults	Oral	25-50mg at bedtime.
Bronchospasm, Severe Acute		Parenteral	12.5-25mg, as needed.
Hypotension	Adults	Subcutaneous or IM	10-50mg. If necessary, a second IM dose of 50mg or an IV dose of 25mg.
		Direct Slow IV	10-25mg; if necessary, additional IV doses in 5-10 minutes; do not exceed 150mg daily.
	Children	Subcutaneous or IV	1.5-3mg/kg daily divided into 4-6 doses.

ADVERSE EFFECTS: Insomnia, headache, sweating, nervousness, anxiety, hypertension.
CONTRAINDICATIONS: May potentiate actions of theophylline or precipitate arrhythmias.

EPIGLOTTITIS, PATHOGENS, TREATMENT
Pathogens: H. influenza may cause fulminant epiglottitis in infants and young children; acute epiglottitis in adults is unusual but not rare (Mayo-Smith, M.F., et al., N. Engl. J. Med. 314, 1133-1139, 1986; Baker, A.S. and Eavey, R.D., ibid, 1185-1186, 1986). There is sudden onset of fever; hyperemia and edema of the epiglottis may lead to respiratory obstruction.

Bacteremia occurs in 65 to 90% of children with acute epiglottitis. The results of culture of the pharynx do not reliably identify the causative organism of the infection of the epiglottis. In 75% of children with H. influenza bacteremia, the same organisms grow from direct culture of the epiglottis (Westmore, R.F. and Handler, S.D., Ann. Otolaryngol. 88, 822-826, 1979; Lewis, J.K., et al., Clin. Pediatr. 17, 494-496, 1978).

In adults, acute epiglottitis with systemic involvement and bacteremia is almost invariably due to H. influenza, type b (Tveteras, K. and Kristensen, S., Clin. Otolaryngol. 12, 337-343, 1987).
Treatment: In any child with epiglottitis; an artificial airway is established immediately at presentation. The use of a prophylactic airway has reduced mortality in children from 6% to under 1% (Cantrell, R.W., et al., Laryngoscope 88, 994-1005, 1978).

Since H. influenza is the predominant organism in acute epiglottitis, I.V. antibiotic therapy is directed against this organism. Ampicillin is the drug of choice for H. influenzae beta-lactamase-negative infection; however, in consideration of the possibility of ampicillin-resistant strains, chloramphenicol is included or a suitable second-generation cephalosporin (Cefuroxime) or third-generation cephalosporin (Cefotaxime, Ceftriaxone) is used in initial antimicrobial coverage. Antibiotics are given for several days (as necessary) in the hospital and then taken orally for 10-14 days at home.
Prevention: H. influenzae type b polysaccharide vaccine is being offered to children; vaccination is begun at two months of age. Most epiglottitis usually occurs between the ages of two and six years; thus, epiglottitis may nearly vanish within a few years (Cochi, S.L. and Broome, C.V., Ped. Inf. Dis. 5, 12-19, 1986).

EPINEPHRINE
(Adrenaline)
USES: **Epinephrine** stimulates alpha (**vasoconstriction**) receptors, beta-1 (increased **myocardial contractility** and **conduction**) receptors, and beta-2 (**bronchodilation** and **vasodilation**) receptors. Uses are given in the next Table:

Uses of Epinephrine
Severe Acute Asthma Attacks
Severe Acute Anaphylactic Reactions and Anaphylactic Shock
Cardiac Arrest and Arrhythmias

Severe Acute Asthma Attacks: Subcutaneously administered epinephrine injection is sometimes used for the treatment of severe acute asthma attacks. Epinephrine relaxes bronchial smooth muscle by stimulation of beta-2 receptors; epinephrine constricts bronchial arterioles by stimulation of alpha receptors. Subcutaneous administration of epinephrine injection in patients with asthmatic attacks may produce bronchodilation within 5-10 minutes and maximal effects in about 20 minutes.
Severe Acute Anaphylactic Reactions and Anaphylactic Shock: Epinephrine is the drug of choice in the emergency treatment of severe acute anaphylactic reactions including anaphylactic shock.
Cardiac Arrest and Arrhythmias: Epinephrine acts on beta-1 receptors producing increased myocardial contractility and can convert asystole to sinus rhythm and makes ventricular fibrillation more susceptible to direct current countershock. Peripheral vasoconstriction (alpha receptors) improves coronary and cerebral perfusion pressure, which is the primary beneficial effect in cardiac arrest. Other cardiovascular effects of epinephrine during resuscitation include increased systemic vascular resistance, arterial blood pressure, heart rate, myocardial contraction, automaticity and myocardial oxygen requirements.
DOSAGE FORMS: Oral Inhalation(Aerosol): 160, 200, 250mcg/metered spray; Parenteral (Sus-Phrine): 5mg/ml (1:200); Parenteral Injection: 0.01mg/ml (1:100,000); 0.1mg/ml (1:10,000); 0.5mg/ml (1:2000); 1mg/ml (1:1000).
DOSAGE: Epinephrine hydrochloride injection (1mg/ml) is preferably administered subcutaneously; it may be administered IM but avoid injection into the buttocks. In emergency situations, epinephrine may be injected very slowly IV as a dilute solution or infused slowly IV. Epinephrine may be injected intracardially or via an endotracheal tube. Dosage is given in the next Table:

Dosage of Epinephrine

Condition	Age	Route	Dosage
Severe Acute Asthma Attacks; Severe Acute Anaphylactic-Reactions and Anaphylactic Shock	Adult	SubQ or IM	0.1-0.5mg (0.1-0.5ml of a 1:1000 injection) Anaphylactic Shock: Repeat at 10 to 15 minute intervals as needed. Asthma: Repeat at 20 min. to 4 h. intervals as needed.
	Child.	SubQ	0.01mg/kg (0.01ml/kg of a 1:1000 injection). Max. single dose, 0.5mg. Repeat at 20 min. to 4 h. intervals as needed. For prolonged effects, 1:200 aqueous suspension in single doses of 0.02-0.025mg/kg (0.004-0.005ml/kg).
Cardiac Arrest	Adult	IV	0.5-1mg (range 0.1-1mg, usually as a 1:10,000 injection). Repeat every 5 min. as needed. **or** initial IV followed by 0.3mg of epinephrine subcutaneously or the drug may be infused IV at an initial rate of 1mcg/min., increasing the rate to up to 4mcg/min. as needed.

EPINEPHRINE (Cont.)

Dosage of Epinephrine

Condition	Age	Route	Dosage
	Child.	IV	0.01mg/kg (0.1ml/kg of a 1:10,000 injection or 1ml/kg of a 1:100,000 injection). IV doses may be repeated every 5 min. as needed. or 0.1mcg/kg/min. initially; then increase rate by increments by 0.1mcg/kg/min. to max. of 1.5mcg/kg/min.
	Adults	Tracheobronchial	1mg (10ml of a 1:10,000 sol'n)
	Child.	Tracheobronchial	2-3 times IV dose.

ADVERSE EFFECTS: Dose-related restlessness, anxiety, tremor, weakness, dizziness, headache, palpitations, hypertension and cardiac arrhythmias. Anginal pain with coronary insufficiency. Cerebral hemorrhage secondary to increase in blood pressure from overdose. Elevation of blood glucose.
CONTRAINDICATIONS: Intra-arterial administration is associated with marked vasoconstriction.
MONITOR: Blood pressure, heart rate, relief of allergic or asthmatic symptoms.
PHARMACOKINETICS: Onset (subcut.): 3-10 min.; duration (subcut.): up to several hours.

EPINEPHRINE RACEMIC
(Vaponefrin, Micronefrin, Asthmanefrin)
USES: **Racemic epinephrine** is used in the treatment of **viral croup** to reduce airway edema. Aerosolized racemic epinephrine is the most effective medication for this purpose. In most patients, the use of racemic epinephrine aerosol is associated with a rapid decrease in stridor, this effect lasts for 1 to 3 hours. Racemic epinephrine is also used to decrease stridor due to airway swelling following endotracheal intubation.

Epinephrine aerosols provide only temporary relief of respiratory distress. If used on an outpatient basis, the patient must be observed for at least 4 hours since rebound or worsening of the patient's underlying condition may occur. Patients that require treatment should be hospitalized. Treatment with racemic epinephrine does not alter the natural course of the disease.
DOSAGE FORMS: Sol'n: 2.25%. The aerosol solution is prepared by mixing 0.5ml of racemic epinehprine solution with 2.5ml of saline. This mixture is then administered by aerosolization in a face mask.
DOSAGE: The aerosols consisting of 0.05ml/kg of racemic epinephrine (max. dose of 0.5ml) in 2.5ml of saline are usually administered every 3 to 4 hours but usually not more frequently than every 2 hours.
ADVERSE EFFECTS: Tachycardia is the most common side effect of these treatments. Other side effects include headache, nausea and palpitations.

ERGOCALCIFEROL
(Drisdol, Calciferol)

USES: **Ergocalciferol** is a **vitamin D analog,** used in the treatment of **hypocalcemia;** it is activated by 25-hydroxylation in liver and 1-hydroxylation in kidney.

DOSAGE FORMS: Oral: Caps: 1.25mg (50,000 units); Sol'n: 200mcg (8000 units) per ml; Tabs: 1.25mg (50,000 units); Parenteral: Inject: 12.5mg (500,000 units) per ml.

DOSAGE: Each mg of ergocalciferol is equivalent to 40,000 USP units; each mcg is equivalent to 40 USP units. Dosage must be individualized to maintain serum calcium of 9-10mg/dl and urinary calcium less than 3mg/kg/day. Conditions and dosage are shown in the next Table:

Vitamin D Deficiency and Dosage of Ergocalciferol

Condition	Dosage
Nutritional Rickets and Osteomalacia	Oral, 25mcg daily results in normal serum calcium and phosphate in about 10 days, radiographic evidence of healing of bone in 2-4 weeks and complete healing in 6 months. 50-125mcg daily for 6-12 weeks for prompt healing. In children with malabsorption, 250-625mcg daily.
Tetany and Rickets	Orally or IV to control tetany. 50-125mcg daily until bones have healed or 250mcg daily for 3 weeks. Patients with tetany should also receive calcium.
Familial Hypophosphatemia (Vit. D-Resistant Rickets)	Oral, 1-2mg daily with phosphate supplements; daily dose is increased in 250-250mcg increments at 3-4 month intervals until adequate response.
Fanconi Syndrome	Oral, child. 625mcg-1.25mg daily; adults 1.25-10mg daily.
Vit. D Dependent Rickets	Oral, child. 75-125mcg and up to 1.5mg daily. Adult 250mcg-1.5mg, up to 12.5mg daily.
Anticonvulsant-Induced Rickets and Osteomalacia	Oral, 50mcg-1.25mg daily; prophylaxis, 25mcg daily or 250mcg weekly.
Hypoparathyroidism & Pseudohypoparathyroidism	Oral, 625mcg-5mg daily and calcium supplements. Prolonged dosages greater than 2.5mg daily results in toxicity.
Renal Osteodystrophy	Oral, Child: 100mcg-1mg/day; Adults: 500mcg-12.5mg/day
Dietary Supplementation	Prevent Rickets: 10mcg daily Premature Infants: 12-20mcg daily Prematures with Hypocalcemia: up to 750mcg daily.

ADVERSE EFFECTS: Monitor serum calcium, serum phosphorus and alkaline phosphatase.

ERGOTAMINE TARTRATE PREPARATIONS
(Ergomar, Ergostat, Cafergot, Migergot, Wigraine, Bellergal)

USES: Uses of ergotamine tartrate are given in the next Table:

Uses of Ergotamine Tartrate
Acute Attacks of Migraine (Drug of Choice)
Alleviate or Prevent Acute Attacks of Cluster Headache

Ergotamine is used in the treatment of acute attacks of migraine and cluster headaches. It is not used for long-term prophylaxis because of the incidence and severity of adverse effects. It may be used for short-term daily use, eg, 10-14 days, for the treatment of cluster headache.

Prophylaxis Ergotamine is not recommended for prophylaxis because its potent peripheral vasoconstrictor action may produce arterial insufficiency and dependence.

Mechanism of Action: Ergotamine causes peripheral **vasoconstriction** especially in the dilated external carotid artery. It acts as a vasoconstrictor if the tonus of the blood vessel is low and as a vasodilator if the tonus is high.

The remarkably specific antimigraine action of ergotamine is thought to be related to its actions on vascular or neuronal serotonin receptors.

ERGOTAMINE TARTRATE PREPARATIONS (Cont.)

DOSAGE FORMS: Dosage forms of ergotamine tartrate are given in the next Table:

Commercial Ergotamine Preparations

Preparation	Form	Ergotamine	Caffeine	Belladonna	Barbiturates
Cafergot(Sandoz)	Tabs	as tartrate, 1mg	100mg		
	Supp.	as tartrate, 2mg	100mg		
Cafergot-PB (Sandoz)	Tabs	as tartrate, 1mg	100mg	0.125mg	Pentobarbital, 30mg
	Supp.	as tartrate, 2mg	100mg	0.25mg	Pentobarbital, 60mg
Wigraine(Organon)	Tabs	as tartrate, 1mg	100mg	-	-
	Supp.	as tartrate, 2mg	100mg	-	-
Ergomar(Fisons)	Sublingual Tabs	as tartrate, 2mg	-	-	-
Ergostat(Parke-Davis)	Sublingual Tabs	as tartrate, 2mg	-	-	-
Medihaler Ergotamine(Riker)	Aerosol	as tartrate, 9mg/ml 360mcg/metered spray	-	-	-
Bellergal-S (Sandoz)	Tablet (Timed-Release)	as tartrate, 0.6mg	-	0.2mg	Phenobarbital, 40mg

DOSAGE: Dosages of the different preparations of ergotamine tartrate for treatment of acute migraine headache are given in the next Table:

Dosage of Ergotamine Tartrate

Route	Dosage
Inhalation: (Medihaler Ergotamine)	Adults: One inhalation(0.36mg) initially, repeated at intervals of no less than 5 min. to a max. of 6 inhalations/day or 15 inhalations/week
Sublingual: (Ergomar or Ergostat)	Adults: 2mg at onset of an attack followed by 2mg every 30 min. if necessary (max., 6mg in 24 hrs. and 10mg in one week).
Oral: (Cafergot, Wigraine, Cafergot PB)	Adults: Two tabs. (1mg/tab.) at onset of migraine attack; then, if needed, one additional tab. every 30 min. Total dose should not exceed 6 tabs./attack or 10/wk. Children: One-half tab. initially (0.5mg); then if needed, one-half tab. every 30 min. (max. 3 tabs)
Suppositories (Cafergot, Wigraine, Cafergot PB)	Adults: Usually one suppository (2 mg) at the beginning of an attack. If needed, repeat dose after 1hr. (max. 2 supps. per attack, or 5 supps. per week).

The Bellergal preparation contains only 0.6mg of ergotamine tartrate compared to 1mg per tablet for other preparations. Bellergal is claimed to be useful in migraine prophylaxis when attacks occur frequently; it is not useful for treatment of acute attacks because the amount of ergotamine is inadequate. Prolonged administration of ergotamine is contraindicated. The oral dosage of Bellergal for adults is as follows: two timed-released tablets daily (one in the morning and one in the evening).

ADVERSE EFFECTS: The most frequent adverse effects are nausea, vomiting, epigastric discomfort, diarrhea, polydipsia, and drowsiness. Other more serious adverse effects are paresthesias of the extremities, cramps and weakness of the legs, myalgia, precordial pain, transient sinus tachycardia and bradycardia. Rarely, gangrene or serious cardiovascular effects have been reported. Rebound headaches can occur during chronic use, possibly leading to escalation of dosage by the patient.

There is a risk of provoking bronchospasm in asthmatic patients when ergotamine is administered by inhalation.

CONTRAINDICATIONS: Hypertension, cerebrovascular disease, coronary artery disease, angina pectoris, severe peripheral vascular disease, thyrotoxicosis, hepatic or renal impairment, sepsis, severe pruritis, malnutrition, pregnancy (category X).

PHARMACOKINETICS: Onset:Oral; 0.5-3 hrs.; Rectal: 1-3 hrs.; Inhalation: 15-30 min.; Bioavailability:Oral:Low (2%); Rectal: Good (5%), Sublingual: Poor; Inhalation: Low and variable; Metabolism: Liver. The low bioavailability is the result of significant degradation (97%) first-pass effect. Half-Life: 96 minutes; Excretion:Bile (90%); urine (3-4%).

ERYTHROMYCIN

(ERYC, E-Mycin, Ery-Tab, Ilotycin, Robimycin, Pediamycin, Wyamycin, PCE, Ilosone, E.E.S, EryPed, Erythrocin, Eramycin, Erypar)

USES: Erythromycin is the drug of choice or alternative therapy to penicillin for bacterial infections as given in the next Table:

Uses of Erythromycin

Erythromycin as Drug of Choice:
- **Atypical pneumonia** caused by **Mycoplasma pneumoniae**, community-based pneumonia, mild or moderate, in older children and adults, when most likely caused by M. pneumoniae or Streptococcus pneumoniae
- **Legionnaire's disease (Legionella pneumophilia)**
- Pittsburgh pneumonia agent (Legionella micdadei)
- **Chlamydia trachomatis** infections in infants (e.g., pneumonia, conjunctivitis) and children (e.g., urethritis, cervicitis secondary to sexual abuse) and pregnant women [cervicitis, pelvic inflammatory disease(PID)]
- **Gastroenteritis** caused by **Campylobacter jejuni.**
- **Erythrasma,** a superficial infection caused by Corynebacterium minutissimum
- **Pertussis** to eliminate B. pertussis carrier (use estolate salt)
- **Corynebacterium** diphtheriae, especially carriers
- **Chancroid**

Erythromycin as Alternate Therapy to Penicillin:
- Acute diphtheria, caused by corynebacterium diphtheriae, as alternate to penicillin G for treatment of pharyngitis scarlet fever, impetigo, cellulitis and erysipelas caused by group A Streptococcus pyogenes
- Pneumonia and bronchitis caused by S. pneumoniae
- Prophylaxis of recurrences of rheumatic fever; sulfadiazine may be preferred
- Prophylactic therapy to prevent endocarditis
- Acute otitis media due to S. pneumoniae or S. pyogenes; a combination of erythromycin and a sulfonamide usually is more effective than erythromycin alone in children with otitis media caused by H. influenzae
- Minor staphylococcal infections, eg, bullous impetigo and carbuncles

Other Infections:
- Anthrax, C.tetani, Vincent's gingivitis, erysipeloid, actinomycosis, Listeria infections, Nocardia, early and late syphilis; pregnant women with syphilis, disseminated gonorrhea (arthritis-dermatitis syndrome)

Pertussis: Pertussis is caused by a toxin; erythromycin estolate (14 day course) eliminates B. pertussis in the nasopharynx and thus reduces infectivity. Erythromycin estolate also is administered prophylactically to exposed persons. The estolate salt is preferred for prophylaxis and treatment of pertussis; estolate is more effective than stearate or ethylsuccinate, possibly due to higher serum and tissue levels achieved with a given dose (Bass, J.W., Pediatr. Inf. Dis. 5, 154-157, 1986).

Mechanism of Action: Erythromycin inhibits bacterial synthesis by binding to the 50S ribosomal subunit which prevents elongation of the peptide chain. It is mainly bacteriostatic but may be bacteriocidal depending on dose and organism.

Erythromycin is classified as a macrolide; macrolides are a group of antibiotics produced by actinomycetes and distinguished by a large lactone ring linked to a sugar in a glycosidic linkage. Erythromycin is the most important antibiotic of this group.

DOSAGE FORMS: The generic name, trade or brand name(s) and dosage forms of erythromycin, are given in the next Table:

Generic, Trade or Brand Name(s) and Dosage Forms of Erythromycin

Generic Name	Trade or Brand Name(s)	Dosage
Erythromycin	ERYC	Caps with Enteric Coated Pellets: 125, 250mg
	E-Mycin, Ery-Tab, Ilotycin, Robimycin	Tabs, Enteric Coated: 250mg

ERYTHROMYCIN (Cont.)

Generic, Trade or Brand Name(s) and Dosage Forms of Erythromycin

Generic Name	Trade or Brand Name(s)	Dosage
	E-Mycin, Ery-Tab	Tabs, Enteric Coated: 330mg
	Ery-Tab	Tabs, Enteric Coated: 500mg
	Erythromycin Base, Filmtab	Tabs, Film Coated: 250, 500mg
	PCE	Particle in Tabs: 333mg.
Erythromycin Estolate	Ilosone	Caps: 250mg Susp: 125, 250mg/5ml; 100mg/ml Tabs: 250mg Tabs, Chewable: 125, 250mg
Erythromycin Ethylsuccinate	E.E.S.	Susp: 100mg/2.5ml; 200mg/5ml
	Ery Ped	Susp: 400mg/5ml
	E.E.S.	Tabs, Chewable: 200mg
	E.E.S.	Tabs, Film-Coated: 400mg
Erythromycin Gluceptate	Ilotycin	Parenteral: 500mg, 1g
Erythromycin Lactobionate	Erythrocin	Parenteral: 500mg, 1g
Erythromycin Stearate	Eramycin	Tabs, Film-Coated: 250mg
	Erypar	Tabs, Film-Coated: 500mg

DOSAGE: Drug should be taken with a full glass of water, 1 h. before or 2 h. after meals. Dosage of erythromycin is given in the next Table:

Dosage of Erythromycin

Generic Name	Age	Route	Dosage
Erythromycin Base	Adult	Oral	250-500mg, every 6 h. to max. of 4g/day
	Child.	Oral	30-50mg/kg/day in 4 divided doses
Erythromycin Estolate	Adult	Oral	250-500mg, every 6 h. to max. of 4g/day
	Child.	Oral	30-50mg/kg/day in 4 divided doses
Erythromycin Ethylsuccinate (400mg EES = 250mg Erythro base)	Adult	Oral	400mg every 6 h. to max. of 4g/day
	Child.	Oral	30-50mg/kg/day in 4 divided doses
Erythromycin Gluceptate	Adult	IV (Infuse >30 min.)	15-20mg/kg/day in 4 divided doses to max. of 4g/day
Erythromycin Lactobionate	Child.	IV (Infuse >30 min.)	20-50mg/kg/day in 4 divided doses
	Neonate <7d	IV (Infuse >30 min.)	20mg/kg/day in 2 divided doses
	Neonate >7d	IV (Infuse >30 min.)	30mg/kg/day in 3 divided doses
Erythromycin Stearate	Adults	Oral	250-500mg every 6 h. to max. 4g/day
	Child.	Oral	30-50mg/kg/day in 4 divided doses

PHARMACOKINETICS: Peak Plasma Conc: Following oral absorption, 30 min (suspension) to 4 h. (coated tablet). Metabolism: Liver; Half-Life: 1-1.5 h; 5-6 h. in anuric patients. Distribution: Erythromycin is not present in the CSF except in patients with meningitis. Excretion: Bile to feces.

ADVERSE EFFECTS: Occ. GI distress with abdominal cramping, nausea, vomiting; also rash and urticaria. IM form is very painful. IV administration frequently produces pain, venous irritation and phlebitis.

Reversible intrahepatic cholestatic jaundice is seen with estolate and ethylsuccinate forms usually in adults after 10-14 days of therapy. Symptoms resolve in 1-2 weeks; serum enzymes return to normal after several months.

MONITOR: Liver function tests in patients who develop symptoms while receiving estolate or ethylsuccinate form.

Check daily for vein irritation and phlebitis in patients receiving IV forms. Some pharmacies buffer the IV solution with sodium bicarbonate to reduce vein irritation.

ERYTHROMYCIN (Cont.)
CONTRAINDICATIONS: Hepatic dysfunction (estolate and ethylsuccinate forms); IM form contraindicated in patients with hypersensitivity to local anesthetics of the para-aminobenzoic acid type, such as procaine.
DRUG INTERACTIONS: The effects of erythromycin on drug levels are given in the next Table:

Effects of Erythromycin on Drug Levels

Drug	Erythromycin Effect
Theophylline	Increase in serum theophylline levels
Carbamazepine (Tegretol)	Carbamazepine can be elevated by erythromycin leading to carbamazepine toxicity
Warfarin	Prolongation of prothrombin time with possible hemorrhage; monitor prothrombin time (PT)
Methylprednisolone	Methylprednisolone levels are increased.
Digoxin	Digoxin levels elevated due to alteration of gut flora and resultant lack of inactivation of digoxin.

Increase in levels of theophyllines, carbamazepine, warfarin and methylprednisolone is probably due to inhibition of hepatic metabolism by erythromycin.

ERYTHROMYCIN and SULFISOXAZOLE
(Pediazole, Eryzole, E.S.P., Sulfimycin)
USES: Pediazole is used to treat **acute otitis media** caused by Streptococcus pneumoniae and Haemophilus influenzae. S. pneumoniae is susceptible to erythromycin and H. influenzae is susceptible to the sulfonamide, sulfisoxazole.

Amoxicillin is the drug that is usually used to treat acute otitis media. However, when amoxicillin-resistant H. influenzae is present, alternate therapy is erythromycin plus a sulfonamide, trimethoprim/sulfamethoxazole, and cefaclor (Ceclor).

Pediazole may also be effective in the treatment of acute bacterial sinusitis.
DOSAGE FORMS OF PEDIAZOLE: Erythromycin (as ethylsuccinate) 200mg, sulfisoxazole, 600mg, per 5ml suspension.
DOSAGE: Pediazole is not recommended for children less than two months.

Dosage of Pediazole may be calculated by weight based on the erythromycin component(50mg/kg/day) or on the sulfisoxazole component(150mg/kg/day) and given in 4 divided doses for 10 days. Maximum dose: sulfisoxazole 6gm/day.
ADVERSE EFFECTS: Blood dyscrasias, hepato-or renal toxicity, Stevens-Johnson syndrome, anaphylaxis, pancreatitis, lupus-like syndrome, pseudomembranous colitis, neuritis, convulsions, ataxia, rash, GI upset, reversible hearing loss.

ERYTHROPOIETIN

(Epogen)

USES: **Erythropoietin** is a **glycoprotein hormone** produced by recombinant DNA techniques which promotes production of erythrocytes. Clinical studies have investigated erythropoietin use in various conditions, as listed in the following Table (Zorsky, P.E., Drug Therapy, 50-57, Sept., 1990):

Uses and Potential Uses of Erythropoietin
Anemia of Renal Failure - FDA Approved
Anemia of AIDS and/or Zidovudine (AZT)
Anemia of Rheumatoid Arthritis
Anemia of Cancer or Chemotherapy
Anemia of Prematurity
Preoperative Autologous Blood Donation

The only condition for which erythropoietin is FDA approved is for treatment of the anemia of renal failure; phase III clinical trial has been completed and demonstrates efficacy in raising hematocrit, elimination of transfusions, reduction in iron overload, and improved quality of life (Eschbach, J.W., et al., Ann. Intern. Med. 111, 992-1000, 1989).

Mechanism of Action: Endogenous erythropoietin is a hormone primarily produced by renal peritubular cells, with small amounts produced by the liver; it contains 166 amino acids and a complex carbohydrate structure which is essential for activity. Biosynthetic (recombinant) erythropoietin has been produced with identical amino acid structure, and equivalence by functional and immunologic assay. Erythropoietin stimulates RBC production (erythropoiesis) by stimulating the proliferation and differentiation of RBC precursors (eg, burst-forming units - erythroid, colony-forming units - erythroid, erythroblasts, and reticulocytes)(Review: Erslev, A.J., N. Engl. J. Med. 324, 1339-1344, 1991; Nissenson, A.R., Ann. Intern. Med. 114, 402-416, 1991).

DOSAGE FORMS: Injection: 2000, 3000, 4000, 10,000 units/ml.

DOSAGE: Erythropoietin is administered IV. The usual goal of therapy is to maintain the hematocrit at 32-38%. Response to erythropoietin is dose-dependent, and a variety of doses have been used. Dosage of erythropoietin for patients with renal failure are given in the following Table (Ad Hoc Committee for the National Kidney Foundation, "Statement on the Clinical Use of Recombinant Erythropoietin in Anemia of End-Stage Renal Disease," Am. J. Kid. Dis. 14, 163-169, 1989; Eschbach, J.W., et al., Ann. Intern. Med. 111, 992-1000, 1989):

Dosage of Erythropoietin

Condition	Dosage
Renal Failure	Initially, 150 units/kg IV 3 times weekly until hematocrit is 35%; expected rise: 1.8% weekly. Maintenance: 50-75 units/kg IV 3 times weekly; adjust by 12.5-25 units/kg as necessary to maintain hematocrit in desired range (Dose range for maintenance: 12.5-525 units/kg).

ADVERSE EFFECTS: In the phase III clinical trial of erythropoietin in 333 patients with renal failure, the following adverse effects were reported: myalgias (5%), headache (17%), flank pain (14%), iron deficiency (43%), increased blood pressure (35%), and seizures (5.4%). Slight increases in creatinine, phosphate and potassium levels were noted (Eschbach, J.W. et al., Ann. Intern. Med. 111, 992-1000, 1989).

MONITORING: Patients with renal failure on erythropoietin should be monitored for response to therapy and possible adverse effects. Monitoring guidelines are suggested in the following Table (Ad Hoc Committee for the National Kidney Foundation, Am. J. Kid. Dis. 14, 163-169, 1989):

Monitoring Guidelines for Erythropoietin Therapy in Renal Failure

Parameter	Frequency
Blood Pressure	3 times/week.
Hematocrit	Weekly for 12 weeks, then every other week.
Reticulocytes	Weekly for 4 weeks, then as needed.
Potassium	Twice a month until stable, then monthly.
Iron/TIBC and Ferritin	Monthly for 3 months, then every other month.

Patients should receive iron supplementation to maintain transferrin saturation (serum iron/TIBC) greater than 20% and serum ferritin greater than 100 nanograms/ml; iron stores should be at least at this level prior to initiating therapy.

ESTRADIOL ETHINYL
(Estraderm [Estradiol], Estinyl, Feminone)

USES: Uses of ethinyl estradiol are given in the next Table:

Uses of Ethinyl Estradiol
Menopausal Vasomotor Symptoms
Replacement Therapy in Female Hypogonadism
Dysfunctional Uterine Bleeding
Palliative Treatment of Advanced, Inoperable Metastatic Carcinoma of the Breast in Selected Postmenopausal Women
Advanced, Inoperable Carcinoma of the Prostate

Ethinyl estradiol is used alone and as a component of some estrogen/progestin oral contraceptives. It is estradiol with a -C≡CH group substituted for hydrogen at the 17 position on ring D of the steroid nucleus. Transdermal form is estradiol without ethinyl group.

DOSAGE FORMS: Dosage forms of ethinyl estradiol are given in the next Table:

Dosage Forms of Ethinyl Estradiol

Trade Name	Forms
Estinyl (Schering)	Tabs: 0.02, 0.05, 0.5mg.
Feminone (Upjohn)	Tabs: 0.05mg.
Estraderm (Ciba)	Transdermal patch 0.05mg/day, 0.1mg/day(Estradiol).

DOSAGE: Take oral medication with food to decrease nausea. Dosage of ethinyl estradiol in different conditions is given in the next Table:

Dosage of Ethinyl Estradiol

Condition	Route	Dosage
Menopausal Vasomotor Symptoms	Oral	Early Menopause: 0.05mg once daily for 21 consecutive days, followed by 7 days without the drug. Late Menopause: Same regimen as above except use 0.02mg daily for the first few cycles;then, dosage may be increased to 0.05mg daily in subsequent cycles.
	Transdermal Patch (Estradiol)	Initially, one 0.05mg/day patch twice a week applied to trunk (avoid breasts). Maintenance: Administer cyclically (3 wks on, 1 wk off). Rotate application sites. Discontinue or taper every 3-6 months.
Surgical Castration	Oral	0.05mg 3 times daily. With clinical improvement (usually several weeks) dosage may be reduced to 0.05mg daily.
Female Hypogonadism	Oral	0.05mg 1-3 times daily given during the first 2 weeks of a theoretical menstrual cycle, followed by progesterone during the last half of the "cycle". Continue for 3-6 months, followed by 2 months without the drugs to determine whether the woman can maintain her menstrual cycle without hormonal therapy. If menstruation does not occur, consider additional courses of ethinyl estradiol.
	Transdermal Patch (Estradiol)	Initially, one 0.05mg/day patch twice a week applied to trunk (avoid breasts). Maintenance: Administer cyclically (3 wks on, 1 wk off). Rotate application sites. Discontinue or taper every 3-6 months.
Metastatic Carcinoma of the Breast in Selected Postmenopausal Women	Oral	1mg 3 times daily for at least 3 months.
Inoperable Carcinoma of the Prostate	Oral	0.15-2mg daily. Monitor by serial determination of acid phosphatase.

ADVERSE EFFECTS: Transdermal: Erythema and irritation at the application site (15% of patients); required discontinuance in 2% of patients.

Take oral medication with food to decrease incidence of nausea. Other adverse reactions include fullness of breasts, edema caused by sodium and water retention, hypertension, depression, hair loss or hirsutism, changes in libido, increased risk of gallbladder disease, endometrial carcinoma, thromboembolism, hepatic tumors.

ESTROGENS, CONJUGATED
(Premarin)

USES: This is a combination of the sodium salts of the sulfate esters of estrogenic substances, principally estrone 50% to 65% and equilin (20% to 35%). Conjugated estrogens are derived wholly or in part from urine of pregnant mares or may be prepared synthetically from estrone and equilin.

Uses of conjugated estrogens are given in the next Table:

Uses of Conjugated Estrogens
Menopausal Vasomotor Symptoms
Prevention of Osteoporosis
Replacement Therapy in Hypogonadism
Female Castration
Dysfunctional Uterine Bleeding due to Atrophic Endometrium
Intravenously for Rapid Cessation of Dysfunctional Uterine Bleeding
Postpartum Breast Engorgement
Breast Carcinoma in Women more than five years after Menopause or in Appropriately Selected Men with Breast Carcinoma
Prostatic Carcinoma
Bleeding Due to Uremia (experimental)

Conjugated estrogens are used for the management of moderate to severe vasomotor symptoms associated with menopause; however, estrogens are not effective for the management of nervous symptoms or depression associated with menopause in patients without vasomotor symptoms.

DOSAGE FORMS: Tabs for Oral Use: 0.3, 0.625, 0.9, 1.25 and 2.5mg; Vaginal Cream: 0.625mg/g in 42.5g containers; IV: 25mg.

DOSAGE: Dosage of conjugated estrogens in different conditions if given in the next Table:

Dosage of Conjugated Estrogens

Condition	Route	Dosage
Menopausal Vasomotor Symptoms, moderate to severe	Oral	0.3-1.25mg once daily for 21 consecutive days followed by 7 days without the drug; if the woman is menstruating, administration of the drug is started on the fifth day of the menstrual cycle. If the woman has not menstruated within the last 2 or more months, administration of the drug is started arbitrarily. Discontinue or taper every 3-6 months.
Atrophic Vaginitis or Kraurosis Vulvae	Oral	0.3-1.25mg once daily for 21 consecutive days followed by 7 days without the drug. Discontinue or taper every 3-6 months.
	Vaginal Cream	2-4g daily intravaginally or topically for 21 consecutive days followed by 7 days without the drug.
Prevention of Osteoporosis	Oral	0.625mg daily for 21 consecutive days followed by 7 days without the drug; repeat as necessary.
Female Hypogonadism	Oral	2.5 to 7.5mg daily in divided doses for 20 days followed by 10 days without the drug. Repeat course if withdrawal bleeding does not occur within 10 days. The number of courses of estrogen therapy required to induce menstruation varies, depending on the individual responsiveness of the endometrium. If bleeding occurs before the end of the 10-day drug free period, begin 20-day estrogen-progestin regimen with conjugated estrogen 2.5-7.5mg daily given in divided doses for 20 days; during the last 5 days of estrogen therapy, an oral progestin is administered. If menstruation begins before this estrogen-progestin regimen is completed, therapy should be discontinued and then reinstituted on the fifth day of menstruation.

ESTROGENS, CONJUGATED (Cont.)

Dosage of Conjugated Estrogens

Condition	Route	Dosage
Female Castration	Oral	1.25mg daily for 20 days followed by 10 days without the drug.
Dysfunctional Uterine Bleeding due to Atrophic Endometrium	Oral	2.5 to 5.0mg daily in divided doses for one week with a progestin added to the regimen.
Emergency Treatment of Dysfunctional Uterine Bleeding due to Atrophic Endometrium	IV or IM	25mg; repeat dose in 6-12 hours; oral treatment with an estrogen progestin combination is then started.
Postpartum Breast Engorgement	Oral	3.75mg every 4 hours for 5 doses or 1.25mg every 4 hours for 5 days.
Breast Carcinoma	Oral	10mg three times daily for at least three months.
Prostatic Carcinoma	Oral	1.25-2.5mg 3 times daily; follow with serum acid phosphatase assays
Uremic Bleeding	IV	Limited data. See Review: Couch, P. and Stumpf, J.L., Clinical Pharmacy 9, 673-681, 1990).

PHARMACOKINETICS: Oral: GI absorption is complete; wide distribution; concentrated in fat. Inactivation mainly in the liver with degradation to less active estrogenic products such as estrone. Metabolites are conjugated with sulfate and glucuronic acid and excreted in urine.

Vaginal creams are readily absorbed and produce plasma levels of extradiol and estrone approaching those attained after oral ingestion (mostly in the form of estrone).

ADVERSE EFFECTS: Nausea, vomiting, breast tenderness and spotting occur frequently. Thromboembolism, thrombophlebitis, diabetes, hypertension and gall bladder disease may occur. Edema, as weight changes, depression, intolerance to contact lenses, hair loss or hirsutism and changes in libido have been observed. Increased risk of endometrial carcinoma and hepatic tumors.

PRECAUTIONS: Pregnancy, lactation, thromboembolic disease.

ETHACRYNIC ACID
(Edecrin)

USES: Ethacrynic Acid is a sulfonamide-type **loop diuretic;** its uses are given in the next Table:

Uses of Ethacrynic Acid

Uses	Condition
Edema	Congestive heart failure(CHF) Renal failure (IV administration preferable) Acute pulmonary edema (IV administration preferable) Nephrotic syndrome Hepatic cirrhosis
Hypertension	Mild to moderate hypertension, especially when complicated by congestive heart failure or renal disease. Note that the thiazide diuretics are usually the initial diuretics of choice in most patients.
Hypercalcemia	Reduces serum calcium concentration by increasing calcium excretion.

Furosemide inhibits the reabsorption of electrolytes in the ascending limb of the loop of Henle. Excessive losses of potassium, hydrogen, and chloride may result in metabolic alkalosis.

HYPERTENSION: Treatment of hypertension with ethacrynic acid is given in the next Table(The 1988 Report of the Joint National Committee on Detection, Evaluation and Treatment of High Blood Pressure, Arch.Intern. Med. 148, 1023-1038, 1988):

Treatment of Hypertension with Ethacrynic Acid

Step 1: Nonpharmacologic Approaches (see **HYPERTENSION**)

↓

Step 2: Ethacrynic acid (Usual Min., 25mg/day; Usual Max., 100 mg/day)
Observe up to 6 months; if ethacrynic acid ineffective then,

↓

Step 3: Add a second drug of a different class
or Increase the dosage of ethacrynic acid
or Substitute another drug

↓

Step 4: Add a third drug of a different class
or Substitute a second drug

↓

Step 5: Consider further evaluation and/or referral
or Add a third or fourth drug

"Step-Down": For patients with mild hypertension, after 1 year of control, consider decreasing or withdrawing ethacrynic acid and other hypotensive drugs.

DOSAGE FORMS: Tabs: 25, 50mg; Inj (ethacrynate sodium): 50mg.

DOSAGE: Ethacrynic acid is administered orally; ethacrynate sodium is administered IV only - not IM or subcutaneously. Dosage is given in the next Table:

Dosage of Ethacrynic Acid

Condition	Age	Route	Dosage
Edema	Adults	Oral	50mg as a single dose on the first day, increase by 25-50mg daily either as a single dose or divided doses 2 times daily. Max. 400mg daily.
	Children	Oral	25mg/dose, once daily. Increase by 25mg every 2-3 days, Max. 2-3mg/kg daily. Dosage by weight: 0.5-1mg/kg/dose.
	Adults	IV	0.5-1mg/kg or 50-100mg.
	Children	IV	1mg/kg.
Hypertension	Adults	Oral	Initially, 25-50mg daily; increase gradually, usual max. 100mg daily in 2 divided doses, occasionally up to 200mg daily is required.

ETHACRYNIC ACID (Cont.)

PHARMACOKINETICS: Onset and duration data are given in the next Table:

Onset and Duration of Furosemide

Route	Onset	Peak	Duration
Oral	30 min.	2 hr.	6-8 hr.
IV	5 min.	15-30 min.	2 hr.

ADVERSE EFFECTS: The most frequent adverse reactions are hypokalemia, dehydration, hypotension and hypochloremic metabolic alkalosis. Hyperglycemia, hyperuricemia, hypocalcemia and hypomagnesemia may occur.

Weakness has been reported.

Adverse GI effects include nausea, vomiting, diarrhea and cramps.

Ototoxicity: Tinnitis, reversible or permanent hearing impairment, usually following IV administration in doses exceeding usual therapeutic dose; most likely to occur in patients with severe renal impairment or in patients receiving other ototoxic drugs, eg, aminoglycosides.

Use with caution in hepatic cirrhosis.

Prolonged use in premature infants may lead to nephrocalcinosis due to increased urinary calcium excretion.

CONTRAINDICATIONS: Anuria, except for a single dose. Pregnancy except when benefits outweigh risks.

MONITOR: Serum potassium, often; other electrolytes, eg, Na^+, Cl^-, CO_2 content, magnesium, and blood glucose, uric acid, BUN and creatinine, occasionally.

DRUG INTERACTIONS: Drug interactions are given in the next Table:

Drug Interactions of Ethacrynic Acid

Drug(s)	Effect
Aminoglycosides	Increased incidence of ototoxicity
Lithium	Decreased renal clearance of lithium possibly resulting in lithium toxicity
Cardiac Glycosides	Possibly fatal cardiac arrhythmias secondary to hypokalemia.
Neuromuscular Blocking Agents, eg, Tubocurarine	Prolonged neuromuscular blockage due to potassium depletion or decreased urinary excretion of the muscle relaxant.
Insulin or Oral Anti-diabetic Agents	Interference with hypoglycemic effects.

ETHAMBUTOL

(Myambutol)

USES: **Ethambutol** is an **antituberculosis agent** administered with at least one other antituberculosis drug.

Uncomplicated T.B.: Isoniazid and rifampin. Use ethambutol if patient resides in or has emigrated from an area with high level of initial drug resistance, or if the patient has a previous history of antituberculosis therapy. Ethambutol is also used in conjunction with other antituberculosis agents in the treatment of diseases caused by other mycobacteria.

Mechanism of Action: Ethambutol inhibits the synthesis of cell metabolites, which inhibits cell metabolism and results in cell death. It is effective only against actively growing bacilli.

DOSAGE FORMS: Tabs: 100, 400mg

DOSAGE: Ethambutol hydrochloride is administered orally. Manufacturer recommends that ethambutol not be used in children younger than 13 years of age but this drug has been used in children as young as 6 years. Dosage is given in the next Table:

Dosage of Ethambutol

Condition	Dosage
No Previous Therapy with Antituberculosis Agent	15mg/kg once daily or 50mg/kg twice weekly in combination for 6-9 months for uncomplicated pulmonary tuberculosis.
Previous Antituberculosis Therapy	25mg/kg daily for 60 days or until bacteriologic smears and cultures become negative, followed by 15mg/kg daily

Dosage should be decreased in severe renal impairment.

ETHAMBUTOL (Cont.)
PHARMACOKINETICS: About 80% of an oral dose is rapidly absorbed. Absorption is not substantially affected when the drug is administered with food; Peak: 2-4 hours; Plasma Protein Binding: 20-30%; Half-Life: 4-6 hr.; Metabolism: Partially metabolized by liver. Red blood cells serve as a depot to allow slow release into plasma.
Excretion: 80% excreted in the urine unchanged and 20% metabolized.
ADVERSE EFFECTS: The most important adverse effect is optic neuritis with decreases in visual acuity. Optic neuritis tends to occur with larger doses or in patients with renal impairment. It appears over several months usually as blurred vision, color blindness and restriction of visual fields. It is usually completely reversible over weeks to months with prompt drug discontinuation (Kahana, L.M., Can. Med. Assoc. J. 137, 213, 1987). Hyperuricemia due to impaired urinary excretion of uric acid may occur. May cause GI disturbances. Other adverse effects include dermatitis, pruritis, joint pain, headache, confusion.
MONITOR: Obtain baseline ophthalmologic studies before beginning therapy and then monthly. Follow visual acuity, visual fields, and (green) color vision. Discontinue if any visual deterioration occurs. Monitor uric acid, liver function, hematologic and renal function.

ETHOSUXIMIDE
(Zarontin)
USES: **Ethosuximide** is **drug of choice** in management of **absence (petite mal) seizures**; these are characterized by transient episodes of loss of awareness without convulsive movements.
DOSAGE FORMS: Caps: 250mg; Syrup: 250mg/5ml
DOSAGE: Ethosuximide is administered orally. Dosage must be carefully and slowly adjusted to individual requirements and response. Dosage is given in the next Table:

Dosage of Ethosuximide

Age	Dosage
3-6 years	250mg/day initially in two divided doses; then adjust every 4-7 days by 250mg/day to optimum effect. Optimal daily dose is usually 20-40mg/kg/day given in 2 divided doses. Max. 1.5g/day
>6 yrs & Adult	500mg/day; then adjust every 4-7 days in 250mg/day increments to optimum effect. Usual maintenance is 20-30mg/kg/day. Max. 1.5g/day

Around puberty, a lower dose is usually required to achieve the same serum level.
PHARMACOKINETICS: Metabolism: Ethosuximide is oxidized to inactive form in the liver; 10-20% is excreted unchanged by the kidneys. See other parameters under Monitoring.
ADVERSE EFFECTS: Frequent dose-related side effects are nausea, vomiting, lethargy, hiccups, drowsiness and dizziness; these may diminish with time. Occasionally, Parkinson-like symptoms, photophobia and agitation are observed. Rarely, a lupus-like syndrome, Stevens-Johnson syndrome, leukopenia, thrombocytopenia, aplastic anemia and ataxia are seen.

Ethosuximide may increase frequency of grand mal seizures in patients with mixed type seizures.

Use with caution in hepatic and renal disease.
MONITOR: Therapeutic: 40-100mcg/ml. Time to Obtain First Serum Specimen (Steady State): Children:6 days, Adults: 12 days. Trough:Immediately prior to the next oral dose. Time to Peak Concentration: 2-4h after an oral capsule; less for syrup. Half-life: Children: 30 h., Adults: 60 h. Toxic: >100mcg/ml. Guidelines for therapy and serum specimen monitoring are given in the next Table:

Guidelines for Therapy and Monitoring

Therapy	Monitoring
Children (<11 yr):15-40mg/kg/day	Children: 6 days
Adults: 15-30mg/kg/day	Adults: 12 days
	Maintenance Monitoring:4-6 mos. intervals provided therapeutic response is good

Periodic complete blood count(CBC) should be performed.

ETOPOSIDE
(VePesid)

USES: Etoposide is a podophyllotoxin derivative used in **cancer therapy**; indications are given in the next Table:

Uses of Etoposide

Cancer	Comments
Lung Carcinoma (particularly Small Cell)	Average response rate, 40%; potential use as a component of combination regimens.
Testicular Cancer (Nonseminomatous)	Cisplatin + etoposide ± bleomycin. Salvage therapy for patients not cured by PVB (cisplatin + vinblastine ± bleomycin)
Choriocarcinoma; Acute Myelogenous Leukemia; Non-Hodgkin's Lymphomas; Childhood Solid Tumors	Active in patients with these tumors

DOSAGE FORMS: IV Solution: 20mg/ml; Capsules: 50mg.

DOSAGE: Etoposide has been given orally; it is usually administered by IV. Refer to specific chemotherapy protocols. Dosage is given in the next Table:

Dosage of Etoposide

50 to 100mg/m^2 infused daily for five days.
Alternatively, 100mg/m^2 daily on days one, three and five every three to four weeks in combination with other drugs.

Doses as high as 800mg/m^2 daily have been used in some protocols.

PHARMACOKINETICS: Absorption, Oral: 20% to 80%; Plasma Protein Binding: 94%; Half-Lives: 2 and 5 hrs.; Excretion: About 45% of a dose is recovered in the urine after 72 hrs., approximately two-thirds as unchanged drug. CSF Concentration: <10% of plasma concentration.

ADVERSE EFFECTS: Leukopenia is dose limiting. Low WBC occurs between 8 and 14 days; recovery by days 16 to 21. Nausea and vomiting are usually mild. Alopecia is common. Fever, chills and palpitations may occur. Peripheral neuropathy may be cumulative with that caused by other neurotoxins e.g. cisplatin. Hypotension may occur with IV push injection and this drug should be given by slow infusion over 30-60 minutes.

EYES (CORNEA AND CONJUNCTIVA), PATHOGENS, TREATMENT

Pathogens: The pathogens that cause infection of the cornea and conjunctiva are given in the next Table (Handbook of Antimicrobial Therapy, The Medical Letter, 1990):

Pathogens Causing Infection of Cornea and Conjunctiva
1. Herpes and other viruses (adenovirus, varicella, etc.)
2. Neisseria gonorrhoeae (in newborn)
3. Haemophilus aegyptius (Koch-Weeks bacillus)
4. Streptococcus pneumoniae
5. Haemophilus influenzae (in children)
6. Moraxella lacunata
7. Staphylococcus aureus
8. Pseudomonas aeruginosa
9. Other gram-negative bacilli
10. Chlamydia trachomatis (trachoma and inclusion conjunctivitis)
11. Fungi

Different pathogens cause acute conjunctivitis in neonates and older children; these are given in the next Table (Eiferman, R.A. et al., Patient Care, pgs. 164-177, Aug. 15, 1986):

Pathogens in Neonates and Older Children	
Age	Common Pathogen(s)
1-5 days	N. gonorrhoeae
first week - first month	Chlamydia trachomatis, H. influenzae, Staphylococcus aureus, and enterococci.
1 month - 18 years	H. influenzae, adenoviruses, S. pneumoniae.

Prevention of N. Gonorrhoeae: Tetracycline ointment (1%) is effective in preventing gonococcal ophthalmia neonatorum (Laga, M. et al., N. Engl. J. Med. 318, 653-657, 1988).Topical erythromycin (Ilotycin Ophthalmic) drops in each eye at birth prevents both gonococcal and chlamydial conjunctivitis and does not irritate the infant's eyes (Hammerschlag, M.R., et al., JAMA 244, 2291, 1980).

Silver nitrate, 1%, drops in each eye at birth has been used in the past to prevent gonococcal conjunctivitis; however, silver nitrate may cause irritation which has been confused with conjunctivitis.

N. gonorrhoeae conjunctivitis may develop in neonates who have not received topical prophylaxis as may occur with home delivery or drops improperly administered.

Treatment: Antimicrobial treatment is given in the next Table:

Antimicrobial Treatment of Infections of Cornea and Conjunctiva	
Organism	Drug Treatment
Neisseria gonorrhoeae	Adults, Children >20kg: Ceftriaxone 1g IM once. Irrigate eyes with saline or ophthalmic solution. Children <20kg, Neonates: Ceftriaxone 25-50mg/kg daily as a single IV or IM dose or Cefotaxime 50mg/kg daily in 2 divided doses IV or IM or Penicillin G 100,000 units/kg daily in 4 divided doses (2 doses if <7d)(susceptible isolates only). Treat for 7 days. Irrigate eyes as above.
Chlamydia	Conjunctivitis: Erythromycin 50mg/kg daily in 4 divided doses orally for 14 days. NOTE: same therapy used for chlamydia pneumonia. Trachoma: Various recommendations. Topical erythromycin, tetracycline or sulfacetamide twice daily for 2 months plus erythromycin 10mg/kg or doxycycline 2.5-4mg/kg once daily orally for 40 days (1991 Red Book, p. 169-170).
H. influenzae or S. pneumoniae S. Aureus E. Coli Pseudomonas	Topical polymyxin B bacitracin or Erythromycin ophthalmic ointment (Ilotycin Ophthalmic) 1%, four times daily. or 10% sodium sulfacetamide (AK-Sulf, Cetamide, Sodium Sulamyd Ophthalmic) or Topical tetracycline; HCl ointment (Achromycin Ophthalmic)
Adenoviral infections	None

Otitis Media and Acute Conjunctivitis: Patients who develop both acute conjunctivitis and otitis media who are treated systemically for otitis media will not require separate treatment for acute conjunctivitis.

FAMOTIDINE
(Pepcid)

USES: Uses of famotidine are given in the next Table:

Uses of Famotidine
Active Duodenal Ulcers
Prophylaxis to Prevent Recurrence of Duodenal Ulcers
Active Gastric Ulcers
Zollinger-Ellison Syndrome

Famotidine healed duodenal ulcers in 70% to 90% over four to six weeks. Famotidine 40mg at night healed 91% to 97% of gastric ulcers after eight weeks. A nightly dose of 20mg is effective in reducing the rate of relapse of duodenal ulcers and controls the manifestations of reflex esophagitis (Weir, D.G., Brit. Med. J. 296, 195-200, Jan. 16, 1988).

The lack of toxic effects makes famotidine a potentially useful drug for treatment of peptic ulcers.

Mechanism of Action: Famotidine competitively inhibits the action of histamine on H_2 receptors of parietal cells, thus reducing acid secretion by parietal cells of the stomach; it acts like the other H_2 receptor antagonists, i.e., cimetidine (Tagamet), ranitidine (Zantac), and nizatidine (Axid).

DOSAGE FORMS: Tabs: 20mg, 40mg; Pepcid Suspension: 40mg/5ml; IV: 10mg/ml.

DOSAGE: Dosage of famotidine is given in the next Table:

Dosage of Femotidine

Condition	Oral Dosage
Active Ulcer	40mg daily at bedtime; or 20mg twice a day both for up to 8 weeks.
Maintenance	20mg daily at bedtime.
Hypersecretory Conditions such as Zollinger-Ellison Syndrome	Initially, 20mg every 6 hours; max. 160mg every 6 hours.

IV dosage is similar to oral dosage. Dosage in renal impairment (CrCl < 10ml/min): 20mg/day or 40mg every other day.

PHARMACOKINETICS: Peak: 1-3.5 hours; Metabolism: Liver to sulphoxide derivative; Half-Life: 2.5-4 hours; Excretion: Urine, 30% recovered unchanged.

ADVERSE EFFECTS: Famotidine apparently has no effect on the elimination of drugs metabolized by the liver. Toxic symptoms include altered bowel habits, dizziness, and headache; patients may experience constipation or diarrhea.

FENOPROFEN
(Nalfon)

USES: **Fenoprofen** is a **nonsteroidal anti-inflammatory drug (NSAID),** chemically and pharmacologically similar to **Ibuprofen;** it has **anti-inflammatory, analgesic,** and **antipyretic properties** and **inhibits** prostaglandin synthesis. Uses are given in the next Table:

Uses of Fenoprofen
Arthritis: Rheumatoid Arthritis, Osteoarthritis, Ankylosing Spondylitis, Psoriatic Arthritis, Reiter's Syndrome
Investigation Drug for Treatment of Gout

Fenoprofen may be used as initial therapy or as an alternative to aspirin in the treatment of rheumatoid arthritis and osteoarthritis.

DOSAGE FORMS: Caps: 200 and 300mg; Tabs: 600mg.

DOSAGE: Dosage for children has not been established; fenoprofen is given orally. Dosage is given in the next Table:

Dosage of Fenoprofen

Condition	Dosage
Rheumatoid Arthritis or Osteoarthritis	300 to 600mg, three or four times daily. Max. 3.2g; after a satisfactory response, adjust dosage to patients needs. If gastrointestinal reactions occur, fenoprofen may be given with meals or milk.
Mild to Moderate Pain	200mg every four to six hours as needed.

FENOPROFEN (Cont.)

PHARMACOKINETICS: Well absorbed; Plasma Peak: 90 minutes; Protein Binding: 99%; does not appear in breast milk, amniotic fluid, cord blood or saliva; Volume of Distribution: 0.08-0.10 liter/kg. Half-Life: 2-3 hours. Excretion: Urine in conjugated form.

ADVERSE EFFECTS: The most common adverse effects are gastrointestinal disturbances; these include dyspepsia, constipation, nausea and vomiting. Gastrointestinal bleeding occurs less often than with aspirin; ulceration has been reported. Central nervous system reactions include drowsiness, dizziness, headache, nervousness, and confusion. Pruritis, rash, palpitations, sweating, tremor, tinnitus, blurred vision, and decreased hearing have been reported. Fenoprofen has caused nephrotic syndrome with interstitial nephritis.

Fenoprofen reduces platelet aggregation and adhesiveness and increases bleeding time.

DRUG INTERACTIONS: Increased activity of anticoagulants and oral hypoglycemic agents.

FENTANYL CITRATE
(Sublimaze)

USES: Fentanyl is an opiate; uses are given in the next Table:

Uses of Fentanyl
Relief of Pain
Preoperative Sedation
General Anesthesia: with or without additional agents

DOSAGE FORMS: Parenteral(inj): 50 micrograms/ml.

DOSAGE: Fentanyl may be given IV or IM. Dosage is given in the next Table:

Dosage of Fentanyl

Condition	Dosage
Relief of Pain	Adults: 50-100 micrograms IV or IM every 30-60 minutes as needed. Children: 1-2 micrograms/kg IV or IM every 30-60 minutes as needed. Continuous Infusion: Initially, 1 microgram/kg/hour, titrate to effect.
Preoperative Sedation	Adults: 50-100 micrograms IM 30-60 minutes prior to surgery. Children: 1-2 micrograms/kg IM 30-60 minutes prior to surgery.
General Anesthesia	Adjunct to General Anesthesia: Low-dose: 2 micrograms/kg; Moderate-dose: 2-20 micrograms/kg; High-dose: 25-50 micrograms/kg. General Anesthesia Without Additional Anesthetics: 50-100 micrograms/kg.

ADVERSE EFFECTS: Addicting. The most serious adverse effect is respiratory depression, which may be reversed with naloxone. Respiratory depression may be delayed in some patients particularly with high dose therapy (100 micrograms/kg)(Caspi, J. et al., Crit. Care Med. 16, 238-240, 1988). Histamine release occurs less frequently than with morphine. Nausea, vomiting, muscle rigidity, laryngospasm, bronchoconstriction, and bradycardia may occur.

Use with caution in infants because pharmacokinetics are unpredictable in the very young.

FLUCONAZOLE
(Diflucan)

USES: Fluconazole is an antifungal agent, structurally related to ketoconazole and miconazole. Uses are given in the following Table (Galgiani, J.N., Ann. Intern. Med. 113, 177-179, 1990):

Uses of Miconazole
Cryptococcal Meningitis
Treatment - Not the Drug of Choice
Prevention of Recurrence
Candidiasis
Oral or Esophageal
Invasive Disease - Not the Drug of Choice
Other Severe Systemic Fungal Infections
Coccidioidomycosis - Data Insufficient
Histoplasmosis - Data Insufficient
Blastomycosis - Data Insufficient

Cryptococcal Meningitis: Amphoterecin B plus flucytosine is superior to fluconazole for treatment of cryptococcal meningitis in AIDS patients (Larsen, R.A. et al., Ann. Intern. Med. 113, 183-187, 1990). However, fluconazole is effective as maintenance therapy to prevent recurrence of cryptococcal meningitis compared to placebo (Bozzette, S.A. et al., NEJM 324, 580-584, 1991).

Candidiasis: Fluconazole is effective therapy for treatment of oral and esophageal candidiasis, and should be considered one of several alternative treatments; usefulness for prophylaxis or treatment of systemic candidiasis has not been established (Galgiani, J.N., Ann. Intern. Med. 113, 177-179, 1990).

Other Severe Systemic Fungal Infections: There is insufficient data to define the role of fluconazole in the treatment of infections caused by coccidioidomycosis, histoplasmosis and blastomycosis.

DOSAGE FORMS: Tabs: 50, 100, 200mg; IV: 2mg/ml.

DOSAGE: Fluconazole is administered orally or intravenously over 2-4 hours. Dosage of fluconazole is given in the following Table:

Dosage of Fluconazole

Condition	Dosage
Cryptococcal Meningitis - Treatment	400mg daily as a single oral (or IV) dose.
Cryptococcal Meningitis - Prevent Recurrence	200mg daily as a single oral (or IV) dose.
Candidiasis - Oral or Esophageal	200mg on day 1 followed by 100mg daily as a single oral (or IV) dose.
Candidiasis - Systemic	400mg on day 1 followed by 200mg daily as a single oral (or IV) dose.
Children 3-13 yrs	Load: 10mg/kg, Maintenance: 3-6mg/kg/day as a single dose beginning 24 hrs after load.

PHARMACOKINETICS: Oral Absorption: 1-2 hrs; Peak serum level: same IV and PO; CSF levels: 50-90% of serum levels; Excretion: 70-80% renal; Half-Life: 30 hrs; Protein binding: 11%.

ADVERSE EFFECTS: Nausea (4%); Other reactions, 1.5-2%: headache, rash, vomiting, abdominal pain, and diarrhea.

FLUCYTOSINE
(Ancobon)

USES: Flucytosine is an **antifungal** agent; uses are given in the following Table:

Uses of Flucytosine
Candida - Sepsis, Endocarditis, Urinary Tract Infection
Cryptococcus - Meningitis, Pneumonia

Flucytosine may be effective for treatment of candida urinary tract infection, but is generally combined with amphotericin B for treatment of systemic candidal or cryptococcal infections.

Mechanism of Action: Flucytosine enters fungal cells where it is converted to fluorouracil. Fluorouracil competes with uracil, disrupting RNA and subsequently, protein synthesis. Another flucytosine metabolite, fluorodeoxyuredylic acid, inhibits thymidylate synthetase, disrupting DNA synthesis.

DOSAGE FORMS: Caps: 250, 500mg.

DOSAGE: Flucytosine is administered orally; dosage is given in the following Table:

Condition	Dosage	
Usual	50-200mg/kg daily in 4 divided doses.	
Renal Impairment	CrCl 20-40ml/min	12.5-37.5mg/kg every 12 h
	10-20ml/min	12.5-37.5mg/kg every 24 h
	<10ml/min	12.5-37.5mg/kg every 24-48 h

PHARMACOKINETICS: Oral Absorption: 75-90%; Peak: within 2 hrs; Protein Binding: 2-4%; Half-Life: 2.5-6 hrs, prolonged in renal impairment; Excretion: Renal.

ADVERSE EFFECTS: Bone marrow: moderate hypoplasia with anemia, leukopenia, thrombocytopenia. GI: nausea, vomiting, diarrhea. Other: Transaminase elevation, BUN and creatinine elevation.

MONITOR: CBC, platelet count, creatinine, alkaline phosphatase AST (SGOT), ALT (SGPT). May cause falsely elevated creatinine determinations by alkaline picrate method.

FLUDROCORTISONE
(Florinef)

USES: Fludrocortisone (9-alpha-fluorohydrocortisone) is used only for **oral mineralocorticoid replacement**; uses are given in the next Table:

Uses of Fludrocortisone
Adrenocortical Insufficiency
Salt-Losing Forms of Congenital Adrenogenital Syndrome, eg, 21-Hydroxylase Deficiency

Fludrocortisone is useful in patients with adrenocortical insufficiency or salt-losing forms of congenital adrenogenital syndrome after electrolyte balance has been restored.

In patients with adrenocortical insufficiency and in patients with salt-losing forms of congenital adrenogenital syndrome, hydrocortisone or cortisone in conjunction with liberal salt intake is administered. In patients with subtle or overt salt wasting, 9-alpha-fluorocortisol or desoxycorticosterone should be given (Miller, W.L. and Levine, L.S., J. Pediatr. 111, 1-17, 1987).

DOSAGE FORMS: Tabs: 0.1mg

DOSAGE: Fludrocortisone acetate is administered orally. Dosage depends on the severity of the disease and response of the patient. Dosage is given in the next Table:

Condition	Dosage
Adrenocortical Insufficiency	0.1mg daily (range: 0.1mg 3 times weekly to 0.2mg daily); if hypertension occurs, 0.05mg is given daily. Cortisone (10-37.5mg daily in divided doses) or hydrocortisone (10-30mg daily in divided doses) is usually given orally concomitantly with fludrocortisone.
Salt-Losing Forms of Congenital Adrenogenital Syndrome	0.1-0.2mg daily.

ADVERSE EFFECTS: The drug is contraindicated in all conditions except those which require a high degree of mineralocorticoid activity. If elevated B.P. develops, decrease dose to 0.05mg/day.

0.1mg 9-alpha-fluorocortisol = 1mg desoxycorticosterone.

FLUNISOLIDE

(Nasalide, Aerobid)

USES: **Flunisolide** is a **fluorinated corticosteroid** that is used as a **nasal spray** for the symptomatic treatment of **seasonal** or **perennial rhinitis** of allergic or nonallergic etiology, when conventional therapy with antihistamines or decongestants is ineffective or produces intolerable adverse effects.

Rhinorrhea, nasal pruritis, erythema, nasal congestion, postnasal drainage and sneezing are reduced. Nasal polyps may be reduced in size and obstruction reduced significantly.

In patients with seasonal or perennial rhinitis, symptomatic relief is usually evident within 2-3 days of intranasal therapy; however, up to 2-3 weeks may be required for optimum effectiveness.

Flunisolide is used by oral inhalation for control of symptoms of asthma in patients who require chronic corticosteroid therapy.

Mechanism of Action: Flunisolide exerts a marked anti-inflammatory effect on the nasal mucosa by inhibiting the release of inflammatory mediators from mast cells and basophils and blocking the inflammatory effects of leukocytes in the nose. The number of surface basophils and eosinophils is reduced and both vasodilation and edema are decreased. Corticosteroids inhibit both immediate and delayed reactions to allergen challenge (Clissold, S.P. and Heel, R. C., Drugs 28, 485-518, 1984).

DOSAGE FORMS: Nasal spray (Nasalide): 25 micrograms/actuation; Inhaler (Aerobid): 250micrograms/spray.

DOSAGE: Dosage of Aerobid in asthma is 500-1000micrograms (2-4 sprays) twice daily. Dosage of Nasalide is given in the next Table:

Dosage of Flunisolide as Nasalide

Age	Dosage
Adults	Initially, two sprays (50 microgram) in each nostril two times daily; if necessary, this dose may be increased to two sprays in each nostril three times daily (max. dose, 400 microgram/day)
Children 6 to 14 yrs.	Initially, one spray (25 microgram) in each nostril three times daily or two sprays in each nostril two times daily (max. dose, 200 microgram/day)

When the maximal response is obtained (usually in one to two weeks), the dose is then reduced to the lowest level that maintains symptomatic control.

PHARMACOKINETICS: Flunisolide is well absorbed; however, flunisolide is rapidly metabolized to less active metabolites by the liver. Thus, there is a low incidence of systemic side effects.

ADVERSE EFFECTS: The most common adverse effects are stinging and burning (40% of patients) that lasts only a few seconds. Sneezing, headache, dry nose and nasal bleeding have been reported. Monitor for suppression of the hypothalamic-pituitary-adrenal axis.

FLUORIDE

(Pediaflor, Karidium, Luride, Flura-Drops, others)

USES: Fluoride is used to **prevent dental caries**, to desensitize exposed root surfaces of teeth, and in various bone diseases to increase bone density and relieve bone pain.

Patients with osteoporosis and at least one vertebral fracture were treated with 25mg of enteric-coated sodium fluoride twice daily, 1g of calcium. and 800 IV of vitamin D; these patients were less likely to develop vertebral fractures than were patients who were not treated with sodium fluoride. The only adverse effect was pain and tenderness around the large joints of the legs (Mamelle, N. et al., Lancet 2, 361-365, 1988).

DOSAGE FORMS: Sol'n: 0.5, 2, 2.25, 5.5, 5.9mg/ml; Chewable Tabs: 0.25, 0.5, 1.0mg

DOSAGE: In the prevention of dental caries, oral fluoride should be administered only when the fluoride concentration in drinking water is 0.7ppm or less. Concentration of fluoride in drinking water (ppm), dose of fluoride and age are given in the next Table:

Dose of Fluoride(mg/day)

Age	Concentration of Fluoride in Drinking Water(ppm) <0.3	0.3-0.7
2 wks-2 yr	0.25mg	0
2-3 yr	0.5mg	0.25mg
3-13 yr	1.00mg	0.50mg

ADVERSE EFFECTS: Chronic: Mottled enamel; Acute: Fatal dose is estimated as 500mg in children and 5-10g in adults. Hypersalivation, epigastric pain, nausea, vomiting, abdominal pain, diarrhea. Shock may occur.

FLUOXETINE

(Prozac)

USES: Fluoxetine is a bicyclic antidepressant which is structurally unique but is no more effective than other antidepressants. However, it has potential for fewer and different side effects as compared to other antidepressants (The Medical Letter 30, 45-48, April 22, 1988).

Fluoxetine usually begins to act about 1-4 weeks after beginning treatment; this is similar to the onset of action with tricyclic antidepressants (Sommi, R.W. et al., Pharmacotherapy 7, 1, 1987).

In clinical trials, up to 80mg fluoxetine is as effective as up to 300mg/day of imipramine (Tofranil; and others) or amitriptyline (Elavil; and others) for treatment of depression (Schatzberg, A.F. et al., J. Clin. Psychopharmacol. 7, 44S, Dec. 1987). Fluoxetine (20-80mg/day) is comparable to 50-200mg/day of doxepin(Sinequan; and others) in relieving symptoms in elderly patients who were moderately depressed (Feighner, J.P. and Cohn, J.B., J. Clin. Psychiatry 46, Sec. 2:20, March 1985).

Fluoxetine may be more effective than other antidepressants for decreasing symptoms of obscessive-compulsive disorder (Fontaine, R. and Chouinard, G., J. Clin. Psychopharmacol. 6, 98, 1986).

Mechanism of Action: Fluoxetine is a selective inhibitor of serotonin reuptake into presynaptic nerve terminals in the central nervous system, with little or no block of the uptake of norepinephrine or dopamine (Fuller, R.W. and Wong, D.T., J. Clin Psychopharmacol 7, 36S, 1987).

The effect of inhibiting serotonin uptake is to increase the concentration of serotonin in critical synaptic areas in the brain. Increased serotonin in these areas of the brain modifies certain affective and behavioral disorders.

Fluoxetine binds only minimally to histaminic (H-1), cholinergic and alpha-1 adrenergic receptors which are belived to be associated with many of the adverse effects of other antidepressants (Stark, P. et al., J. Clin. Psychiatry 46, Sec. 2.7, March 1985).

Chemical Structure: Fluoxetine is a phenylpropylamide bicyclic, chemically distinct from currently available tricyclic and second generation antidepressants.

DOSAGE FORMS: 20mg capsules.

DOSAGE: Effective doses of fluoxetine range from 20mg to 80mg daily, given orally once a day (in the morning) or in divided doses twice a day (morning and noon). Twenty mg daily is as effective in most patients as higher doses and results in fewer adverse effects (Sommi, R.W. et al., Pharmacotherapy 7, 1-15, 1987).

Dosage is initiated with 20mg daily and as necessary, titrated after several weeks in 20mg/day increments to a maximum of 80mg daily.

FLUOXETINE (Cont.)
PHARMACOKINETICS: Absorption: Well-absorbed and not influenced by food; Peak: 6-8 hours; Metabolism: Fluoxetine is demethylated in the liver to norfluoxetine which is also active; Half Life: Fluoxetin, 1-3 days; norfluoxetin, 7 days. However, the plasma half-life of fluoxetin increases with long-term administration, from 2 to 5.1 days in subjects given 60mg daily (Sommi, R.W. et al., Pharmacotherapy 7, 1-15, 1987). The half-life is similar in elderly and young patients(Benfield, P. et al., Drugs, 32, 481-508, 1986). Excretion: Only 2.5% excreted unchanged in the urine; other inactive metabolites excreted in the urine.
ADVERSE EFFECTS: Approximately 14% of patients discontinued therapy due to adverse reactions (Sommi, R.W. et al., Pharmacotherapy 7, 1-15, 1987).

As already mentioned, fluoxetine has minimal effect on norepinephrine or acetylcholine function. Thus, there are infrequent cardiovascular side effects such as tachycardia, and orthostatic hypotension. or anticholinergic side effects, such as dry mouth, constipation, or urinary retention.

There is a lack of weight gain as occurs with tricyclic antidepressants; in fact, fluoxetine use is associated with weight loss.

Adverse effects, arranged in decreasing order of incidence, are as follows: nausea/vomiting, headache, somnolence, rhinitis, back pain, insomnia, dry mouth, constipation, anxiety/nervousness, diarrhea and edema (Debus, J.R. etal., J. Clin. Psychiatry 49, 422-426, 1988). Other adverse effects include tremor, asthemia and dizziness.

About 4% of patients develop urticaria or some other rash, fever, leukocytosis, arthralgias, respiratory distress and transaminase elevations.

Fluoxetine, like tricyclics, may precipitate mania or hypomania (Lebegue, B., Am. J. Psychiatry 144, 1620, Dec. 1987).

It is necessary to wait 5 weeks after discontinuation of fluoxetine before initiating treatment with a monoamine oxidase inhibitor (MAOI) (Sternbach, H., Lancet 2, 850-851, Oct. 8, 1988)
Overdose: Agitation, vomiting and seizures.

FLURAZEPAM
(Dalmane)
USES: **Flurazepam** is a **benzodiazepine** sharing the actions of other benzodiazepines and is used as a **hypnotic agent** in the short term treatment of **insomnia** for periods up to 4 weeks.
Mechanism of Action: The hypnotic effect is probably related to its facilitation of gamma aminobutyric acid-mediated neurotransmission.
DOSAGE FORMS: Caps: 15, 30mg
DOSAGE: Flurazepam is administered orally at bedtime; it is not recommended in children under 15 years. 30mg initial dose is preferred for young healthy patients; elderly patients, especially those over 70 years, should be given an initial dose of 15mg.
PHARMACOKINETICS: Clinical effect increases on the second and third night of continuous use and persists for several nights after drugs discontinuation. Metabolism: Liver; Half-Life: 50-100 hr.; Steady State: 7-10 days.
ADVERSE EFFECTS: Morning drowsiness or hangover in about 5%; occasionally, impairment of motor function and intellectual performance, dry mouth, nightmares, delirium and confusion. Rarely, hematologic abnormalities and hepatic dysfunction. Withdrawal may occur with abrupt discontinuation of this drug.
PRECAUTIONS: Safety and efficacy of flurazepam in children younger than 15 years of age have not been established.

FUROSEMIDE

(Lasix, Furomide, Lo-Aqua)

USES: **Furosemide** is a sulfonamide-type **loop diuretic;** its uses are given in the next Table:

Uses of Furosemide

Uses	Condition
Edema	Congestive heart failure(CHF) Renal failure (IV administration preferable) Acute pulmonary edema (IV administration preferable) Nephrotic syndrome Hepatic cirrhosis
Hypertension	Mild to moderate hypertension, especially when complicated by congestive heart failure or renal disease. Note that the thiazide diuretics are usually the initial diuretics of choice in most patients.
Hypercalcemia	Reduces serum calcium concentration by increasing calcium excretion.

Furosemide inhibits the reabsorption of electrolytes in the ascending limb of the loop of Henle. Excessive losses of potassium, hydrogen, and chloride may result in metabolic alkalosis.

HYPERTENSION: Treatment of hypertension with furosemide is given in the next Table(The 1988 Report of the Joint National Committee on Detection, Evaluation and Treatment of High Blood Pressure, Arch.Intern. Med. 148, 1023-1038, 1988):

Treatment of Hypertension with Furosemide

Step 1: Nonpharmacologic Approaches (see **HYPERTENSION)**

↓

Step 2: Furosemide (Usual Minimum, 20-40mg/day; Usual Maximum, 320 mg/day)
Observe up to 6 months; if furosemide ineffective then,

↓

Step 3: Add a second drug of a different class
or Increase the dosage of furosemide
or Substitute another drug

↓

Step 4: Add a third drug of a different class
or Substitute a second drug

↓

Step 5: Consider further evaluation and/or referral
or Add a third or fourth drug

"Step-Down": For patients with mild hypertension, after 1 year of control, consider decreasing or withdrawing furosemide and other hypotensive drugs.

DOSAGE FORMS: Tabs: 20, 40, 80mg; Inj: 10mg/ml; Oral Liquid: 8, 10mg/ml

DOSAGE: Furosemide may be administered orally, IV or IM. Dosage is given in the next Table:

Dosage of Furosemide

Condition	Age	Route	Dosage
Edema	Adults	Oral	20-80mg as single dose, preferably in the morning. If no response, dose may be increased by 20 to 40mg increments every 6-8 h. Effective dose may be given once or twice daily thereafter or 2-4 consecutive days each week. Max. 600mg daily.
	Infants and Children	Oral	1mg/kg as a single dose. If no response, increase dose by 1 or 2mg/kg increments every 6-8 hrs. Max. 6mg/kg/dose.
	Adults	IV or IM	20-40mg as a single injection. If no response, increase dose by 20mg increments not more often than every 2 h. until diuretic response obtained. Effective single dose may be given once or twice daily.

FUROSEMIDE (Cont.)
(Table Cont.)

Condition	Age	Route	Dosage
Acute Pulmonary Edema	Adults	IV Slowly over 1-2 minutes	40mg. If no satisfactory response in 1 h., dose may be increased to 80mg. In adults with hypertensive crisis, plus pulmonary edema or renal failure, give 100-200mg.
	Infants or Children	IV or IM	1mg/kg. If necessary, the initial dose may be increased by 1mg/kg no more often than every 2 hours. Max. 6mg/kg/dose.
Hypertension	Adults	Oral	40mg twice daily initially and for maintenance.

PHARMACOKINETICS: Onset and duration data are given in the next Table:

Onset and Duration of Furosemide

Route	Onset	Peak	Duration
Oral	30-60 min.	1-2 hr.	6 hr.
IV	15 min.	30-60 min.	1-2 hr.

Duration may be prolonged in severe renal insufficiency. Absorption: 70%; Half-Life: 50 min; 120 min. in CHF; several hrs. in renal insufficiency. Protein binding: 95%; Metabolism: 30% metabolized; 70% excreted unchanged by tubular secretion.

ADVERSE EFFECTS: The most frequent adverse reactions are hypokalemia, dehydration, hypotension and hypochloremic metabolic alkalosis. Hyperglycemia, hyperuricemia, hypercholesterolemia and hypertriglyceridemia may occur as with thiazides. Hypomagnesemia may occur.

Sexual dysfunction may be psychologically debilitating.

Weakness has been reported.

Adverse GI effects include nausea, vomiting, diarrhea and cramps.

Ototoxicity: Tinnitis, reversible or permanent hearing impairment, usually following IV or IM administration in doses exceeding usual therapeutic dose; most likely to occur in patients with severe renal impairment or in patients receiving other ototoxic drugs, eg, aminoglycosides.

Allergic interstitial nephritis has been reported. Hepatic cirrhosis: Use with caution.

Prolonged use in premature infants may lead to nephrocalcinosis due to increased urinary calcium excretion.

CONTRAINDICATIONS: Sulfa allergy, Anuria, except for a single dose. Pregnancy except when benefits outweigh risks.

MONITOR: Serum potassium, often; other electrolytes, eg, Na^+, Cl^-, CO_2 content, magnesium, and blood glucose, uric acid, BUN and creatinine, occasionally.

DRUG INTERACTIONS: Drug interactions are given in the next Table:

Drug Interactions of Furosemide

Drug(s)	Effect
Aminoglycosides	Increased incidence of ototoxicity
Lithium	Decreased renal clearance of lithium possibly resulting in lithium toxicity
Cardiac Glycosides	Possibly fatal cardiac arrhythmias secondary to hypokalemia.
Neuromuscular Blocking Agents, eg, Tubocurarine	Prolonged neuromuscular blockage due to potassium depletion or decreased urinary excretion of the muscle relaxant.
Insulin or Oral Antidiabetic Agents	Interference with hypoglycemic effects.

GAMMA BENZENE HEXACHLORIDE
(Kwell, Lindane)

USES: Uses of gamma benzene hexachloride are given in the next Table:

Uses of Gamma Benzene Hexachloride
Treatment of **Scabies** (Sarcoptes Scabiae) and Eggs
Treatment of **Lice** (Pediculosis): Head Louse (Pediculus Capitis), Body Louse (Pediculus Corporis) and **Crab Louse** (Phthirius Pubis) and their Nits.

Gamma benzene hexachloride is used in the topical treatment of scabies (parasitic arthropod Sarcoptes scabiae) and in treatment of pediculosis (lice). **It is a drug of choice for the treatment of scabies.** It is toxic to Sarcoptes scabiae (the causative agent of scabies and their eggs); also toxic to Pediculus capitis (head lice), Pediculus corporis (body louse) and Phthirus pubis (crab louse) and possibly their nits.

Do not use in infants, young children, and during pregnancy because of potential CNS toxicity; the CDC currently recommends alternative therapy for children <10 years. Some clinicians use gamma benzene hexachloride as young as 1-2 years of age. Alternative treatment for scabies and lice in infants, young children, and pregnant or lactating women are given in the next Table:

Alternative Therapy for Scabies and Lice in Children <10 Years, Pregnancy and Lactating Women

Condition	Treatment
Scabies	10% Crotamiton (Eurax) or 6% Sulfur in Petrolatum
Lice	Pyrethrins with Piperonyl Butoxide

DOSAGE FORMS: Shampoo: 1%; Lotion: 1%; Cream: 1%

DOSAGE: Thoroughly machine wash and dry clothing and bed sheets after starting treatment. Treat family members.

Scabies: Up to 20g to 30g of lotion or cream is applied to all parts of the body except the face. Avoid eyes, eyelashes and mucous membranes. The medication is washed off thoroughly following overnight exposure (8-12 hours). It can be applied again after a seven-day interval, but usually only one treatment is required.

Head Lice: Up to 30ml of shampoo is massaged into the hair for four minutes. The hair is then thoroughly rinsed with warm water and towel dried. Treatment is repeated in one week.

Pubic Lice: The shampoo is applied to the affected and adjacent hairy areas, particularly the pubic mons and perianal region, and is removed after four minutes; in hairy individuals, the thighs, trunk, and axillary regions also should be shampooed. When the hair is dry, any remaining nits or nit shells should be removed with a fine-toothed comb and tweezers. Retreatment in seven days is indicated only if gross signs of infestation (new nits, living lice) are present.

Body Lice: Apply a thin layer of lotion or cream to infested and adjacent hairy areas, leave on for 8 to 12 hours, and remove by showering or bathing.

ADVERSE EFFECTS: Irritant contact dermatitis when used in excess, too frequently or for extended periods.

It is systemically absorbed and CNS toxicity may occur, especially in the young. CNS toxicity is usually manifested as stimulation progressing to convulsions; treat with I.V. diazepam or barbiturates.

GANCICLOVIR
(Cytovene)

USES: Ganciclovir is a synthetic purine analog with antiviral activity against various herpes viruses including cytomegalovirus (CMV), herpes simplex types 1 and 2, Epstein-Barr Virus, and Varicella-Zoster virus. The principal use of ganciclovir is in treatment of cytomegalovirus infections in immunocompromised patients (eg, acquired immunodeficiency syndrome and organ or bone marrow transplant recipients) as listed in the next Table:

Uses of Ganciclovir
CMV Infections:
Retinitis
GI infections (colitis, esophagitis, gastritis and rectal disease)
Pneumonitis
Hepatobiliary Disease

Ganciclovir is most effective against CMV retinitis, but retinal detachment may occur during healing. Ganciclovir is also effective against CMV GI infections and hepatobiliary disease; results in patients with CMV pneumonitis have been variable, possibly due to the presence of other pathogens. Prophylactic ganciclovir is effective in preventing CMV interstitial pneumonia in allogeneic bone marrow transplant recipients with asymptomatic CMV infection (Schmidt, G.M. et al., N. Engl. J. Med. 324, 1005-1011, April, 1991).

The indications for ganciclovir therapy have not been fully defined.

Mechanism of Action: Ganciclovir is a purine analog of guanine which inhibits viral DNA chain elongation. Ganciclovir itself does not have antiviral activity, but is converted intracellularly to the active compound, ganciclovir triphosphage, which is virustatic.

DOSAGE FORM: Parenteral: 500mg.

DOSAGE: Ganciclovir is administered by slow IV infusion over 1 hr.; dosage is given in the next Table:

Dosage of Ganciclovir	
CMV Retinitis Induction	5mg/kg IV over 1 hr every 12 hrs
CMV Retinitis Maintenance	5mg/kg IV daily or 6mg/kg daily for 5 days weekly
Other CMV Infections	5mg/kg every 12 hrs or 2.5mg/kg every 8 hrs for 14-21 days

Dosage Adjust in Renal Failure: If creatinine clearance is 25-49ml/min, dose is 2.5mg/kg every 24 hrs; if CrCl is less than 25, dose is 1.25mg/kg every 24 hrs.

ADVERSE EFFECTS: Retinal detachment may occur during resolution of retinitis. CNS effects include headaches, confusion, seizures and coma. Hematologic effects, particularly neutropenia (25-50%) and thrombocytopenia (20%) due to myelotoxic effects may be severe and occur frequently.

DRUG INTERACTIONS: Concomitant use of other antiviral or antineoplastic drugs may increase the risk of hematologic toxicity.

GEMFIBROZIL
(Lopid)

USES: Gemfibrozil is approved by the FDA primarily for **triglyceride lowering** to reduce the risk of **pancreatitis** and not for routine use in lowering cholesterol. The effect of gemfibrozil on serum lipids is given in the next Table:

Effect of Gemfibrozil on Serum Lipids

Trigly.	VLDL	Chol.	LDL-Chol.	HDL-Chol.	HDL Chol./Tot.Chol.
Marked Decrease	Marked Decrease	Mild Decrease	5-15% Decrease	Increase	Increase

Gemfibrozil is primarily and highly effective in **lowering triglycerides,** and there is an associated increase on HDL-cholesterol. It may be considered for the treatment of adult patients with very high serum triglycerides (750mg)(types IV and V hyperlipoproteinemias) who present a risk for pancreatitis; it is not useful for treatment of the hypertriglyceridemia of type I hyperlidemia.

Mechanism of Action: Gemfibrozil inhibits peripheral lipolysis and decreases the hepatic extraction of free fatty acids, thus reducing hepatic triglyceride production. It inhibits the synthesis and increases the clearance of VLDL carrier apolipoprotein B, leading to a decrease in VLDL production.

DOSAGE FORM: Caps: 300mg; Tabs: 600mg.

DOSAGE: The usual dosage of gemfibrozil is 1200mg daily, taken in two divided doses 30 minutes before the morning and evening meal.

ADVERSE EFFECTS: The more common adverse effects are gastrointestinal symptoms; adverse effects of gemfibrozil are given in the next Table:

Adverse Effects of Gemfibrozil

System	Effect(s)
Gastrointestinal	Abdominal pain (6%), epigastric pain (5%), diarrhea (5%), nausea (4%), vomiting (2%), flatulence (1%).
Integumentary	Rash, dermatitis, pruritus, urticaria.
CNS	Headache, dizziness, blurred vision.
Musculoskeletal	Painful extremities.
Hematopoietic	Anemia, eosinophilia, leukopenia.

DRUG INTERACTIONS: Gemfibrozil potentiates the effects of oral anticoagulants; the dosage of the anticoagulant should be reduced to maintain the prothrombin time at desired level to prevent bleeding complications. Frequent prothrombin determinations should be done until the prothrombin level has stabilized.

CONTRAINDICATIONS: Hepatic or severe renal dysfunction, including primary biliary cirrhosis; pre-existing gall bladder disease.

WARNINGS: Gemfibrozil may increase cholesterol excretion into the bile leading to cholelithiasis. Therapy should be discontinued if gallstones are found. Gemfibrozil combined with lovastatin has been associated with rhabdomyolysis.

PHARMACOKINETICS: Absorption: Well absorbed; Peak: 1 to 2 hours; Half-Life: 1.5 hours; Excretion: Urine (70%).

MONITOR: Monitor triglycerides and cholesterol prior to initiation of therapy and at four week intervals.

GENTAMICIN

(Garamycin and Others)

USES: Gentamicin is an **aminoglycoside antibiotic** (gentamicin, streptomycin, amikacin, tobramycin, kanamycin, netilmicin, sisomicin) and is used frequently in hospitals for parenteral treatment of patients who have serious infections caused by **aerobic gram-negative bacilli** (eg, a number of the Enterobacteriaceae, P. aeruginosa). Its major advantage over other aminoglycosides is its low cost due to expiration of its patent; activities of gentamicin are given in the next Table (Pancoast, S.J., Med. Clin. No. Am. 72, 581-612, May, 1988; Adams, H.G., Personal Comm.):

Activities of Gentamicin

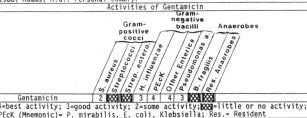

	Gram-positive cocci			Gram-negative bacilli				Anaerobes	
	S. aureus	Streptococci	Strep. entero.	H. influenzae	PEcK	Other Enterics	Pseudomonas a.	B. fragilis	Res. Anaerobes
Gentamicin	2	▩	▩	3	4	4	3	▩	▩

4=best activity; 3=good activity; 2=some activity; ▩=little or no activity; PEcK (Mnemonic)= P. mirabilis, E. coli, Klebsiella; Res.= Resident

The major useful bacterial spectrum of gentamicin is given in the next Table:

Bacterial Spectrum of Gentamicin

Enterobacteriaceae: Escherichia coli, Klebsiella, Enterobacter and Serratia species, Proteus mirabilis, indole-positive Proteus (Providencia rettgeri, Morganella morganii, Proteus vulgaris), Providencia stuartii and Citrobacter species. Salmonella and Shigella species are usually susceptible but other effective and less toxic antibiotics are used.

Pseudomonas aeruginosa: Aminoglycosides are usually combined with a penicillin, eg, carbenicillin, or cephalosporin, eg, ceftazidime.

Enterococci, eg, Streptococcus faecalis: Gentamicin plus penicillin G or ampicillin is frequently treatment of choice for enterococcal endocarditis.

Prophylaxis of Endocarditis: Gentamicin plus ampicillin is the standard parenteral regimen for high risk patients.

Staphylococci, eg, S. aureus and S. epidermidis

Gentamicin is used to treat susceptible organisms involving the following tissue: lower respiratory tract, intra-abdominal, soft tissue, bone or joint, wound, and complicated urinary tract infections; bacteremias; and meningitis. It is the preferred aminoglycoside with ampicillin for the prophylaxis of endocarditis. Gentamicin does not penetrate into CSF.

Mechanism of Action: The mechanism of action of gentamicin is like other aminoglycosides in that it binds to the bacterial 30S ribosomal subunit to produce a non-functional 70S initiation complex that results in the inhibition of bacterial cell protein synthesis and misreading of the genetic code.

DOSAGE FORMS: Inj. (IV or IM): 10mg/ml, 40mg/ml; Intrathecal: 2mg/ml; Ophth. Oint.: 3mg/g; Ophth. Sol'n:3mg/ml; Topical Oint.: 0.1%.

GENTAMICIN (Cont.)

DOSAGE: Gentamicin sulfate is administered by IM injection or IV infusion. It is administered intrathecally or intraventricularly in treatment of CNS infections. IM and IV dosage is identical. Dosage is given in the next Table:

Dosage of Gentamicin

Condition	Age	Route	Dosage
Usual	Adults	IM or IV	3-5mg/kg daily in equally divided doses at 8-hour intervals; max. 5mg/kg daily.
	Children	IM or IV	6-7.5mg/kg daily in equally divided doses at 8-hour intervals.
	Term Infant	IM or IV	2.5mg/kg/dose; <7d, 12 hr dosing; >7d, 8 hr dosing.
	28-34 weeks	IM or IV	2.5mg/kg/dose; <7d, 18 hr dosing; >7d, 12 hr dosing.
	<28 weeks	IM or IV	2.5mg/kg/dose; <7d, 24 hr dosing; >7d, 18 hr dosing.
Prophylaxis of Bacterial Endocarditis secondary to Dental Procedures; Minor Upper Respiratory Tract Surgery or Instrumentation (Parenteral regimen for high risk patients)	Adults and Child. >26kg	IM or IV	1.5mg/kg of gentamicin and 2g ampicillin given separately IM or IV 30 min. prior to procedure and 1.5g Amoxicillin orally 6 hours later or repeat half parenteral regimen 8 hours later.
	Children <27kg	IM or IV	2mg/kg of gentamicin and 50mg/kg ampicillin given separately IM or IV 30 min. prior to procedure and 25mg/kg amoxicillin orally 6 hours later or instead of oral follow-up dose, repeat parenteral regimen, half doses, 8 hrs later.
Prophylaxis of Bacterial Endocarditis secondary to GI, Biliary or GU Tract Surgery or Instrumentation (Parenteral regimen)	Adults and Child. >26kg	IM or IV	1.5mg/kg of gentamicin and 2g ampicillin given separately IM or IV 30-60 min. prior to procedure and half doses 8 hrs later or amoxicillin 1.5g orally 6 hrs later.
	Child. <27kg	IM or IV	2mg/kg of gentamicin and 50mg/kg ampicillin given separately IM or IV 30 min. prior to procedure and half doses 8 hrs later or amoxicillin 25mg/kg 6 hrs later.
Central Nervous System (CNS)	Adults	Intrathecal or Intraventricular	4-8mg as single daily dose plus IM or IV.
	Children >3 months	Intrathecal or Intraventricular	1-2mg as single daily dose plus IM or IV. Continue for at least 1 day after CSF culture and/or stained smears become negative.

Dosage Adjustment in Renal Failure: When serum gentamicin concentrations cannot be measured, dosage guidelines based on predictive nomograms are used (Sarubbi, F.A., Jr. and Hull, J.H., Ann. Intern. Med. 89, 612-618, 1978).

(1) Loading Dose: The usual loading dose for gentamicin is 1.5 to 2.0mg/kg (ideal weight) for expected peak serum level of 4 to 10mcg/ml.

(2) Calculate creatinine clearance using the formula:

$$\text{Creatinine Clearance(Male)} = \frac{\text{Wt. } (140 - \text{age})}{(72)(\text{serum creatinine})}; \quad \text{Wt.=Lean Body Weight}$$

$$\text{Creatinine Clearance(Female)} = \frac{\text{Wt. } (140 - \text{age})}{(72)(\text{serum creatinine})} \times 0.85$$

(3) Select maintenance dose (as percentage of chosen loading dose) to continue peak serum concentrations indicated above according to desired dosing interval and the patients corrected creatinine clearance as given in the next Table:

GENTAMICIN (Cont.)

Percentage of Loading Dose Required for Dosage Interval Selected

C(c)cr (ml/min)	Half-Life* (hours)	8 hours	12 hours	24 hours
90	3.1	84%	-	-
80	3.4	80	91%	-
70	3.9	76	88	-
60	4.5	71	84	-
50	5.3	65	79	-
40	6.5	57	72	92%
30	8.4	48	63	86
25	9.9	43	57	81
20	11.9	37	50	75
17	13.6	33	46	70
15	15.1	31	42	67
12	17.9	27	37	61
10**	20.4	24	34	56
7	25.9	19	28	47
5	31.5	16	23	41
2	46.8	11	16	30
0	69.3	8	11	21

*Alternatively, one-half of the chosen loading dose may be given at an interval approximately equal to the estimated half-life.
**Dosing for patients with C(c)cr<10 ml/min should be assisted by measured serum levels. From Sarubbi, F.A., Jr. and Hull, J.H., Ann. Intern. Med. 89, 612-618, 1978.

ADVERSE EFFECTS: Toxicity and untoward effects are listed in the next Table (Edson, R.S. and Keys, T.F., Mayo Clin. Proc. 58, 99-102, 1983):

Toxicity of Gentamicin

Major:
- **Renal Toxicity**
- **Vestibular Toxicity**
- **Auditory Toxicity**
- **Neuromuscular Blockade**

Minor: Skin Rash, Drug-Induced Fever

The three main toxic side effects of gentamicin are ototoxicity, nephrotoxicity, and neuromuscular blockage (Smith, C.R. et al., N. Engl. J. Med. 302, 1106, May 15, 1980); it is important to control the dose given by monitoring peak and troughlevels of the drug, particularly in patients with any degree of renal failure. As renal function declines, drug half-life increases to up to 50 hours.

Nephrotoxicity is usually mild. Irreversible ototoxicity may occur; both the hearing (cochlear) and equilibrium (vestibular) functions may be affected.

Electrolyte disturbances are given in the next Table:

Electrolyte Disturbances

Hypomagnesemia
Hypocalcemia
Hypokalemia

Hypomagnesemia (<1.6mg/dl) is observed in almost 40% of patients; hypocalcemia and hypokalemia may also occur. It may be advisable to monitor serum magnesium and use replacement therapy (Zaloga, G.P. et al., Surg. Gynecol. Obstet. 158, 561-565, 1984).

PHARMACOKINETICS: Therapeutic: 4-10mcg/ml; Toxic: >12mcg/ml; Peak Values: 4-10mcg/ml; Trough: <2mcg/ml.; Half-Life: 2 hours; Time to Steady State: Adults (<30 years), 2.5-15 hours; Adults (>30 years), 7.5-75 hours; Children, 2.5-12.5 hours; Neonates, 10-45 hours. Time to steady state and time to peak concentration may be significantly prolonged in patients with renal dysfunction.

Gentamicin is eliminated exclusively by renal excretion; excessive serum concentrations may occur and lead to further renal impairment. The renal damage is to the renal proximal tubules and is usually reversible if discovered early.

GENTAMICIN (Cont.)
MONITOR: Monitor the parameters given in the next Table:

Monitor Parameters, Gentamicin Treatment

Parameter	Comment
Serum Gentamicin Levels	Initially and every 2-3 days during therapy
Serum Creatinine or BUN	Before and every 2-3 days during therapy
Audiograms	Baseline and weekly in patients with pre-existing renal, auditory or vestibular impairment or in patients who receive prolonged, high-dose therapy
Tinnitus or Vertigo	Daily

Serum Gentamicin Levels: Red top tube, separate serum and freeze. Obtain serum specimens as follows:
(1) 24-48 hours after starting therapy if loading dose is not given.
(2) 5 to 30 minutes before I.V. gentamicin (trough).
(3) 30 minutes after a 30 minute I.V. infusion of gentamicin (peak).
I.M. administration: 30 minutes to one hour.

Heparinized tubes should not be used to collect specimens.

The first serum level of gentamicin is obtained when gentamicin has reached steady-state serum concentrations; steady-state is reached in 24 to 48 hours after starting therapy if the patient has not received a loading dose (steady state = 5-7 drug half-lives; half-life of gentamicin is 2 to 4 hours). The following times should be recorded on the laboratory requisition form and on the patient's chart:

Trough Specimen Drawn ______(Time) (5 to 30 minutes before Gentamicin)
Gentamicin Started ______(Time)
Gentamicin Completed ______(Time) (30 minutes I.V. infusion)
Peak Specimen Drawn ______(Time) (30 minutes after I.V. Gentamicin)

To minimize risk of toxicity, it has been recommended that peak levels not exceed 10mcg/ml and that trough levels should fall between 1 and 2mcg/ml. High concentrations of beta-lactam antibiotics inactivate aminoglycosides (gentamicin, streptomycin, amikacin, tobramycin & kanamycin); to reduce this interaction, specimens containing both classes of antibiotics should either be assayed immediately using a rapid method or stored frozen.

DRUG INTERACTIONS: Drug interactions with gentamicin are given in the next Table:

Drug Interactions with Gentamicin

Drug	Effect
Other Aminoglycosides, Amphotericin B, Bacitracin, Cephalosporins, Colistin, Cisplatin, Methylflurane, Polymyxin B, Vancomycin	Drugs associated with renal toxicity, ototoxicity and neurotoxicity may be additive with similar toxic effects of gentamicin.
General Anaesthetics and Neuromuscular Blocking Agents, eg, Succinylcholine and Tubocurarine	May potentiate neuromuscular blockage of gentamicin and cause respiratory paralysis.

GLIPIZIDE
(Glucotrol)

USES: **Glipizide** is a "second" generation **sulfonylurea** compound which is used to lower glucose levels in patients with **non-insulin dependent diabetes mellitus** (NIDDM; Type II diabetes mellitus). Glipizide is only used following dietary management; dietary management is continued during therapy with glipizide.

Mechanism of Action: Sulfonylureas act by stimulating the release of insulin from pancreatic islets by **increasing the sensitivity of the beta cells to glucose,** which stimulates insulin secretion. Sulfonylureas may suppress the secretion of glucagon and the production of hepatic glucose and potentiate insulin-stimulated glucose transport in adipose tissue and across skeletal muscle membrane.

DOSAGE FORMS: Tabs: 5,10mg

DOSAGE: Take drug approximately 30 minutes prior to a meal. Initially, 5mg before breakfast. Increase if needed per blood glucose by 2.5-5mg every few days. Max. 15mg once daily dose. Max. 50mg daily in divided doses 30 minutes before meals.

In elderly or debilitated patients, initially, 2.5mg daily; minimize increments.

PHARMACOKINETICS: Absorption: Rapid; Protein Binding: 98.4%, Peak: 1-3.5 hrs; Metabolism: Liver; Half-Life: 3.3 hrs. Duration: 6-12 hrs.

ADVERSE EFFECTS: Adverse effects are relatively uncommon in that only 1.5% of patients discontinue glipizide because of adverse reactions. Gastrointestinal disturbances: 1.7% to 3.7%; skin rashes: up to 1.4%. Hypoglycemia may occur. Sulfa-allergy: use with caution or not at all.

MONITOR: Blood glucose is monitored every one to two weeks until the dosage of glipizide is established and monthly thereafter; therapy is continued if the response is satisfactory.

GLUCAGON

USES: **Glucagon** is a **peptide hormone** secreted by pancreatic islets of Langerhans. Uses of glucagon are given in the following Table:

Uses of Glucagon
Hypoglycemia - Emergency Treatment
Radiologic Examination of the GI Tract

Hypoglycemia: Glucagon is used for emergency treatment of hypoglycemia, usually diabetic patients. Patients may also require IV dextrose. Glucagon is only effective if hepatic glycogen stores are adequate. Patients should respond within 5-20 minutes; failure to awaken may indicate glucose response (eg, patients with inadequate glycogen stores) or CNS damage secondary to prolonged hypoglycemia.

Radiologic Examination of the GI Tract: Glucagon causes smooth muscle relaxation of the stomach, small intestine, and colon which facilitates radiologic examination in certain settings.

Mechanism of Action: Glucagon stimulates hepatic glycogenolysis leading to increased blood glucose. Other effects include smooth muscle relaxation of the GI tract and a positive inotropic and chronotropic effect.

DOSAGE FORMS: Parenteral: 1, 10mg. 1mg = 1 unit.

DOSAGE: Glucagon may be administered IM, IV, or subcutaneously. Dosage of glucagon is given in the following Table:

Dosage of Glucagon

Condition	Age	Dosage
Hypoglycemia	Adult	0.5-1mg every 5-20 min as needed.
	Children	0.03-0.1mg/kg/dose every 5-20 min as needed; max: 1mg.
	Neonates	0.3mg/kg/dose every 4 hrs as needed.
Radiologic GI Exam	Adult	0.25-2mg prior to the procedure.

PHARMACOKINETICS: Maximum Effect: within 30 min; Duration of Action: 1-2 hrs. Half-Life: 3-10 min; Degradation: liver and kidneys

ADVERSE EFFECTS: Generally well tolerated. Glycogen must be available for therapeutic effect.

GLYBURIDE
(DiaBeta, Micronase)
USES: **Glyburide** is a "second" generation **sulfonylurea** compound which is used to lower glucose levels in patients with **non-insulin dependent diabetes mellitus** (NIDDM; Type II diabetes mellitus). Glyburide is only used following dietary management; dietary management is continued during therapy with glyburide.
Mechanism of Action: Sulfonylureas act by stimulating the release of insulin from pancreatic islets by **increasing the sensitivity of the beta cells to glucose,** which stimulates insulin secretion. Sulfonylureas may suppress the secretion of glucagon and the production of hepatic glucose and potentiate insulin-stimulated glucose transport in adipose tissue and across skeletal muscle membrane (Review: Amer. J. Med. Suppl. 2A, August 20, 1990).
DOSAGE FORMS: Tabs: 1.25, 2.5, 5mg
DOSAGE: Glyburide is taken with breakfast. Initially, 2.5-5.0mg daily. Increase by 2.5mg at weekly intervals if needed as a function of blood glucose. Maintenance dose: 1.25-20mg daily in single or divided doses. Max. 20mg daily.
PHARMACOKINETICS: Absorption: Rapid; Peak: 4-5.3 hours. Protein Binding: 97%; Metabolism: Liver; Half-Life: 10 hours; Duration: 10-15 hours.
ADVERSE EFFECTS: Gastrointestinal disturbances: 1.8%; Skin rashes occur in 1.5% of patients and may disappear with continued use. FDA Pregnancy Category B. Hypoglycemia may occur. Sulfa-allergy: use with caution or not at all.
MONITOR: Blood glucose is monitored every one to two weeks until the dosage of glyburide is established and monthly thereafter; therapy is continued if the response is satisfactory.

GLYCOPYRROLATE
(Robinul)
USES: Glycopyrrolate is an anticholinergic antispasmodic; uses are given in the next Table:

Uses of Glycopyrrolate
Peptic Ulcer Disease
Respiratory Antisecretory:
Salivation and Excessive Secretions of Respiratory Tract
Prevent Cholinergic Effects during Surgery, eg, Cardiac arrhythmias, Hypotension and Bradycardia
Postoperative Medication: Administered concurrently with Anticholinesterase Agents, e.g., Neostigmine, Pyridostigmine

Peptic Ulcer Disease: Glycopyrrolate is used as an adjunct in the treatment of peptic ulcer disease; it reduces the volume of gastric secretion. Glycopyrrolate injection is used in patients with peptic ulcer disease when rapid reduction in gastric secretion is desired or oral therapy is not tolerated. Benefit in treatment of peptic ulcer disease is unproven.
Respiratory Antisecretory: Glycopyrrolate injection has been used as a preoperative medication to inhibit salivation and excessive secretions of the respiratory tract. Note thiopental or halothane do not stimulate these secretions. Glycopyrrolate may be used in other situations as a respiratory antisecretory agent.
Prevent Cholinergic Effects: Glycopyrrolate injection may be used to prevent cholinergic effects during surgery, eg, cardiac arrhythmias, hypotension, and bradycardia, which may result from traction on viscera with resultant vagal stimulation, stimulation of the carotid sinus, or administration of drugs, eg, succinylcholine.
Postoperative Medication: Glycopyrrolate may be injected concurrently with anticholinesterase agents, eg, neostigmine; pyridostigmine, to block the adverse muscarinic effects of these agents when they are used after surgery to terminate non-depolarizing muscle blockade (Tubocurarine, Pancuronium, Vecuronium, Atracurium, etc.).

GLYCOPYRROLATE (Cont.)
DOSAGE FORMS: Tabs:1, 2mg; Inject: 0.2mg/ml.
DOSAGE: Glycopyrrolate is administered orally, IM or direct IV injection. Safety in children younger than 12 years of age is not established. Oral dose is approximately 10 times IV dose. Dosage is given in the next Table:

Dosage of Glycopyrrolate

Condition	Age	Route	Dosage
Peptic Ulcer Disease	Adults	Oral	Initially, 1-2mg, 3 times daily (morning, early afternoon, bedtime); maintenance: 1mg 2 times daily. Max. 8mg daily.
		IM or IV	0.1-0.2mg, every 4 hours, 3-4 times daily.
Respiratory Antisecretory	Adults	IM or IV	0.1-0.2mg, 30-60 min. prior to induction of anesthesia or at time of other preanesthesia medications (opiates, sedatives). Repeat doses every 4-8 h as needed.
	Child <2 yr.	IM or IV	0.004-0.010mg/kg/dose every 4-8 h as needed.
Intraoperative (Prevent Cholinergic Effects)	Adults	IV	0.1mg; if necessary, repeat at 2-3 minute intervals.
	Children	IV	0.0044mg/kg (max. 0.1mg); if necessary, repeat at 2-3 min. intervals.
Block Adverse Muscarinic Effects of Anticholinesterase Agents, e.g., Neostigmine Pyridostigmine	Adults or Children	IV	0.2mg for each 1mg of neostigmine or 5mg of pyridostigmine; glycopyrrolate is administered concurrently in the same syringe with or a few min. before the anticholinesterase agent.

ADVERSE EFFECTS: Arrhythmias, tachycardia, xerostomia (dry mouth), mydriasis, dry hot skin, blurred vision, restlessness, fatigue, hyperthermia. Use with caution in hepatic and renal disease, ulcerative colitis and asthma.
PHARMACOKINETICS: Onset: IV, 1 min.; IM or subcut.,15-20 min.; Vagal blocking effects: persists 2-3 hours after parenteral administration; Inhibition of salivation: persists up to 7 hours after parenteral administration; Oral Administration: anticholinergic effects persists up to 8-12 hours; Excretion: mainly unchanged in feces via biliary elimination and in urine.

GONORRHEA

More than 1 million cases of gonorrhea have been reported in the U.S. annually from 1980-1984; there are probably over 2 million actual cases per year. The highest rates of infection are found in ages 15-24; one of every 30 teen-agers (15-19 age group) will contact gonorrhea each year. In 1981, over 250,000 cases of gonorrhea were reported among American teenagers (Mascola, L. et al., Pediatric Infect. Dis. 2, 302-303, 1983). An increased prematurity rate has been associated wtih maternal infection by N. gonorrhoeae.

Sexual partners, men and women, should be examined, cultured, and treated at once. All patients treated for gonorrhea should have a serologic test for syphilis. All patients treated with spectinomycin should have a serologic test for syphilis three months later.

Follow-up cultures should be obtained from the infected site(s) 4-7 days after completion of treatment. Cultures should be obtained from the rectum of all women who have been treated for gonorrhea.

The clinical manifestations of N. gonorrhoeae closely resembles those of chlamydia trachomatis. The two organisms commonly occur together in the same patient, and it is usually not possible to distinguish gonococcal from chlamydial infections clinically. The conditions caused by Neisseria gonorrhoeae are given in the next Table:

Neisseria Gonorrhoeae in Men, Women and Infants

Men and Women	Women	Men	Infants
Conjunctivitis	Barthinolitis	Urethritis	Conjunctivitis
Proctitis	Vaginitis(Pre-Pubertal Girls)	Epididymitis	Oropharyngitis
Pharyngeal Infection			
Disseminated Gonococcal Infection	Acute Pelvic Inflammatory Disease(PID): Cervicitis, Endometritis, Salpingitis, Peritonitis, Perihepatitis		

Gonococcal Conjunctivitis: Gonococcal conjunctivitis is transmitted in the same way as chlamydial infection, that is, direct inoculation into the neonate's eye, during passage of the newborn through the vagina at time of birth. Conjunctivitis begins 1 to 7 days after rupture of membranes; the differential diagnosis includes chemical conjunctivitis due to silver nitrate that develops within the first 24 hours of life; chlamydial conjunctivitis that usually appears from 1 to 4 weeks after birth; and conjunctivitis due to other bacterial pathogens.

Oropharynx: N. gonorrhoeae has been cultured from the throat in 10 percent or more of patients with genital gonorrhea; patients who participate in orogenital sex, particularly male homosexuals, are at increased risk.

In most cases, colonization of the oropharynx with Neisseria gonorrhoeae is asymptomatic; occasionally pharyngitis and tonsillitis occurs. The mucosal surfaces are swollen, erythematous, often with areas of whitish gray superficial exudate; severe cases can result in ulceration (Wright, J.M. et al., Pediatric Infect. Dis. 3, 80-88, 1984). Diagnosis is established by throat culture; do not use Gonozyme (Abbott) assay nor Gram stain. Nonpathogenic, commensural Neisseria in the pharynx of most people prevent use of the Gram stain for diagnosis of pharyngeal gonorrhea.

Cervical Specimens: Eighty to ninety percent of women with endocervical gonorrhea have cultures positive for N. gonorrhoeae (Handsfield, H.H., Hosp. Pract. 17, 99-116, 1982).

Salpingitis: An estimated 12 to 20% of females with untreated gonorrhea eventually develop salpingitis (Weisner, P.J., DM, 26, 6-10, 1980). Adolescent females may be more susceptible to upper genital tract infection than older females.

Gonorrhea in Pregnancy: Ascending gonococcal infection during pregnancy may cause pelvic inflammation disease(PID) including septic abortion before the 12th week of gestation. After the 12th week of gestation, the chorion attaches to the endometrial decidua, obliterating the intrauterine cavity; and after the 16th week, the chorioamnion occludes the endocervix, obstructing the route for ascending intraluminal spread. Ascending gonococcal infection after the 16th week may cause chorioamnionitis, a major cause of premature rupture of membranes and premature labor.

GONORRHEA (Cont.)

Urethral Specimens from Males: Gonococcal urethritis is usually accompanied by urethral exudate.

Disseminated Gonococcal Infection: The usual clinical manifestations of disseminated gonococcal infection and nongonococcal bacterial arthritis are given in the next Table; (Goldenberg, D.L. and Reed, J.I., N. Engl. J. Med. 312, 764-771, 1985:

Differential Features of Disseminated Gonococcal Infection and Nongonococcal Bacterial Arthritis

Disseminated Gonococcal Infection	Nongonococcal Bacterial Arthritis
Generally in Young, Healthy Adults	Often in Very Young, Elderly, or Immunocompromised Persons
Initial Migratory Polyarthralgias Common	Polyarthralgias Rare
Tenosynovitis in Majority	Tenosynovitis Rare
Dermatitis in Majority	Dermatitis Rare
>50% Polyarthritis	>85% Monoarthritis
Positive Blood Culture in <10%	Positive Blood Culture in 50%
Positive Joint-Fluid Culture in 25%	Positive Joint-Fluid Culture in 85-90%

The most common initial manifestation of disseminated gonococcal infection is a migratory polyarthralgia (O'Brien, J. P. et al., Medicine 62, 395-406, 1983). Fever, dermatitis and tenosynovitis occur in about two-thirds of patients. Polyarthritis is present in approximately 50% of patients. Skin lesions are usually small papules located in the trunk or extremities.

About 30-40% of patients with disseminated gonococcal infection present with hot, swollen, purulent joint; the knees are most frequently involved. The synovial-fluid leukocyte count is usually over 50,000 cells per cu mm. Meningococcal arthritis is often misdiagnosed as disseminated gonococcal infection (Hook, E.W. and Holmes, K.K., Ann. Int. Med. 102, 229-243, 1985).

Laboratory Diagnosis: The usual specimens and diagnostic methods for diagnosis of gonorrhea are given in the next Table:

Test Sites and Diagnostic Methods for Diagnosis of Gonorrhea

Test Site	Gram Stain	Culture	Gonococcal Antigen Assay Gonozyme, Abbott
Urethra	Yes	Yes	Yes
Cervix	No	Yes	Yes
Throat	No	Yes	No
Joint Fluid	Yes	Yes	Yes
Rectum	Yes	Yes	No
Conjunctivitis	Yes	Yes	Yes

Gram Stain: A gram-stained specimen is considered positive for gonorrhea if gram-negative diplococci with typical structure are seen within polymorphonuclear leukocytes; negative if gram-negative diplococci are not seen; and equivocal if typical organisms are seen only extracellularly or atypical gram-negative cocci are seen in polymorphonuclear leukocytes.

Treatment of Gonorrhea: Treatment of gonococcal infection has been influenced by the emergence of antibiotic resistant strains including penicillinase-producing N. Gonorrhoeae (PPNG) and tetracycline resistant N. Gonorrhoeae (TRNG)(Schwarcz, S.K. et al., JAMA 264, 1413-1417, 1990). The high frequency of chlamydial infections and difficulty with diagnosis make concomittant therapy necessary.

Treatment of adult gonococcal infections is given in the next Table MMWR 38, 85, Sept. 1, 1989):

Treatment of Adult Gonococcal Infections

Type	Therapeutic Regimen
Uncomplicated Urethral, Endocervical, or Rectal Infections	Ceftriaxone 250mg IM once plus Doxycycline 100mg orally 2 times a day for 7 days. Alternatively, Spectinomycin 2g IM once (followed by Doxycycline)
Pharyngeal Gonococcal Infection	Ceftriaxone 250mg IM once. Alternatively, Ciprofloxacin 500mg orally as a single dose. Repeat culture in 4-7 days
Treatment of Gonococcal Infection in Pregnancy	Ceftriaxone 250mg IM once plus Erythromycin base 500mg orally 4 times a day for 7 days. Alternatively, Spectinomycin 2g IM once (followed by Erythromycin)

GONORRHEA (Cont.)

Type	Therapeutic Regimen
Disseminated Gonococcal Infections	Ceftriaxone 1gm IM or IV, every 24 hrs or Ceftizoxime 1gm IV every 8 hrs or Cefotaxime 1gm IV every 8 hrs. Alternatively, Spectinomycin 2g IM every 12 hrs. If organism penicillin-sensitive, Ampicillin 1g IV every 6 hours. Discharge reliable patients 24-48 hrs after symptoms resolve, complete 7 day course of antibiotics with Cefuroxime axetil 500mg 2 times a day or amoxicillin 500mg with clavulanic acid 3 times a day or Ciprofloxacin 500mg 2 times a day
Meningitis or Endocarditis	Ceftriaxone 1-2g IV every 12 hrs, 10-14 day course for meningitis, at least 4 weeks for endocarditis
Ophthalmia	Ceftriaxone 1g IM once

Treatment of pediatric gonococcal infections is given in the next Table (MMWR 38, 85, Sept. 1, 1989):

Treatment of Pediatric Gonococcal Infections

Type	Therapeutic Regimen
Infants Born to Mothers with Gonococcal Infection	Ceftriaxone 50mg/kg IV or IM once (max. 125mg). Use alternative therapy in hyperbilirubinemic infants
Infants with Gonococcal Infection	Ceftriaxone 25-50mg/kg/day IV or IM in a single daily dose or Cefotaxime 25mg/kg IV or IM every 12 hrs. If organism penicillin-sensitive, Crystalline Penicillin G, 100,000units/kg/day in 2 equal doses, 4 equal doses for infants more than 1 week old. Meningitis, 150,000units/kg/day.
Children <45kg with uncomplicated vulvovaginitis, cervicitis, urethritis, pharyngitis, or proctitis	Ceftriaxone 125mg IM once. Alternatively, Spectinomycin 40mg/kg IM once.
Children <45kg with bacteremia, arthritis, or meningitis	Ceftriaxone 50mg/kg (max. 1gm) once daily for 7 days for bacteremia or arthritis. Meningitis should be treated for 10-14 days, max dose 2g.
Children >45kg	Use adult regimens

Children, like adults, should be treated for concurrent chlamydial infection. Children ≥ 8 years of age should be treated with doxycycline 100mg 2 times a day for 7 days. Children less than 8 years are treated with erythromycin. Gonorrhea infection in children less than 8 years of age and pregnant females are not treated with tetracycline.

GRAM-NEGATIVE SEPTICEMIA - In Adults with Cancer, Fever and Neutropenia: Antibiotic therapy for patients with cancer, fever and neutropenia remains controversial (Bodey, G.P., Arch. Intern. Med. 144, 1845-1851, 1984).

Response rate in gram-negative septicemia is given in the next Table (Anaissie, E. et al., N. Engl. J. Med. 318, 1694-1695, June 23, 1988):

Response Rate in Gram-Negative Septicemia

Regimen	% Response	Reference
Ceftazidime	92	Fainstein, V. et al., J. Antimicrob. Chemother. 12, Suppl A, 101-110, 1983.
Ceftazidime and Tobramycin	86	
Aztreonam	86	Jones, P.G. et al., Am. J. Med. 81, 243-248, 1986.
Aztreonam and Amikacin	87	
Cefoperazone	73	Piccart, M. et al., Antimicrob. Agents Chemother. 26, 870-875, 1984.
Cefoperazone and Amikacin	50	
Ceftazidime	89	Pizzo, P.A. et al., N. Eng. J. Med. 315, 552-558, 1986.
Cephalothin, Gentamicin and Carbenicillin	91	
Timentin (Ticaricillin and Clavulanic Acid)	76	Fainstein, V. et al., Am. J. Med. 79, Suppl 5B, 62-66, 1985.
Ceftazidime plus Full-Course Amikacin (>8 days)	81	N. Engl. J. Med. 317, 1692-1698, 1987.
Ceftazidime plus Short-Course Amikacin (3 days)	48	

GRAM-NEGATIVE SEPTICEMIA (Cont.)

Some of these data indicate that single agent therapy with selected beta-lactams (ceftazidime, cefoperazone, aztreonam) is as effective as a combination of the same agent with an aminoglycoside. In two studies using imipenem and ceftazidime, there was no difference in response in patients with profound and persistent neutropenia, whether or not an aminoglycoside was included in the regimen (Wade, J. et al., In Program and Abstracts of the 27th Interscience Conference on Antimicrobial Agents and Chemotherapy, N.Y., Oct. 4-7, 1987. Wash., D.C., Am. Soc. Microbiology, 1987; Anaissie, E. et al., Am. J. Med. (in press).

However, some members of the European Organization for Research and Treatment of Cancer (EORTC) are insistent that ceftazidime be given in combination with a full course (>8 days) of amikacin (N. Engl. J. Med. 317, 1692-1698, 1987; Calandra, T. et al., N. Engl. J. Med. 318, 1695-1696, June 23, 1988).

GRISEOFULVIN

(Grisactin, Grifulvin V, Fulvicin-U/F)

USES: Griseofuvin is an oral fungistatic antibiotic used in the treatment of **tineas (ringworm infections)** of the skin, hair, and nails including tinea corporis, tinea pedis, tinea cruris, tinea barbae, tinea capitis, and tinea unguium (onychomycosis) caused by susceptible species of Trichophyton, Microsporum or Epidermophyton. Griseofulvin should be reserved for infections not amenable to topical antifungal agents. The drug is not effective against other fungal infections; thus, the infecting organism should be identified as a dermatophyte before initiating therapy.

DOSAGE FORMS: Griseofulvin (Microsize): Oral: Caps: 125mg, 250mg; Susp.: 125mg/5ml; Tabs: 250mg, 500mg. Griseofulvin Ultramicrosize: Oral: Tabs: 125mg, 165mg, 250mg, 330mg.

DOSAGE: Griseofulvin is administered orally as a single daily dose or in 2-4 equally divided doses. Divided dosage regimens usually are indicated only if the patient cannot tolerate a single daily dose or large initial doses are required. Griseofulvin should be taken with milk or other fat-containing foods to maximize absorption. Dosage, in terms of the microcrystalline forms and ultramicrocrystalline forms, is given in the next Table:

Dosage of Griseofulvin

Form	Age	Dosage
Microcrystalline	Adults	500mg daily for minor infections; 750mg to 1g daily for severe infections.
	Children	10-15mg/kg daily.
	<2 years	Dosage not established.
Ultramicro-crystalline	Adults	330mg daily for milder infections of tinea corporis, tinea cruris and tinea capitis. 660-750mg daily for severe infections and for difficult infections such as tinea pedis and tinea unguium.
	Children	7mg/kg/day
	<2 years	Dosage not established

Representative treatment periods are given in the next Table:

Representative Treatment Periods

Disease	Treatment Period
Tinea Corporis	2-4 weeks
Tinea Capitis	4-6 weeks or longer
Tinea Pedis	4-8 weeks or longer
Tinea Unguium	At least 3-4 months for fingernail infections; at least 6 months for toenail infections.

ADVERSE EFFECTS: Headache, nausea and vomiting occasionally occur; rare photosensitivity reactions, peripheral neuritis, and leukopenia; may exacerbate acute intermittent porphyria.

PHARMACOKINETICS: Absorption: 50%; Peak: 4-8 hours; Half-Life: 17.5 hours.

CONTRAINDICATIONS: Hepatocellular failure; porphyria

MONITOR: Periodic hematologic, hepatic and renal function tests if long-term therapy.

H_2 ANTAGONISTS

H_2 antagonists inhibit the action of histamine on the H_2 receptors of gastric parietal cells. Gastric acid secretion at basal level and with stimulation is reduced; pepsin secretion is indirectly reduced since the volume of gastric juice is reduced. The effects of H_2 antagonists are listed in the following Table:

Effects of H_2 Antagonists
Reduces Basal Gastric Acid Secretion
Reduces Stimulated Gastric Acid Secretion
Reduces Pepsin Secretion (Indirectly)

USES: H_2 antagonists have been used for treatment and prevention of peptic ulcers, prophylaxis for stress ulcer bleeding, symptomatic relief of gastroesophageal reflux, and treatment of pathologic GI hypersecretory conditions (Lipsy, R.J. et al., "Clinical Review of Histamine 2 Receptor Antagonists," Arch. Intern. Med. 150, 745-751, 1990). Clinical uses of H_2 antagonists are given in the following Table:

Uses of H_2 Antagonists
Peptic Ulcer Disease (Gastric and Duodenal)
Treatment
Prevention of Recurrence
Stress Ulcer Bleeding Prophylaxis
Gastroesophageal Reflux - Symptomatic Relief
Pathologic GI Hypersecretory Conditions
Zollinger-Ellison Syndrome
Systemic Mastocytosis
Multiple Endocrine Adenomas

DOSAGE: All H_2 antagonists block the histamine receptor site on the parietal cell reducing acid secretion. Oral adult dosage of H_2 antagonists in various conditions is given in the next Table (Feldman, M. and Burton, M.E., N. Engl. J. Med. 323, 1672-1680, Dec. 1990):

Dosage of H_2 Antagonists

Generic (Brand) Name	Heal duodenal Ulcer(mg)	Prevent Recurrence(mg)	Heal Gastric Ulcer(mg)
Cimetidine (Tagamet)	300qid or 400bid or 800hs	400hs	300qid or 400 bid or 800hs
Ranitidine (Zantac)	150bid or 300hs	150hs	150bid
Nizatidine (Axid)	150bid or 300hs	150hs	Not approved
Famotidine (Pepcid)	40hs	20hs	40hs

Qid means four times a day, bid means twice a day, hs means at bedtime.

All H_2 antagonists are excreted by the kidneys and dose adjustments are necessary for patients with impaired renal function. See individual agents for additional information.

ADVERSE EFFECTS: Although all of these agents have similar activity against H_2 receptors, pharmacology and side effects provide the basis for selection. The most common side effects (1-3% of patients) include diarrhea, headache, drowsiness, fatigue, muscle pain, and constipation. Transient elevation of transaminases and adverse hematologic effects (leukopenia, thrombocytopenia, anemia) occur rarely. Cardiac effects including bradycardia and hypotension may occur due to antagonism of cardiac H_2 receptors; this effect may be seen with rapid IV administration, especially in hemodynamically unstable patients, but is rarely of clinical consequence (Feldman, M. and Burton, M.E., N. Engl. J. Med. 323, 1672-1680, Dec. 1990). Weak antiadrenergic effects of cimetidine and to a lesser extent ranitidine, may produce side effects including impotence, gynecomastia, and low sperm count. Interference with the hepatic oxidative enzyme system may prolong the half-life of diazepam, phenytoin, theophylline, warfarin, lidocaine, Beta-adrenergic blocking agents, and other drugs. This effect occurs most frequently with cimetidine and to a lesser extent ranitidine. Adverse effects of H_2 antagonists are listed in the following Table (Friedman, G., Clinical Symposia 40, No. 5, 1988):

Adverse Effects of H_2 Antagonists

Drug	Antiadrenergic	Hepatic Oxidative Enzyme
Cimetidine	++	++
Ranitidine	+(*)	+
Famotidine	0	0
Nizatidine	0	0

(*)Causes increased prolactin levels but not gynecomastia or galactorrhea.

HALOPERIDOL
(Haldol)

USES: **Haloperidol** is used primarily to treat **psychotic disorders;** uses are given in the next Table:

Uses of Haloperidol
Acute Active Psychosis
Schizophrenia
Schizoaffective Disorder
Paranoid Syndrome
Ballismus
Tourette's Syndrome (Drug of Choice)
Adjunctive Therapy in Mental Retardation
Chorea of Huntington's Disease
Antiemetic

The **antiemetic action** is achieved mainly through inhibition of stimuli at the chemoreceptor trigger zone. Haloperidol is used to alleviate nausea and vomiting associated with narcotics, anesthesia and surgery, radiation therapy, cancer chemotherapy and gastrointestinal disorders.

Haloperidol is a antidopaminergic butyrophenone derivative which is pharmacologically, but not chemically, related to the high-potency piperazine phenothiazines.

DOSAGE FORMS: Haloperidol occurs in three forms, haloperidol for oral use; haloperidol lactate for both oral and IM injection and haloperidol decanoate for IM injection. The dosage forms of these preparations are given in the next Table:

Dosage Forms of Haloperidol

Drug	Route	Dosage Forms
Haloperidol	Oral	Tabs: 0.5, 1, 2, 5, 10, 20mg
Haloperidol Lactate	Oral IM, IV	Solution: 2mg/ml Injection: 5mg/ml
Haloperidol Decanoate	IM Depot Form	Injection: 50mg/ml, 100mg/ml

DOSAGE: Dosage of haloperidol in different conditions is given in the next Table:

Dosage of Haloperidol

Condition	Age	Route and (Preparation)	Dosage
Acute Psychoses with Marked Agitation	Adults >12yrs	IM (Lactate)	Initially, 2-5mg. Subsequent doses every 4-8 hours or if required, every hour until symptoms controlled. Usual daily dose, 10mg Oral dose is then started.
Acute Psychoses	Adults	IV (Lactate)	IV administration not FDA approved Suggested dose: mild agitation, 0.5-2mg; moderate agitation, 5-10mg; severe agitation, 10mg or more (Martinez, K.M. et al., Samaritan Medicine 4, 22-27, 1986).
Chronic Psychoses	Adults	IM Decanoate Depot Form	First, stabilize patient on antipsychotic medication before use of decanoate. Give oral haloperidol first to exclude sensitivity to haloperidol. Initial IM dose in depot form is 10-15 times the previous daily dose in oral haloperidol equivalents with a max. initial dose of 100mg (2ml). Administer by deep IM every 4 weeks max. 300mg.

HALOPERIDOL (Cont.)
Table Cont.

Dosage Forms of Haloperidol

Condition	Age	Route and (Preparation)	Dosage
Acute Active Psychoses	Adults >12yrs	Oral (Haloperidol; Lactate)	Initially for moderate symptoms, 0.5 to 2mg and for severe symptoms, 3-5mg every 8-12 hrs until symptoms controlled. Usual daily dose, 10mg. After control has been obtained, reduce dose gradually to minimum effective level (usually 2-8mg daily).
	Elderly or Debilitated	Oral (Haloperidol; Lactate)	Initially, 0.5-2mg 2 or 3 times daily, gradually increased in increments of 0.5mg daily at 5 to 7 day intervals.
	Children (6-12yrs)	Oral (Haloperidol; Lactate)	Initially, 0.5-1.5mg daily; increase by 0.5mg/day to a maintenance dose of 0.05-0.1mg/kg/day.
Agitation or Hyperkinesia in Disturbed Children	Children (3-6yrs)	Oral (Haloperidol; Lactate)	0.01-0.03mg/kg/day given once daily.
Chronic Schizophrenia	Adults >12yrs	Oral (Haloperidol; Lactate)	Initially, 6-12mg daily in divided doses, gradually increased until control is achieved and then gradually decreased to maintenance levels (usually 15-20mg daily).
	Elderly or Debilitated	Oral (Haloperidol; Lactate)	Initially, 0.5-1.5mg daily increased gradually to the usual maintenance dose of 2-8mg daily.
	Children 3-12yrs	Oral (Haloperidol; Lactate)	Initially, 0.5mg daily, increased by 0.5mg at 5-7 day intervals until desired therapeutic effect is obtained; give in two or three divided doses. Maintenance doses 0.05 to 0.15mg/kg/day.
Tourette's	Adults	Oral (Haloperidol; Lactate)	Initially, 0.5-2mg 2 or 3 times daily. Increase dose as needed.
	Children 3-12yrs	Oral (Haloperidol; Lactate)	Dose range 0.05-0.075mg/kg daily in 2 or 3 divided doses.
Antiemetic	Adults	IM (Haloperidol; Lactate)	1,2 or 5mg every 12 hrs as needed.
		Oral (Haloperidol; Haloperidol Lactate)	1, 2, or 5mg twice daily

PHARMACOKINETICS: Oral: Absorption: Well absorbed; Time to Peak: 1-3 hours; Volume of Distribution: 20 liter/kg. Metabolism: Liver, N-dealkylation and glucuronidation; Plasma Half-Life: 12 to 38 hours.
I.V.:Oral bioavailability is 60% of intravenous bioavailability. Haloperidol Decanoate: This is a depot preparation that depends on the enzymatic hydrolysis of the ester to haloperidol. Haloperidol decanoate is given once monthly in amounts approximately 10-20 times the daily oral maintenance dose. Steady-state plasma concentrations of 2-8ng/ml are reached by the third monthly injection.

ADVERSE EFFECTS: Akathisia and acute dystonias may occur; tardive dyskinesia, extrapyramidal symptoms, orthostatic hypotension. Lowers seizure threshold. Neuroleptic Malignant Syndrome occurs in 0.5-1% of patients treated with neuroleptics.

HEADACHE

The major types of headache are given in the next Table:

Major Types of Headache
Muscle-Contraction (Tension) Headache
Cluster Headache
Migraine Headache

Muscle-Contraction (Tension) Headache: Muscle-contraction (tension) headaches are characterized by mild to moderate nonthrobbing pain, tightness or pressure around the head and neck unassociated with autonomic disturbances. This type of headache often develops in response to stress. The pain is usually steady, nonpulsatile, unilateral or bilateral, and often suboccipital often referring to the frontal region and the face.

Cluster Headache: Cluster headaches is related to migraine headaches; the typical form is classified as **episodic** or **periodic**, characterized by 30-40 minutes of excruciating, nonthrobbing, unilateral, oculofrontal or oculotemporal pain, occurring in a series or "cluster" of closely spaced attacks, often at night. The pain is associated with flushing, increased lacrimation, sweating and rhinorrhea. In **chronic cluster headache**, the periods of remission are diminished.

Migraine Headache: Migraine is thought to be due to vasoconstriction of cranial blood vessels with concomitant decrease in the amplitude of pulsations. Headache pain is commonly unilateral in onset, most severe in the temporal and frontal regions, frequently occurring at night or on awakening, sometimes accompanied by nausea, vomiting, photophobia, irritability and constipation or diarrhea. Some patients experience prodromal symptoms, such as sensory, mood, or motor disturbances.

Treatment of different types of headache is given in the next Table:

Treatment of Headache

Type	Treatment
Muscle-Contraction (Tension)Headache Acute	Mild to Moderate Pain: **Nonopiate analgesic:** Aspirin, acetaminophen, ibuprofen or other NSAIDs. or **Antidepressant:** Amitriptyline (Elavil) or **Antianxiety Drug:** Diazepam (Valium) alone or with an analgesic. or **Fiorinal:** Aspirin, butalbital and caffeine or other **Sedative;** Meprobamate(Micrainin) with an analgesic
Cluster Headache Prophylaxis	Prophylactic drugs are as follows: **Methysergide or lithium carbonate or corticosteroids**
Cluster Headache Acute	**Ergotamine tartrate,** sublingual or inhalation or **Ergotamine/caffeine suppositories** or **Dihydroergotamine,** IV or IM. **Inhalation of 100% oxygen** (8 to 10 liter/minute for 5 to 10 minutes)(Kudrow, L., Headache, 21, 1-4, 1981). **Ergotamine tartrate,** 1mg or 2mg an hour or so before an anticipated attack. If a patient is awakened by headache bouts during the night, consider giving 1-5mg ergotamine tartrate at bedtime.
Cluster Headache (Chronic Paroxysomal Hemicrania)	**Indomethacin,** oral, 25 to 50mg, three times daily.
Migraine, Acute	Nonspecific symptomatic relief of mild attacks: **Mild analgesics:** Aspirin or acetaminophen **Stronger analgesic:** Aspirin with codeine, propoxyphene (Darvon) or **Sedative:** Barbiturates or **Antianxiety drug:** Diazepam (Valium) or **Sedative and analgesic:** Fiorinal, Midrin Metoclopramide:These drugs may be ineffective if given after the attack has begun because of gastric stasis. Metoclopramide (Reglan),(10-20mg) is recommended to restore gastric motility, permit absorption of analgesics and prevent nausea and vomiting (Kunkel, R.S., Cleveland Clinic Quarterly 52, 95-101, 1985). Give metoclopramide, 10-20mg, 10 to 20 minutes prior to analgesic. Do not give metoclopramide to young children.

HEADACHE (Cont.)
Table (Cont.)

Type	Treatment
	Moderate to severe symptoms: **Dihydroergotamine,** IM or IV for patients with severe headache; dihydroergotamine is the drug of choice in physician's offices and hospital emergency rooms. Ergotamine, sublingual and inhalation forms, is a second choice in these situations. Caffeine increases the absorption and enhances vasoconstrictor effect of ergotamine. Give metoclopramide to prevent nausea and vomiting caused by ergotamine or the migraine attack and enhance ergotamine's absorption. It may be desirable to give an antiemetic rectally or intramuscularly; the phenothiazine antiemetics, eg, prochlorperazine (Compazine) or promethazine (Phenergan) may be given. Cafergot P-B (ergotamine tartrate, pentobarbital, belladonna alkaloids, caffeine) may prevent nausea and vomiting. Alternative to Ergotamine is **Midrin** for patients who cannot tolerate ergotamine. Midrin is a mixture of isometheptene mucate, dichloralphenazone, and acetaminophen. Severe Headache that fails to respond to Ergot preparations may be relieved by analgesic, eg, meperidine (Demerol).
Status Migrainosus	Persistent migraine headache may be intractable to ergotamine and strong analgesics; **dexamethasone acetate,** 16mg IM has produced improvement. or **Prednisone,** oral, 60mg-80mg for first two days and then reduced gradually over a few days. or **Combined** intravenous administration of **dihydroergotamine,** 0.5mg and metoclopramide 10mg every eight hours (Raskin, N.H. and Raskin, K.E., Neurology 34, 245, 1984).
Migraine in Children	Biofeedback, **cyproheptadine** or **aspirin;** when these steps are not effective, ergotamine is used.
Migraine, Prophylaxis	**Beta-blockers** ,eg, propranolol, atenolol, metoprolol, nadolol, timolol (Turner, P., Postgrad. Med. J. 60, suppl. 2, 51-55, 1984; Steiner, T.J. and Joseph, R., Postgrad. Med. J. 60, suppl. 2, 56-60, 1984). Other drugs used as prophylaxis are as follows: **tricyclic antidepressants, amitriptylline, phenelzine, calcium channel blocking drugs,** (Meyer, J.S., Ann. Intern. Med. 102, 395-397, 1985) and **nonsteroidal anti-inflammatory drugs, eg, naproxen.** Long-term prophylactic use of ergotamine is inadvisable because of its potential adverse effects.
Combined Headache (Migraine plus Muscle-Contraction), Chronic Prophylaxis	It may be necessary to hospitalize some patients and **withdraw** all analgesics. A **phenothiazine,** eg, **chlorpromazine** has been given during analgesic withdrawal. An antianxiety drug, eg, diazepam, may be useful. **Beta-Blocker, eg, propranolol.** **Anti-depressant, eg, amitriptyline.** **Monamine oxidase inhibitor (MAOI).**
Combined Headache (Migraine plus Muscle Contraction) Acute	Treat symptoms of dominant headache type(eg, **ergotamine** for **migraine** and **analgesics or antidepressant for muscle contraction** or combination of ergotamine and simple analgesics.

HEADACHE (Cont.)

ERGOTAMINE PREPARATIONS: Some of the commercial ergotamine preparations that are available are given in the next Table:

Commercial Ergotamine Preparations

Preparation	Form	Ergotamine	Caffeine	Belladonna	Barbiturates
Cafergot(Sandoz)	Tabs	as tartrate, 1mg	100mg		
	Supp.	as tartrate, 2mg	100mg		
Cafergot-PB (Sandoz)	Tabs	as tartrate, 1mg	100mg	0.125mg	Pentobarbital, 30mg
	Supp.	as tartrate, 2mg	100mg	0.25mg	Pentobarbital, 60mg
Wigraine(Organon)	Tabs	as tartrate, 1mg	100mg	-	-
	Supp.	as tartrate, 2mg	100mg	-	-
Ergomar(Fisons) Ergostat(Parke-Davis)	Sublingual Tabs	as tartrate, 2mg	-	-	-
Medihaler Ergotamine(Riker)	Aerosol	as tartrate, 9mg/ml 360mcg/metered spray	-	-	-
Bellergal-S (Sandoz)	Tablet (Timed-Release)	as tartrate, 0.6mg	-	0.2mg	Phenobarbital, 40mg
DHE 45(Sandoz) Dihydroergotamine	IM or IV	Dihydroergotamine mesylate, 1mg/ml	-	-	-

Caffeine: Caffeine increases the absorption and enhances the vasoconstrictor effect of ergotamine. However, caffeine may interfere with sleep.

Belladonna Alkaloids: Belladonna alkaloids are thought to allay the nausea and vomiting associated with migraine attack or with ergotamine.

Barbiturate: Barbiturate is used as a sedative (depression of the CNS). The barbiturates that are used are pentobarbital, a short-to-intermediate acting barbiturate and phenobarbital, a long-acting barbiturate.

PREPARATIONS FOR MUSCLE-CONTRACTION (TENSION) AND MIGRAINE HEADACHE

Commercial preparations for treatment of muscle-contraction (tension) and migraine headache are given in the next Table:

Preparations for Treatment of Muscle-Contraction(Tension)and Migraine Headache

Preparation	Form	Butalbital	Aspirin	Acetaminophen	Caffeine	Other
Axotal(Adria)	Tabs	50mg	650mg	-	-	-
Esgic(Gilbert)	Tabs	50mg	-	325mg	40mg	-
Fiorinal(Sandoz)	Caps, Tabs	50mg	325mg	-	40mg	-
Phrenilin Phrenilin Forte	Caps or Tabs	50mg	-	325mg or 650mg (Forte)	-	-

"Other" drugs that are used to treat migraine and other headaches are given in the next Table:

"Other" Drugs to Treat Migraine and Other Headaches

Drug	Uses
Beta-Blockers, eg, **Propranolol**, Atenolol, Timolol, Metoprolol and Nadolol.	Prevention (prophylaxis) of migraine headache. **Propranolol** is considered by some authorities to be the drug of choice (Olsson, J.E. et al., Acta Neurol. Scand. 70, 160-168, 1984).
Calcium Channel Blocking Drugs, eg, Verapamil and others	Verapamil has been effective in the **prophylaxis of migraine** in those patients who did respond to ergotamine, propranolol or amitriptyline (Markley, H.G. et al., Neurology 34, 973-976, 1984). Dosage: For migraine prophylaxis, 80mg 3 or 4 times daily.
Cyproheptadine	Cyproheptadine, an antihistamine has nonspecific calcium channel blocking activity. It is used for **migraine prophylaxis.**
Antidepressants Amitriptyline	Prophylaxis of migraine in some studies (Couch, J.R. and Hassanein, R.S., Arch. Neurol. 36, 695-699, 1979) and muscle-contraction headaches. Dosage: Migraine Prophylaxis: 25mg at bedtime; increase by 25mg every 1-2 weeks to a daily dose of 100 to 200mg in 3-4 divided doses. Muscle-Contraction Headache: 50 to 75mg at bedtime; increase every 2-3 weeks to 200-250mg daily in 3-4 divided doses. Discontinue after patient is symptom free for 1-2 months.
Lithium Carbonate	**Prevention of chronic cluster headache** (Ekbom, K., Headache 21, 132-139, 1981). Dosage: 300mg, 2-4 times daily or timed-release tablets, twice daily.

HEPARIN, CALCIUM OR SODIUM

USES: Heparin is used in the prophylaxis and management of **thromboembolic disease** on the venous side of the circulation, that is, **venous thrombosis** and **pulmonary embolism.** In heparin therapy, the APTT is usually maintained at from 1.5 to 2.0 times the upper limits of normal (50 to 65 seconds). In another approach, the APTT is maintained at from 1.5 to 2.5 times the patient's admission APTT. The uses of heparin are given in the next Table (Hirsh, J., N. Engl. J. Med. 324, 1565-1574, May, 1991):

Uses of Heparin
Prophylaxis and treatment of **venous thrombosis** and its extension
Prophylaxis and treatment of **pulmonary embolism**
Treatment of patients with **unstable angina** and **acute myocardial infarction**
Prevention of **mural thrombosis** after **myocardial infarction**
Prevention of **coronary-artery rethrombosis** after **thrombolysis**
Treatment of selected cases of **disseminated intravascular coagulopathy(DIC)**
Prevent activation of the coagulation mechanism as blood passes through an **extracorporeal circuit** in **dialysis procedures** and during arterial and cardiac surgery.

Mechanism of Action: Heparin first interacts with antithrombin III, converting antithrombin to its active form as illustrated in the next Figure:

Interaction of Heparin with Antithrombin III

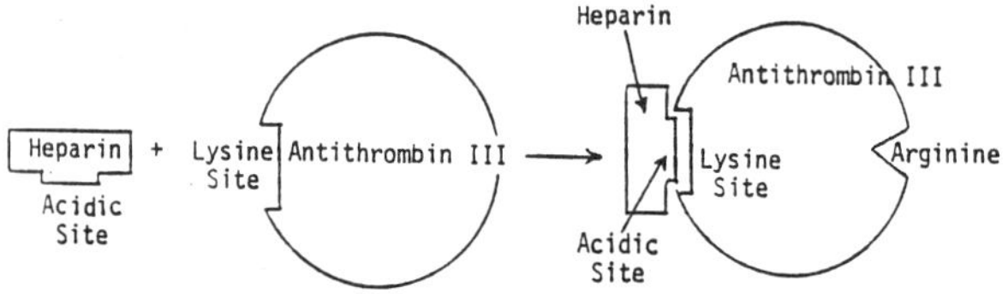

Heparin is a negatively charged heterogeneous group of mucopolysaccharide, derived from mast cells of animal tissues, that reacts with basic amino acid lysine of the antithrombin III molecule; following this interaction, another basic amino acid, arginine is exposed. This complex inhibits the active site of the activated coagulation factors XIIa, XIa, IXa, Xa, and thrombin.

The coagulation cascade is shown in the next Figure:

Coagulation Cascade

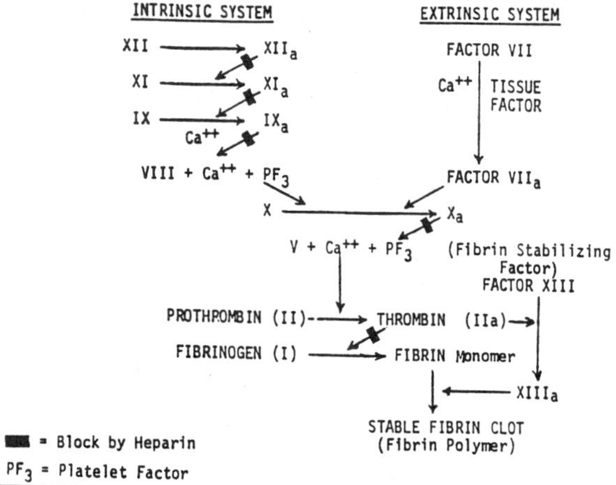

HEPARIN, CALCIUM OR SODIUM (Cont.)

Heparin also inhibits plasmin, the active serine protease of the fibrinolytic system.

DOSAGE FORMS: Calcium: 25,000units/ml; Sodium: 2, 10, 50, 100, 1,000, 2,000, 2,500, 5,000, 7,500, 10,000, 15,000, 20,000, 40,000 units/ml.

DOSAGE: The route of administration is given in the next Table:

Route of Administration

Therapy	Route
Full-Dose	IV infusion; intermittent IV injection or deep subcutaneous (intrafat) injection.
Low-Dose	Deep subcutaneous injection.
Fixed-Combination Prep. (Dihydroergotamine mesylate and Heparin Sodium)	Only by deep subcutaneous injection.

Heparin should not be administered IM because of irritation, pain, and hematoma at the injection site.

Subcutaneous Administration: Use a 25- or 26-gauge 1/2 or 5/8 inch needle above the iliac crest or into the abdominal fat layer to minimize tissue trauma; abdominal injections should not be made within 2 inches of the umbilicus. Do not massage injection sites before or after injection. Change site for each dose.

Dosage of heparin calcium or heparin sodium is expressed in USP units and is identical for the calcium and the sodium salts. Dosage is given in the next Table:

Dosage of Heparin

Route	Age	Dosage
Intravenous, Continuous	Adults	Initially: 5,000 units or 75-100u/kg then 17.5 units/kg/hr. Adjust as needed. Usual range: 12.5-25 units/kg/hr.
	Child.	Initially: 50 units/kg followed by 15-25U/kg/hr
Intravenous, Intermittent	Adults	Initially:10,000 units followed by 5,000 to 10,000 units every four to six hrs or 100units/kg/dose
	Child.	100 u/kg/dose every 4 hours.
Subcutaneous, Low-Dose Prophylaxis Before Surgery	Adults	5,000 units two hours before surgery and every 8-12 hrs thereafter until patient is discharged or is fully ambulatory.
Subcutaneous Full-Dose Effects	Adults	5,000 units IV and 10,000-20,000 units SC followed by 8,000-10,000 units every 8 hrs or 15,000-20,000 units every 12 hrs.

Dosage of heparin for specific clinical indications is given in the next Table (Hirsh, J., N. Engl. J. Med. 324, 1565-1574, May, 1991):

Dosage of Heparin

Condition	Dosage
Prophylaxis of Deep Venous Thrombosis and Pulmonary Embolism	5000 units SC every 8-12 hrs or 3500 units SC every 8 hrs; adjust to keep APTT upper normal range.
Treatment of Deep Venous Thrombosis	5000 units IV bolus followed by 30,000-35,000 units/day IV or 35,000-40,000 units/day SC; adjust to keep APTT 1.5-2.5 times control.
Unstable Angina	5000 units IV bolus followed by 24,000units/day IV; adjust to keep APTT 1.5-2.5 times control
Prevention of Mural Thrombosis after Myocardial Infarction	12,500 units SC twice daily.
Prevention of Mortality and Reinfarction	2000 units IV bolus followed by 12,500 units SC twice daily.
Maintain Patency after Thrombolysis (t-PA used)	5000 units IV bolus followed by 24,000 units/day IV; adjust to keep APTT 1.25-2.5 times control
Reduce Mortality after Thrombolysis (Streptokinase used)	2000 units IV bolus followed by 12,500 units SC twice daily.

In an extensive review of 70 randomized trials involving 16,000 patients, perioperative use of subcutaneous heparin can prevent half of all pulmonary emboli and two-thirds of all deep vein thromboses (Collins, R. et al., NEJM 318(18), 1162-1173, 1988).

HEPARIN, CALCIUM OR SODIUM (Cont.)

Duration of therapy for thrombophlebitis or pulmonary embolus is 5-10 days. A coumarin derivative is generally used for follow-up anticoagulant therapy after the effects of full-dose heparin therapy have been established and when long-term anticoagulant therapy is indicated. Overlap heparin and coumarin for a short period of time (see ANTICOAGULATION). A five-day course of heparin with warfarin begun on the first day is as effective as a 10-day course with warfarin begun on the fifth day in preventing recurrent venous thromboembolism in patients with proximal venous thrombosis (Hull, R., et al., NEJM 322(18), 1260-1264, 1990).

ADVERSE EFFECTS: The incidence of heparin-induced hemorrhage is 3-10%. It is usually confined to soft-tissue bleeding or hematuria and is not life-threatening. CNS hemorrhage may be life threatening.

The remedy for mild bleeding is dosage reduction. If a PTT done one hr following reduction shows heparin response in the therapeutic range, continue with lower rate (Hirsh, J. et al., Patient Care, pgs. 43-61, Dec. 15, 1988).

Thrombocytopenia occurs in 5-10% of patients in association with heparin therapy; 10-20% of these patients may develop thrombosis, primarily on the arterial side of the circulation, and may necessitate amputation of the involved limb. This effect is not dose related (Bell, W.R., J. Lab. Clin. Med. 111(6), 600-605, 1988).

A platelet count every three days allows this complication to be detected early (Stein, P.D. and Willis, P.W., Arch. Intern. Med. 143, 991-994 1983). Osteoporosis with prolonged use of large doses.

Fear of hemorrhage may inhibit physicians from using sufficient heparin soon enough to protect the patient (Wheeler, A.P. et al., Arch. Intern. Med. 148, 1321-1325, 1988).

CONTRAINDICATIONS: Active bleeding or bleeding tendencies; threatened abortion; subacute bacterial endocarditis, suspected intracranial hemorrhage, regional or lumbar block anesthesia; severe hypertension; shock; and after eye, brain, or spinal cord injury; uremia; recent neurologic or ophthalmic surgery; thrombocytopenia. Heparin does not cross the placenta.

PRECAUTIONS: When cephalosporins are given with heparin, there is possible increased bleeding risk with moxalactam (additive); avoid concurrent use of over 20,000U/day of heparin with moxalactam (The Medical Letter 26, 11-14, Feb. 3, 1984). Do not give heparin IM.

PHARMACOKINETICS: Onset: Immediate after IV administration. Half-Life: 93 mins. (deep venous thrombosis); 52 mins. (pulmonary embolus). Metabolism: Heparin is metabolized in the liver; Protein Binding: 95%; Excretion: Up to 55% excreted unchanged by kidney.

MONITOR: Laboratory tests to monitor for heparin toxicity are given in the next Table:

Laboratory Tests to Monitor for Heparin Toxicity
Activated Partial Thromboplastin Time (APTT)
Platelet Count (every 3 days)
Hematocrit
Stool Guaiac
Urine for Hematuria

Activated partial thromboplastin time(APTT) is the most commonly used and generally accepted laboratory method for monitoring heparin therapy. The APTT is maintained at 1.5 to 2.5 times the patient's admission APTT or 1.5 to 2.0 times control.

Before starting heparin therapy, obtain a specimen for PTT; then check PTT after 6 hours of therapy; a 6-hour PTT reflects the effect of continuous IV heparin after the bolus effect has diminished. Then, check the PTT every 6 hours until a therapeutic level is attained. Afterward, once daily determination of PTT is adequate.

HEPARIN, CALCIUM OR SODIUM (Cont.)

A suggested protocol for continuous IV heparin is to begin with 5000 units IV bolus, followed by 31,000 units/day. First APTT determination, 6 hrs after bolus. Adjust heparin dosage as given in the following Table (Hirsh, J., N. Engl. J. Med. 324, 1565-1574, May, 1991):

Protocol for Adjusting IV Heparin Dose

APTT (sec)*	Repeat bolus (units)	Stop Infusion (min.)	Change rate ml/hr(U/day)**	Next APTT
<50	5000	-	+3 (+2880)	6hr
50-59	-	-	+3 (+2880)	6hr
60-85	-	-	-	Next AM
86-95	-	-	-2 (-1920)	Next AM
96-120	-	30	-2 (-1920)	6hr
>120	-	60	-4 (-3840)	6hr

*APTT normal range 27-35 sec (Dade-Actin PS reagent)
**Concentration of heparin: 40 units/ml.

Activated coagulation time(ACT) is especially convenient for monitoring the degree of anticoagulation in patients undergoing extracorporeal circulation because the test can be performed at bedside. The ACT is maintained at 2-3 times the control value in seconds.

ANTIDOTE: Protamine sulfate (1mg per 100 U heparin in previous 4 h.) Administer IV protamine very slowly over 1-3 minutes; do not give more than 50mg of protamine in a 10 minute period or more than 100mg at once unless absolutely necessary.

DRUG INTERACTIONS: Drug interactions with heparin are given in the next Table:

Drug Interactions with Heparin

Drug(s)	Comment
Drugs Affecting Platelet Function (Aspirin, other NSAIDs, Dipyridamole, Dextran)	These drugs may increased the risk of hemorrhage; use these drugs with caution in patients receiving heparin.
Thrombolytic Agents (Streptokinase or Urokinase)	These drugs may increase the risk of hemorrhage. Heparin therapy should not be started following streptokinase or urokinase therapy until the thrombin time has returned to less than twice the normal control. Streptokinase or urokinase therapy should not be started following heparin therapy until the thrombin time has returned to less than twice the normal control
Dihydroergotamine Mesylate	Potentiates the antithrombogenic effects of heparin.

HEPATITIS B IMMUNE GLOBULIN
(HBIG, Hep-B-Gammagee, HyperHep)

USES: Hepatitis B immune globulin(HBIG) is used to provide **passive immunity** to hepatitis B infection in the prophylactic treatment of individuals exposed to hepatitis B virus or HBsAg-positive materials, e.g., blood, plasma, serum. HBIG contains antibodies specific to HBsAg; these antibodies combine with HBsAg and neutralize the hepatitis B virus so that its infective or pathogenic properties are inhibited.

Uses of HBIG are given in the next Table:

Uses of Hepatitis B Immune Globulin(HBIG) Following Exposure to Hepatitis B
Percutaneous (eg, needlestick) or **bite exposure**
Direct **mucous membrane contact (eg, oral, ophthalmic)**, or **ingestion** (eg, pipetting accident)
Neonates born to HBsAg-Positive and/or HBeAg-positive women
Sexual or intimate contact
Homosexual males exposed by sexual or intimate contact

Following administration of HBIG to individuals exposed to HBsAg-positive blood, clinically apparent hepatitis B infection, that is, serologic markers and clinical symptoms, develop in only 2% of HBIG treated individuals, and subclinical infection, that is presence of serologic markers only, develop in 10% of treated individuals. In some patients, postexposure administration of HBIG may delay development of hepatitis B infection.

When hepatitis B infection becomes clinically apparent and/or serologic testing indicates the presence of HBsAg, the antibody probably does not neutralize the virus. However, HBIG may modify the course of infection.

When HBIG is administered with **hepatitis B vaccine,** the active immune response produced by hepatitis B vaccine is not suppressed.

Combined HBIG and hepatitis B virus **vaccine** should be given in all of the conditions listed in the previous Table. However, combined passive (HBIG) and active (vaccine) immunization currently is not routinely recommended for susceptible heterosexual individuals exposed by sexual or intimate contact to an HBsAg-positive individual; give HBIG alone. But use combined approach for susceptible heterosexual individuals who are regular sexual contacts of a known HBsAg carrier.

DOSAGE: Recommendations for neonates, born to HBsAg-positive mothers, and sexual contacts to HBsAg-positive individuals are given in the next Table; (Morbid. Mortal. Week. Rep. (MMWR) 34, 313-335, 1985):

Hepatitis B Virus Postexposure Recommendations

	Hepatitis B Immune Globulin (HBIG)		Hepatitis B Vaccine	
Exposure	Dose	Recommended Timing	Dose	Recommended Timing
Perinatal	0.5ml IM	Within 12 hours of birth	0.5ml IM	Within 12 hours of birth; repeat at 1 and 6 months
Sexual	0.06ml/kg IM (max. 5ml)	Single dose within 14 days of sexual contact	See Note	

For neonates, HBIG and the vaccine can be given at the same time but at a different site.

Note: Vaccine is recommended for homosexual men and for regular sexual contacts of HBV carriers and is optional in initial treatment of heterosexual contacts of persons with acute HBV.

HEPATITIS B IMMUNE GLOBULIN (Cont.)

A summary of postexposure prophylaxis of percutaneous eg, needlestick, exposures to sources that contain or might contain HBsAg is given in the next Table; (Morbid, Mortal. Week. Rep. (MMWR) 34, 313-335, 1985):

Recommendations for Hepatitis B Prophylaxis Following Percutaneous Exposure

Source	Exposed Person: Unvaccinated	Exposed Person: Vaccinated
HBsAg-positive	1. HBIG x 1 immediately (0.06ml/kg IM) 2. Initiate HB vaccine series: First dose within 1 week; second and third doses, 1 and 6 months later.	1. Test exposed person for anti-HBs. 2. If inadequate antibody, HBIG (x1) immediately plus HB vaccine booster dose.
Known source **High-risk** **HBsAg-positive**	1. Initiate HB vaccine series 1. 2. Test source for HBsAg. If positive, HBIG x 1.	1. Test source for HBsAg only if exposed is vaccine nonresponder; if source is HBsAg-positive, give HBIG x 1 immediately plus HB vaccine booster dose.
Low-risk **HBsAg-positive** **Unknown source**	Initiate HB vaccine series.	1. Test exposed person for anti-HBs. 2. If inadequate antibody, give HB vaccine booster dose

Inject IM into deltoid muscle or into the anterolateral aspects of the thigh.

In neonates and small children, IM injections with HBIG should be made into the anterolateral aspect of the thigh.

The usual dose of HBIG in children and adults is 0.06ml/kg (adults usually 3-5ml).

Neonates: 0.5ml; administer no later than 12 hours after birth.

CONTRAINDICATIONS: Contraindicated in patients with allergy to human Ig, coagulopathies, IgA deficiency, thrombocytopenia.

ADVERSE EFFECTS: Adverse effects include local pain and tenderness at the injection site, urticaria and angioedema.

HEPATITIS B VACCINE
(Heptavax-B)

USES: Hepatitis B vaccine is a noninfectious formalin-inactivated preparation derived from the surface antigen (HBsAg) of hepatitis B virus. It is prepared from HBsAg-positive blood donated by carriers of hepatitis B virus. Hepatitis B vaccine is indicated for immunization against infection caused by all known B virus subtypes. Uses are given in the next Table:

Uses of Hepatitis B Vaccine
All Newborns of HBs Positive Mothers
Children belonging to an **Ethnic Group at High Risk** for the Disease (see below) or if his Parents are at High Risk for the Disease (see below)
Ethnic Groups at High Risk: **Alaskan Eskimos, Indochinese Refugees, Haitian Refugees.**
Individuals at High Risk:
Health Care Personnel
Hematology and Hemodialysis Patients and Staff
Patients and Staff of Institutions for the Mentally Retarded
Morticians and Embalmers
Blood Bank and Fractionation Workers
Recipients of Blood Clotting Factor Concentrates
Homosexual Males
Household and Sexual Contacts of HBV Carriers
Prostitutes
Heterosexually Active Persons with Multiple Sexual Partners
IV Drug Abusers
Prisoners
International Travelers who will be in highly Endemic Areas for more than Six Months

DOSAGE FORMS: Heptavax-B, 10 microgram per 0.5ml (Pediatric); Heptavax-B, Adult Formulation, 20 microgram per ml (Adult). Recombinant vaccine produced in yeast is available: Recombivax HB 5 microgram per 0.5ml (Pediatric), 10 microgram per ml (Adult), 40 microgram per ml (Dialysis); Engerix-B 10 microgram per 0.5ml (Pediatric), 20 microgram per ml (Adult).

DOSAGE: The sites and dosage that should be used for injection of hepatitis B vaccine are given in the next Table:

Sites and Dosage for Injection of Hepatitis B Vaccine

Age/Condition	Site and Dosage
Neonates	IM into anterolateral thigh for neonates and infants; 0.5ml (10 microgram) within 12 hours of birth; repeat at 1 and 6 months. Use 0.5ml (5 microgram) if using Recombivax HB. The vaccine and and hepatitis B immune globulin should not be injected at the same site or with the same syringe.
Children to Age 10	IM into deltoid; 0.5ml (10 microgram) and 1 month and 6 months later. Use 0.5ml (5 microgram) if using Recombivax HB.
Adults and Children Older than 10 years	IM into deltoid; 1ml (20 microgram) and 1 month and 6 months later. Use 1ml (10 microgram) if using Recombivax HB.
Individuals Undergoing Hemolysis and Individuals who are Immunsuppressed	IM into deltoid; 2ml (40 microgram); the 40 microgram dose should be divided into two 20 microgram doses and administered at different sites; then, 1 month and 6 months later. Same dose of Recombivax HB.
Individuals with Bleeding Disorders, eg, Thrombocytopenia or Hemophilia	Subcutaneous injections

The three-dose regimen stimulates production of neutralizing antibodies in 85% to 95% of vaccinees; immunity probably lasts five years. A single booster injection may then be necessary to maintain immunity. Pregnancy is not a contraindication to use of the vaccine.

Serologic Confirmation: Serologic confirmation is recommended for the following individuals: dialysis patients and staff, immunosuppressed individuals and individuals who have received the vaccine in the buttocks.

CONTRAINDICATIONS: Previous systemic allergic reaction; Recombinant vaccine is contraindicated in patients allergic to yeast.

ADVERSE EFFECTS: Local soreness, headache, respiratory symptoms, GI upset, fatigue, fever.

HETASTARCH

(Hespan)

USES: Hetastarch is a synthetic polymer of **glucose** which acts as a colloid. The molecular weight of at least 80% of the polymer units ranges from 10,000 to 2,000,000. The colloidal properties of a 6% hetastarch solution resemble those of albumin. Uses of hetastarch are given in the next Table:

Uses of Hetastarch
Hypovolemia
Shock or Impending Shock
Sedimentary Agent in Preparation of Granulocytes by Leukapheresis (Continuous and Intermittent Flow Cytapheresis)

Hetastarch is used to expand plasma volume in the treatment of hypovolemia, shock, or impending shock caused by hemorrhage, burns, surgery, sepsis or other trauma. The use of hetastarch for the treatment of shock not accompanied by hypovolemia may be hazardous because of the danger of volume overloading.

Each 500ml of hetastarch contains 6% hetastarch, 0.9% sodium chloride, provides 77mEq of sodium and 77mEq of chloride, pH 5.5(4.5 to 7.0), and osmolality of 310mOsm/liter.

Hetastarch is not a substitue for whole blood or plasma and has no oxygen-carrying capacity.

DOSAGE FORMS: Sol'n 6% in 0.9% sodium chloride solution in 500ml containers

DOSAGE: Hetastarch is administered by IV infusion; discard partially used bottles. No data are available on the safety of hetastarch in children, however, up to 20ml/kg has been given to pediatric patients for volume expansion. Dosage is given in the next Table:

Dosage of Hetastarch

Condition	Age	Dosage
Plasma Volume Expansion	Adults	Usual dosage, 500 to 1000ml; total dosage does not usually exceed 1500ml daily or approximately 20ml/kg for the typical 70kg patient; doses of 3-4 liters are not uncommon in severe hypovolemia, eg, trauma.
Acute Hemorrhagic Shock	Adults	20ml/kg/hr; in burn or septic shock, rate is usually slower.

Leukapheresis: In continuous-flow centrifugation(CFC) leukapheresis procedures, 250-700ml of hetastarch 6% solution is usually infused at a constant fixed ratio, 1:8 to venous whole blood. Multiple CFC procedure of up to two per week to a total of 7-10 have been reported to be safe.

PHARMACOKINETICS: Excretion: 40% in urine in 24 hrs.; usually, in 2 weeks, intravascular concentration of the drug is less than 1% of the total dose administered.

ADVERSE EFFECTS: Nausea, vomiting, mild febrile reactions, chills, pruritis, and urticaria. Rarely, anaphylactoid reactions have occurred. Excessive doses decrease hematocrit, dilute plasma proteins and interfere with platelet function. Prolongation of bleeding time may occur with doses greater than 20ml/kg.

CONTRAINDICATIONS: Severe congestive heart failure and renal failure with oliguria or anuria due to possible hypervolemia.

HYDRALAZINE

(Apresoline)

USES: Hydralazine is a vasodilator, used in the management of moderate to severe **hypertension.** Treatment of hypertension with hydralazine is given in the next table (The 1988 Report of the Joint National Committee on Detection, Evaluation, and Treatment of High Blood Pressure, Arch. Intern. Med. 148, 1023-1038, 1988):

Treatment of Hypertension with Hydralazine

Step 1: Nonpharmacologic Approaches (see **HYPERTENSION**)

↓

Step 2: **Diuretic** or **Beta-Blocker** or **Calcium Antagonist** or **ACE Inhibitor**
Observe up to 6 months; if treatment ineffective then,

↓

Step 3: Add a second drug of a different class, eg, hydralazine
or Increase the dosage of the first drug
or Substitute another drug, eg, hydralazine

↓

Step 4: Add a third drug of a different class, this could be hydralazine depending on drug in Step 3
or Substitute a second drug; this could be hydralazine depending on drug in Step 3

↓

Step 5: Consider further evaluation and/or referral
or Add a third or fourth drug, this could be hydralazine

Mechanism of Action: Hydralazine is an antihypertensive agent which reduces peripheral resistance and blood pressure as a result of a direct vasodilatory effect on vascular smooth muscle; the effect on arterioles is greater than on veins. The hydralazine-induced decrease in blood pressure is accompanied by increased heart rate, cardiac output, and stroke volume, probably because of a reflex response due to decreased peripheral resistance. The drug has no direct effect on the heart.

DOSAGE FORMS: Tabs: 10, 25, 50, 100mg; Amps: 20mg/ml.

DOSAGE: Hydralazine hydrochloride is usually administered orally; in patients who are unable to take the drug orally or when a rapid decrease in blood pressure is required, the drug may be given IM or IV. Hydralazine is usually the third agent in the regimen for treatment of chronic hypertension. Dosage is given in the next Table:

Dosage of Hydralazine

Condition	Age	Route	Dosage
Chronic Hypertension	Adults	Oral	10-25mg, two or three times daily; dosage may be increased by 10 to 25mg until b.p. is reduced to desired level; Max. daily dose, 300-400mg.
	Child.	Oral	0.75mg/kg daily in four divided doses; dosage may be increased gradually over 3-4 weeks to a max. of 7.5mg/kg daily.
Hypertensive Crisis	Adults	IV(Slow) or IM	5-20mg, increased to 40mg if necessary; repeat as required.
	Pregnancy	IV(Slow)	5-20mg
	Child.	IV(Slow) or IM	0.1-0.5mg/kg/dose titrate to desired effect with doses every 20-30 minutes, then every 4-6 hrs.

When patients are on IV or IM therapy, oral hypertensive therapy should be instituted while the blood pressure is being stabilized.

PHARMACOKINETICS: Onset: 20-30 min. (Oral); 5-20 min.(IV); 10-30 min.(IM); Duration: 2-4 hours (Oral); 2-6 hours(IV); 2-6 hours(IM); Bioavailability: 30%-50%; Protein Binding: 87%; Volume of Distribution: 1.6 liter/kg; Half-Life: 2.4 hours; Metabolism: Acetylation. Fast acetylators have lower plasma levels than slow acetylators. Elimination: Kidney.

HYDRALAZINE (Cont.)

ADVERSE EFFECTS: Adverse effects of hydralazine and methods to counteract these effects are given in the next Table:

Adverse Effects and Methods to Counteract these Effects

Adverse Effects	Counteract
Sodium and Water Retention	Diuretic
Headache and Tachycardia	Increase dose gradually
Tachycardia	Prior and concomitant use of an antiadrenergic drug, eg, beta-blocker
Myocardial Ischemia	Beta-blocker plus diuretic

G.I. Disturbances: Anorexia, nausea, vomiting, diarrhea.

Hematologic: Reduction in hemoglobin concentration, erythrocyte count, leukopenia, agranulocytosis and thrombocytopenia.

Sensitivity Reactions: Hydralazine may produce an acute rheumatoid syndrome simulating systemic lupus erythematosus(SLE); the condition is characterized by a positive antinuclear antibody(ANA) test, L.E. cells in peripheral blood, fever, myalgia, arthalgia, splenomegaly, and edema. This syndrome is most common in slow acetylators receiving 200mg daily or more, occurs more frequently in women, and is less prevalent in blacks. Renal disease is rare. The effects are reversible when the drug is withdrawn.

Other Adverse Reactions: Rarely, hydralazine has caused peripheral neuropathy, hepatotoxicity, and acute cholangitis. The peripheral neuropathy is caused by pyridoxine deficiency which can be corrected by administration of pyridoxine.

CONTRAINDICATIONS: Coronary artery disease; mitral valvular rheumatic diseases.

MONITOR: Blood pressure(b.p.); obtain baseline and periodic CBC and ANA titers if indicated.

HYDROCHLOROTHIAZIDE

(Aquazide-H, Esidrix, Hydro-D, Hydrodiuril, Oretic)

USES: Hydrochlorothiazide is a **thiazide diuretic** that is used in the treatment of **edema** and **hypertension**. Uses of hydrochlorothiazide are given in the next Table:

Uses of Hydrochlorothiazide

Condition	Comment
Hypertension	Preferred diuretic in patients with normal renal function
Edema	
Chronic Congestive Heart Failure(CHF)	Used in patients with normal renal function
Nephrotic Syndrome	
Renal Calculi	Decreased urinary calcium excretion
Diabetes Insipidus Nephrotic & Central Forms	Reduces urine volume by mild sodium and extracellular volume depletion which increased sodium and water reabsorption in the proximal tubules and thus reduces delivery of glomerular filtrate to the diluting segment.

Hypertension: Diuretics initially lower blood pressure by reducing the plasma volume; during long-term therapy, peripheral resistance also is decreased. Treatment of hypertension with hydrochlorothiazide is given in the next Table (The 1988 Report of the Joint National Committee on Detection, Evaluation, and Treatment of High Blood Pressure, Arch. Intern Med. 148, 1023-1038, 1988):

Treatment of Hypertension with Hydrochlorothiazide

Step 1: Nonpharmacologic Approaches (see **HYPERTENSION**)

↓

Step 2: Hydrochlorothiazide (Usual Minimum, 12.5-25 mg/day; Usual Maximum, 50 mg/day);
Observe up to 6 months; if ineffective then,

↓

Step 3: Add a second drug of a different class
or Increase the dosage of hydrochlorothiazide
or Substitute another drug

↓

Step 4: Add a third drug of a different class
or Substitute a second drug

↓

Step 5: Consider further evaluation and/or referral
or Add a third or fourth drug

"Step-Down": For patients with mild hypertension after 1 year of control, consider decreasing or withdrawing hydrochlorothiazide and other hypotensive drugs.

HYDROCHLOROTHIAZIDE (Cont.)
Mechanism of Action: Hydrochlorothiazide, like other thiazide diuretics, act on the cortical thick ascending loop of Henle and proximal distal tubule where it inhibits sodium chloride reabsorption. The urinary excretion of sodium chloride and water is increased.
DOSAGE FORMS: Tabs: 25, 50, and 100mg; Sol'n.: 50mg/5ml.
DOSAGE: Hydrochlorothiazide is administered orally; it is not effective as a diuretic when creatinine clearance is <20-30ml/min. Dosage is given in the next Table:

Condition	Age	Dosage
Edema	Adults	Initial: 25-200mg daily in 1-3 divided doses; after several days or when nonedematous weight is attained, maintenance dose of 25-100mg daily or intermittently. Max. 200mg/day.
Hypertension	Adults	Initial: 12.5-50mg daily as a single dose in the morning or in 2 divided doses. Maintenance dose: 12.5-100mg daily in a single dose. Max.200mg/day. Use minimum effective dose.
	Child	2-3mg/kg daily in 2 divided doses.

PHARMACOKINETICS: Onset of Diuresis: <2 hours; Peak: 3-6 hours; Duration: 6-12 hours. Onset of Hypotensive Effect: 3-4 days. Duration of Hypotensive Effect after Discontinuation:One week or less. Metabolism: No; Excretion:Urine
ADVERSE EFFECTS: Adverse effects are given in the next Table:

Adverse Effects of Hydrochlorothiazide

Effect	Comment
Hyperuricemia	Treatment unnecessary unless prior personal history or family history of gout.
Hyperglycemia	Loss of diabetic control occurs occasionally
Hyponatremia	Dilutional; restrict fluid intake and withdraw diuretic
Hypokalemia	Occurs in most patients. Give KCl supplementation or potassium-sparing diuretic therapy to the following: older patients; cirrhotics; patients on digitalis; serum potassium <3mmol/liter; those on other potasssium-wasting drugs.
Hypercalcemia	
Hypomagnesemia	
Increased serum Low Density Lipo-protein(LDL) and Triglyceride	
Thrombocytopenia	

Hypochloremic metabolic alkalosis may occur secondary to increased sodium delivered to renal distal tubular lumen, increased activity of aldosterone on the renal distal lining cells with absorption of sodium from the lumen in exchange for potasssium ions and hydrogen ions.

Other conditions that are associated with hydrochlorothiazide include pancreatitis, depression and allergic reactions.
CONTRAINDICATIONS: Anuria; pregnancy unless associated wtih severe edema; allergy.
PRECAUTIONS: Liver disease; diabetes; gout; significant renal function impairment.
MONITOR: Monitor parameters as follows:

Parameters to Monitor

Parameter	Comments
Serum Electrolytes: Potassium, Sodium, Chloride, Bicarbonate	Baseline values; then weekly to monthly initially; then every 3-6 months when stable
Serum Calcium & Magnesium	Periodically

Electrolytes should be monitored more closely if the patient develops diarrhea or vomiting. In selected patients, monitor serum uric acid, glucose, calcium, magnesium and cholesterol.

HYDROCHLOROTHIAZIDE AND AMILORIDE
(Generic brands, Moduretic)

USES: Moduretic is a drug with a fixed combination of diuretics, hydrochlorothiazide and amiloride; uses are given in the next Table:

Uses of Moduretic
Hypertension to Prevent or Treat Hydrochlorothiazide-Induced Hypokalemia
Edema to Prevent or Treat Hydrochlorothiazide-Induced Hypokalemia

Hydrochlorothiazide may induce **hypokalemia; amiloride** has **potassium-sparing effect** and is especially useful in treating or preventing the potassium losing effects of hydrochlorothiazide.

Hypertension: Treatment of hypertension with moduretic is given in the next Table (The 1988 Report of the Joint National Committee on Detection, Evaluation, and Treatment of High Blood Pressure, Arch. Intern Med. 148, 1023-1038, 1988):

Treatment of Hypertension with Moduretic

Step 1: Nonpharmacologic Approaches (see **HYPERTENSION**)

↓

Step 2: Moduretic should not be used initially. Dosage should first be adjusted by administering each drug, hydrochlorothiazide and amiloride, separately. If the optimum maintenance dosage corresponds to the ratio in the commercial combined preparation, the fixed combination may be used.

↓ Observe up to 6 months; if ineffective then

Step 3: Add a drug of a different class
or Increase the dosage of Moduretic
or Substitute another drug

↓

Step 4: Add a third drug of a different class
or Substitute a second drug

↓

Step 5: Consider further evaluation and/or referral
or Add a third or fourth drug

"Step-Down": For patients with mild hypertension, after 1 year of control, consider decreasing or withdrawing moduretic and other hypotensive drugs.

Edema: Moduretic should not be used initially. Dosage should first be adjusted be administering each drug, hydrochlorothiazide and amiloride, separately. If the optimum maintenance dosage corresponds to the ratio in the commercial combined preparation, the fixed combination may be used.

Mechanism of Action: Amiloride, like spironolactone and triamterene, acts on the renal distal tubular cells, interfering with the exchange of sodium ions from the tubular lumen for hydrogen and potassium ions from the distal tubular lining cells. Amiloride is not a potent antihypertensive agent.

The antihypertensive effect of amiloride and hydrochlorothiazide (Moduretic) is comparable to that of triamterine and hydrochlorothiazide (Dyazide or Maxzide) but Moduretic causes greater potassium loss due to the larger dose of thiazide.

DOSAGE FORMS: Each tablet of Moduretic contains hydrochlorothiazide, 50mg and amiloride hydrochloride, 5mg.

DOSAGE: Moduretic is not used for children; it is administered orally. Dosage of Moduretic is given in the next Table:

Dosage of Moduretic

Condition	Dosage
Hypertension	Initially, one tablet daily. Dosage should be adjusted in accordance with the blood pressure and serum potassium level
Edema	One or two tablets daily; serum potassium should be monitored

PHARMACOKINETICS: Pharmacokinetics are similar to the individual components

ADVERSE EFFECTS: Adverse effects are similar to the individual components. Hyperkalemia may occur despite concomitant hydrochlorothiazide therapy. Other adverse effects include orthostatic hypotension, hyperuricemia, hyperglycemia, headache, weakness, rash, dizziness, jaundice, blood dyscrasias.

PRECAUTIONS: Diabetes,gout,hepatic dysfunction,systemic lupus erythematosus.

CONTRAINDICATIONS: Hyperkalemia, renal insufficiency,diabetic nephropathy, lactation.

MONITOR: Serum potassium

HYDROCHLOROTHIAZIDE AND TRIAMTERINE
(Dyazide, Maxzide)

USES: This combination, **hydrochlorothiazide and triamterine** is a diuretic antihypertensive principally due to its hydrochlorothiazide component; the triamterine component reduces the excessive potassium loss which may occur with hydrochlorothiazide. Uses of hydrochlorothiazide, triamterine are given in the next Table:

Uses of Hydrochlorothiazide, Triamterine
Hypertension
Edema: Congestive Heart Failure, Cirrhosis, Nephrotic Syndrome

Hypertension or Edema: Hydrochlorothiazide, triamterine is indicated for the treatment of hypertension or edema in patients who develop hypokalemia on hydrochlorothiazide alone. The combination is also indicated for those patients who require a thiazide diuretic and in whom the development of hypokalemia cannot be risked, eg, patients on concomitant digitalis preparations, or with a history of cardiac arrhythmias.

Hypertension: Treatment of hypertension with Dyazide or Maxzide is given in the next table (The 1988 Report of the Joint National Committee on Detection, Evaluation, and Treatment of High Blood Pressure, Arch. Intern Med. 148, 1023-1038, 1988):

Treatment of Hypertension with Dyazide or Maxzide

Step 1: Nonpharmacologic Approaches (see **HYPERTENSION**)

↓

Step 2: Dyazide or Maxzide
Observe up to 6 months; if ineffective then,

↓

Step 3: Add a drug of a different class
or Increase the dosage of Dyazide or Maxzide
or Substitute another drug

↓

Step 4: Add a third drug of a different class
or Substitute a second drug

↓

Step 5: Consider further evaluation and/or referral
or Add a third or fourth drug

"Step-Down": For patients with mild hypertension, after 1 year of control, consider decreasing or withdrawing hypotensive drugs.

Mechanism of Action: Hydrochlorothiazide is a diuretic that increases the urinary excretion of sodium chloride and water by inhibiting sodium reabsorption in the cortical thick ascending limb of Henle's loop and the adjacent distal tubules (cortical diluting segment).

Triamterene is a diuretic that acts on renal distal tubular cells; it interferes with the exchange of sodium ion from the tubular lumen with potassium and hydrogen ion from the lining cells. Triamterine is used primarily for its potassium-sparing effect.

DOSAGE FORMS: Dosage forms of Dyazide and Maxzide are given in the next Table:

Dosage of Dyazide and Maxzide

Product	Triamterine	Hydrochlorothiazide
Dyazide (Capsules)	50mg	25mg
Maxzide (Tablets)	75mg	50mg
Maxzide-25 (Tablets)	37.5mg	25mg

DOSAGE: Dosage of Dyazide and Maxzide in adults is based on the desired dosage of hydrochlorothiazide. Adjust dosage in accordance with b.p. and serum potassium levels. Usual dosage of hydrochlorothiazide is 25-50mg daily in single or divided doses.

PHARMACOKINETICS: See hydrochlorothiazide. Triamterine: Rapidly absorbed; Bioavailability: 50%; Onset: One hour. Peak: 2-3 hours; diuresis declines in 7-9 hours. Half-Life: 1.5-2 hours.

ADVERSE EFFECTS: Similar to individual components. Orthostatic hypertension, fluid electrolyte imbalance, hyperuricemia, renal stones, hyperglycemia, muscle cramps, dizziness, G.I. disturbances, headache, rash, blood dyscrasias, jaundice.

CONTRAINDICATIONS: Anuria; progressive renal or hepatic dysfunction, hyperkalemia, sulfonamide allergy, lactation.

HYDROCORTISONE

(Cortisol, A-hydroCort, Cortef, Solu-Cortef)

USES: Hydrocortisone (Cortisol) is a **corticosteroid** secreted by the adrenal cortex; uses are given in the next Table:

Uses of Hydrocortisone
Acute (Addisonian Crisis) or Chronic Adrenocortical Insufficiency
Congenital Adrenal Hyperplasia, Salt-Losing Form
eg, 21-Hydroxylase Deficiency
Replacement Therapy for Major Surgery

Hydrocortisone has both **glucocorticoid** and **weak mineralocorticoid activities;** it is identical to cortisol, the endogenous glucocorticoid.

DOSAGE FORMS: Dosage forms of hydrocortisone are given in the next Table:

Dosage Forms of Hydrocortisone

Generic Name	Trade Name	Dosage Forms
Hydrocortisone	Cortef	5, 10, 20mg (Oral)
Hydrocortisone Cypionate	Cortef	10mg/5ml (Oral)
Hydrocortisone Acetate	Hydrocortone Acetate	25,50mg/ml (Parenteral)
Hydrocortisone Sodium Phosphate	Hydrocortone Phosphate	50mg/ml (Parenteral)
Hydrocortisone Sodium Succinate	A-HydroCort Solu-Cortef	100, 250, 500mg, 1g (Parenteral)

The oral preparations (base and cypionate salt) are often used for replacement therapy. The water-soluble forms (acetate, sodium phosphate, sodium succinate) are given intravenously or intramuscularly in emergencies.

DOSAGE: Hydrocortisone is given orally, IM or IV. The oral preparations (hydrocortisone and cypionate form) are used for replacement therapy. IM or IV therapy (water soluble forms, sodium phosphate, sodium succinate) is used for patients who are unable to take the drug orally or in emergency situations. Dosage is given in the next Table:

Dosage of Hydrocortisone

Condition	Route	Drug	Dosage
Chronic Adrenocortical Insufficiency (Addison's Dis.)	Oral	Hydrocortisone; or Hydrocortisone Cypionate	12 to 15mg/M^2 daily; two-thirds in the morning, one-third in afternoon.
Congenital Adrenal Hyperplasia	Oral	Hydrocortisone; or Hydrocortisone Cypionate	25mg/M^2 daily; one-third is given in the morning, two-thirds in the evening. Higher doses (30-36mg/M^2 daily) may be required initially.
Acute Adrenocortical Insufficiency (Addisonian Crisis); Emergencies, Shock; or Congenital Adrenal Hyperplasia(CAH), Salt-Losing Crisis	IV	Hydrocortisone Sodium Phosphate; or Hydrocortisone Sodium Succinate	Emergencies: 100mg, repeat if necessary. Shock: 50mg/kg Congenital Adrenal Hyperplasia(CAH), Salt-Losing Crisis: 50 to 100mg for one to two days until crisis is controlled. Child: 2-4x physiologic replacement or 1-2mg/kg/dose IV bolus then 25-150 mg/day for infants and 150-250mg/day for older child.
	IM	Hydrocortisone Sodium Phosphate; or Hydrocortisone Sodium Succinate	100 to 250mg; repeat if necessary. Child: 2-4x physiologic replacement.
Asthma	IV	Hydrocortisone Sodium Phosphate; or Hydrocortisone Sodium Succinate	4-8mg/kg/dose (max. 250mg) load followed by 8mg/kg/day in 4 divided doses.

The adrenal cortex normally secretes 20mg of hydrocortisone daily. Hydrocortisone therapy varies greatly, depending on the underlying condition, acute events, and patient response; dose must be individualized based on the clinical situation.

HYDROCORTISONE (Cont.)
ADVERSE EFFECTS: There are a wide variety of adverse effects, both acute and chronic, associated with use of steroids, including hydrocortisone.
Acute Withdrawal: Hypotension, shock, hypoglycemia, arthralgia, myalgia, fever.
Chronic Use: Chronic use of hydrocortisone may simulate findings in Cushing's syndrome as given in the next Table:

Adverse Effects of Chronic Use of Hydrocortisone

System Involved	Effect
Immunological Suppression	Increased susceptibility to infection
Fluid and Electrolyte Disturbances	Hypokalemia; metabolic alkalosis; salt and water retention; hypertension; congestive heart failure(CHF)
Endocrine	Cushing's syndrome; glucose intolerance, negative nitrogen blance; decreased protein anabolism; growth retardation; menstrual abnormalities
Musculoskeletal	Weakness; decreased muscle mass; myopathy; osteoporosis; pathologic fractures
Gastrointestinal Tract	Peptic ulcers; esophageal ulcers; pancreatitis
Dermatologic	Acne, poor wound healing; facial erythema; petechiae; ecchymoses
Ophthalmic	Cataracts

PHARMACOKINETICS: Half-Life: 1.5 hours. Parenteral forms should be dosed every 4-6 hours to maintain constant high concentrations in stress situations.

HYDROCORTISONE ACETATE ANORECTAL PREPARATION
(Anusol-HC)
USES: This preparation is used to treat **hemorrhoids, anorectal irritation** or **pruritis ani**; hydrocortisone is included for its anti-inflammatory effect.
DOSAGE FORM: Ointment and suppositories. Hydrocortisone, 0.5%, and other ingredients.
DOSAGE: Suppositories: One rectally morning and at bedtime for 3-6 days or until inflammation subsides. Ointment: Apply externally to cleansed dried area, or internally with applicator. Use 3-4 times daily for 3-6 days until inflammation subsides.
ADVERSE EFFECTS: Adrenal suppression if used to excess for prolonged period of time; dermal and epidermal atrophy; poor wound healing; local irritation; folliculitis; hypertrichosis; acne-form eruptions; hypopigmentation; secondary infections.
PRECAUTIONS: Tuberculosis; diverticulitis; exacerbation of infections; children; pregnancy; lactation.

HYDROCORTISONE, NEOMYCIN, POLYMYXIN B

(Cortisporin Otic)

USES: Cortisporin Otic contains two **antibacterial agents**, **neomycin** and **polymyxin B** and the **corticosteroid**, **hydrocortisone** and is used to treat **acute external otitis**. The most common bacterial isolate in external otitis is pseudomonas. Topical preparations containing neomycin and polymyxin B are the drugs of choice for empiric therapy of acute external otitis.

The antibacterial spectrum includes both gram-positive and gram-negative organisms. Neomycin is an aminoglycoside antibiotic. It is effective against Escherichia, Enterobacter aerogenes and most species of Klebsiella, Salmonella, Shigella and Proteus; many strains of Staphylococcus aureus also are sensitive. However, it has only weak activity against many strains of Pseudomonas. Polymyxin B has anti-pseudomonal activity.

Hydrocortisone is useful in treating severe inflammation which may complicate otitis; it is also used to treat allergic dermatitis.

DOSAGE FORMS: The composition of Cortisporin Otic Solution and Suspension (Burroughs Wellcome) is given in the next Table:

Composition of Cortisporin Otic Solution and Suspension

Preparation	Antibiotics	Corticosteroid	Other Ingredients
Cortisporin Otic Sol. (BW).	Neomycin sulfate (equilvalent to 3.5 mg base) polymyxin B sulfate 10,000 units/ml.	Hydrocortisone 1%.	Cupric sulfate, glycerin, propylene glycol, potassium metabisulfite, 0.1%
Suspension (BW).	Neomycin sulfate (equilvalent to 3.5 mg base) polymyxin B sulfate 10,000 units/ml.	Hydrocortisone 1%.	Cetyl alcohol, propylene glycol, polysorbate 80, thimerosal, 0.01%

DOSAGE: Adults: Clean ear; then administer 4 drops in ear canal every 6-8 hours; max. 10 days. Children: Clean ear; then administer 3 drops in ear canal every 6-8 hours; max. 10 days.

ADVERSE EFFECTS: Neomycin an aminoglycoside, may cause cutaneous hypersensitivity. The prevalence of hypersensitivity to topical neomycin is about 1% when neomycin is used on undamaged skin for seven days; the prevalence is much higher in patients with contact dermatitis or chronic dermatoses. If irritation or sensitivity develops, use an otic preparation which does not contain neomycin.

PRECAUTIONS: Do not use in patients with fungal, tuberculosis, or viral otic conditions. Suspension should be used in patients with perforation of the tympanic membrane to avoid the burning sensation associated with the solution.

HYDROXYZINE

(Atarax, Vistaril)

USES AND DOSAGE: The uses and dosage of hydroxyzine are given in the next Table:

Uses and Dosage of Hydroxyzine

Use	Children	Adults
Anxiety and tension assoc. with psychoneuroses; and adjunct in patients with organic dis. who have assoc. anxiety	Oral: 2mg/kg daily in divided doses every 6 hours	Oral:50-100mg, 4 times daily
Disturbed or hysterical patients and management of agitation caused by alcohol withdrawal		50-100mg, IM, repeat every 4-6h as needed
Pruritis caused by allergic conditions, eg, chronic urticaria or atopic or contact dermatoses or histamine-medicated pruritis	Oral: 2mg/kg daily in divided doses every 6 hours	Oral:25mg, 3 or 4 times daily.
Sedation before and following general anesthesia	0.5mg/kg orally or 0.5-1.0mg/kg IM	50-100mg, orally or 25-100mg, IM
Nausea and vomiting (excluding nausea and vomiting of pregnancy	0.5-1.0mg/kg IM	25-100mg, IM

DOSAGE FORMS: Tabs (HCl): 10, 25, 50, 100mg; Caps (pamoate): 25, 50, 100mg; Syrup (HCl): 10mg/5ml; Susp. (pamoate): 25mg/5ml; Vials (HCl): 25, 50mg/ml.

ADVERSE EFFECTS: May potentiate barbiturates, meperidine and other depressants. May cause dry mouth, drowsiness, tremor and convulsions.

HYPERCALCEMIA, TREATMENT

Management of hypercalcemia is given in the next Table(Bilezikian, J.P., Disease-a-Month 34, Dec. 1988):

Management of Hypercalcemia

General	Specific
Rehydration	Therapy for underlying etiology
Saline administration	Plicamycin
Diuresis with furosemide	Bisphosphonates (eg, Etidronate)
Dialysis	Calcitonin
Mobilization	Phosphate
	WR2721 (Ethiofos)(not generally available)
	Gallium nitrate
	Glucocorticoids

Rehydration: The fluid of choice is saline because, in addition to rehydration, the salt in the IV solution induces a saliuresis which is accompanied by an obligatory loss of urinary calcium.

Diuresis with Furosemide: Furosemide, a loop diuretic, may be useful especially in older individuals to help to guard against overhydration and to induce the loss of urinary calcium.

Hemodialysis or Peritoneal Dialysis: Dialysis may be necessary in severely hypercalcemic patients.

Mobilization: The patient should be mobilized as soon as possible.

Therapeutic agents used in the treatment of acute hypercalcemia are given in the following Table (Schaiff, R.A.B. et al., Clin. Pharm. 8, 108-121, 1989):

Therapy of Acute Hypercalcemia

Therapy	Onset	Dosage
0.9% Saline Administration	Rapid	100-250 (up to 500)ml/hr. Most useful to correct volume depletion. May cause volume overload or hypokalemia.
Furosemide	<4h	80-120mg IV every 2-6h. May cause hypovolemia, hypokalemia, hypomagnesemia.
Calcitonin	<2-4h	Test dose: 1 IU, then 4-8 IU IM or SC every 6-12h. May cause nausea, vomiting, hypersensitivity reactions.
Etidronate	24-48hrs	7.5mg/kg IV daily. Infuse in 250ml of fluid over at least 2h. Very effective for treatment of hypercalcemia of malignancy (Singer, F.R. et al., Arch. Intern. Med. 151, 471-476, 1991). Chronic therapy, 10-20mg/kg daily given orally. Nephrotoxic
Plicamycin	<24h	25 micrograms/kg IV every 48-72h. 12.5 micrograms/kg in renal or hepatic disease. May cause hemorrhage, hepatotoxicity, nephrotoxicity. Infuse in 1 liter of fluid over 4-6h.
Gallium Nitrate	2-7days	100-200mg/m^2 body surface area daily for 5 days via continuous infusion (Warrell, R.P. et al., Ann. Intern. Med. 108, 669-674, 1988). Approved for marketing as an orphan drug 1/17/91. Nephrotoxic.

HYPERTENSION,TREATMENT

Classification: The follow-up criteria for initial blood pressure measurement and classification of blood pressure are given in the next Table (The 1988 Report of the Joint National Committee on Detection, Evaluation, and Treatment of High Blood Pressure, Arch. Intern. Med. 148, 1023-1038, 1988):

Follow-Up Criteria for Initial B.P. Measurement and Classification

BP Range, mm Hg	Follow-Up	Classification
Diastolic B.P.		
<85	Recheck within 2 yr.	Normal B.P.
85-89	Recheck within 1 yr.	High-Normal B.P.
90-104	Confirm within 2 mo.	Mild Hypertension
105-114	Evaluate or refer within 2 wks.	Moderate Hypertension
>114	Evaluate or refer immediately	Severe Hypertension
Systolic B.P. when Diastolic B.P. <90 mmHg		
<140	Recheck within 2 yr.	Normal B.P.
140-199	Confirm with 2 mo.	
140-159		Borderline Isolated Systolic Hypertension
>159		Isolated Systolic Hypertension
>199	Evaluate or refer promptly to source of care within 2 wks.	

Classification of hypertension in children is given in the next Table (Report of the second Task Force on Blood Pressure Control in Children, 1987, Pediatrics 79, 1-25, 1987):

Classification of Hypertension in the Young

Age Groups	> 94th Percentile Systolic B.P.	> 94th Percentile Diastolic B.P.	> 98th Percentile Systolic B.P.	> 98th Percentile Diastolic B.P.
Newborns:				
up to 8 days	>95		>105	
8-30 days	>103		>109	
Infants (<2 yr.):	>111	>73	>117	>81
Children:				
3-5 years	>115	>75	>123	>81
6-9 years	>121	>77	>129	>85
10-12 years	>125	>81	>133	>89
13-15 years	>135	>85	>143	>91
Adolescent(16-18yr):	>141	>91	>149	>97

Treatment: In the treatment of chronic essential hypertension, a stepped-approach is recommended as illustrated in the next Table (The 1988 Report of the Joint National Committee on Detection, Evaluation, and Treatment of High Blood Pressure, Arch. Intern. Med. 148, 1023-1038, 1988):

Treatment of Hypertension

Step 1: **Nonpharmacologic Approaches:** Sodium and alcohol restriction, weight control, tobacco avoidance, exercise, modification of dietary fats.

↓

Step 2: **Diuretic** or **Beta-Blocker** or **Calcium Antagonist** or **ACE Inhibitor**
Observe up to 6 months; if treatment ineffective,

↓

Step 3: **Add a second drug of a different class:**
Diuretic or **Beta-Blocker** or **Calcium Antagonist** or **ACE Inhibitor**
or Alpha-Blockers, or Centrally Acting Alpha-2-Adrenergic Agonists or Rauwolfia Serpentia or Vasodilators
or **Increase the dosage of the first drug.**
or **Substitute a second drug**

↓

Step 4: **Add a third drug of a different class.**
or **Substitute a second drug**

↓

Step 5: **Consider further evaluation and/or referral.**
or **Add a third or fourth drug**

"Step-Down": For patients with mild hypertension, after 1 year of control, consider decreasing or withdrawing medication.

HYPERTENSION, TREATMENT (Cont.)

The drugs that are used to treat hypertension are given in the next Table (The 1988 Report of the Joint National Committee on Detection, Evolution and Treatment of High Blood Pressure, Arch. Intern.Med. 148, 1023-1038, 1988):

Treatment of Hypertension

Diuretics
Thiazide and Related Sulfonamides:
Hydrochlorothiazide (Hydrodiuril and others)
Chlorothiazide (Diuril)
Metolazone (Zaroxolyn)
Chlorthalidone (Hygroton)
Indapamide (Lozol)
Loop Diuretics:
Furosemide (Lasix)
Bumetamide (Bumex)
Ethacrynic Acid (Edecrin)
Potassium Sparing:
Spironolactone (Aldactone)
Triamterene (Dyrenium)
Amiloride (Midamor)
Combinations:
Hydrochlorothiazide with Triamterene (Dyazide, Maxzide)
Hydrochlorothiazide with Amiloride (Moduretic)
Adrenergic Inhibitors
Beta-Adrenergic Blockers:
Nadolol (Corgard)
Timolol (Timoptic)
Propranolol (Inderal)
Atenolol (Tenormin)
Metoprolol (Lopressor)
Pindolol (Visken)
Combination Drugs:
Atenolol, Chlorthalidone
Propranolol, Hydrochlorothiazide (Inderide)
Centrally Acting Alpha Blockers:
Clonidine (Catapres)
Methyldopa (Aldomet)
Guanabenz (Wytensin)
Combination Drugs:
Methyldopa, Hydrochlorothiazide (Aldoril)
Peripheral-Acting Adrenergic Antagonists:
Guanethidine (Ismelin)
Rauwolfia Alkaloids
Reserpine
Alpha-1 Adrenergic Blockers:
Prazosin hydrochloride (Minipress)
Terazosin hydrochloride
Combined Alpha-Beta Adrenergic Blocker:
Labetalol (Normodyne, Trandate)
Combination Drugs:
Labetalol with Hydrochlorothiazide (Normozide)
Direct-Acting Vasodilators:
Hydralazine (Apresoline)
Minoxidil (Loniten)
Angiotensin-Converting Enzyme Inhibitors:
Captopril (Capoten)
Enalapril (Vasotec)
Lisinopril (Prinivil)
Combination Drugs:
Captopril plus Hydrochlorothiazide (Capozide)
Enalapril plus Hydrochlorothiazide (Vaseretic)
Calcium Channel Blocking Drugs:
Nifedipine (Procardia, Adalat)
Verapamil (Calan, Isoptin)
Diltiazem (Cardizem)

HYPERTENSION, TREATMENT (Cont.)

Step 1: Nonpharmacologic Approaches: Nonpharmacologic therapies to reduce blood pressure should be tried first in some patients prior to drug therapy. Successful nonpharmacologic approaches may reduce the level of drug needed to achieve control in hypertensive patients. Nonpharmacologic therapy is given in the next Table (Arch. Intern. Med. 148, 1023-1038, 1988):

Nonpharmacologic Approaches to Control of Blood Pressure

Nonpharmacologic Therapy	Comments
Sodium Restriction	Restrict sodium to 70 to 100mEq/day (approx. 1.5 to 2.5g of sodium or 4 to 6g of salt).
Alcohol Restriction	Limit alcohol intake to 30ml (1oz.) of ethanol daily [60ml(2oz.) of 100-proof whiskey, 240ml(8oz.) of wine, or 720ml(24oz.) of beer].
Weight Control	Obesity and blood pressure closely related.
Tobacco Avoidance	
Exercise	Facilitates weight control.
High Intake, Polyunsaturated Fat and Low Intake, Saturated Fat	Lowers cholesterol and reduces risk of coronary artery disease.

Step 2: In the most recent revision, the choices for initial drug therapy have been expanded to include calcium antagonists and angiotensin-converting enzyme (ACE) inhibitors, in addition to the previously recommended diuretics and beta-blockers. Approximately 50 percent of patients with mild hypertension are successfully treated with one of these drugs. The objective of therapy is blood pressure of 140/90mmHg or lower.

First-step drug therapy for patients with mild hypertension is shown in the next Table (Cloher, T.P., Whelton, P.K., Arch. Intern. Med. 146, 529-533, 1986):

Drugs Recommended for First-Step Therapy of Patients with Mild Hypertension

	Family/ General Practice,(%)	Internal Medicine Practice,(%)	Specialty Medicine Practice,(%)
Diuretics	92	89	87
Beta-Blockers	5	9	10
Others	3	2	1

Others: Reserpine, Methyldopa, Hydralazine, and Guanethidine.

Seventy-five percent of physicians used initial treatment with an unsupplemented thiazide diuretic: hydrochlorothiazide, 25mg/day (12% of physicians); 50mg/day (72% of physicians); 100mg/day (9% of physicians). The remainder recommended a thiazide-potassium-sparing agent combination, a long-acting thiazide-like agent or a loop diuretic. When beta-blockers are used, propranolol or atenolol are the preferred drugs.

Beta-blockers should be avoided in asthmatic patients and in patients with congestive heart failure. Beta-blockers may be particularly useful in hypertensive patients following myocardial infarct and angina pectoris. Angiotensin-converting enzyme(ACE)inhibitors (captopril, enalapril, and lisinopril) may be selected in patients with congestive heart failure or diabetic patients with renal disease (Working Group on Management of Patients with Hypertension and High Blood Cholesterol, Ann. Intern. Med. 114, 224-237, Feb. 1991).

Consideration should also be given to the effects of antihypertensive drugs on serum lipid levels. Not all patients are sensitive to hyperlipemic effects of diuretics (Ames, R.P. and Hill, P., Am. J. Med. 61, 748-756, 1976) and these effects may be transient (Veterans Administration Cooperative Study Group on Antihypertensive Agents, JAMA 248, 2004-2011, 1982), but consideration should be given to these effects. The effects of antihypertensive drugs on serum lipid profile is given in the following Table (Schoenberger, J.A., Amer. J. Med. 90 (suppl.4B), 3S-7S, April, 1991):

Effects of Antihypertensive Drugs on Lipid and Lipoprotein Levels

Drug Class	Total Cholesterol	LDL Cholesterol	Triglycerides	HDL Cholesterol
Ideal drug	Dec	Dec	Dec	Inc
Thiazides	Inc	Inc	Inc	Dec-Unch
Beta-blockers	Unch	Unch-Inc	Inc	Dec
Alpha-blockers	Dec-Unch	Dec	Dec-Unch	Inc
Sympatholytics	Unch	Dec	Inc	Dec
ACE Inhibitors	Dec-Unch	Dec-Unch	Dec-Unch	Unch-Inc
Calcium Antag.	Unch	Unch	Unch	Unch

HYPERTENSION, TREATMENT (Cont.)

Some authors contend that blacks and older patients tend to respond better to diuretics or calcium antagonists than to beta-blockers or ACE inhibitors (Working Group on Management of Patients with Hypertension and High Blood Cholesterol, Ann. Intern. Med. 114, 224-237, February, 1991), other authors contest this idea (Schoenberger, J.A., Amer. J. Med. 90 (Suppl. 4B), 3S-7S, April, 1991). Gender has not been found to be a significant determinant of the response to drugs.

Numerous options exist for antihypertensive therapy; choice of agent(s) will depend on individual circumstances. Some of the options for monotherapy, substitution therapy and combined therapy are given in the following Table (Schoenberger, J.A., Amer. J. Med. 90 (Suppl. 4B), 3S-7S, April, 1991):

Treatment of Hypertension: Monotherapy, Substitution

Monotherapy	Substitution	Combination
Diuretic	Calcium Antag.	Add ACE inhib.
Beta-blocker	ACE inhib.	Add Diuretic
ACE inhib.	Beta-blocker	Add Diuretic
Calcium antag.	Diuretic	Add Alpha-blocker
Alpha-blocker	ACE inhib.	Add Beta-blocker

HYPERTENSIVE EMERGENCIES

HYPERTENSIVE EMERGENCIES: Hypertensive emergency is defined as a severe elevation of systemic blood pressure with acute end-organ injury (eg, Encephalopathy, papilledema, pulmonary edema, or acute renal failure). Suggested treatment in such cases should be with IV sodium nitroprusside or in milder cases, IV diazoxide or oral or sublinqual nifedipine. However, in patients with asymptomatic moderate to severe hypertension, potential benefits must be weighed against the chance of adverse consequences (Editorials: Ferguson, R.K. and Vlasses, P.H., Arch. Intern. Med. 149, 257-258, 1989; Fagan, T.C., Arch. Intern. Med. 149, 2169-2170, 1989; Weber, M.A., Arch. Intern. Med. 149, 2635-2637, 1989).

Drug options for **hypertensive emergencies** are given in the next Table (Patient Care, pgs. 118-119, April 15, 1986; The 1988 Report of the Joint National Committee on Detection, Evaluation, and Treatment of High Blood Pressure Arch. Intern. Med. 148, 1023-1038, May 1988; Calhoun, D.A. and Oparil, S., N. Engl. J. Med. 323, 1177-1183, 1990):

Drug Options for Hypertensive Emergencies

Drug (Dosage Form)	Dosage	Onset & Action	Adverse Effects
Direct Vasodilators			
Diazoxide (Hyperstat IV) (15mg/ml)	IV Single Dose: 1-3mg/kg to max 150mg. Repeat doses every 5-15 minutes as needed or IV Continuous Infusion: 7.5-30mg/min titrate to desired effect.	1-2min	Chest pain, flushing, hyperglycemia, hyperuricemia, hypotension, nausea, tachycardia, vomiting
Hydralazine HCl (Apresoline) (20mg/ml ampule)	IV Single Dose: Adult: 10-20mg in at least 20ml of normal saline; max infusion: 0.5ml/min; interrupt frequently when blood pressure starts to fall. IM: 10-50mg Pregnancy: 5-20mg Child: 0.1-0.5mg/kg	10-20 min	Chest pain, flushing, headache, palpitations, tachycardia, vomiting.
Minoxidil (Loniten)	2.5-5mg orally, repeat after 2-3 hrs. Child: 0.2mg/kg (max. 5mg) (Strife, C.F. et al., Pediatrics 78, 861-864, 1986).		
Nitroglycerin	5-100microgram/min as IV infusion Child: 0.5-5microgram/kg/min	2-5min	Headache, tachycardia, vomiting, methemoglobinemia.
Sodium Nitroprusside (Nipride, Nitropress) (50mg/5ml vial; 50mg/2ml vial)	IV Continuous Infusion: 0.5-10microgram/kg/min.	Instantaneous	Apprehension, muscle twitching, nausea, vomiting, sweating, thiocyanate or cyanide intoxication

HYPERTENSIVE EMERGENCIES (Cont.)

Sympathetic Blocking Drugs			
Clonidine HCl (Catapres) (0.1, 0.2, 0.3mg tabs.)	Oral or Sublingual: 0.1-0.2mg Use every hour as required	10-20 min	Drowsiness occurs very commonly(59%)(Jaker, M. et al., Arch. Intern. Med. 149, 260-265, 1989). Dry mouth
Labetalol HCl (Normodyne, Trandate) (100mg/ 20ml ampule)	IV Single Dose: 20-80mg bolus every 10 min. or IV Continuous Infusion: 0.5-2mg/min; 300mg maximum Child: 1-3mg/kg/hr (Balfe, J.W., et al., Adv. Pediatr. 36, 201-246, 1989).	5-10 min	Orthostatic hypotension, paresthesias (eg, scalp tingling), bronchospasm, nausea, vomiting, pain at injection site.
Methyldopate HCl (Aldomet) (250mg/ 5ml vial)	IV Single Dose: 250-500mg diluted in up to 100ml of 5% dextrose injection. Child: 20-40mg/kg/day in 4 doses.	30-60 min	Drowsiness
Trimethaphan camsylate (Arfonad) (500mg/10ml ampule)	IV Continuous Infusion: 0.5-5mg/min	1-5 min	Blurred vision, dry mouth, orthostatic hypotension, paresis of bowel and bladder.
Alpha-Receptor Blocking Drug			
Phentolamine mesylate (Regitine) (5mg/vial)	IV Single Dose: 5-15mg. Repeat every 5-15 min as needed or 1-5mg/min. Child: 0.05-0.1mg/kg/dose IV or IM	1-2 min	Flushing, tachycardia, orthostatic hypotension
Calcium Entry Blocker			
Nifedipine (Procardia) (10mg caps.)	Oral or Sublingual: 10mg; repeat after 30 min or 20mg once orally (Jaker, M., et al., Arch. Intern. Med. 149, 260-265, 1989) Child: 0.2-0.5mg/kg	5-15 min	Flushing, headache, orthostatic hypotension.
Angiotensin-Converting Enzyme Inhibitor			
Captopril (Capoten) (12.5, 25.0, 50.0, 100mg tablets).	Oral or Sublingual: 25mg (Range: 6.25-50mg); repeat as required. Child: <6 mo.: 0.05-0.5mg/kg; >6 mo.: 0.5-2.0mg/kg("Report of the Second Task Force on Blood Pressure Control in Children-1987," Pediatr. 79(1),1-25, 1987).	15-20 min	Hypotension
Diuretic			
Furosemide (Lasix) (10mg/ml in 2, 4, 10ml ampules)	IV Single Dose: 20-100mg injected over 1-2min. Child: 1mg/kg/dose IV Continuous Infusion: Equal to or less than 4mg/min; 400mg max.	10-20 min.	Excessive diuresis, hyperuricemia, hypokalemia, hypovolemia, ototoxicity.

IM: Start with the smallest dose and adjust subsequent doses and dosing interval according to the response in blood pressure.
IV Infusion: Start slowly and adjust the rate and concentration of the drug according to the blood pressure response.

IBUPROFEN

(Advil, Haltran, Medipren, Motrin, Nuprin, Rufen, Trendar)

USES: Ibuprofen is a **nonsteroidal anti-inflammatory drug** (NSAID); its pharmacologic actions are similar to those of other NSAIDs such as aspirin, **phenylbutazone**, & **indomethacin** in that it has **anti-inflammatory**, **antipyretic**, and **analgesic activity**.

Mechanism of Action: The anti-inflammatory action may be due to inhibition of synthesis and/or release of prostaglandins. Ibuprofen produces antipyresis by acting on the hypothalamus, with heat dissipation being increased as a result of vasodilation and increased peripheral blood flow.

All cells, except nonnucleated erythrocytes, are capable of synthesizing prostaglandins which are released in response to trauma of any kind. The pathological release of prostaglandins which contribute to inflammation, fever, and pain is inhibited by ibuprofen. The synthesis of prostaglandins and the inhibition by ibuprofen is illustrated in the next Figure (Vane, J. and Botting, R., FASEB J. 1, 89-96, 1987):

Synthesis of Prostaglandins and Inhibition by Ibuprofen

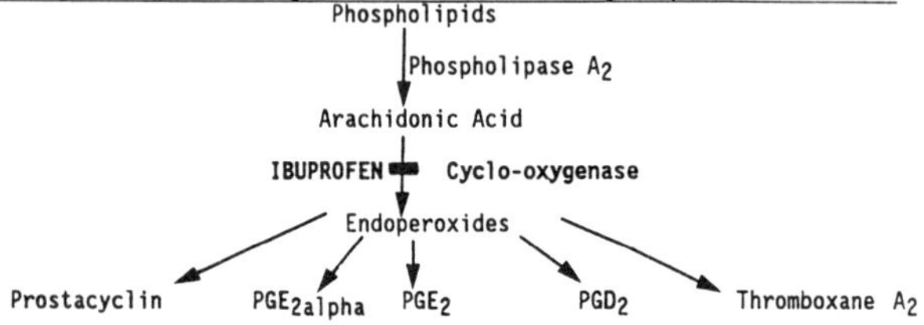

Ibuprofen irreversibly aceylates and inactivates cyclo-oxygenase, an enzyme which catalyzes the formation of prostaglandin precursors (endoperoxides) from arachidonic acid.

PGE_2 may be especially important in the inflammatory process.

In the development of fever, endogenous pyrogen is released from leukocytes and acts directly on the thermoregulatory center in the hypothalamus. This effect is associated with a rise in prostaglandins in the brain. Ibuprofen prevents the temperature-rising effects of pyrogens and the rise in brain prostaglandin levels.

DOSAGE FORMS: Tabs: 200, 300, 400, 600, 800mg; Susp: 100mg/5ml.

DOSAGE: Administer orally. If GI symptoms develop, administer ibuprofen with meals or reduce dosage.

Conditions and Dose

Condition	Dose
Inflammatory Conditions: Acute and Chronic Rheumatoid Arthritis and Osteoarthritis	Adult: 400-800mg, 3 or 4 times daily. Do not exceed 3.2g daily. Optimal therapeutic response within 2 weeks.
Juvenile Rheumatoid Arthritis	Children: 30-70mg/kg/day in 3-4 divided doses.
Pain (mild to moderate)	Adult: 200-400mg every 4-6h; max., 2.4g daily; max. 10 days
Fever	Adult: 200-400mg every 4-6h; max., 2.4g daily; max. 3 days Children: 20mg/kg/day in 3-4 divided doses.
Dysmenorrhea	Adult: 200-400mg every 4h as necessary to relieve pain. Max. 2.4g daily

IBUPROFEN (Cont.)

ADVERSE EFFECTS: The incidence of adverse effects are low; ibuprofen may be better tolerated than most other NSAIDs.

Adverse effects of ibuprofen are given in the next Table:

Adverse Effects of Ibuprofen

System	Effects
Gastrointestinal	Nausea, vomiting, diarrhea, constipation, heartburn, and epigastric pain. There is less GI bleeding with ibuprofen than with aspirin.
Central Nervous System	Headache, lightheadedness and dizziness.
Renal	Acute renal failure, acute interstitial nephritis, nephrotic syndrome, possibly, renal papillary necrosis.
Eye	Amblyopia.
Platelets	Inhibits platelet aggregation less than aspirin or indomethacin.
Other Hematologic Effects	Lymphopenia, agranulocytosis, hemolytic anemia are rare.
Liver	Hepatitis.
Skin	Rashes
Hypersensitivity Reactions	Hypersensitive reactions have occurred, including bronchospasm and anaphylaxis.

CONTRAINDICATIONS: Do not use ibuprofen in patients known to be hypersensitive to NSAIDs. Do not use in patients with nasal polyps or angioedema. Use with caution in patients with renal impairment.

PHARMACOKINETICS: Absorption: Rapid; Protein-Binding: 99%; Peak: 1-2 hours; Half-Life: 1.8 to 2.6 hours.

DRUG INTERACTIONS: Drug interactions are given in the next Table:

Drug Interactions of Ibuprofen

Drug	Effect
Warfarin	Not affected with doses up to 2.4g daily; larger doses may displace warfarin from protein binding sites.

IMIPENEM AND CILASTATIN

(Primaxin)

USES: This is a combination antibiotic that combines imipenem, a carbapenem, with cilastatin, an inhibitor of renal dihydropeptidase. Cilastatin has no antimicrobial activity but is present solely to prevent degradation of imipenem by this renal enzyme. The spectrum of antimicrobial activity is broader than any other approved class of antibiotics with coverage including gram-negative and gram-positive, aerobic and anaerobic bacteria; activities of imipenem are given in the next Table (Lipman, B. and Neu, H.C., Med. Clin. No. Am. 72, 567-579, May 1988; Adams, H.G., Personal Comm.):

Activities of Imipenem

	Gram-positive cocci			Gram-negative bacilli				Anaerobes	
	S. aureus	Streptococci	Strep. entero.	H. influenzae	PEcK	Other Enterics	Pseudomonas a.	B. fragilis	Res. Anaerobes
Imipenem	4	4	3	4	4	4	4	4	4

4=best activity; 3=good activity; 2=some activity; ▩=little or no activity; PEcK (Mnemonic)= P. mirabilis, E. coli, Klebsiella; Res.= Resident

Gram-Positive Cocci: Imipenem is active against virtually all gram positive cocci except the enterococcus, Streptococcus faecium, some coagulase-negative staphylococci and methicillin-resistant Staphylococcus aureus.

Gram-Positive Bacilli: Imipenem has only moderate activity against Clostridium difficile but has good activity against Listeria monocytogenes.

Gram-Negative Bacilli: Imipenem is active against virtually all gram negative bacilli except Pseudomonas maltophilia and Pseudomonas cepacia. Emergence of imipenem-resistant Pseudomonas isolates has been observed during the course of therapy of patients with cystic fibrosis and other diseases.

Gram-Negative Cocci: Imipenem is active against gram negative cocci: Neisseria gonorrhea (gonococcus), Neisseria meningitidis (meningococcus), and Moraxella (Branhamella) catarrhalis.

Anaerobes: Imipenem is active against virtually all anaerobes; its activity approaches that of metronidazole, clindamycin and chloramphenicol. It has only moderate activity against Clostridium difficile.

Chlamydiae and Mycoplasma: Imipenem is not reliably active against Chlamydia trachomatis or Mycobacterium fortuitum.

Mechanism of Action: Imipenem binds to penicillin-binding protein(PBP)1 and PBP2 to cause elongation and subsequent lysis of bacteria.

Structure: See **BETA-LACTAM ANTIBIOTICS.**

DOSAGE FORMS: Powder: 250 and 500mg.

DOSAGE: Imipenem is infused intravenously. Dosage is given in the next Table:

Dosage of Imipenem

Type or Severity of Infection	Gram-Pos.; Anaerobes; Highly Susceptible Gram-Neg. Organisms	Other Gram-Negative Organisms
Mild	250mg every 6 hours	500mg every 6 hours
Moderate	500mg every 8 hours or 500mg every 6 hours	500mg every 6 hours or 1g every 8 hours
Severe, Life-Threatening	500mg every 6 hours	1g every 8 hours or 1g every 6 hours
Uncomplicated Urinary Tract Infection	250mg every 6 hours	250mg every 6 hours
Complicated Urinary Tract Infection	500mg every 6 hours	500mg every 6 hours

Maximum daily dosage not to exceed 50mg/kg daily or 4g daily, whichever is lower.

Pediatric experience is limited but doses of 50-100mg/kg/day divided in 3 or 4 doses has been used.

IMIPENEM AND CILASTATIN (Cont.)

Impaired Renal Function: The dosage for adults (body weight 70kg) with impaired renal failure is given in the next Table:

Dosage for Adults (Body Wt 70kg) with Impaired Renal Failure

Creatinine Clearance ($ml/min/1.73m^2$)	Less Severe Infections or Presence of Highly Susceptible Organisms	Life Threatening Infections-Maximum Dosage
30-70	500mg every 8 hours	500mg every 6 hrs.
20-30	500mg every 12 hours	500mg every 8 hrs.
0-20	250mg every 12 hours	500mg every 12 hrs.

A supplemental dose of imipenem/cilastatin should be given after each hemodialysis session unless the next dose is scheduled within four hours.

PHARMACOKINETICS: Protein-Binding: 20%; Half-Life: 1 hour; Excretion: Kidney; 70% excreted unchanged. Both imipenem and cilastatin are removed by hemolysis; Distribution: Penetrates into inflamed meninges.

ADVERSE EFFECTS: Imipenem has most of the toxic effects of other beta-lactam antibiotics; adverse effects are given in the next Table:

Adverse Effects of Imipenem

System	Effect
Gastrointestinal	Nausea and vomiting in 4 percent of patients; diarrhea in 3 percent of patients.
Systemic	Hypersensitivity in 3 percent of patients.
Central Nervous System	Seizures in 1.5 percent of patients. Predisposing factors are renal failure and high doses (>2g daily.)
Hematologic	Eosinophilia (4%), neutropenia, thrombocytopenia, positive Coombs test without hemolysis (2%).
Hepatic	Elevated transaminases (2-6%).

Hypersensitivity: Penicillins and imipenem are beta-lactam antibiotics. Almost 50% of individuals who have penicillin-positive skin tests demonstrate reactivity to one or more of the imipenem determinants. It is concluded that imipenem should not be administered to patients with a known or presumed history of immediate hypersensitivity reactions to penicillin, except under the same circumstances and with the same precautions as when administering penicillin itself (Saxon, A. et al., J. Allergy Clin. Immunol. 82, 213-217, 1988).

IMIPRAMINE
(Tofranil)

USES: Imipramine is a tricyclic antidepressant; imipramine is used to treat depressive affective (mood) disorders and functional enuresis (bed wetting) in children.

DOSAGE FORMS: Tabs: 10, 25, 50mg; Caps: 75, 100, 125, 150mg; Vial: 12.5mg/ml

DOSAGE: Administer orally and IM.

Conditions and Dose

Condition	Dose
Depressive Affective (Mood) Disorders	Initially, 75-100mg daily up to 200mg daily for outpatients and 300mg daily for inpatients: maintenance adult dose of 50-150mg daily. Do not terminate drug abruptly. Dosage in adolescent and geriatric patients should be lower; initially, 30-40mg daily; the optimal dosage rarely exceed 100mg daily. Maximum antidepressant effects may not occur for 2 or more weeks after therapy is begun. Child: Initially, 1.5mg/kg daily, increase by 1mg/kg every 3-4 days to maximum 5mg/kg daily. Safety and efficacy in children younger than 12 years has not been established.
Functional Enuresis (Bed Wetting) in Children	Not recommended in children younger than 6 years. Initially, 10-25mg nightly at 1 hr prior to bedtime. If a satisfactory response is not obtained within 1 week, increase dosage gradually to maximum dosage recommended for age (6-8 yrs: 50mg; 8-10yrs: 60mg; 10-12yrs: 70mg; 12-14yrs: 75mg). For early-night bedwetters, 25mg at midafternoon and again at bedtime. After satisfactory response of many weeks, gradually reduce treatment.

ADVERSE EFFECTS: Caution in presence of MAO inhibitors, arrhythmias, glaucoma. May effect sensorium. Use cautiously in patients with cardiovascular diseases, urinary retention, or seizure disorders.

IMMUNE GLOBULIN,IV(IGIV)
(Gamimune N, Sandoglobulin, Gammagard, Venoglobulin-I)

USES: IGIV is used when an immediate increase in circulating immunoglobulin levels is required. It contains at least 90% gamma globulin, IgG; the distribution of the IgG subclasses corresponds to that of normal serum. There are only trace amounts of IgA and IgM. Uses and recommended regimen of IGIV are given in the next Table (Stiehm, E.R., Patient Care, 87-97, Nov.15, 1987; "Innovative Uses of Intravenous Immunoglobulins in Clinical Hematology", Am. J. Med. 83(suppl. 4A), 1-56, Oct. 23, 1987; Berkman, S.A. et al., "Clinical Uses of Intravenous Immunoglobulins," Ann. Int. Med. 112, 278-292, 1990):

Uses and Recommended Regimen of Immune Globulin,IV(IGIV)

Condition	Recommended Regimen
Immunodeficiencies: **Primary antibody deficiencies:** X-linked agammaglobulinemia; Common variable immunodeficiency,etc. **Combined antibody and cellular deficiencies:** Severe combined immunodeficiency; Wiskott-Aldrich syndrome, etc. **Secondary antibody deficiencies:** Nephrotic syndrome; Protein-losing enteropathy, Iatrogenically Induced or Disease-Associated Immunodepression, eg, Major Surgery (Bone Marrow or Cardiac Transplants) or Patients with Hematologic Malignancies, Extensive Burns or Collagen-Vascular Diseases.	Gammagard, 200-400mg/kg once monthly or Gamimune N, 100-200mg/kg once monthly, or max. 400mg/kg; or if necessary more frquently then once monthly or Sandoglobulin, 200mg/kg once monthly, or more frequently. If recurrent infections are present use 400-600mg/kg/month. Venoglobulin-I, 200mg/kg once monthly or more frequently. Increase dose to 300-400mg/kg/month as necessary.
Pediatric AIDS	200-400mg/kg/month
Autoimmune disorders Acute childhood or adult idiopathic thrombocytopenic purpura(ITP)	Gamimune N or Sandoglobulin 400mg/kg/day for 5 days, as needed thereafter; may be used with corticosteroid therapy
Chronic ITP	Same as above; repeat courses as often as needed for up to 6 months
Kawasaki syndrome* (Review: Rowley, A.H. and Shulman, S.T., "What is the Status of IV Gamma-Globulin for Kawasaki Syndrome in the United States and Canada?" Pediatr. Infect. Dis. 7, No.7, 463-466, 1988)	Single dose of 2g/kg more effective than 400mg/kg/day for 4 days, both regimens used aspirin 100mg/kg/day concomitantly (Newburger, J.W. et al., N. Engl. J. Med. 324, 1633-1639, 1991).
Neonatal sepsis* (Clapp, D.W. et al., J. Pediatr., 115, No.6, 973-978, 1989; Noya, F. and Baker, C.,"Intravenously Administered Immune Globulin for Premature Infants: A Time To Wait," J. Pediatr., 115, No.6, 969-971, 1989).	Under investigation; IGIV may be of therapeutic value in certain high-risk, low-birth-weight infants
Cytomegalovirus (CMV) pneumonia* during bone marrow transplant	Several studies indicate IGIV containing CMV antibodies reduces CMV infection and CMV pneumonia during transplant; IGIV not indicated for established CMV infection

*This is not an FDA-recognized indication for this drug.

The chief use of IGIV is in the management of antibody deficiency.

IMMUNE GLOBULIN, IV(IGIV) (Cont.)
DOSAGE FORMS: Immune globulin is a solution, prepared by cold alcohol fractionation of pooled plasma from the blood of at least 1000 individuals. Dosage forms of immune globulin IV are given in the next Table (Stiehm, E.R., Patient Care, pgs. 87-97, Nov. 15, 1987):

Dosage Forms of Immune Globulin IV

Name	Company	Product Form	Comments
Sandoglobulin	Sandoz	3% or 6% in sucrose; 1, 3, or 6g powder*	Introduced in 1984
Gammagard	Hyland Therapeutics	5% in glycine; 2.5 or 5g powder	Introduced in 1986; lowest in IgA
Gamimune N	Cutter Biological	5% in maltose; 10-, 50-, or 100-ml vials	Introduced in 1986

*Lyophilized, reconsitute before use with diluent provided.
DOSAGE: See Table on Uses and Recommended Regimen of Immune Globulin IV.
PHARMOKINETICS: Half-life of IgG: 21-24 days with individual variation.
ADVERSE EFFECTS: Adverse reactions occur in 10% or less of individuals and less than 1% of patients who are not immunodeficient. Most adverse reactions appear to be related to the rate of administration rather than the dose and may be relieved by decreasing the rate of administration or by temporarily stopping the infusion. Mild chest, hip, or back pain; nausea; vomiting; chills; fever; malaise; fatigue; a feeling of faintness or lightheadedness; headache; chest tightness; and dyspnea have been reported.
CONTRAINDICATIONS: Contraindicated in patients who have had an anaphylactic reaction or severe systemic reaction to IGIV and in individuals with selective IgA deficiencies or specific anti-IgA.
PARAMETERS TO MONITOR: Monitor serum IgG levels. The reference range of IgG by age is given in the next Table (Bakerman, S., ABC's of Interpretive Laboratory Data, Interpretive Laboratory Data, Inc., P.O. Box 7066, Greenville, N.C., 27835-7066):

Reference Range for IgG by Age

Age	IgG(mg/dl)
Newborn	1,031±200
1-3 mo.	430±119
4-6 mo.	427±186
7-12 mo.	661±219
13-24 mo.	762±209
25-36 mo.	892±183
3-5 yr.	929±228
6-8 yr.	923±256
9-11 yr.	1,124±235
12-16 yr.	946±124
Adults	1,158±305

IMMUNIZATION

Prior to immunization, informed consent must be obtained from the parent or patient.

The recommended schedule for active immunization of normal infants and children is given in the next Table (MMWR 38, 205-227, 1989; Report of the Committee on Infectious Diseases, American Academy of Pediatrics, 1991 Red Book):

Recommended Immunization Schedule for Normal Infants and Children

Age	Vaccines	Comments
2mo*	DTP-1, OPV-1 HbOC-1 or PRP-OMP-1	Can be given earlier in areas of high endemicity
4mo	DTP-2, OPV-2 HbOC-2 or PRP-OMP-2	6wk to 2mo interval desired between OPV doses to avoid interference.
6mo	DTP-3	An additional dose of OPV at this time is optional for use in high-risk areas.
	HbOC-3	Unnecessary if using PRP-OMP
12mo	PRP-OMP-3	Unnecessary if using HbOC
15mo**	MMR-1, DTP-4, OPV-3	Completion of primary series of DTP and OPV
	HbOC-4	Fourth dose unnecessary if patient has received 3 doses of PRP-OMP. May substitute PRP-OMP or PRP-D for HbOC-4.
4-6yr	DTP-5, OPV-4 MMR-2***	Preferably at or before school entry.
14-16yr	Td#	Repeat every 10yr throughout life.

DTP= Diphtheria and Tetanus Toxoids and Pertussis Vaccine.
OPV= Oral Poliovirus Vaccine.
HbOC=HibTITER (Lederle-Praxis): Haemophilus influenza conjugate vaccine.
PRP-OMP=Pedvax HIB (Merck Sharp and Dohme): Haemophilus influenza conjugate vaccine
PRP-D=ProHIBit (Connaught): Haemophilus influenza conjugate vaccine
MMR=Measles, Mumps and Rubella
*This and other recommended ages should not be considered absolute; 2 months can be 6-10 weeks, for instance.
**Provided at least 6 months have elapsed since DTP-3 or, if fewer than 3 DTPs have been given, at least 6 weeks since last previous dose of DTP or OPV. MMR vaccine should not be delayed just to allow simultaneous administration with DTP and OPV. Administering MMR at 15 months and DTP-4 and OPV-3 at 18 months continues to be an acceptable alternative. During outbreaks, high risk infants may receive measles vaccination as early as 6 months of age with repeat vaccination at 15 months.
***Second MMR vaccine is recommended at 4-6 yrs by the Immunization Practices Advisory Committee (ACIP)(MMWR 38, No. 5-9, 1-18, 1989); Second MMR is recommended at 11-12 yrs by the Committee on Infectious Diseases of The American Academy of Pediatrics (Pediatrics 84, 1110-1113, 1989). Either alternative is acceptable.
#Td=Tetanus and Diphtheria Toxoids Adsorbed (for adult use).

Diphtheria, Tetanus, Pertussis (DTP) Vaccine: DTP is administered to children concomitantly with polio vaccine; for DTP, give five intramuscular doses of 0.5ml each, beginning at two months of age, with succeeding doses at 4, 6, and 15 months and at 4-6 years of age.

Reaction to Diphtheria, Tetanus, Pertussis (DTP) Vaccine: Inadvertent subcutaneous injection can cause local irritation, pain or sterile abscess.

Systemic reactions to DTP vaccine result largely from its pertussis component (whole killed pertussis bacteria, Bordetella pertussis). Some children develop an intense, systemic reaction within 48 hours of vaccine administration; there is persistent crying or screaming, fever and rarely, convulsions and encephalopathy. Children who have a history of these reactions should not be given a booster shot of DTP; booster shots for these children should be diphtheria and tetanus toxoid. About 50% of children develop a local reaction including group A streptococcal abscesses following DTP vaccination (Stetler, H.C. et al., Pediatrics 75, 299-303, 1985); there is no increase in the risk of sudden infant death syndrome (SIDS) after immunization with DTP vaccine (Griffin, M. et al., N. Engl. J. Med. 319, 618-623, 1988).

IMMUNIZATION (Cont.)

Diphtheria toxoid: Diphtheria toxoid (formalin-inactivate corynebacterium diphtheria toxin) causes few adverse reactions; inadvertent subcutaneous injection can cause local irritation, pain or sterile abscess.

Tetanus: Tetanus (formalin-inactivated toxin of Clostridium tetani) seldom results in local reactions. Recurrent abscess formation has been associated with hypersensitivity to tetanus toxoid (Church, J.A. and Richards, W., Pediatrics 75, 899-900, May 1985).

Oral Polio Vaccine (OPV): The oral polio vaccine (OPV), which consists of the attenuated live polioviruses, types I, II, III, is taken orally at the same scheduled times as the DTP shots except the 6 month dose is optional (see schedule in previous Table). Avoid giving OPV to hospitalized patients since virus is shed and could spread to immunocompromised patients.

OPV has gained wider acceptance, as compared to killed virus parenteral formulation, because OPV is cheaper, more easily administered and it was believed that local secretory antibody (IgA) in the gut provided a barrier to infection; however, it has been reported that persistence of circulating antibody is not essential for long-term protection against paralytic poliomyelitis (Cairns Smith, W., Lancet 1, 174, 1985).

Poliomyelitis in the United States is associated with the oral polio vaccine (0.5 to 3.4 cases per million) (Editorial, The Lancet 2, 1309-1310, Dec. 8, 1984).

Measles, Mumps, Rubella (MMR) Vaccine: Measles, mumps, rubella (MMR) vaccine, which consists of live, attenuated vaccines, is reconstituted and 0.5ml (the entire contents of the single-dose vial) is injected subcutaneously at 15 months of age (MMR-1), and a second dose (MMR-2) is recommended at 4-6 yrs by the Immunization Practices Advisory Committee (ACIP)(MMWR 38, No. 5-9, 1-18, 1989) or at 11-12 years of age by the Committee on Infectious Diseases of the American Academy of Pediatrics (Pediatrics 84, 1110-1113, 1989). Either alternative is acceptable.

There has been outbreaks of measles on college campuses. The American College Health Association recommends that colleges and universities require all students born after 1956 to present documentation of immunity to measles and other vaccine-preventable diseases as a prerequisite to matriculation or registration. Outbreaks of measles have also involved preschool age and school age children. These outbreaks involve children who are too young to be vaccinated or have not been vaccinated for other reasons, but may also involve vaccinated individuals who do not mount an appropriate immunologic response (primary vaccine failure)(Markowitz, L.E. et al., "Patterns of Transmission in Measles Outbreaks in the United States, 1985-1986," NEJM 320, No. 2, 75-81, 1989). Secondary vaccine failure is rare (Miller, C., "Live Measles Vaccine: A 21 Year Follow Up," British Med. J. 295, 22-24, 1987). During epidemics of measles, infants as young as 6 months may be vaccinated with repeat vaccination at 15 months. Local health departments should determine when such measures are necessary.

MMR vaccine is associated with local irritation at the site of injection, malaise, sore throat, headache, and low-grade fever.

Measles vaccine is associated with subacute sclerosing panencephalitis (one per million), rashes and local reaction.

Reactions associated with the mumps vaccine are uncommon; they include parotitis, allergic reactions, and rare nervous system manifestations.

Rubella or German measles may cause birth defects in fetuses carried by women who become infected during the first trimester of pregnancy. Rubella vaccine is prepared in human diploid cell culture. The vaccine is produced in different forms: monovalent form (rubella only) and in combinations: measles-rubella (MR); rubella-mumps; and measles, mumps, rubella (MMR). Antibody develops in at least 95% of those vaccinated. Because of the theoretical risk to the fetus, females of childbearing age should receive vaccine only if they are not pregnant and are counseled not to become pregnant for 3 months after vaccination. There were about 225 reported rubella cases in the U.S. and 6 cases of congenital rubella syndrome in 1988. Colleges and universities have become a primary focus for rubella vaccination.

Rubella vaccine is associated with joint pain (40%), lymphadenopathy and, less commonly, a rash; arthritis and arthralgias (30% in children) occur more commonly in adults. (Immunization Practices Advisory Comm., CDC in Ann. Intern. Med. 101, 505-513, 1984).

IMMUNIZATION (Cont.)

Mumps cases in the adult population have increased recently. Although generally a benign disease, a recent study of an outbreak on college campuses (123 cases) reported meningeal involvement (17%) and orchitis (19%) and a hospitalization rate of 6% (Sosin, D.M. et al., Pediatr. 84, No. 5, 779-784, 1989).

Haemophilus Influenza, Type B (Hib) Vaccine: Haemophilus influenzae type B (Hib) is the most common cause of meningitis and epiglottitis, and a leading cause of other infections in children under age 2. Eachyear in the U.S. about one in 1,000 children under 5 years of age develops systemic H. flu disease due to type b; thus, a child's cumulative risk over the first 5 years of life is one in 200. Attack rates peak between 6 months and 1 year of age, and decline thereafter. Epiglottitis occurs mostly in children over the age of 2.

A Haemophilus influenza type b vaccine, derived from the capsular polysaccharide (HbPV), has initially developed. This vaccine was recommended for children 18 months of age and older and four of five studies demonstrated efficacy in the range of 41-88%; one study did not show benefit. This vaccine has been replaced by Haemophilus influenza conjugate vaccines (HbCV) in which the capsular polysaccharide is linked to a protein carrier. This linkage makes the vaccine effective, even when given at 2 months of age. Characteristics and dosing schedules for Haemophilus influenza type b conjugate vaccines is given in the following Table (Committee on Infectious Diseases of the American Academy of Pedatrics, March, 1991):

Characteristics and Dosage of H. Influenza Type b Conjugate Vaccines

Trade Name (Manufacturer)	Carrier Protein	Age-First dose(mo.)	Primary Series	Booster*
HibTITER	CRM197 (non-	2-6	3 doses, 2 mo. apart	15mo.
(Lederle-	toxic mutant	7-11	2 doses, 2 mo. apart	15mo.
Praxis)	diphtheria	12-14	1 dose	15mo.
Abbrev: HbOC	toxin)	15-59	1 dose	None
Pedvax HIB	Neisseria	2-6	2 doses, 2 mo. apart	12mo.
(Merck)	meningitidis	7-11	2 doses, 2 mo. apart	15mo.
Abbrev: PRP-OMP	outer membrane	12-14	1 dose	15mo.
	protein complex	15-59	1 dose	None
ProHIBIT (Cannaught) Abbrev: PRP-D	Diphtheria Toxoid	15-59	1 dose	None

* Booster dose should be at least 2 months after previous dose.

The efficacy of HbCV varies with the particular vaccine used and the population studies. Results of 4 studies estimate efficacy rate of 35-100% (Review: MMWR, "Haemophilus b Conjugate Vaccines for Prevention of Haemophilus Influenzae Type b Disease Among Infants and Children Two Months of Age and Older," 40, No. RR-1, 1-7, January 11, 1991).

Tetanus Prophylaxis in Wound Management: Tetanus prophylaxis in wound management is given in the next Table (Kizer, K.W. and Hawkins, C., Family Practice Reports 3, 149-156, 1984):

Tetanus Prophylaxis in Wound Management

History of Tetanus Immunization (Doses)	Clean Minor Wounds: Tetanus & Diphtheria	Clean Minor Wounds: Tetanus Immune Globulin (TIG)	All Other Wounds: Tetanus & Diphtheria	All Other Wounds: Tetanus Immune Globulin (TIG)
Uncertain	Yes	No	Yes	Yes
0-1	Yes	No	Yes	Yes
2	Yes	No	Yes	No (Yes, if Wound > 24hrs)
3 or More	No(Yes, if >10 yrs. since last dose).	No	No(Yes, if >5 yrs. since last dose).	No

IMMUNIZATION (Cont.)

Immunization for Children Not Immunized in Early Infancy: A schedule for immunization for children not immunized in early infancy is given in the next Table (Report of the Committee on Infectious Diseases, American Academy of Pediatrics, 1991 Red Book, p. 16):

Immunization for Children Not Immunized in Early Infancy

Age	Vaccine	First Visit	2 Months	4 Months	10-16 Months	4-6 Years	11-12 Years
Under 7 yrs. of Age	DTP	Yes	Yes	Yes	Yes	Yes	-
	OPV	Yes	Yes	-	Yes	Yes	-
	MMR	Yes	-	-	-	-	Yes**
	HbCV	Yes	Yes*	-	-	-	-
		First Visit	2 Months	8-14 Months	11-14 Years	17 Years	Every 10 yrs.
7 Years and Over	Td	Yes	Yes	Yes	-	Yes	Yes
	OPV	Yes	Yes	Yes	-	-	-
	MMR	Yes	-	-	Yes**	-	-

* Second HbCV indicated only if first dose received at <15 months.
**Second MMR recommended at 4-6 yrs by Immunization Practices Advisory Committee (ACIP)(MMWR 38, No. 5-9, 1-18, 1989) - see text.
DTP=Diphtheria, Tetanus, Pertussis; OPV=Oral Polio Vaccine; MMR=Measles, Mumps Rubella; Td = Adult tetanus toxoid (full dose) and diphtheria toxoid (reduced dose) for adult use.

Note that pertussis vaccine is not given to children over the age of seven because of adverse effects.

Special Problems in Immunization: Special problems in immunization occur in conditions listed in the next Table (Kizer, K.W. and Hawkins, C., Family Medicine Reports 2, 141-148, 1984):

Conditions Associated with Special Problems in Immunization

Condition	Contraindications	Explanation
Immunosuppression: Medication or Treatment: Corticosteroids; Alkylating Drugs; Antimetabolites & Radiation. Disease(eg, Leukemia, Lymphoma, Generalized Malignancy). Pregnancy	Live Attenuated Vaccines: Polio; Measles, Mumps, Rubella (MMR); Yellow Fever; Vaccinia.	Live Attenuated Vaccine: Induce Immunity by Replicating in the Body and Cause Active Infection; Immunosuppressed Patients may Develop an Uncontrolled Infection; during Pregnancy, Intrauterine Infection may occur with Live Attenuated Vaccines.
Allergies: Eggs	Patients Allergic to Chicken: Influenza Yellow Fever Vaccine, Measles and Mumps Vaccines.	Influenza and Yellow Fever are Grown on Embryonic Eggs; Measles and Mumps Vaccines are Prepared in Chick Cell Cultures.
Neomycin	Patients Allergic to Neomycin: Influenza, Measles, Mumps and Rubella vaccine	Neomycin is used to Prevent Bacterial Contamination During Growth in Culture: Measles, Mumps, and Rubella Vaccine (MMR); Influenza Vaccine
Intercurrent Febrile Illnesses	Intercurrent Febrile Illness	Avoid Additional Adverse Effects
History of Past Immunizations	Previous Reaction	Avoid Serious Reaction

IMMUNIZATION (Cont.)

Immunization of Children with Human Immunodeficiency Virus (HIV) Infection: Recommendations for Immunization of children with HIV infection is given in the next Table (MMWR 37, 181-186, 1988):

Recommendations for Immunization of Children with HIV Infection

Children with symptomatic HIV infection
- Do not give live virus (eg, OPV) or live bacterial (eg BCG) vaccines.
- Do give Adult Td or DTP(diphtheria, tetanus, pertussis), IPV(inactivated polio vaccine)and Hemophilus influenzae type b vaccines as recommended
- Is advisable to give inactivated influenza virus vaccine each year to children over 6 months of age.
- Due to the severity of measles in symptomatic HIV infected individuals and the lack of reported serious adverse effects from MMR vaccination, the World Health Organization (WHO) recommends that this vaccine be administered and Immunization practices Advisory Committee (ACIP) suggest that this vaccine be considered.
- For measles exposure, passive immunization with normal immunoglobulin (IG) is indicated; and for varicella exposure, hyperimmune varicella-zoster immune globulin (VZIG).

Children with asymptomatic HIV infection
- Acceptable to give live MMR vaccine.
- For polio vaccination, use IPV (rather than OPV) since family members may have symptomatic HIV infection.

Children not known to be infected with HIV
- Vaccinate according to standard recommendations of the Immunization Practices Advisory Committee (ACIP).

Children living with someone infected with HIV
- Do not use OPV since the recipient excretes the vaccine viruses, which could be transmitted to the person immunosuppressed by HIV.
- MMR is acceptable because these vaccine viruses cannot be transmitted to household contacts.

National Childhood Vaccine Injury Act; Requirements for Permanent Vaccination Records and for Reporting of Selected Events After Vaccination: Since March 21, 1988, health-care providers who administer certain vaccines and toxoids are required by law to record permanently certain information and to report certain events; reportable events are shown in the next Table (MMWR 37, 197-200, April 8, 1988; JAMA 259, 2527-2528, 1988):

Reportable events following vaccination

Vaccine/Toxoid	Event	Interval from Vaccination
DTP, P, DTP/Polio Combined	A. Anaphylaxis or anaphylactic shock.	24 hours
	B. Encephalopathy (or encephalitis)*.	7 days
	C. Shock-collapse or hypotonic-hyporesponsive collapse*.	7 days
	D. Residual seizure disorder*.	(See Aids to Interpretation*)
	E. Any acute complication or sequela (including death) of above events.	No limit
	F. Events in vaccinees described in manufacturer's package insert as contraindications to additional doses of vaccine#(such as convulsions).	(See package insert)
Measles, Mumps, and Rubella; DT, Td, Tetanus Toxoid	A. Anaphylaxis or anaphylactic shock.	24 hours
	B. Encephalopathy (or encephalitis)*.	15 days for measles, mumps and rubella vaccines; 7 days for DT, Td and T toxoids
	C. Residual seizure disorder*.	(See Aids to Interpretation)
	D. Any acute complication or sequela (including death) of above events.	No limit
	E. Events in vaccinees described in manufacturer's package insert as contraindications to additional doses of vaccine#.	(See package insert).

IMMUNIZATION (Cont.)

Vaccine/Toxoid	Event	Interval from Vaccination
Oral Polio Vaccine	A. Paralytic poliomyelitis	
	- in a non-immunodeficient recipient.	30 days
	- in an immunodeficient recipient	6 months
	- in a vaccine-associated community case.	No limit
	B. Any acute complication or sequela	No limit
	C. Events in vaccinees described in manufacturer's package insert as contraindications to additional doses of vaccine#	(See package insert)
Inactivated Polio Vaccine	A. Anaphylaxis or anaphylactic shock	24 hours
	B. Any acute complication or sequela (including death) of above event.	No limit
	C. Events in vaccinees described in manufacturer's package insert as contraindications to additional doses of vaccine#	

*Refer to original recommendations for Aids to Interpretation.
#The health-care provider must refer to contraindications section of the manufacturer's package insert for each vaccine.

Reportable events applicable to these vaccines are shown in the next Table (MMWR 37, 197-200, April 8, 1988; JAMA 259, 2527-2528, 1988):

Reporting of Events Occurring After Vaccination

	Vaccine Purchased with Public Money	Vaccine Purchased with Private Money
Who Reports:	Health-care provider who administered the vaccine.	Health-care provider who administered the vaccine.
What Products To Report:	DTP, P, Measles, Mumps, Rubella, DT, Td, T, OPV, IPV, and DTP/Polio Combined.	DTP, P, Measles, Mumps Rubella, DT, Td, T, OPV, IPV, and DTP/Polio Combined.
What Reactions To Report:	Events listed in Table 1 including contraindicating reactions specified in manufacturers' package inserts.	Events listed in Table 1 including contraindicating reactions specified in manufacturers' package inserts.
How to Report	Initial report taken by local, county, or state health department. State health department completes CDC form 71.19.	Health-care provider completes Adverse Reaction Report-FDA form 1639 (include interval from vaccination, manufacturer, and lot number on form).
Where to Report:	State health departments send CDC form 71.19 to: MSAEFI/IM (E05) Centers for Disease Control Atlanta, GA 30333	Completed FDA form 1639 is sent to: Food and Drug Administration (HFN-730) Rockville, MD 20857
Where to Obtain Forms:	State health departments.	FDA and publications such as FDA Drug Bulletin.

IMMUNIZATION (Cont.)

Special Circumstances Immunizations: Vaccines, other than those normally give in childhood immunization schedules, are listed in the next Table (Kizer, K.W and Hawkins, C., Family Medicine Reports 2, 149-156, 1984; Eickhoff, T.C., Patient Care, pgs. 137-147, Mar., 30, 1988):

Special Circumstances Immunizations

Vaccine	Indications and Contraindications	Dose/Rate
Hepatitis B Heptavax, an inactivated virus. (Recombivax HB) recombinant vaccine derived from HB_sAg produced in yeast cells.	Indications: All newborn of HBsAg positive mothers; child belonging to an ethnic group at high risk of the disease or if his parents are at high risk, I.V. drug users, homosexual men, hemophiliacs, health care workers (physicians, dentists, nurses, laboratory technicians), inmates and staff members of mental institutions, kidney dialysis patients, heterosexuals with sexually transmitted diseases and natives of Alaska, the Pacific Islands, eastern Asia, and sub-Sahara Africa. Contraindications: None.	All Patients: IM Inject. (upper arm or shoulder) at 0, 1, and 6mos. Adults: 1ml (20mcg) each dose; immunocompromised patients: 2ml (40mcg) each dose. Children: <10 0.5ml (10mcg) each dose.
Influenza Inactivated virus (Fluogen, Fluzone, Influenza Virus Vaccine, Trivalent) whose composition varies form year to year.	Indications: Indicated in patients with chronic cardiovascular or pulmonary disease (eg, asthma), residents of chronic care homes, and medical personnel in contact with high-risk groups; also healthy patients >65 and patients with other chronic diseases including diabetes mellitus, renal dysfunction, hemoglobinopathies or immunosuppression (including AIDS); patients 6 mo.-18 yrs on long-term aspirin therapy due to risk of Reye Syndrome after influenza (MMWR, 39, 1-15, 1990). Contraindications: Egg sensitivity; avoid in first trimester of pregnancy.	<6 mo. - not recommended 6-35mo.-0.25ml split virus IM 1 or 2 doses 3-8 yr.-0.5ml split virus IM 1 or 2 doses >8 yr.-0.5ml whole or split virus IM 1 dose.
Pneumococcal Disease Pneumococcal inactivated-bacteria polysaccharid vaccine containing materials from 23 types of Streptococcus pneumoniae (Pneumovax 23, Pnu-Imune 23)	Indications: Adults with chronic cardiovascular or pulmonary disease; those at increased risk for pneumococcal disease, including patients with anatomic or functional asplenia, cirrhosis, alcoholism, renal failure, nephrotic syndrome, diabetes mellitus, immunocompromised host (including HIV-symptomatic or asymptomatic) and healthy adults age 65 or older (MMWR 38, 64-77, 1989). Contraindications: Pregnancy	0.5ml subcutaneous, or IM should be given to patients 2 yr of age or older. Routine revaccination is not recommended, but should be considered in high risk children and adults (Report of the Committee on Infectious Diseases, Amer Acad. of Pedia. Red Book 376-378, 1991.
Meningococcal Polysaccharide vaccines, against disease caused by Neisseria Meningitidis, A, C, Y and W-135	Indications: Recommendations for vaccine use (MMWR 34, 255-259, May 10, 1985): Control of epidemics due to serogroups represented in the vaccine; high risk groups, eg, individuals with terminal complement component deficiencies and those with anatomic or functional asplenia; travelers to countries recognized as hyperendemic or epidemic disease, eg, Sub-Sahara Africa.	0.5ml subcutaneously

IMMUNIZATION (Cont.)

Vaccinia (Smallpox)	Indications: Laboratory workers occupationally exposed to orthopox viruses.	
Varicella (Chicken Pox) Live attenuated varicella virus	Possible Indications: Healthy children at 12-18 months of age simultaneously administered with MMR and/or susceptible children with cancer, leukemia, or who are undergoing chemotherapy (Isaacs, D. and Menser, M., Lancet 335, 1384-1387, 1990).	Not available

Influenza: In 1990-1991, the prevalent influenza types and strains are expected to be similar to A/Taiwan/1/86(H1N1), A/Shanghai/16/89(H3N2), and B/Yamagata/16/88 vaccine. Amantadine hydrochloride is recommended to reduce the duration and severity of influenza A infection in unvaccinated individuals to control outbreaks in institutions and for prophylaxis in high risk patients (MMWR 39, No. RR-7, 1-15, May 11, 1990).

Varicella (Chicken Pox): Varicella is caused by Herpes virus varicellae, or varicella-zoster virus. Life-threatening complications may occur in patients with varicella (Fleisher, G. et al., Am. J. Dis. Child. 135, 896-899, 1981). A live-virus, attenuated vaccine for varicella has been studied since 1973, but is not currently (August 1990) licensed in the United States. Results in healthy and immunocompromised patients has generally demonstrated good seroconversion rates (94-100%) with persistence of antibody for 10 years. However, leukemic patients on maintenance chemotherapy have had significant reactions, 40% of 372 patients developed a rash, 16 were treated with acyclovir, 4 of whom had a severe febrile reaction (Gershon, A.A. et al., N. Engl. J. Med. 320, 892-897, 1989). Virus in certain lots were less-attenuated and clinical trials with new lots are currently underway. Varicella vaccine is currently being considered for immunization of healthy children, most likely in combination with MMR at 12-18 months of age (Review: Isaacs, D. and Menser, M., Lancet 335, 1384-1387, 1990).

Other Vaccines: Other vaccines, some of which are in various stages of development, are given in the next Table:

Other Vaccines
Bacille Calmette-Guerin (BCG) Vaccine
Malaria (Patarroyo, M. et al., Nature 332, 158, 1988).
Leprosy
Meningococcal Vaccine Serogroup B
Herpes Vaccine
Japanese Encephalitis Vaccine (Hoke, C.H., et al., N. Engl. J. Med. 319, 608-614, 1988; Monath, T.P., N. Engl. J. Med. 319, 641-643, 1988).
Typhoid Vaccine
Cholera Vaccine (Levine, M.M. et al., Lancet 2, 467-470, Aug. 27, 1988).
Yellow Fever Vaccine (MMWR 39, No. RR-6, 1-5, May 4, 1990)
Smallpox Vaccine
Plague Vaccine
Rotavirus (Wright, P.F. et al., Pediatr. 80, 473-480, 1987).

Future vaccines will involve recombinant and synthetic antigens; emphasis will be on control of many different infections with single polyvalent vaccines directed against individual epitopes rather than complex antigens (Hilleman, M.R., Ann. Int. Med. 101, 852-858, 1984).

INDOMETHACIN
(Indocin)

USES: **Indomethacin** is a **nonsteroidal, anti-inflammatory drug** (NSAID); its pharmacologic actions are similar to those of other NSAIDs such as aspirin, phenylbutazone and ibuprofen in that it has **anti-inflammatory**, **antipyretic** and **analgesic activity**.

Indomethacin is also used to close a persistently **patent ductus arteriosus** in premature neonates. Its ability to constrict the patent ductus arteriosus is believed to be due to inhibition of prostaglandin synthesis.

Mechanism of Action: All cells, except nonnucleated erythrocytes, are capable of synthesizing prostaglandins which are released in response to trauma of any kind. The pathological release of prostaglandins which contribute to inflammation, fever, and pain is inhibited by indomethacin. The synthesis of prostaglandins and the inhibition by indomethacin is illustrated in the next Figure (Vane, J. and Botting, R., FASEB J. 1, 89-96, 1987):

Synthesis of Prostaglandins and Inhibition by Indomethacin

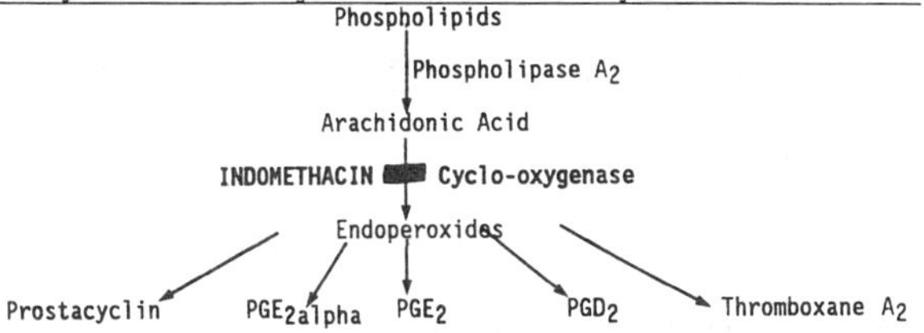

Indomethacin irreversibly aceylates and inactivates cyclooxygenase, an enzyme which catalyzes the formation of prostaglandin precursors (endoperoxides) from arachidonic acid.

PGE_2 may be especially important in the inflammatory process.

In the development of fever, endogenous pyrogen is released from leukocytes and acts directly on the thermoregulatory center in the hypothalamus. This effect is associated with a rise in prostaglandins in the brain. Indomethacin prevents the temperature-rising effects of pyrogens and the rise in brain prostaglandin levels.

DOSAGE FORMS: Caps: 25, 50mg; Extended Release Caps: 75mg; Susp.: 25mg/5ml; Rectal Suppositories: 50mg; IV (for Patent Ductus Arteriosus): 1mg.

DOSAGE: Administer orally or rectally.

Conditions and Dose

Condition	Dose
Inflammatory Conditions: **Rheumatoid Arthritis (moderate to severe); Osteoarthritis; Ankylosing Spondylitis**	Initial, 25mg, 2 or 3 times daily; if well tolerated, may increase dose by 25 or 50mg daily at weekly intervals to max. of 150-200mg daily For extended-release capsules: Initial, 75mg capsules, morning or bedtime; if well tolerated, increase to 75mg twice daily. Expect symptomatic improvement from 4-6 days to up to 1 month
Acute Exacerbations of Chronic Arthritis	Initial, 25 or 50mg daily; if well tolerated, may increase dose by 25 or 50mg daily at weekly intervals to max. of 150-200mg daily
Symptomatic Treatment of Acute Gouty Arthritis	50mg, 3 times daily. When symptoms subside, reduce drug. Relief: Pain, 2-4h; tenderness and heat, 24-36 hrs. swelling, 3-5 days. Extended-release capsules are recommended.
Acute Painful Shoulder (Bursitis and/or Tendinitis)	75-150mg daily in 3 or 4 divided doses. Usual duration of treatment is 7-14 days.
Pericarditis following Myocardial Infarction	75-200mg daily in 3 or 4 divided doses

INDOMETHACIN (Cont.)

Indomethacin in children should be used with great caution; hepatotoxicity has occurred in children being treated for juvenile rheumatoid arthritis. For the management of juvenile rheumatoid arthritis, children 2-14 years of age: initial dose, 2mg/kg daily in divided doses, max. 4mg/kg daily; do not exceed 150-200mg daily.

Treatment of Patent Ductus Arteriosus: Indomethacin sodium trihydrate by IV injection, is used to treat patent ductus arteriosus; the treatment of patent ductus arteriosus is given in the next Table:

Indomethacin Treatment of Patent Ductus Arteriosus in Neonates

First Course:

Initial dose 0.2mg/kg regardless of the neonate's age.

Second dose 12-24 h later; dose depends on age of neonate at time of administration of first dose. For neonates younger than 48 h of age at the time of the first dose, second and third doses of 0.1mg/kg each are used. For neonates 2-7 days of age at the time of the first dose, second and third doses of 0.2mg/kg each are used. For neonates older than 7 days of age at the time of the first dose, second and third doses of 0.25mg/kg each are used.

Third dose 12-24 h later.

If anuria or oliguria, i.e., urine output less than 0.6ml/kg per hour, is present at the time of a second or third dose, the dose should be withheld.

Second Course:

If the ductus remains patent, a second course of indomethacin should be given.

In neonates, monitor renal and hepatic function before and during use.

ADVERSE EFFECTS: Adverse effects of indomethacin are given in the next Table:

Adverse Effects of Indomethacin

System	Effect
Gastrointestinal	Nausea, vomiting, abdominal distress, indigestion, epigastric burning, constipation in 3% to 9% of patients; these effects are decreased by taking the drug with food. Also, single or multiple ulcers of the esophagus, stomach or small intestine with bleeding may occur.
Central Nervous System	Headaches (10% of patients, usually in the morning), vertigo, dizziness, somnolence, depression and fatigue are common. Other adverse effects that occur less commonly are convulsions, peripheral neuropathy, lightheadedness, syncope, confusion, coma and behavior disturbances.
Eye	Corneal deposits and retinal disturbances with prolonged use.
Hematological	Leukopenia, hemolytic or aplastic anemia, purpura, bone marrow depression, agranulocytosis, and thrombocytopenia have rarely occurred. Inhibits platelet aggregation which may lead to bleeding.
Liver	Hepatitis; may be fatal. Monitor AST (SGOT) and ALT (SGPT).
Renal	Acute interstitial nephritis; In neonates, transient decrease in urine output is common.
Electrolytes	Increased serum potassium (occasionally more than 1meq/L increase).
Skin	Rash, pruritis, urticaria
Hypersensitivity Reactions	Dyspnea, acute respiratory distress, hypotension.

PHARMACOKINETICS: Absorption: Rapid and almost complete; Protein-Binding: 90%; Metabolism: Liver; Peak: 3 hours; Half-Life: 5 to 10 hours.

DRUG INTERACTIONS: Drug interactions are given in the next Table:

Drug Interactions of Indomethacin

Drug	Effect
Probenecid	May increase plasma levels of indomethacin
Furosemide	Reduces natriuretic and antihypertensive effect

INSOMNIA, TREATMENT

Hypnotics (Greek,hypnotikos,sleepy,causing sleep) induce sleep. Treatment of insomnia is given in the next Table:

Treatment of Insomnia

Problem	Treatment
Mild Temporary Insomnia	Consider diphenhydramine, e.g. Benadryl 25-50mg at bedtime.
Initiating Sleep	Triazolam (Halcion): 0.25-0.5mg at bedtime; for elderly or debilitated, 0.125-0.25mg. Not recommended for children under 18. Max. one month
Prevent Repeated Awakening During Sleep	Flurazepam (Dalmane):30mg at bedtime; for elderly or debilitated, 15mg. Short-term use only. Not recommended for children under 15.
	Temazepam (Restoril): 15-30mg at bedtime; for elderly or debilitated, 15mg. Short-term use only. Not recommended for children.

The Drugs that are used to treat insomnia are listed in the next Table:

Drugs Used to Treat Insomnia

Over the Counter Drugs: Antihistamines(Non-prescription) Diphenhydramine (Benadryl,Nervine,Nytol,Sleep-Eze3,Sominex2); Doxylamine(Unisom); Pyrilamine(Dormarex)

Benzodiazepines: Triazolam(Halcion); Lorazepam(Ativan); Flurazepam(Dalmane) Temazepam(Restoril); Quazepam(Doral)

Hypnotic Drugs(Prescription): Chloral Hydrate(Noctec and others); Ethchlorvynol(Placidyl); Ethinamate(Valmid); Glutethimide(Doriden); Methyprylon (Noludar)

Barbiturates: Phenobarbital; Amobarbital(Amytal); Pentobarbital(Nembutal) Secobarbital(Seconal)

Antihistamines: Antihistamines, such as diphenhydramine(Benadryl) are also used as hypnotics; they are present in most over-the-counter sleep preparations such as Nervine, Nytol, Sominex. Antihistamines do not cause tolerance or physical dependence.

Benzodiazepines: Benzodiazepines are usually the **drugs of choice** when an antianxiety, sedative or hypnotic action is needed. When drug therapy is indicated to alleviate problems of **initiating sleep** ,triazolam(Halcion) is most effective because of its rapid onset of action and ability to decrease sleep latency. Flurazepam(Dalmane) and temazepan (Restoril) are most effective in **preventing repeated awakenings during sleep** because of the longer duration of their hypnotic effect. Triazolam(Halcion) and temazepam(Restoril) minimize impairment of daytime skills; however, rebound insomnia may occur upon abrupt discontinuance of therapy, especially with triazolam(Halcion) (Bixler, E.O. et al., J. Clin., Pharmacol. 25, 115-124, 1985). Rebound insomnia may be lessened by tapering triazolam (eg, 0.5mg for seven nights, 0.25mg for two nights, 0.125mg for two nights, then off) (Greenblatt, D.J. et al., N. Engl. J. Med. 317, 722-728, 1987). The most widely used benzodiazepine hypnotics arranged in descending order of usage, are as follows: triazolam(Halcion); lorazepam (Ativan); flurazepam(Dalmane); temazepam (Restoril).

Hypnotics: The prescription hypnotics tend to lose their effectiveness with continued use and can cause severe toxicity with overdose. None of these drugs are included in the list of the top 200 prescription drugs.

Barbiturates: Barbituates tend to lose their effectiveness with continued use and can cause severe toxicity.

INSULINS

USES: Insulin is used to control blood glucose levels in patients with insulin-dependent diabetes mellitus (IDDM). Insulin is used to control blood glucose in patients with non-insulin dependent diabetes mellitus (NIDDM) in the conditions listed in the next Table:

Use of Insulin in Non-Insulin Dependent Diabetes Mellitus (NIDDM)
Severely Impaired Renal Function
Severely Impaired Hepatic Function
Stress, eg, Infection; Surgery; Use of Corticosteroid Therapy Concomitantly
During Pregnancy when Blood Glucose Regulation is Required.

Insulin Preparations: Insulin products that are usually available from a hospital pharmacy are given in the next Table; (Physician Bulletin, Pharmacy and Therapeutics Committee, 1/87):

Insulin Products Available at Hospital Pharmacies

Manufacturer	Species	Type	Trade Name
I. HUMAN (purity ≤ 1ppm proinsulin)			
Lilly	Human	Regular	Humulin-R
Lilly	Human	NPH	Humulin-N
Lilly	Human	Lente	Humulin-L
Squibb-Novo	Human	Lente	Novolin-L
II. PURIFIED (purity ≤ 10ppm proinsulin)			
Squibb-Novo	Pork	Regular	Purified Pork
Lilly	Beef	Regular	Iletin II
Squibb-Novo	Pork	NPH	Purified Pork
Lilly	Beef	NPH	Iletin II
Squibb-Novo	Pork	Lente	Purified Pork
Squibb-Novo	Pork	Semilente	Purified Pork
Squibb-Novo	Beef	Ultralente	Purified Beef
Lilly	Pork	PZI	Iletin II
III. CONVENTIONAL (purity ≤ 25ppm proinsulin)			
Lilly	Beef-Pork	Regular	Iletin I
Lilly	Beef-Pork	NPH	Iletin I
Lilly	Beef-Pork	Lente	Iletin I
Lilly	Beef-Pork	Semilente	Iletin I
Lilly	Beef-Pork	PZI	Iletin I

All orders for insulin require the information as listed in the next Table:

Information Required when Ordering Insulin
Manufacturer (Squibb-Novo or Lilly)
Species (Pork, Beef, Beef-Pork, Human)
Type (Regular, NPH, Lente, etc.)
Dose (The word "units" should be spelled out)

Structure of Insulin: Insulin is synthesized as a single-chain precursor, pre-proinsulin which is converted to proinsulin and stored in the beta cells of the islets of Langerhans. Proinsulin has a molecular weight of 9000; it contains 86 amino acids. The structure of proinsulin is shown in the next Figure;

Structure of Proinsulin

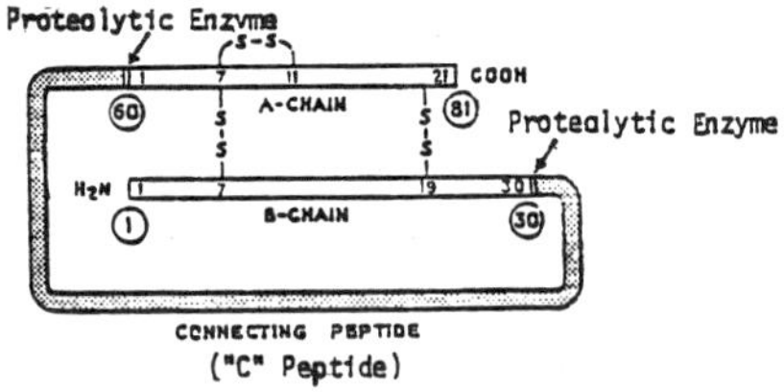

Proinsulin: Proinsuln consists of insulin and a connecting peptide, sometimes called the "C"peptide. This peptide has 31 amino acids. The connecting peptide connects the A and B chains of insulin. The A chain has 21 amino

INSULINS (Cont.)
acids and the B chain has 30 amino acids; thus insulin has a total of 51 amino acids and a molecular weight of 6000. The A and B chains of insulin are held together by disulfide bonds.

Porcine (Pork) Insulin: Porcine insulin differs from human insulin by one amino acid; the C terminal amino acid of the B chain in the human insulin molecule is threonine, while it is alanine in the pig.

Beef Insulin: Beef insulin differs from human insulin by three amino acids: alanine at B30, valine instead of isoleucine at A10 and alanine instead of threonine at A8.

Human Insulin: Human insulin is made either by (1) enzymatic removal of the C-terminal amino acid, alanine, of the B chain of pork insulin and replacing it with threonine which is found in human insulin, or (2) recombinant DNA techniques using E. coli. In the technique of recombinant DNA, synthetic genes for insulin A and B chains are spliced to E. coli genes for beta-galactosidase and joined with sulfide bonds to form the insulin molecule. Alternately, the proinsulin gene may be introduced into E. coli and the resulting proinsulin is then converted to insulin.

Advantages of Human Insulins: The advantages of human insulins are listed in the following Table (Raptis, S. and Dimitriadis, G., "Human Insulin" Clin. Physiol. Biochem. 3, 29-42, 1985):

Advantages of Human Insulin
Lower titers of circulating antibodies are induced
Fewer skin reactions
Absorption more rapid
Degradation at injection site is less

Preparations of human insulins, comparable to conventional insulins, are given in the next Table:

Human Insulins Comparable to Conventional Insulins

Human Insulins	Comparable Conventional Insulins
Humulin R; Novolin R	Regular Iletin I (Lilly); Reg. Insulin (Squibb-Novo); Purified Pork Insulin (Squibb-Novo); Reg. Iletin II (Lilly); Velosulin (Nordisk-USA).
Humulin N; Novolin N	NPH Iletin I (Lilly); NPH Insulin (Squibb-Novo); NPH Iletin II, (Beef or Pork) (Lilly); NPH Purified Pork Isophane Insulin (Squibb-Novo); Insulated NPH (Nordisk-USA); Mixtard (70% NPH Isophane, 30% Reg.) (Nordisk-USA).
Humulin L; Novolin L	Lente Iletin I (Lilly); Lente Insulin (Squibb-Novo); Beef Lente Iletin II (Lilly); Pork Lente Iletin II (Lilly); Lente Purified Pork Insulin (Squibb-Novo).
Humulin U	Ultralente Iletin I (Lilly); Ultralente Insulin (Squibb-Novo); Ultralente Purified Beef Insulin (Squibb-Novo).

When patients do not know what insulin they are taking, human insulin should be prescribed. When switching from non-human to human insulin, dosage should not change unless insulin resistance is suspected.

Flocculation of Human NPH Insulin: Humulin NPH insulin (Lilly) may precipitate in its vial; this occurred in 1 in 72 vials. Flocculation is associated with loss of potency of up to 30%. The manufacturer has changed its procedure for production and the problem may not be as common as reported in this article (Benson, E.A. et al., Diabetes Care 11, 563-566, 1988).

Preparations of insulin available differ by onset, peak effects, and duration of activity. Although insulin preparations vary somewhat, they are generally classified as rapid-, intermediate- or long-acting. Hypoglycemic effects following a single subcutaneous dose are given in the next Table:

Hypoglycemic Effects of Insulin Preparations

Preparation	Onset(hr)	Max. Effect(hr)	Duration(hr)
Rapid Acting			
Insulin (Regular)	0.5-1	2-4	6-8
Prompt Insulin Zinc (Semilente)	1-2	4-10	12-16
Intermediate Acting			
Isophane Insulin (NPH)	1-2	4-12	18-24
Insulin Zinc (Lente)	2-4	6-12	18-24
Long Acting			
Protamine Zinc Insulin	4-8	14-24	28-36
Extended Insulin Zinc (Ultralente)	4-8	10-30	28-36

INSULINS (Cont.)
DOSAGE: Insulin therapy must be individualized. In diabetic ketoacidosis, pediatric dosage is 0.1units/kg/hr (usual range: 0.05-0.14 units/kg/hr) regular insulin IV; adult dosage is generally 5-10units/hr by infusion. Serum glucose values must be monitored to maintain a correction rate of not greater than 100mg/dl hourly.

Maintenance dosage of insulin must be individualized to maintain premeal blood glucose levels of 80-140mg/dl (100-200mg/dl for children <5 years). The usual dose range is 0.5-1 unit/kg/day for children and adults, 0.8-1.2 units/kg/day for adolescents during growth spurt. One method of determining insulin doses in a newly diagnosed diabetic is to calculate a total daily dose, of which two-thirds is given in the morning. Morning dose should be one-third regular and two-thirds NPH. Evening dose is one-third of the total daily dose, of which half is regular and half is NPH.

IODINATED GLYCEROL, CODEINE
(Tussi-Organidin, Others)

USES: **Tussi-Organidin** is used in the treatment of nonproductive **cough.** It contains two components, iodinated glcerol, which acts peripherally, and codeine phosphate which acts centrally.

Iodinated glycerol appears to liquefy thick, tenacious sputum in the same manner as inorganic iodides.

Codeine causes suppression of the cough reflex by a direct effect on the cough center in the medulla of the brain; it appears to have a drying effect on respiratory tract mucosa and increases viscosity of bronchial secretions. It also has mild analgesic and sedative effects.

DOSAGE FORMS: Iodinated glycerol, 30mg and codeine phosphate, 10mg per 5ml.

DOSAGE: Adults: 5-10ml every 4 hours; Children: 2.5-5ml every 4 hours. Do not exceed recommended antitussive dose of codeine: Child: 1.0-1.5mg/kg/day.

ADVERSE EFFECTS: Nausea, vomiting, constipation, drowsiness, acne. Iodism and hypothyroidism may occur with prolonged therapy.

CONTRAINDICATIONS: Pregnancy (Cat.X), lactation, neonates

PRECAUTIONS: Thyroid disease, cystic fibrosis, adolescent acne, increased intracranial pressure, head injury.

INTERACTIONS: Potentiates antithyroid drugs; codeine potentiates alcohol, CNS depressants.

IODINATED GLYCEROL, DEXTROMETHORPHAN
(Tussi-Organidin DM)

USES: **Tussi-Organidin DM** is used in the treatment of nonproductive **cough.** It contain two components, iodinated glycerol which acts peripherally and dextromethorphan which acts centrally.

Iodinated glycerol appears to liquefy thick, tenacious sputum in the same manner as inorganic iodides.

Dextromethorphan depresses the cough reflex and has no expectorant action.

DOSAGE FORMS: Iodinated glycerol 30mg and dextromethorphan HBr 10mg per 5ml.

DOSAGE: Adults: 5-10ml every 4 hours; Children: 2.5-5ml every 4 hours.

ADVERSE EFFECTS: Nausea, vomiting, constipation, drowsiness, acne. Iodism and hypothyroidism may occur with prolonged therapy.

CONTRAINDICATIONS: Pregnancy (Cat.X), lactation, neonates, MAOIs.

PRECAUTIONS: Thyroid disease, cystic fibrosis, adolescent acne.

INTERACTIONS: Potentiates antithyroid drugs.

IPECAC SYRUP

USES: **Ipecac** syrup is used to induce **vomiting** in the early management of acute oral drug overdose and in certain cases of oral poisoning.

Activated charcoal will absorb syrup of ipecac; therefore induce vomiting with ipecac before administering activated charcoal.

Ipecac is contraindicated in patients with depressed level of consciousness due to the risk of aspiration. Ipecac should not be administered to patients who have ingested hydrocarbons (eg, gasoline, kerosene, paint thinner), strong alkali (eg, lye, Drano) or strong acid. Prolonged emesis may occur in some patients with resultant delay in administration of activated charcoal. A poison control center (eg, Rocky Mountain Poison Control Center, 1-800-332-3073), should generally be consulted prior to administration of ipecac.

Mechanism of Action: Ipecac produces emesis by stimulation of the medullary chemoreceptor trigger zone (CTZ) and by irritation of the gastric mucosa. The drug produces regurgitation of the contents from the stomach and upper intestinal tract.

DOSAGE: Dosage of Ipecac is given in the next Table:

Dose of Ipecac by Age

Age	Dose(ml)
6 months-1 year	5-10
1 year-11 years	15
12 years and older	30

Emesis will occur only if stomach is distended with fluid.

ADVERSE EFFECTS: Cardiac toxicity (arrhythmias) GI irritation, prolonged emesis. Chronic abuse, as seen in patients with eating disorders may lead to electrolyte disturbances, myopathy, Mallory-Weiss Syndrome, and other manifestations of chronic vomiting.

IPRATROPIUM

(Atrovent)

USES: Ipratropium is a synthetic analogue of **atropine** and is the first **anticholinergic** drug to be approved by the FDA as a **bronchodilator;** uses are given in the next Table (Gross, N.J., N. Engl. J. Med. 319, 486-494, 1988):

Uses of Ipratropium
Bronchospasm associated with Chronic Bronchitis and Emphysema
Adjunct to other Bronchodilator Therapy, particularly in Status Asthmaticus

Bronchospasm Associated with Chronic Bronchitis and Emphysema: Ipratropium is at least as potent a bronchodilator as adrenergic drugs in the treatment of patients with chronic bronchitis and emphysema. It increases FEV_1 and decreases functional residual capacity (Tashkin, D.P. et al., Am. J. Med. 81, Suppl. 5A, 81-89, 1986; Easton, P.A. et al., N. Engl. J. Med. 315, 735-739, 1986).

Adjunct to Other Bronchodilator Therapy in Status Asthmaticus: The use of adrenergic drugs and ipratropium, either simultaneously or in sequence usually results in greater improvement in airflow than the use of either agent given alone (Bryant, D.H., Chest 88, 24-29, 1985; Ward, M.J. et al., Br. J. Dis. Chest. 79, 374-378, 1985).

Mechanism of Action: Ipratropium is an **anticholinergic bronchodilator;** it is a specific **competitive antagonist of acetylcholine.** Release of acetylcholine at large and medium-sized airways results in smooth-muscle contraction and release of secretions from submucosal glands stimulated by their muscarinic receptors.

Structure of Ipratropium Bromide: The structure of ipratropium bromide is identical to that of atropine except ipratropium is a quaternary ammonium compound while atropine is a tertiary ammonium compound as illustrated in the next Figure:

Ammonium Structures of Ipratropium Bromide and Atropine

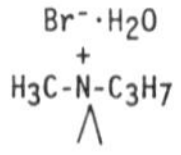

Ipratropium Bromide
Quaternary Ammonium Compound

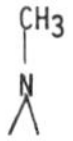

Atropine
Tertiary Ammonium Compound

In atropine, nitrogen has a valence of 3 while in ipratropium bromide, nitrogen has a valence of 5 and carries a positive charge. Therefore, ipratropium is insoluble in lipids but soluble in water as opposed to atropine which is soluble in both lipids and water; ipratropium is nonabsorbable and remains in the airways.

DOSAGE FORMS: The only form in which ipratropium bromide is available in the United States is as a solution delivered by a metered-dose inhaler (18 micrograms per inhalation). Ipratropium is water soluble but insoluble in lipids. Therefore, it acts locally and is not absorbed.

DOSAGE: Adults: Two inhalations (36 micrograms) 4 times daily; max. 12 inhalations/day. Children: Not recommended.

ADVERSE EFFECTS: Ipratropium has minimal side effects because of its relative nonabsorbability due to lipid insolubility. It does not affect respiratory mucociliary clearance, urinary flow, or intraocular tension (Gross, N.J., N. Engl. J. Med. 319, 486-494, 1988). Worsening of narrow-angle glaucoma has been reported.

IRON DEXTRAN
(Imferon)

USES: **Iron** dextran is used in IM or IV treatment of **iron-deficiency anemia.** It is a colloidal solution of ferric hydroxide.

Parenteral iron therapy is rarely necessary as opposed to oral therapy. Parenteral iron therapy may be required in iron-deficient patients in whom administration of oral iron is not feasible or is ineffective. Conditions that may require parenteral iron include oral iron intolerance, poor absorption, G.I. disease, refusal or inability to take oral medication, or when rapid replenishment of iron stores is necessary as in iron deficiency anemia of infancy or the last trimester of pregnancy.

DOSAGE: Dosage of iron dextran is expressed in terms of mg of elemental iron; iron dextran injection contains the equivalent of 50mg of elemental iron per ml. The formula that is used to calculate the iron replacement is as follows:

Wt (kg) x 4.5 x (13.5 - pt's Hg) = mg of Iron
As an example: Wt., 150lbs (68kg); Hg, 6 gms.
68 x 4.5 x (13.5 - 6) = 2295 mg of Iron

For iron replacement secondary to blood loss, that is, patients with hemorrhagic diatheses or patients on long-term renal hemodialysis, the formulas above are not applicable; instead, the following formula, based on the approximation that one ml of normocytic normochronic erythroctyes contains one mg of elemental iron, may be used.

Blood Loss in ml x Hematocrit (as a Decimal Fraction) = mg of Iron.

IV Dosage: Give test dose of 25mg of iron slowly over 5 minutes. Anaphylactic reactions are usually evident within minutes; however, wait for at least one hour after test dose before giving initial dose.

Iron dextran may be injected at a rate not exceeding 50mg of iron per minute (1ml/min). If there are no adverse reactions, subsequent doses may be increased to 100mg of iron daily after 2 or 3 days until the calculated dose has been administered. The total replacement dose has been given over several hours, but increased frequency of adverse effects has been reported, especially delayed reactions such as fever, arthralgia, and myalgia.

IM Dosage: Give test dose of 25mg of iron dextran. Anaphylactic reactions are usually evident within minutes; however, wait for at least one hour before giving initial dose.

Iron dextran may be injected IM daily or less frequently until the calculated amount is given. Use "Z-track" technique for IM administration. The weight of the patient and maximum IM dose are given in the next Table:

Weight and Maximum IM Dose of Iron Dextran

Weight	Dose(mg)
<5.0kg (10 lbs)	25
5.0-10kg (12-20 lbs)	50
10-50kg (20-110 lbs)	100
>50kg (>110 lbs)	250

ADVERSE EFFECTS: Anaphylaxis, sweating, dyspnea, urticaria, itching, arthralgia, myalgia, and febrile episodes, headache, transient paresthesia, faintness, syncope, hypotension, dizziness, seizures, nausea, vomiting, shivering, tachycardia, regional lymphadenopathy, malaise, metallic taste in the mouth, and transient loss of taste perception.

Local reactions are common at the site following IM injection.

Laboratory Test Interferences: Large IV doses (greater than 100mg of iron) may color the serum brown and may cause false elevations of serum bilirubin and false decreases in serum calcium. Serum iron concentrations and total iron-binding capacity are unreliable for 3 weeks following administration of iron dextran. Examination of the bone marrow is not reliable for up to several months following administration of iron dextran.

IRON SALTS

USES: Iron salts are used for the prevention and treatment of **iron deficiency. Causes of iron deficiency** anemia are given in the next Table:

Causes of Iron Deficiency Anemia
Nutritional Iron Deficiency
Chronic Blood Loss, eg, G.I., Uterine, Hookworm
Achlorhydria and Gastrectomy
Defective Absorption, eg, Sprue or Steatorrhea
Increased Demands, eg, Pregnancy

In infants whose diet consists largely of milk, dietary intake of iron is inadequate and prophylactic iron therapy is required. In normal full-term infants, iron stores are usually adequate during the first few months of life, but prophylactic iron therapy should be initiated when the infant is about 3 months of age. In low birthweight infants (less than 3.5kg), prophylactic iron therapy should be started soon after birth. Iron supplemented formulas are usually used for this purpose.

Pregnant women need supplemental iron because of increased physiologic needs.

The laboratory findings in iron deficiency anemia are given in the next Table:

Laboratory Findings in Iron Deficiency Anemia

Test	Finding in Iron Deficiency Anemia
Serum Iron	Decreased
Serum Iron Binding Capacity	Increased
Percent Saturation of Transferrin	Decreased
Serum Ferritin	Decreased

DOSAGE FORMS: (Oral) **Ferrous Fumarate** (33% iron) Susp.; Drops (Feostat): 45mg (15mg iron) per 0.6ml; Susp. (Feostat): 100mg (33mg iron) per 5ml; Tabs: 60mg (20mg iron); 200mg (66mg iron); 325 (107mg iron); Chewable Tabs:100mg (33mg iron); Caps, Extended-Release: 325mg (107mg iron) **Ferrous Gluconate** (12% iron) Caps (Fergon): 435mg (50mg iron); Sol'n. (Fergon): 300mg(35mg iron) per 5ml; Tabs(Fergon): 320mg (37mg iron) **Ferrous Sulfate** (20% iron) (Fergon) Elixir: 300mg(60mg iron)/5ml; 90mg(18mg iron)/5ml(Fer-In-Sol); Tabs: 325mg(65mg iron); Caps (Sustained-release): 250mg (50mg iron); Multiple other preparations.

DOSAGE: Iron salts are given only orally; deaths have occurred on parenteral use of iron salts. Dose of iron in prophylaxis and therapy are given in the next Table:

Dose of Elemental Iron in Prophylaxis and Therapy

Condition	Dose of Elemental Iron
Iron Def. Anemia in Adults	50-100mg daily
Iron Def. Anemia in Children	3-9mg/kg daily in 3 divided doses
Prophylaxis, Pregnant Women	30mg daily
Prophylaxis, Normal Term Infant	1-2mg/kg daily birth until 3 years old
Prophylaxis, Low Birth Weight Infant	2-4mg/kg daily soon after birth

Less G.I. irritation occurs when iron is given with meals. Vitamin C, 200mg per 30mg iron, enhances absorption of iron.

The landmarks in successful treatment with iron deficiency anemia are given in the next Table:

Landmarks in Successful Treatment with Iron of Iron Deficiency Anemia

Landmark	Time
Symptoms	Improve within a few days
Peak Reticulocytosis	5-10 days
Hemoglobin Concentration	Rises after 2-4 weeks
Normal Blood Hemoglobin Level	2 months

In treatment of severe deficiencies, iron therapy should be continued for 6 months.

ADVERSE EFFECTS: Constipation, diarrhea, dark stools, nausea, and/or epigastric pain in approximately 5-20% of patients. G.I. intolerance is a function of the total amount of elemental iron per dose; effects usually subside in a few days. G.I. effects are decreased by ingesting iron after meals instead of between meals. Dilute liquid iron in water or juice to prevent staining of teeth.

IRON SALTS (Cont.)

DRUG INTERACTIONS: Inhibits absorption of tetracyclines from G.I. tract and vice versa; tetracycline should be given 3 hours after or 2 hours before oral iron administration.

Laboratory Test Interferences: Iron preparations cause black feces and may interfere with tests used for detection of occult blood in the stools. Guaiac test occasionally yields false positive test results; benzidine test are usually not affected.

IRON POISONING: Iron is an important cause of accidental poisoning death in children. Contact poison control center immediately (eg, Rocky Mountain Poison Control Center, 1-800-332-3073). Obtain studies as shown in the next Table:

Studies in Iron Poisoning

Laboratory Studies:
- Complete Blood Count(CBC)
- Glucose
- Serum Iron
- Electrolytes
- Urea Nitrogen(BUN)
- Liver Function Tests: SGOT(AST), SGPT(ALT), Serum Bilirubin, Alkaline Phosphatase, Gamma Glutamyl Transpeptidase(GGTP) Prothrombin Time(PT) and Partial Thromboplastin Time(PTT)
- Blood Type and Cross-Match

Radiologic Studies:
- Plain Film of Abdomen

If serum iron is not available, other criteria are used to reflect elevated serum iron level: Significiant vomiting or diarrhea during the first six hours postingestion, a white blood cell count(WBC) greater than 15,000/cu mm, or a serum glucose level greater than 150 mg/dl and the presence of radiopaque material on plain film of the abdomen all correlate highly with an elevated serum iron level (Lacouture, P.G. et al., J. Pediatr. 99, 89-91, 1981).

Ingestion levels (mg of iron ingested/kg body weight) and probable toxicity of iron are given in the next Table:

Ingestion Level of Iron and Probable Toxicity

Ingestion Level(mg/kg Body Weight)	Probable Toxicity
< 20	Non-Toxic
> 20	Potentially toxic

The average lethal dose is about 200 to 250 mg/kg body weight.

The percent elemental iron in the three major forms of iron salts are 33 percent for ferrous fumarate, 20 percent for ferrous sulfate and 12 percent for ferrous gluconate. An estimate of milligrams of elemental iron ingested per kilogram body weight is given by the following formula:

$$\text{Dose(mg/kg of Iron)} = \frac{\text{(No. of Tablets x Iron Salt/Tablet x \%Iron)}}{\text{Wt.(kg)}}$$

Example: 10kg child; 70 Tablets Ferrous Sulfate, 325mg each;
Dose(mg/kg of Iron) = (70 Tablets x 325mg/Tablet x 0.20)/10kg
Dose(mg/kg of Iron) = 455mg of Iron/kg Body Weight

Correlation of peak serum iron levels with potential seriousness of intoxication is given in the next Table; (Henretig, F.M. and Temple, A.R., Clin. Lab. Med. 4, No. 3, 575-586, Sept. 1984):

Serum Iron Levels and Potential Seriousness of Intoxication

Serum Iron(microgram/dl)	Potential Severity
Under 100	Normal
100-350	Minimum Toxicity
>350 or symptomatic	Start Chelation Immediately, call Poison Center.

Peak serum iron levels after ingestion usually occur between two and six hours.

Iron causes a necrotizing gastroenteritis with bleeding and accumulation of blood in the intestinal lumen and bloody diarrhea. After 16-24 hours, the patient may develop metabolic acidosis and shock.

Typically, ingestions occur when 2 year old children get into mother's perinatal vitamins. These pills bear a resemblance to candy, and life-threatening ingestions are not uncommon. Therapy should include gastric lavage and rapid institution of chelation therapy with deferoxamine under the direction of a poison control center (eg, Rocky Mountain Poison Control Center, 1-800-332-3073).

ISOETHARINE

(Bronkosol, Bronchometer, Others)

USES: **Isoetharine** is used as a **bronchodilator** in the symptomatic treatment of bronchial **asthma** and reversible **bronchospasm** which may occur in association with chronic obstructive pulmonary diseases such as chronic bronchitis, pulmonary emphysema and bronchiectasis.

Isoetharine is a synthetic sympathomimetic drug that is similar to isoproterenol, metaproterenol, terbutaline, and albuterol in chemical structure and pharmacologic action. Isoethrane has largely been replaced by terbutaline and albuterol which have a longer duration of action and fewer cardiovascular side effects.

Mechanism of Action: Isoetharine stimulates the beta-receptors to relax bronchial smooth muscle and the smooth muscle of peripheral vasculature; isoetharine has little or no effect on alpha-adrenergic receptors.

DOSAGE FORMS: Aerosol (10, 20ml dispensers): 20 metered doses/ml; each dose contains 340mcg isoetharine; Sol;n: 1% (10mg/ml); other preparations are available.

DOSAGE: Adults: 340-680mcg (1 or 2 inhalations) as often as every 4 hours, more often under medical advice or supervision; Oxygen nebulization:0.25-0.5ml of 1% solution in 2ml of Normal Saline.

ADVERSE EFFECTS: Cardiovascular effects (tachycardia, arrhythmias) and CNS effects (anxiety, tremor, headache) predominate. Paradoxical bronchoconstriction occurs occasionally.

ISOMETHEPTENE MUCATE

(Midrin, Isocom)

USES: Midrin or Isocom is used in the treatment of **migraine headaches**; the manufacturer indicates it may be useful in the treatment of tension and vascular headache.

Isometheptene acts as a cerebral vasoconstrictor and reduces regional cerebral blood flow in migraine patients. Isometheptene is currently classified as "possibly effective" for treatment of migraine headaches by the FDA.

DOSAGE FORMS: Caps. containing isometheptene mucate, 65mg;dichloralphenazone, 100mg and acetaminophen, 325mg.

DOSAGE: Dosage is given in the next Table:

Dosage of Midrin

Condition	Dosage
Migraine Headache	Initially, 2 capsules followed by 1 every hour; max. 5 per 12 hours
Tension Headache	1-2 caps. every 4 hours; max. 8 daily

ADVERSE EFFECTS: Drowsiness, dizziness, weakness, palpitations, rash.

CONTRAINDICATIONS: Hypertension, heart disease, peripheral vascular disease, glaucoma, hepatic disease.

DRUG INTERACTIONS: Coumarin anticoagulants may be potentiated initially. Contraindicated in patients on MAOI therapy.

ISONIAZID
(INH, Lanlazid, Nydrazid)

USES: **Isoniazid** is active only against **Mycobacterium**, e.g., M. tuberculosis, M. bovis, and some strains of M. kansasii.

Isoniazid is used in conjunction with at least one other antituberculosis agent in the treatment of clinical tuberculosis. It is also used in conjunction with other antituberculosis agents in the treatment of diseases caused by other mycobacteria.

For tuberculosis preventive therapy, isoniazid is given alone.

Mechanism of Action: Isoniazid inhibits the synthesis of mycolic acid, a component of mycobacterial cell wall. Isoniazid is bacteriostatic or bactericidal and is active against susceptible bacteria only when they are undergoing cell division.

DOSAGE FORMS: Oral: Sol'n.: 50mg/5ml; Tabs: 50, 100, 300mg; Amp. 100mg/ml

DOSAGE: Usually orally; may be given by IM injection when oral therapy is not possible. The dose of isoniazid, in combination with other antituberculosis drug, is given in the next Table:

Dosage of Isoniazid in Treatment and Prevention of Tuberculosis

Condition	Age	Dosage
Prophylaxis	Adults	5mg/kg/day as a single daily dose; max. 300mg/day; give for 6-12 months. Twelve months is recommended for HIV infected patients and persons with abnormal chest radiographs consistent with past tuberculosis (Advisory Committee for Elimination of Tuberculosis, MMWR 39(RR-8), 1-12, 1990).
Prophylaxis	Infants or Children	10mg/kg/day as a single daily dose; max. 300mg/day; give for 6-9 months (Grossman, M. et al., "Consensus: Management of Tuberculin-Positive Children without Evidence of Disease," Pediatr. Infect. Dis. J. 7(4), 243-246, 1988).
Treatment	Adults	300mg/day; plus rifampin 600mg/day; plus pyrazinamide 30mg/kg body wt. for 8 weeks followed by isoniazid 300mg plus rifampin 600mg for 16 weeks. Ethambutal 15mg/kg is added if patient has had previous isoniazid therapy or had emigrated from a country where drug resistance is common (Combs, D.L., et al., Ann. Int. Med. 112(6), 397-406, 1990) Alternatively, a 62-dose, four-drug, 6-month therapy, much of which is twice weekly(weeks 3-26) is efficacious in patients in whom compliance cannot be assured (Cohn, D.L. et al., Ann. Int. Med. 112(6), 407-415, 1990).
Treatment	Children	INH 10mg/kg/day (max. 300mg) with rifampin 15mg/kg/day (max. 600mg/day) for 4-8 weeks, followed by INH 20-40mg/kg (max. 900mg) and rifampin 10-20mg/kg (max. 600mg) twice weekly with careful supervision for the remainder of 9 month regimen.
		or INH, Rifampin (doses as above) and pyrazinamide 15-30mg/kg with or without a fourth drug depending on extent of disease, for 2 months followed by 4 months of INH and Rifampin. Meningitis should be treated for 9-12 months (Snider, D.E. et al., "Tuberculosis in Children," Pediatr. Infect. Dis. J., 7(4), 271-278, 1988).

PHARMACOKINETICS: Peak: 2 hours. Metabolism: Isoniazid is acetylated. Half-Life: Slow acetylators, 3 hours; fast acetylators, 1 hour.

ADVERSE EFFECTS: CNS: peripheral neuritis usually preceded by paresthesia of the feet and hands. Neurotoxic effects may be prevented or relieved by the administration of 10-50mg of pyridoxine hydrochloride daily during isoniazid therapy; pyridoxine should be administered in malnourished patients.

ISONIAZID (Cont.)
Hepatic: Mild and transient increase in AST(SGOT), ALT(SGPT) and bilirubin occur in approximately 10-20% of patients. The risk of developing hepatitis is <1 per 1000 for patients less than 20 years old; the risk increases with age to 23 per 1000 for patients 50 to 64 years old and 45 per 1000 for patients more than 65 years old (Stead, W.W. et al., Ann. Intern. Med. 107, 843, 1987). Isoniazid should be stopped if patients develop symptoms of hepatitis or when transferase activity increases to three times the upper limit of the reference range.
Sensitivity Reactions: Hypersensitivity reactions have occurred rarely, usually 3-7 weeks following initiation of therapy. If hypersensitivity occurs, discontinue isoniazid immediately. If isoniazid is reinstituted, start with low dose and gradually increase doses; if hypersensitivity reaction occurs, discontinue immediately.
CONTRAINDICATIONS: Liver disease; "active" alcoholism.
LABORATORY TESTS: Liver function tests periodically. Periodic ophthalmologic examinations in patients who develop visual symptoms.
INTERACTIONS: Inhibits metabolism of phenytoin and carbamazepine resulting in elevated serum levels.

ISOPHANE INSULIN SUSPENSION
(NPH Insulin)
USES: **Isophane insulin** is an **intermediate-acting preparation.** Absorption is delayed because the insulin is conjugated with protamine in a complex of reduced isoelectric solubility. This preparation is useful in all forms of diabetes except the initial treatment of diabetes ketoacidosis or in emergencies.
DOSAGE FORMS: 40 Units/ml; 100 Units/ml.
DOSAGE: Subcutaneous (never IV): Dosage must be individualized. Initially, 10 to 20 units (often in combination with regular insulin) 30 to 60 minutes before breakfast. Morning insulin dose (Regular + NPH) usually provides two-thirds of total daily insulin requirements; two-thirds of the A.M. dose is given as NPH, one-third as regular. If needed, a combination of this preparation and regular insulin may be given to provide approximately one-third of the daily amount 30 minutes before the evening meal; PM dose is often half regular, half NPH.
PHARMACOKINETICS: The pharmacokinetics of isophane insulin suspensions are given in the next Table:

Pharmacokinetics of Isophane Insulin Suspensions

			Hours After Subcut. Injection		
Preparation	Source	Purified	Onset	Max. Effect	Duration
Isophane (NPH) 70%, Regular Insulin 30% Mixtard	Porcine	Yes	0.5	4-8	24
NPH Iletin I	Bovine-Porcine	No	2	6-12	18-26
NPH Insulin	Bovine	No	1.5	4-12	24
Beef NPH Iletin II	Bovine	Yes	2	6-12	18-26
Pork NPH Iletin II	Porcine	Yes	2	6-12	18-26
NPH Purified Pork Isophane Insulin	Porcine	Yes	1.5	4-12	24
Insulatard NPH	Porcine	Yes	1.5	4-12	24
Humulin N	Human		1-2	6-12	18-24
Novolin N	Human		1.5	4-12	24

ISOPROTERENOL
(Isuprel and others)

USES: **Isoproterenol** is a synthetic **sympathomimetic** drug which is structurally related to epinephrine but which differs pharmacologically. Isoproterenol is a beta (beta-1 and beta-2) agonist; uses are given in the next Table:

Uses of Isoproterenol
Bronchospasm
Cardiac Arrhythmias, especially bradycardia and complete heart block

Bronchospasm: Isoproterenol stimulates beta-2 receptors of smooth muscle of bronchioles causing bronchodilation; it prevents and relieves brqnchoconstriction. It is used as a bronchodilator in the symptomatic treatment of asthma and reversible bronchospasm which may occur in association with chronic obstructive pulmonary diseases, such as chronic bronchitis, pulmonary emphysema and bronchiectasis.

Cardiac Arrhythmias and Cardiopulmonary Resuscitation: Isoproterenol stimulates beta-1 receptors in the heart causing increasing heart rate and myocardial contractility, enhancing automaticity and conduction velocity.

Isoproterenol is used in patients with second-or third-degree A-V block; it used to maintain heart rate and cardiac output prior to insertion of a pacemaker. It is especially useful for the emergency treatment of Stokes-Adams attacks and is indicated for severe myocardial depression induced by beta-blockers. It is indicated for hemodynamically significant bradycardia resistant to atropine.

DOSAGE FORMS: Inhalation: Isoproterenol is formulated as the hydrochloride or sulfate salt. Preparations are given in the next Table:

Preparations of Isoproterenol for Inhalation

Compound	Preparation	Solution and Concentration
Hydrochloride	Aerosol	120mcg/metered spray 131mcg/metered spray
	Solution for Nebulization	0.25% (1:400)(2.5mg/ml) 0.5% (1:200)(5mg/ml) 1.0% (1:100)(10mg/ml)
Sulfate	Aerosol	0.2% providing 0.080mg/dose

Injection: Isoproterenol Hydrochloride: Solution, 1:5000 (0.2mg/ml) or 1:50,000 (0.02mg/ml).

DOSAGE: Dosage of isoproterenol is given in the next Table:

Dosage of Isoproterenol

Condition	Age	Method	Dosage
Bronchospasm during Acute Asthma Attack	Adults	Metered Dose Inhaler	1 or 2 inhalations of 120 or 131mcg/metered spray 4-6 times daily.
		Nebulizer	2.5-5mg (0.5-1ml of 0.5% solution) in 2-2.5ml Normal Saline Administered over 10-20 minutes.
		IV Bolus	0.01-0.02mg (0.5-1.0ml of 1:50,000 solution). Used rarely due to risk of arrhythmias.
	Children	Metered Dose Inhaler	Used in older children; same as adult dosage.
		Nebulizer	0.05mg/kg/dose diluted to 2-3ml total volume with Normal Saline, administered over 10-20 min.
		IV Drip	0.05-1.5microgram/kg/min. Use lowest dose possible, usually 0.1-0.8microgram/kg/min.
Cardiac Arrhythmias	Adults	IV	2-20microgram/min.
Bradycardia A-V Block	Children	IV	0.05-1.5microgram/kg/min.

ISOPROTERENOL (Cont.)
PHARMACOKINETICS: Inhalation: Onset: 2min; Peak: 3-5 min.; Duration: 30-60 min. Metabolism: Most of the dose is deposited in the oropharynx, swallowed, and metabolized in the gut.

IV Injection: Onset: Immediate; Duration: 8 min. for low dose to 50 min. on high dose. Metabolism: 50% excreted unchanged in urine; 25-35% metabolized by catechol-O-methyltransferase (COMT).
ADVERSE EFFECTS: Sinus and ventricular tachycardia and other arrhythmias, hypotension, tremor, headache and nervousness; refractory bronchial obstruction. Hypokalemia, hyperglycemia and leukocytosis may occur.

Isoproterenol has been noted to cause acute myocardial ischemia in some asthmatic children when administered intravenously. Therefore, continuous monitoring of the ECG and prompt attention to complaints of chest pain or ischemic ECG changes is mandatory whenever this agent is used by an intravenous rate.
DRUG INTERACTIONS: Additive with other sympathomimetics and theophylline.
PRECAUTIONS: Diabetes mellitus, hypertension, coronary insufficiency. Isoproterenol turns red on exposure to air, and patient's saliva and sputum may appear red after oral inhalation. Preparations may contain sulfites which can cause allergic reactions in certain individuals. Isoproterenol may cause potentially fatal reactions in certain patients due to arrhythmias and myocardial insufficiency. Close monitoring is absolutely essential.

ISOSORBIDE DINITRATE
(Isordil, Sorbitrate, Others)
USES: **Isosorbide dinitrate** acts like other nitrates as a **direct-acting vasodilator.** Uses are given in the next Table:

Uses of Isosorbide Dinitrate

Acute Symptomatic Relief of Angina Pectoris
Prevent Acute Attacks of Angina Pectoris
Long-Term Prophylaxis of Angina Pectoris
Refractory Heart Failure
Achalasia or Diffuse Esophageal Spasm

See Nitroglycerine preparations
DOSAGE FORMS: Oral: Caps (extended-release): 40mg; Tabs: 5, 10, 20, 30, 40mg; Tabs (chewable): 5, 10mg; Tabs(extended-release): 40mg; Sublingual (intrabuccal): 2.5, 5, 10mg.
DOSAGE: Dosage of isosorbide dinitrate is given in the next Table:

Dosage of Isosorbide Dinitrate

Condition	Route	Dosage
Acute relief of Angina Pectoris or **Prophylactic Management** in Conditions likely to provoke Angina	Sublingual or Intrabuccally or Chewable Tablet	2.5-10mg. If relief is not attained, additional doses at 5-10 min. intervals; max. is 3 doses in 15-30 min.
Prophylactic Management of Angina	Oral	10-20mg, 3-4 times daily on empty stomach. If headache occurs & cannot be controlled, take oral dose with meals.
	Extended-Release	20 or 40mg every 6-12 hours or 80mg every 8-12 hours.
Heart Failure	Sublingual	5-10mg every 3-4 hours.
	Orally or Chewable Tabs	20-40mg every 4 hours.
Esophageal Spasm	Oral	10-30mg, 4 times daily

PHARMACOKINETICS: The approximate onset and duration of isosorbide dinitrate are given in the next Table:

Onset and Duration of Isosorbide

	Antianginal Effects		Hemodynamic Effects	
Dosage Forms	Onset	Duration	Onset	Duration
Sublingual	within 3 min.	2 hours	within 15-30 min.	1.5-4 hour
Chewable	within 3 min.	0.5-2 hours	5 min.	2-3 hours
Oral	1 hour	5-6 hours	within 20-60 min.	4-6 hours
Extended-Release	30 min.	6-8 hours		

Bioavailability: Tablet: 58%; Extended-Release: 47%; Sublingual: 100%.
ADVERSE EFFECTS: Serious adverse effects are uncommon; adverse effects are mainly cardiovascular, e.g., hypotension and tachycardia; bradycardia is occasionally associated with hypotension and responds to atropine; transient cerebral ischemia may occur. Headache and dizziness may occur.
PRECAUTIONS: Recent myocardial infarction, hypotension, volume depletion, hypertrophic cardiomyopathy. Reduce dose if severe headaches occur. Withdraw gradually. Pregnancy (Cat. C), Lactation.

ISOTRETINOIN
(Accutane)

USES: Isotretinoin the cis form of retinoic acid (vitamin A), is used to treat an especially severe form of cystic or nodular acne designated as acne conglobata or cystic acne.

Acne occurs mainly in puberty and more often in boys than girls; there is a familial tendency.

Acne lesions develop from the sebaceous glands associated with hair follicles; they develop on the face, external auditory meatus, chest, back, and anogenital area. The sebaceous gland contains halocrine cells that secrete triglycerides, fatty acids and sterols; these secretions are known as "sebum."

The main changes in acne are: an increase in sebum secretion; an increase in Propionibacterium acnes bacteria in the duct; an increase in free fatty acids; and inflammation around the sebaceous gland, probably as a result of the release of bacterial enzymes (Buxton, P.K., Brit. Med. J. 296, 41-45, 1988).

The underlying causes of these changes in acne are thought to be hormones and fluid retention. Androgenic hormones increase the size of sebaceous glands and the amount of sebum in both male and female adolescents. In some women with acne, there is lowering of the concentration of sex hormone binding globulin and a subsequent increase in free testosterone concentrations. The premenstrual exacerbation of acne is thought to be due to fluid retention leading to increased hydration of and swelling of the sebaceous duct.

Isotretinoin causes a dramatic reduction in the oiliness of the skin within a month of starting treatment. A four month course of treatment leads to a significant reduction in the number and size of lesions. After treatment has stopped, the benefit continues, resulting in most instances to 80% improvement by about two months afterwards. Rates of relapse are low but some patients require more prolonged treatment or second courses.

Mechanism or Action: Isotretinoin markedly reduces the production of sebum and reduces the size of sebaceous glands by 90% in the first month of treatment. It alters keratinization of the hair follicle, resulting in the reduced formation of comedones. Its anti-inflammatory action is proposed to be due to inhibition of superoxide production and beta-glucuronidase release neutrophiles.

DOSAGE FORMS: Caps: 10, 20 and 40mg.

DOSAGE: Discontinue topical agents, benzoyl peroxide, tretinoin and sulfur; discontinue vitamin A supplements. Give 0.5 to 1mg/kg daily in two divided doses for 15 to 20 weeks. Patients who weigh more than 70kg may require the maximum recommended doses of 2mg/kg/day. The drug should be taken during or after meals.

If the total cyst count has been reduced by more than 70% before 15 to 20 weeks, the drug may be discontinued. If there is recurrence of acne, a second course may be started in two months.

ADVERSE EFFECTS: Teratogenicity: It is estimated that isotretinoin caused 900-1300 birth defects, 700-1000 spontaneous abortions, and 5000 to 7000 induced abortions were performed among women concerned that the drug might have caused malformations of the fetus, since the drug went on the market in 1982 in the United States (JAMA 259, 3225, June 10, 1988). Children born to women who used Accutane during pregnancy have a 25% chance of suffering birth defects; in a study of women who became pregnant while undergoing Accutane treatment, 20% aborted spontaneously; 20% of the remaining gave birth to babies who had at least one major birth defect (Science 240, 714-715, 1988).

Some countries have greater controls on distributions in the United Kingdom, only dermatologists are certified to prescribe the drug. Sweden requires doctors to submit a special request to the government to prescribe it.

Several proposals have been made to better control distribution of the drug in the United States; these include making the drug available only through Board-certified dermatologists or particular medical centers; informed consent by patient, and arrangements for patients to visit an obstetrician - gynecologist to rule out pregnancy and receive contraception counseling are necessary prior to initiating therapy.

ISOTRETINOIN (Cont.)

Other adverse effects of isotretinoin are given in the next Table (Murphy, G.M. and Greaves, M.W., Brit. Med. J. 296, 546-548, Feb. 20, 1988).

Adverse Effects of Isotretinoin Other than Teratogenecity

Mucocutaneous	Musculoskeletal	Ophthalmological	Miscellaneous
Cheilitis	Arthralgia	Papilledema, intracranial hypertension	Hepatotoxicity
Dryness of mucous membranes	Disseminated idiopathic skeletal hyperostosis	Night blindness	Hyperlipidemia
Epistaxis	Premature fusion of epiphyses		
Blepharoconjunctivitis	Muscle stiffness		
Dermatitis			
Palmoplantar desquamation			
Photosensitivity			
Paronychia, shedding of nails			
Diffuse hair loss			

CONTRAINDICATIONS: The drug is contraindicated in women who are pregnant or unwilling to prevent pregnancy while under treatment. Report exposures in pregnant women by calling collect to Roche (201) 235-3021.

PHARMACOKINETICS: Peak: 1-4 hours; Protein Binding: 100% to plasma albumin; Half-Life: 10 hours; Excretion: biliary tract.

JOINTS, PATHOGENS, TREATMENT

Pathogens: The pathogens that are most likely to cause infection of joints are given in the next Table (Handbook of Antimicrobial Therapy, The Medical Letter, 1990; Goldenberg, D.L. and Reed, J.I., N. Engl. J. Med. 312, 764-771, 1985):

Pathogens Causing Infection of Joints

1. Staphlococcus aureus
2. Streptococcus pyogenes (Group A)
3. Neisseria gonorrhoeae
4. Gram-negative bacilli
5. Streptococcus pneumoniae
6. Neisseria meningitidis
7. Haemophilus influenzae (in children)
8. Mycobacterium tuberculosis and other Mycobacteria
9. Fungi
10. Borrelia burgdorf (Lyme Disease)

Viral causes include rubella, hepatitis B, mumps, parvovirus, and lymphocytic choriomeningitis virus (Smith, J.W., Inf. Dis. Clin. N.A. 4, 523-539, 1990).

Acute bacterial arthritis is most often the result of bacteremia; the causes of septic arthritis, with age of patient, are given in the next Table (Parker, R.H. in Infectious Diseases, Hoeprich, P.D., ed., Harper and Row, Publishers, N.Y., First Ed., 1972, pg. 1204):

Bacterial Causes of Bacterial Arthritis and Age

Organism	Age(years) <2 (%)	2-15 (%)	16-50 (%)	>50 (%)
Staphylococcus Aureus	40	50	15	75
Streptococcus Pyogenes	15	25	5	5
Streptococcus Pneumoniae	10	10		5
Haemophilus Influenzae	30	2		
Neisseria Gonorrhoeae		5	75	
Enterobacteriaceae and Pseudomonas	3	5	5	10
Other	2	3	-	5

In children, the most common causes of septic arthritis are Staphylococcus aureus, Streptococcus pyogenes, Streptococcus pneumoniae and H. influenzae. In adults, the most common cause of septic arthritis is Neisseria gonorrhoeae. In older adults the most common cause is Staphylococcus aureus.

Tuberculous Arthritis: Tuberculous arthritis is usually associated with osteomyelitis.

In the elderly, patients with septic arthritis usually have preexisting joint disease, eg, osteoarthritis, rheumatoid arthritis, or prior trauma to the joint (McGuire, N.M. and Kaufman, C.A., J. Am. Ger. Soc. 33, 170, 1985).

JOINTS, PATHOGENS, TREATMENT (Cont.)
Treatment: Antimicrobial treatment based on etiology is given in the next Table:

Antimicrobial Therapy of Arthritis Based on Etiology

Organism	Drug Treatment
Staphylococcus aureus	Parenteral nafcillin or oxacillin plus aminoglycoside. Vancomycin is used in patients allergic to penicillin.
Neisseria gonorrhoeae	Parenteral 3rd generation cephalosporin: ceftriaxone, cefotaxime or ceftizoxime. Allergic patients should be treated with spectinomycin. Penicillin-sensitive organisms may be treated with ampicillin.
Streptococcus pyogenes or pneumoniae	Penicillin G, parenterally
Haemophilus influenzae	Third-generation cephalosporins, eg, cefotaxime, or ceftriaxone

Empiric antimicrobial treatment based on clinical presentation is given in the next Table (Smith, J.W., Inf. Dis. Clin. N.A. 4, 523-539, 1990):

Antimicrobial Therapy of Arthritis Based on Clinical Presentation

Condition	Drug Treatment
Adult, underlying joint or other disease	Cefuroxime 1.5g IV q8h or Nafcillin 2g IV q6h.
End stage renal disease on dialysis	Vancomycin 1g IV every 7 days.
Recent surgery in hospital with known MRSA	Vancomycin 1g IV q12h.
Urinary tract infection and sepsis	Cefotaxime 2g IV q6h or ceftazidime 2g IV q8h.

MRSA = Methicillin-resistant staphylococcus aureus.

KANAMYCIN

(Kantrex)

USES: **Kanamycin** is an **aminoglycoside** antibiotic(gentamicin, streptomycin, amikacin, tobramycin, kanamycin, netilmicin, sisomicin) and is used in hospitals for parenteral treatment of patients who have serious infections caused by **aerobic gram-negative bacilli** (eg, a number of the Enterobacteriaceae, P. aeruginosa). Activities of kanamycin are given in the next Table (Pancoast, S.J., Med. Clin. No. Am. 72, 581-612, May, 1988; Adams, H.G., Personal Comm.):

Activities of Kanamycin

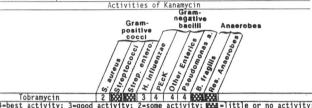

	Gram-positive cocci			Gram-negative bacilli				Anaerobes	
	S. aureus	Streptococci	Strep. entero.	H. influenzae	PEcK	Other Enterics	Pseudomonas a.	B. fragilis	Res. Anaerobes
Tobramycin	2	▩	▩	3	4	4	4	▩	▩

4=best activity; 3=good activity; 2=some activity; ▩=little or no activity;
PEcK (Mnemonic)= P. mirabilis, E. coli, Klebsiella; Res.= Resident

The major useful bacterial spectrum of kanamycin is given in the next Table:

Bacterial Spectrum of Kanamycin

Enterobacteriaceae: Escherichia coli, Klebsiella, Enterobacter and Serratia species, Proteus mirabilis, indole-positive Proteus (Providencia rettgeri, Morganella morganii, Proteus vulgaris), Providencia stuartii and Citrobacter species. Salmonella and Shigella species are usually susceptible but other effective and less toxic antibiotics are used.

Pseudomonas aeruginosa: (Note: Tobramycin is most effective). Aminoglycosides are usually combined with a penicillin, eg, carbenicillin, or cephalosporin, eg, ceftazidime.

Enterococci, eg, Streptococcus faecalis: Gentamicin plus penicillin G or ampicillin is frequently treatment of choice for enterococcal endocarditis (synergistic effect).

Prophylaxis of Endocarditis: Gentamicin plus ampicillin is the standard parenteral regimen for high risk patients.

Staphylococci, eg, S. aureus and S. epidermidis

Kanamycin is used to treat susceptible organisms involving the following tissue: lower respiratory tract, intra-abdominal, soft tissue, bone or joint, wound, and complicated urinary tract infections, bacteremias, and meningitis. Kanamycin may be used parenterally in combination with at least one other antituberculosis agent for treatment of tuberculosis or other mycobacterial diseases, but streptomycin is more commonly used. As with other aminoglycosides, kanamycin's penetration of CSF is unpredictable. Kanamycin has been used orally for preoperative intestinal antisepsis.

Mechanism of Action: The mechanism of action of kanamycin is like other aminoglycosides in that it binds to the bacterial 30S ribosomal subunit to produce a non-functional 70S initiation complex that results in the inhibition of bacterial cell protein synthesis and misreading of the genetic code.

DOSAGE FORMS: Oral: Caps: 500mg; Inj (IV or IM): 37.5, 250, 333mg/ml.

KANAMYCIN (Cont.)

DOSAGE: When kanamycin is administered by IM injection or IV infusion, the dosage is identical. IV infusion should be administered over 30-60 minutes. Dosage is given in the next Table:

Dosage of Kanamycin

Condition	Age	Route	Dosage
Usual	Adults	IM or IV	15mg/kg daily in equally divided doses at 8- or 12-hour intervals max. 1.5gm daily.
	Infants Children	IM or IV	15-30mg/kg daily in equally divided doses at 8- or 12-hour intervals max. 1.5gm daily.
	Neonates <2kg; <7d	IM or IV	15mg/kg daily in equally divided doses at 12-hour intervals.
	Neonates <2kg; >7d	IM or IV	22.5mg/kg daily in equally divided doses at 8-hour intervals.
	Neonates >2kg; <7d	IM or IV	20mg/kg daily in equally divided doses at 12-hour intervals.
	Neonates >2kg; >7d	IM or IV	30mg/kg daily in equally divided doses at 8-hour intervals.
Hepatic Encephalopathy	Adults	Oral	8-12gm daily in divided doses.
Intestinal Antisepsis	Adults	Oral	1gm orally every hour for 4 hours, then 1gm every 6 hours for 36-72 hours.
	Children	Oral	150-250mg/kg daily in equally divided doses every 6 hours; max. 4gm daily

Dosage Adjustment in Renal Failure: When serum kanamycin concentrations cannot be measured, dosage guidelines based on predictive nomograms are used (Sarubbi, F.A., Jr. and Hull, J.H., Ann. Intern. Med. 89, 612-618, 1978).

(1) Loading Dose: The usual loading dose for kanamycin is 5-7.5mg/kg (ideal weight) for expected peak serum level of 15 to 30mcg/ml.

(2) Calculate creatinine clearance using the formula:

$$\text{Creatinine Clearance(Male)} = \frac{\text{Wt. } (140 - \text{age})}{(72)(\text{serum creatinine})};\quad \text{Wt.=Lean Body Weight}$$

$$\text{Creatinine Clearance(Female)} = \frac{\text{Wt. } (140 - \text{age})}{(72)(\text{serum creatinine})} \times 0.85$$

(3) Select maintenance dose (as percentage of chosen loading dose) to continue peak serum concentrations indicated above according to desired dosing interval and the patients corrected creatinine clearance as given in the next Table:

KANAMYCIN (Cont.)

Percentage of Loading Dose Required for Dosage Interval Selected				
C(c)cr (ml/min)	Half-Life* (hours)	8 hours	12 hours	24 hours
90	3.1	84%	-	-
80	3.4	80	91%	-
70	3.9	76	88	-
60	4.5	71	84	-
50	5.3	65	79	-
40	6.5	57	72	92%
30	8.4	48	63	86
25	9.9	43	57	81
20	11.9	37	50	75
17	13.6	33	46	70
15	15.1	31	42	67
12	17.9	27	37	61
10**	20.4	24	34	56
7	25.9	19	28	47
5	31.5	16	23	41
2	46.8	11	16	30
0	69.3	8	11	21

*Alternatively, one-half of the chosen loading dose may be given at an interval approximately equal to the estimated half-life.
**Dosing for patients with C(c)cr<10 ml/min should be assisted by measured serum levels. From Sarubbi, F.A., Jr. and Hull, J.H., Ann. Intern. Med. 89, 612-618, 1978.

ADVERSE EFFECTS: Toxicity and untoward effects are listed in the next Table (Edson, R.S. and Keys, T.F., Mayo Clin. Proc. 58, 99-102, 1983):

Toxicity of Kanamycin

Major:
- **Renal Toxicity**
- **Vestibular Toxicity**
- **Auditory Toxicity**
- **Neuromuscular Blockade**

Minor: Skin Rash, Drug-Induced Fever

The three main toxic side effects of kanamycin are ototoxicity, nephrotoxicity, and neuromuscular blockage (Smith, C.R. et al., N. Engl. J. Med. 302, 1106, May 15, 1980); it is important to control the dose given by monitoring peak and trough levels of the drug, particularly in patients with any degree of renal failure. As renal function declines, drug half-life increases to up to 50 hours.

Nephrotoxicity is usually mild. Irreversible ototoxicity may occur; both the hearing (cochlear) and equilibrium (vestibular) functions may be affected.

Electrolyte disturbances are given in the next Table:

Electrolyte Disturbances

Hypomagnesemia
Hypocalcemia
Hypokalemia

Hypomagnesemia (<1.6mg/dl) is observed in almost 40% of patients; hypocalcemia and hypokalemia may also occur. It may be advisable to monitor serum magnesium and use replacement therapy (Zaloga, G.P. et al., Surg. Gynecol. Obstet. 158, 561-565, 1984).

PHARMACOKINETICS: Peak Values: 15-30mcg/ml; Trough: <5-10mcg/ml; Half-Life: 2-4 hours. Time to steady state and time to peak concentration may be significantly prolonged in patients with renal dysfunction.

Kanamycin is eliminated exclusively by renal excretion; excessive serum concentrations may occur and lead to further renal impairment. The renal damage is to the renal proximal tubules and is usually reversible if discovered early.

KANAMYCIN (Cont.)

MONITOR: Monitor the parameters given in the next Table:

Monitor Parameters, Kanamycin Treatment

Parameter	Comment
Serum Kanamycin Levels	Initially and every 2-3 days during therapy
Serum Creatinine or BUN	Before and every 2-3 days during therapy
Audiograms	Baseline and weekly in patients with pre-existing renal, auditory or vestibular impairment or in patients who receive prolonged, high-dose therapy
Tinnitus or Vertigo	Daily

Serum Kanamycin Levels: Red top tube, separate serum and freeze. Obtain serum specimens as follows:
(1) 24-48 hours after starting therapy if loading dose is not given.
(2) 5 to 30 minutes before I.V. kanamycin (trough).
(3) 30 minutes after a 30 minute I.V. infusion of kanamycin (peak).
I.M. administration: 30 minutes to one hour.

Heparinized tubes should not be used to collect specimens.

The first serum level of kanamycin is obtained when kanamycin has reached steady-state serum concentrations; steady-state is reached in 24 to 48 hours after starting therapy if the patient has not received a loading dose (steady state = 5-7 drug half-lives; half-life of kanamycin is 2 to 4 hours). The following times should be recorded on the laboratory requisition form and on the patient's chart:

Trough Specimen Drawn ______(Time) (5 to 30 minutes before Kanamycin)
Kanamycin Started ______(Time) (30 minutes I.V. infusion)
Kanamycin Completed ______(Time)
Peak Specimen Drawn ______(Time) (30 minutes after I.V. Kanamycin)

DRUG INTERACTIONS: High concentrations of beta-lactam antibiotics inactive aminoglycosides (gentamicin, streptomycin, amikacin, tobramycin & kanamycin); to reduce this interaction, specimens containing both classes of antibiotics should either be assayed immediately using a rapid method or stored frozen. Drug interactions with kanamycin are given in the next Table:

Drug Interactions with Kanamycin

Drug	Effect
Other Aminoglycosides, Amphotericin B, Bacitracin, Cephalosporins, Colistin, Cisplatin, Methylflurane, Polymyxin B, Vancomycin	Drugs associated with renal toxicity, ototoxicity and neurotoxicity may be additive with similar toxic effects of kanamycin.
General Anaesthetics and Neuromuscular Blocking Agents, eg, Succinylcholine and Tubocurarine	May potentiate neuromuscular blockage of kanamycin and cause respiratory paralysis.

KETAMINE

(Ketalar)

USES: Ketamine is a **dissociative anesthetic agent.** Although ketamine has been largely replaced by other agents, it may be used in particular circumstances such as emergency surgery, dressing changes, radiologic procedures in children, and some cardiac surgical procedures (eg, cardiac catheterization). The major disadvantage of ketamine is that emergence reactions (see Adverse Effects) and psychological manifestations occur in nearly half of adults over 30 years old. Ketamine provides good analgesia and amnesia. The major advantage of ketamine is that respiration is not usually depressed, and may be stimulated. Pharyngeal and laryngeal reflexes are preserved; hypoxic and hypercarbic stimulation of respiration is not affected. Pulmonary vascular resistance and hypoxic pulmonary vasoconstriction are not affected. Children and the elderly are less prone to emergence reactions.

DOSAGE FORMS: Injection: 10, 50mg/ml; 100mg/ml must be diluted 1:1.

DOSAGE: Ketamine is administered parenterally. Dosage is given in the next Table:

Dosage of Ketamine

Age	Route	Dosage
Adults Children	IV	2-3mg/kg over 1 minute; repeat half of induction dose as needed.
	IM	5-7mg/kg; up to 13mg/kg may be required.

PHARMACOKINETICS: Half-Life: 1.8-2.8 hours; Onset of Action: IV: 1 minute; IM: 3-4 minutes; Duration of Analgesia: up to 40 minutes.

ADVERSE EFFECTS: CNS: Emergence reactions occur more commonly in adults over 30 years, less commonly in children and geriatric patients. Reactions range from nightmares to delirium to hallucinations and may recur up to weeks later. Minimize reactions by prior administration of a benzodiazepine. Cardiovascular: Ketamine causes myocardial depression in vitro, but increased sympathetic activity leading to increased blood pressure, heart rate, and cardiac output in vivo. Use with caution or not at all in patients with underlying cardiovascular disease. Hypotension may occur in hypovolemic patients. Musculoskeletal: Increased muscle tone may resemble seizures.

KETOCONAZOLE

(Nizoral)

USES: Ketoconazole is an **antifungal agent** with a broad spectrum of activity. It is not useful for treatment of meningitis since CSF concentrations are unpredictable. Uses of ketoconazole are given in the following Table:

Uses of Ketoconazole
Coccidioidomycosis - Pulmonary or Disseminated
Paracoccidioidomycosis - Pulmonary or Disseminated
Histoplasmosis - Pulmonary or Disseminated
Candidiasis - Oral and/or Esophageal, Candiduria, or Chronic Mucocutaneous Candidiasis
Chromomycosis
Blastomycosis
Cryptococcosis(?)
Dermatophyte Infections - Tinea corporis, T. cruris, T. pedis, etc.

Ketoconazole is generally considered a second-line or adjunct therapy to amphotericin B.

Mechanism of Action: Ketoconazole may be fungistatic or fungicidal. Ketoconazole alters cell membranes leading to changes in permeability with secondary metabolic effects, as well as growth inhibition.

DOSAGE FORMS: Tabs: 200mg.

DOSAGE: Ketoconazole is administered orally. Dosage is given in the following Table:

Dosage of Ketoconazole

Condition	Dosage
Usual	200mg daily as a single dose
Severe Infections	400mg-1.6g daily
Children >2 years	3.3-6.6mg/kg/day

Patients with achlorhydria (eg, AIDS gastropathy) absorb ketoconazole poorly; in these patients, the drug should be taken with 200ml of 0.1N hydrochloric acid.

KETOCONAZOLE (Cont.)
PHARMACOKINETICS: Oral Absorption: 1-4 hrs; increased pH decreases absorption; CNS Penetration: unpredictable; Protein Binding: 85-99%; Half-Life: initial, 2 hrs; terminal, 8 hrs; Metabolism: liver; Elimination: bile.
ADVERSE EFFECTS: GI(3-10%): nausea, vomiting; rarely, GI bleeding; transient transaminase elevation and rarely, hepatotoxicity. Endocrine: gynecomastia, adrenocortical insufficiency occurs rarely.
DRUG INTERACTIONS: Severe hypoglycemia may occur with concomitant oral sulfonylurea hypoglycemic agents; phenytoin metabolism may be affected; cyclosporin levels are increased coumarin effects are increased. Drugs which increase gastric acidity (antacids, H_2 antagonists, antimuscarinics) may decrease ketoconazole absorption.

Rifampin may interfere with ketoconazole absorption and increase its metabolism; the manufacturer recommends against concomitant administration of these drugs.

KETOROLAC TROMETHAMINE
(Toradol)
USES: **Ketorolac tromethamine** is a **nonsteroidal anti-inflammatory drug** with analgesic, anti-inflammatory, and antipyretic activities and inhibits prostaglandin synthesis. Ketorolac tromethamine is a relatively new drug and clinical applications have not been fully defined. Uses based on limited clinical trials are given in the next Table:

Uses of Ketorolac Tromethamine
Moderate to Severe Pain Following Surgery
Post Gynecologic Surgery
Post Orthopedic Surgery
Post Abdominal Surgery

Ketorolac tromethamine compares favorably to morphine for pain relief following major surgery (Yee, J.P. et al., Pharmacotherapy 6, 253-261, 1986; O'Hara, D.A. et al., Clin. Pharmacol. Ther. 41, 556-561, 1987).
DOSAGE FORMS: Intramuscular Injection: 15, 30mg/ml.
DOSAGE: Although ketorolac can be given orally, this dosage form is not currently available. Ketorolac is available for intramuscular administration. Dosage is given in the following Table:

Dosage of Ketorolac

Condition	Dosage
Moderate to Severe Pain	Initially 30-60mg IM, followed by 15-30mg IM every 6 hours as needed. Max. daily dose: 150mg on the first day, 120mg on subsequent days.

PHARMACOKINETICS: Absorption: 100% bioavailability after IM administration; Time to Peak Plasma Level: 30-60 minutes; Half-Life: 3.8-6.3 hours (young adults), 4.7-8.6 hours (elderly); Plasma Protein Binding: 99%; Metabolism: Liver; Excretion: Kidney.
ADVERSE EFFECTS: Adverse effects are similar to other NSAIDs. Respiratory depression does not occur. Gastrointestinal effects (3-9%): nausea, dyspepsia, abdominal pain; CNS effects: drowsiness, dizziness, headache; Liver effects (15%): mild elevation of transaminases. Hematologic: Bleeding time may be prolonged. GI tract ulceration occurs occasionally.
DRUG INTERACTIONS: Drug interactions have not been fully described. Ketorolac does not alter warfarin or digoxin binding to a significant extent.

LABETALOL

(Normodyne, Trandate)

USES: **Labetalol** is used to treat patients with **hypertension;** it is a **Step 2** drug. Its antihypertensive effect may be equivalent to that of a beta blocker and vasodilator combined and thus may obviate the need for a third drug.

Mechanism of Action: Labetalol is a competitive antagonist at both alpha- and beta-adrenergic receptor sites but the beta-blocking action predominates. The alpha or beta-1 blocking properties of labetalol varies with route of administration; oral therapy results in an alpha:beta-1 ratio of 1:3 whereas with IV therapy, this ratio is 1:6. The physiologic response to oral and IV therapy may differ.

Blockage of cardiac (beta-1) receptors reduces heart rate and myocardial contractility, thus reducing cardiac output. The atrioventricular (AV) conduction time is slowed and automaticity is suppressed.

Following short-term administration, the antihypertensive effect of labetalol is largely due to vasodilation; vasodilation is secondary to blockage of alpha receptors on smooth muscle of blood vessels.

DOSAGE FORMS: Tabs: 100, 200 and 300mg; Solution for IV Use: 5mg/ml.

DOSAGE: Dosage of labetalol is given in the next Table:

Dosage of Labetalol

Condition	Route	Dosage
Mild to Severe Hypertension	Oral	Initially, 100mg twice daily. Usual maintenance dose for mild to moderate hypertension: 400-800mg daily. Maintenance dose for severe hypertension: up to 1.2-2.4g daily in two to three divided doses. Concomitant diuretic therapy enhances the therapeutic response.
Hypertensive Crisis	IV	Patient supine; monitor blood pressure; avoid rapid reduction of systolic or diastolic b.p. Initially, give 20mg by slow IV injection over a two-minute period. Additional injections of 40 or 80mg can be given at 10-minute intervals until the desired supine blood pressure is achieved or to a total dose of 300mg. Alternately, give labetalol by slow continuous IV at a rate of 0.5-2.5mg/min. Adjust rate of infusion according to blood pressure response.
Pediatric Usage	Oral	Initially, 2.0-3.0mg/kg daily in two to three divided doses. Maximum 10-12mg/kg daily.
	IV	Initially, 1mg/kg/hr; maximum 3mg/kg/hr. (Balfe, J.W. et al., "Hypertension in Childhood," Adv. Pediatr. 36, 201-246, 1989).

PHARMACOKINETICS: Bioavailability is **25%** due to extensive first-pass metabolism. Bioavailability is increased by food, in the elderly, in patients with liver disease and in those taking cimetidine; Protein Binding: 50%; Volume of Distribution: 9.4 liter/kg; Elimination Half-Life: 6-8 hours and is not affected by impaired renal function.

ADVERSE EFFECTS: The major adverse effects of labetalol are due to alpha blockage (orthostatic hypotension) or beta blocking, eg, bronchospasm.

Other adverse effects include hepatitis, nausea, vomiting, paresthesias, sweating, dizziness, flushing, headache, dryness of the mouth, tingling of the scalp and fluid retention.

CONTRAINDICATIONS: Congestive heart failure, heart block, sinus tachycardia.

LACTULOSE

(Chronulac, Cephulac, Others)

USES: Lactulose is used as an adjunct to protein restriction and supportive therapy for the prevention and treatment of **portal-systemic encephalopathy** (PSE) including hepatic pre-coma and coma. Lactulose is also used as a laxative in patients with chronic constipation.

Mechanism of Action: Lactulose reduces the blood ammonia concentration and thus tends to improve the mental state of the patient and improved EEG tracings.

Lactulose is useful as a laxative in the treatment of chronic constipation in adults and the elderly. The drug has been used in the treatment of chronic constipation in children; however, its safety and efficacy in children has not been established.

DOSAGE FORMS: Chronulac(Oral) 3.33g/5ml; Cephulac(Oral or Rectal) 3.33g/5ml

DOSAGE: Usually administered orally. Drug dosages for the prevention and treatment of portal-systemic encephalopathy are given in the next Table:

Drug Dosages for the Prevention and Treatment of Portal-Systemic Encephalopathy(PSE)

Patient	Dosage
Infants	1.67-6.67g (2.5-10ml) daily given in 3-4 divided doses
Children and Adolescents	27-60g (40-90ml) daily, given in 3-4 divided doses
Adults	20-30g(30-45ml) daily, given in 3-4 divided doses
Acute Episodes of Portal-Systemic Encephalopathy (PSE): Adults	20-30g (30-45ml) at 1-to 2-hour intervals, then lactulose is reduced to produce 2-3 soft stools.

For infants, children and adolescents and adults, dosage is adjusted every 1-2 days as necessary to produce 2-3 soft stools.

Drug dosages for the treatment of chronic constipation are given in the next Table:

Drug Dosages for the Treatment of Chronic Constipation

Patient	Dosage
Children	At least 5g(7.5ml) daily, usually as single dose after breakfast (not approved by U.S. Food and Drug Admin.)
Adults	10-20g (15-30ml) daily; dosage may be increased to 40g (60ml) daily, if necessary

ADVERSE EFFECTS: G.I. Symptoms: Discomfort with abdominal cramps, diarrhea.
Drug Interactions: Do not administer additional laxatives.

LABORATORY MONITORING: Serum potassium, especially if diarrhea develops.

LAXATIVE-CATHARTICS

The types of laxative-cathartic effect and latency are given in the next Table (Bruton, L.L. in Gilman, A.G. et al.,(eds.) The Pharmacological Basis of Therapeutics, ed. 8, N.Y. Macmillan, 1990, 914-932):

Type of Laxative-Cathartic Effect		
Softening of Formed Stool (1 to 3 days)	Soft-Semifluid Stool (6 to 8 Hours)	Watery Stool (1 to 3 Hours)
Bulk Forming Products Dietary fiber Methylcellulose Psyllium Preparations	Saline Laxatives (low dose) Milk of Magnesia Magnesium Sulfate	Saline Laxatives (high dose) Milk of Magnesia Magnesium Citrate Magnesium Sulfate Sodium Phosphates Sodium Sulfate
Ducosate Salts Sodium, Potassium or Calcium Salts of Dioctylsulfosuccinate	Diphenylmethane Derivatives Phenolphthalein Bisacodyl	Castor Oil
Lactulose	Anthraquinone Derivatives Senna Cascara Sagrada	Polyethylene Glycol-Electrolyte Prep.

Recommended used of laxatives are given in the next Table:

Condition	Laxative
Empty bowel prior to procto-scopic or colonoscopic procedures.	Polyethylene glycol (Colyte, GoLYTELY). Bisacodyl (Dulcolax, Fleet Bisacodyl). Kits: Dulcolax Bowel Prep Kit, Evac-Q-Kit; Evac-Q-Kwik. Saline Laxatives Fleet Enema Castor Oil Neoloid.
Fecal impaction	Mineral oil (Kondremul).
Portal systemic encephalopathy	Lactulose (Chronulac)
Chronic watery diarrhea	Bulk forming agents: Methylcellulose (Cologel).
Diverticulosis or irritable bowel syndrome; patients with hemorrhoids to relieve painful defecation.	Psyllium hydrophilic colloid: Effersyllium; Konsyl; Metamucil; Naturacil; Perdiem Plain.
Severe constipation	Senna preparations.

LEUCOVORIN CALCIUM
(Wellcovorin)

USES: **Leucovorin calcium** is the calcium salt of **folinic acid**, an active metabolite of folic acid. Uses of leucovorin are given in the next Table:

Uses of Leucovorin
Leucovorin "Rescue" with High-Dose Methotrexate
Antidote for Folic Acid Antagonists:
Methotrexate
Trimethoprim
Pyrimethamine
Megaloblastic Anemia Secondary to Folic Acid Deficiency

Leucovorin "Rescue" with High-Dose Methotrexate: Leucovorin is used in conjunction with high-dose methotrexate to control the duration of exposure of sensitive cells to methotrexate. Leucovorin is administered 6-24 hours after methotrexate infusion.

Antidote for Folic Acid Antagonists: Leucovorin is used as an antidote to diminish the toxicity and counteract the effect of overdosage of the folic acid antagonists, methotrexate, trimethoprim and pyrimethamine.

Megaloblastic Anemia Secondary to Folic Acid Deficiency: Leucovorin is used in the treatment of folate deficiency megaloblastic anemias of infancy, pregnancy, sprue and nutritional deficiencies when oral folic acid therapy is not feasible. Folic acid is much less expensive and is preferred.

DOSAGE FORMS: Tabs: 5,10,15,25mg; Inj: 25,50,100,350mg; 3mg/ml; 5mg/ml.

DOSAGE: Leucovorin calcium is administered orally, or by IM or IV injection. When leucovorin "rescue" is used, there is a possibility that the patient may vomit and not absorb oral leucovorin; then, the drug should be administered parenterally. Dosage is given in the next Table:

Dosage of Leucovorin

Condition	Route	Dosage
"Rescue" in High-Dose Methotrexate Therapy	Orally or Parenterally	Therapy must begin within 24 hours. $10mg/m^2$ orally or parenterally followed by $10mg/m^2$ orally every 6 hours for 72 hrs. If, at 24 hrs. following methotrexate administration, the patient's serum creatinine is 50% or greater than the serum creatinine prior to methotrexate, or methotrexate level is greater than $5x10^{-6}M$ at 24 hrs or $9x10^{-7}M$ at 48 hrs, leucovorin dosage should be increased immediately to $100mg/m^2$ every 3 hrs. until the serum methotrexate concentration is less than $10^{-8}M$. Leucovorin rescue should only be administered under the direction of an oncologist in centers where rapid, reliable methotrexate levels are available.
Antidote for Folic Acid Antagonists: Methotrexate, Trimethoprim, Pyrimethamine	IM or IV	Leucovorin is given in amounts equal to the weight of the antagonist preferably within the first hour. With large overdoses of methotrexate, leucovorin can be administered by IV infusion in doses up to 75mg within 12 hours, followed by 12mg IM every 6 hrs. for 4 doses.

PHARMACOKINETICS: Oral Absorption: Rapid; Metabolism: Metabolized in liver to 5-methyltetrahydrofolate. Onset: 20-30 min (oral); 10-20 min (IM); Peak: 1.5-2 hrs.; Duration: 3-6 hrs. Elimination: renal (80%-90%)

ADVERSE EFFECTS: Hypersensitivity reactions (e.g., urticaria, rash, pruritus, wheezing).

LEVODOPA/CARBIDOPA

(Sinemet)

USES: Sinemet, a combination of levodopa with carbidopa, is the most effective drug available in the United States for the treatment of **Parkinson's disease.**

Approximately 95% of an oral dose of levodopa is decarboxylated in peripheral tissue leaving only 5% for diffusion across the blood-brain barrier. Carbidopa is an inhibitor of peripheral decarboxylation of levodopa; carbidopa does not pass the blood brain barrier. By preventing the extra-cerebral metabolism of levodopa, the amount of levodopa available in the brain is increased.

Mechanism of Action: Parkinson's disease is characterized by greatly decreased levels of dopamine in the basal ganglia. Replacement therapy in Parkinsonism with dopamine is not possible because it does not pass the blood-brain barrier. However, its precursor, l-dopa (levodopa) does penetrate the blood-brain barrier and is decarboxylated in the brain to dopamine.

DOSAGE FORMS: The tablets of Sinemet are available in the forms listed in the next Table:

Forms of Sinemet

Commercial Product	Levodopa(mg)	Carbidopa(mg)
Sinemet 10-100	100	10
Sinemet 25-100	100	25
Sinemet 25-250	250	25

DOSAGE: Sinemet should be given with food to minimize the possible occurrence of nausea and vomiting.

Initial Therapy: Half-tablet of Sinemet 25-100 formulation 2-4 times daily; every 2-3 days, increase dosage by one-half to one tablet daily. If a larger daily dose of levodopa is needed, give one tablet of Sinemet 25-100 three or four times daily. If necessary, this may be increased by one-half to one tablet daily or every other day. Usual Maintenance Dosage: 3-8 tablets of Sinemet 25-250 daily in divided doses.

When a patient is being treated with levodopa and it is desirable to start therapy with Sinemet, then levodopa should be discontinued for at least 12 hours. The initial daily dose of Sinemet should provide approximately 25% of the previous amount of levodopa. The suggested initial dosage is one tablet of Sinemet 10-100 or Sinemet 25-100 three or four times daily for patients who have been maintained on less than 1.5g of levodopa daily; patients may eventually require one tablet of Sinemet 25-250 three or four times daily.

PHARMACOKINETICS: Half-Life of L-Dopa: 1-3 hours.

ADVERSE REACTIONS: Persistent nausea and vomiting (2-5%); frequent abnormal involuntary movements; "bradykinetic episodes", depression, dementia, convulsions, unpleasant dreams, hallucinations, hypotension, tachycardia and arrhythmias. Temporary withdrawal of the drug may cause a dangerous recrudescence of the symptoms of Parkinsonism. Abrupt withdrawal may precipitate neuroleptic malignant syndrome. Excessive doses may cause choreoathetosis.

DRUG INTERACTIONS: The effectiveness of levodopa may be reduced by methyldopa, phenothiazines, butyrophenones, thioxanthenes, rauwolfia alkaloids, phenytoin, papaverine and metoclopramide. Pyridoxine, in diet or vitamins, will negate the effects of carbidopa by inducing peripheral decarboxylation by dopa decarboxylase.

CONTRAINDICATIONS: A hypertensive crisis may occur if levodopa is given with a nonspecific monoamine oxidase inhibitor (MAO-I); these drugs must be discontinued 2 weeks before starting Sinemet. Also, Sinemet is contraindicated in patients with narrow angle glaucoma.

LEVOTHYROXINE SODIUM
(Synthroid, Levothyroid, Levoxine)

USES: Levothyroxine sodium is the monosodium salt of the levoisomer of thyroxine, the principal secretion of the thyroid gland. Levothryroxine is used to replace thyroxine in the following conditions: functional deficiency, primary hypothyroidism, partial or complete absence of the gland, effects of surgery, radiation or antithyroid agents, secondary (pituitary) or tertiary (hypothalamic) hypothyroidism, thyroiditis associated with hypothyroidism.

Thyroid values in euthyroidism and hypothyroidism are given in the next Table:

Thyroid Values in Euthyroidism and Hypothyroidism

Condition	T-4	Free T-4 Dialysis	Free T-4 Index	T-3	Reverse T-3	TSH	TRH Test
Normal	N	N	N	N	N	N	N (Doubling of baseline level of TSH)
Hypothyroid, Primary	Dec.	Dec.	Dec.	Dec.	Dec.	Inc.	Hyperresponsiveness
Hypothyroid, Secondary	Dec.	Dec.	Dec.	Dec.	Dec.	Dec.	No Response
Hypothyroid, Tertiary	Dec.	Dec.	Dec.	Dec.	Dec.	Dec.	Variable, Blunted Response

DOSAGE FORMS: Tabs: 12.5, 25, 50, 75, 100, 112, 125, 150, 175, 200, 300mcg; Injection: 200, 500mcg per vial

DOSAGE: The daily oral dose of levothyroxine in hypothyroidism, by age, is given in the next Table:

Daily Oral Dose of Levothyroxine in Hypothyroidism, by Age

Age	Oral Daily Dose	Comment
Premature Neonates, <2kg	25mcg	Dosage may be increased to 50mcg in 4-6 weeks
Neonate at Risk of Cardiac Failure	25mcg	Dosage may be increased to 50mcg in 4-6 weeks
Full-Term Neonate	37.5mcg(25-50mcg)	
0-6 months	25-50mcg or 8-10mcg/kg	
6-12 months	50-75mcg or 6-8mcg/kg	
1-5 years	75-100mcg or 5-6mcg/kg	
6-12 years	100-150mcg or 4-5mcg/kg	
Older than 12 years	>150mcg or 2-3mcg/kg	
Adults, Mild Hypothyroidism	Initial, 50mcg daily; dosage is increased by increments of 25-50mcg daily at intervals of 2-4 weeks until desired response obtained; usual maintenance dose, 100-200mcg daily. or Healthy adult with relatively recent hypothyroidism, initial dose, 100-200mcg daily.	
Adult, Severe Hypothyroidism	Initial, 12.5-25mcg daily as single dose; dosage is increased by increments of 25-50mcg daily at intervals of 2-4 weeks until desired response is obtained; usual maintenance dose, 100-200mcg daily.	
Geriatric Patients with Hypothyroidism	Initial, 12.5-50mcg daily as single dose; dosage is increased by increments of 12.5-50mcg every 3-8 weeks until desired response is obtained; usual maintenance dose, 75-150mcg daily.	

The usual plasma half-life of thyroxine is 6-7 days; the plasma half-life of thyroxine is increased in hypothyroidism.

IM or IV Injection: The IV route is preferred since an absorption may be variable following IM administration. IV dose is 75% of oral dose.

ADVERSE EFFECTS: Use with extreme caution and reduced dosage in patients with angina pectoris or other cardiovascular disease, including hypertension.

DRUG INTERACTIONS: Potentiates hypoprothrombinemic effect of warfarin and other oral anticoagulants; may increase requirement dosage of insulin or oral antidiabetic agents in diabetics.

LABORATORY EVALUATION: Infants on thyroid replacement therapy for congenital hypothyroidism should be evaluated at 6 weeks, 6 months, 12 months, and yearly thereafter with thyroid function tests: T-4, Free T-4, and TSH. Do not use normal TSH as the sole criterion of the adequacy of dose since TSH concentrations may remain elevated for several months even when therapy is adequate.

LIDOCAINE
(Xylocaine and others)

USES: The uses of lidocaine are given in the next Table:

Uses of Lidocaine
Treatment of **Ventricular Arrhythmias** caused by **Acute Myocardial Infarction, Digitalis Intoxication** and **Cardiac Surgery.**
Treatment for **Status Epilepticus**
Local Anesthetic

Treatment of Ventricular Arrhythmias: **Lidocaine** is the **drug of choice** for the treatment of **ventricular premature contractions** associated with myocardial infarction. Besides ventricular arrhythmias following acute myocardial infarction, lidocaine is used for treatment of ventricular arrhythmias during cardiac manipulative procedures such as cardiac surgery or catheterization.

Therapy with lidocaine should be initiated if ventricular premature contractions associated with myocardial infarction or other cardiac condition show the characteristics as shown in the next Table:

Indications for Therapy with Lidocaine
Interruption of T-Wave
Ventricular Premature Contractions exceed 5 Beats/Minute
Multifocal
Ventricular Premature Contractions Occur in Runs of Two or More (If Bradycardia is Absent)

Lidocaine has been used to prevent recurrence of ventricular fibrillation after cardioversion and to treat ventricular tachycardia before cardioversion.

Lidocaine may be used in the treatment of digitalis-induced ventricular arrhythmias which persist following discontinuance of the glycoside and treatment with potassium chloride.

Status Epilepticus: IV lidocaine has been used for the treatment of status epilepticus.

Local Anesthetic: Lidocaine is used for infiltration anesthesia and for nerve block techniques for peripheral, sympathetic epidural (including caudal) and spinal block anesthesia.

Mechanism of Action: Lidocaine controls ventricular arrhythmias by suppressing automaticity in the His-Purkinje system and by suppressing spontaneous depolarization of the ventricles during diastole. It does not act on the SA node.

DOSAGE FORMS: IV: 10mg/ml, 20mg/ml; IM: 100mg/ml; Prefilled Syringes:10mg/ml, 20mg/ml; Cream: 30mg/ml; Ointment: 25mg/ml, 50mg/ml; Jelly: 20mg/ml

DOSAGE: Lidocaine is administered IM or IV for the treatment of ventricular arrhythmias; monitor using ECG. The deltoid muscle is the preferred site for IM injection.

The dose of lidocaine for ventricular fibrillation is given in the next Table (American Heart Association, Advanced Cardiac Life Support 1987, Pediatric Advanced Life Support, 1988):

Dosage of Lidocaine

Condition	Age	Dosage
Ventricular Arrhythmias	Adults	IV bolus: 50-100mg at a rate of 25-50mg/min; or 1mg/kg. A second dose of 0.5mg/kg may be administered 2-5 minutes after completion of the first injection, max. 3mg/kg. Maintenance if necessary 2-4mg/min for 24-30hours.
	Children	IV bolus: 1mg/kg every 10-15 minutes. Maintenance: 20-50 microgram/kg per minute via infusion pump.
	>69 years, or CHF or Cardiogenic Shock or Hepatic Disease	IV bolus: 25-50mg; maintenance 1 to 2 mg/min. Monitor levels.
Prophylaxis after Acute Myocardial Infarction	Adults	IV bolus of 200mg given as four 50mg injections five minutes apart; each bolus is given over 1-2 min. or IV bolus of 20mg/min for 10 min. Simultaneously with the loading dose, maintenance dose is started at a rate of 3mg/min, continued for 24 hrs

LIDOCAINE (Cont.)

When lidocaine is used for several days as for prophylaxis, dosage should be decreased on the second or third day as clearance decreases.

When used as a local anesthetic, maximum dose in a 2 hour period is 7mg/kg (with epinephrine) or 4-5mg/kg (without epinephrine)(Max dose: 500mg).

PHARMACOKINETICS: Therapeutic: 2-5mcg/ml. Time to Steady State (Sampling Time): 12 hours after beginning lidocaine. Half-life: 74-140 min. Cardiac Failure: 115 min. Uremia: 77 min. Cirrhosis: 296 min. Toxic: >5mcg/ml.

Metabolism: Liver

ADVERSE EFFECTS: The majority of lidocaine's adverse effects involve the central nervous or circulatory systems. Milder adverse reactions, such as drowsiness, dizziness, confusion, transient paresthesias, muscle twitching, and nausea, are common after loading doses or can occur at plasma levels greater than 5mcg/ml. More severe reaction may occur. Central nervous system (CNS) depression, stimulation, or seizures may develop. Cardiac conduction abnormalities, decreased contractility, heart block and hypotension can occur in patients with pre-existing conduction defects or high plasma concentrations.

Plasma levels and signs or symptoms of toxicity need to be closely monitored in patients with altered drug elimination such as cardiac failure, acute myocardial infarction, liver disease and prolonged intravenous infusion.

DRUG INTERACTION: Propranolol and cimetidine reduce the systemic clearance of lidocaine by reducing hepatic blood flow and hepatic metabolism of lidocaine; thus, serum concentration of lidocaine may increase.

When lidocaine is administered with other antiarrhythmic drugs such as procainamide, quinidine, phenytoin or propranolol, the cardiac effects may be additive or antagonistic and toxic effects may be additive.

Concurrent use of tocainide can cause seizures, possibly from additive neurotoxicity.

CONTRAINDICATIONS: Lidocaine is contraindicated in patients with Adams-Stokes syndromes or with severe degrees of SA, AV, or intraventricular heart block in the absence of an artificial pacemaker.

GUIDELINES FOR MONITORING: Guidelines for monitoring serum specimens are given in the next Table:

Guidelines for Monitoring Lidocaine
12 hours after beginning lidocaine infusion; at least every 12 hours in patients with signs or symptoms of cardiac or hepatic insufficiency.
Obtain specimen whenever toxicity is suspected.
Monitor whenever ventricular arrhythmias occur despite lidocaine administration.

Specimen: Red top tube, separate serum and refrigerate; or green (heparin) top tube.

Spuriously low plasma lidocaine concentrations may be obtained when blood is collected in certain commercial rubber-stoppered collection tubes. Use all-glass tubes or test any commercial collecting tube thoroughly before use.

LITHIUM SALTS

(Eskalith, Lithonate, Lithate)

USES: Lithium carbonate and **lithium citrate** are antimanic agents used in the treatment of a variety of psychiatric disorders, as given in the next Table:

Uses of Lithium Salts
Acute Mania
Major Depression
Bipolar Disorder Prophylaxis
Schizophrenic Disorders
Psychiatric Disorders in Children:
Mixed bipolar disorder
Hyperactivity with psychotic or neurotic components
Aggressive behavior

Lithium salts have also been used to treat alcohol dependence, neutropenia secondary to chemotherapy, and chronic cluster or migraine headaches.

Mechanism of Action: Lithium competes with potassium, sodium, calcium and magnesium at the cell level in body tissues. Lithium decreases intracellular cAMP and decreases plasma cGMP. Although many effects have been described, the mechanism of action has not been fully elucidated.

DOSAGE FORMS: Lithium carbonate: Caps: 150, 300, 600mg (4.06, 8.12, 16.24mEq lithium); Tabs: 300mg (8.12mEq lithium); Tabs (extended release): 300, 450mg (8.12, 12.18mEq lithium); Lithium citrate: Solution: 8mEq lithium/5ml.

DOSAGE: Lithium salts are administered orally. Dosage is given in the next Table:

Dosage of Lithium Salts

Age	Dosage
Adults	Initial: Lithium carbonate 1.8g (48mEq lithium) daily in 2 or 3 divided doses; or Lithium carbonate 20-30mg/kg in 2 or 3 divided doses. or Lithium carbonate 600-900mg daily in 2 or 3 divided doses, increase dosage slowly to minimize adverse effects.
	Maintenance: Lithium carbonate 900mg-1.2g (24-32mEq lithium) daily in 2-4 divided doses. Usual max. 2.4g of lithium carbonate daily; occasionally up to 3.6g of lithium carbonate daily. Maintain therapeutic level (0.6-1.2mEq/L).
Children	Initial: Lithium carbonate 15-60mg/kg (0.4-1.6mEq/kg lithium) daily in 2 or 3 divided doses.
	Maintenance: Same dose range as above, maintain therapeutic level (0.6-1.2mEq/L).

PHARMACOKINETICS: Absorption: Caps, tabs, solution: 95-100%; Tabs (extended release): 60-90%; Peak: 0.5-3 hours; 4-12 hours for extended release; Protein binding: none; Metabolism: none; Excretion: urine.

ADVERSE EFFECTS: Lithium has many adverse effects, even at therapeutic levels. These effects primarily involve the CNS, GI tract, and kidneys.

CNS Effects: Headache, minor memory impairment, mental confusion and decreased ability to concentrate occurs in 40% of patients. Hand tremor (45-50%) and transient muscle weakness (30%) occur frequently. Symptoms improve with time in many patients. Seizures have occurred at therapeutic levels, but are usually associated with toxicity.

GI Effects: Nausea, anorexia, bloating, diarrhea, vomiting or abdominal pain occur in 10-30% of patients initially; only 1-10% of patients have persistent symptoms beyond 1-2 years. Dry mouth occurs in 20-50% of patients and is related to polyuria (see below).

Renal Effects: Nephrogenic diabetes insipidus occurs in 30-50% of patients and persists in 10-25%. Clinical manifestations include polyuria and polydipsia.

Other Effects: Hypothyroidism (1-4%) and goiter (5%) may occur. Cardiovascular effects include benign, reversible ECG T-wave depression (20-30%), sinus node dysfunction, and blocks. Hypotension and cardiovascular collapse is seen in severe lithium toxicity. Most patients develop a reversible leukocytosis.

DRUG INTERACTIONS: ACE inhibitors, furosemide, thiazide diuretics and nonsteroidal anti-inflammatory drugs increase lithium concentrations. Concomitant use of antipsychotic agents result in unpredictable pharmacokinetic interactions and adverse neurologic effects may occur (eg, acute encephalopathy or extrapyramidal reactions).

LITHIUM SALTS (Cont.)

Administration of any drug with lithium should be thoroughly investigated beforehand.

MONITOR: Lithium level should be maintained between 0.6-1.2mEq/L. Check level 3-4 days after initiating therapy and every 1-2 months during maintenance. Laboratory studies which should be performed before lithium administration include urinalysis, serum creatinine or BUN, serum sodium, thyroid studies (thyroxine, TSH and thyroid microsomal antibody titers), white blood cell count and ECG.

LOPERAMIDE

(Imodium)

USES: Loperamide is used to treat diarrhea and is used to reduce the volume of discharge from ileostomies. Uses are listed in the next Table:

Uses of Loperamide
Acute and Chronic Diarrhea
Prophylaxis and Treatment of Traveler's Diarrhea
Acute and Chronic Infectious Diarrhea
Possibly Useful in Some Infants with Severe Prolonged Diarrhea Unresponsive to Other Treatment
Control Chronic Diarrhea in Patients with Irritable Bowel Syndrome, Colostomy, Ileostomy and Malabsorption
Control Liquidity in Patients who have Undergone Colectomy for Ulcerative Colitis.

Mechanism of Action: Loperamide is an opioid; it is a derivative of haloperidol and resemble meperidine structurally. It is believed to act by interfering with the cholinergic and noncholinergic mechanisms involved in peristalsis.

DOSAGE FORMS: Caps: 2mg; Liquid: 1mg/5ml

DOSAGE: Loperamide is administered orally;dosage is given in the next Table:

Dosage of Loperamide

Condition	Age	Dosage
Acute Diarrhea	Adults	Initially, 4mg, then 2mg after each unformed stool; max 16mg/day. Stop after 48 hours if ineffective.
Chronic Diarrhea	Adults	Initially as for acute; maintenance 4-8 mg daily as single or divided dose. Discontinue in 10 days if ineffective.
Diarrhea	Child	0.4-0.8mg/kg daily in two to four divided doses. In patients with chronic diarrhea, initially, 0.5-1.5mg/kg daily in two to four divided doses; Maintenance, 0.25-1mg/kg daily in two to four divided doses.
	2-5 yrs. (13-20kg)	First day, 1mg, 3 times daily
	5-8 yrs. (20-30kg)	First day, 2mg, 2 times daily
	8-12 yrs. (>30kg)	First day, 2mg, 3 times daily
		Then give only after loose stool up to max. for first day.

PHARMACOKINETICS: Peak: 2.5 hours (oral solution); 4-5 hours (capsules); Half-Life: 11 hours. Excretion: 30% of dose excreted in feces.

ADVERSE EFFECTS: No significant adverse effects or drug interactions have been reported. Abdominal pain, distention or discomfort, constipation, drowsiness, nausea, vomiting.

CONTRAINDICATIONS: Acute dysentery and when constipation must be avoided.

LORAZEPAM
(Ativan)

USES: **Lorazepam** is a **benzodiazepine;** uses are given in the next Table:

Uses of Lorazepam
Anxiety
Insomnia
Preanesthetic Medication
Alcohol Withdrawal*
Seizure Disorders*

*Investigational

Lorazepam is used to treat anxiety and insomnia associated with anxiety or transient situational stress (Ameer, B. and Greenblatt, D.J., Drugs 21, 161-200, 1981). It is given parenterally when used as a preanesthetic medication because of its amnestic action. It may be useful in the treatment of status epilepticus (Leppik, I.E. et al, JAMA 249, 1452-1454, 1983), the acute alcohol abstinence syndrome (Solomon, J. et al, Clin. Therapeut, 6, 52-58, 1983) and neuroleptic-induced catatonia (Fricchione, G.L. et al, J. Clin. Psychopharmacol. 3, 338-342, 1983).

DOSAGE FORMS: Tabs: 0.5, 1, 2mg; Parenteral: 2,4mg/ml.

DOSAGE: Lorazepam is administered orally, IM or IV injection. Dosage is given in the next Table:

Dosage of Lorazepam

Condition	Age	Dosage
Anxiety	Adult	Initially, 1-2mg, two or three times daily; usual range, 2-6mg daily. The dose can be increased gradually if needed to a max. of 10mg daily in 2 or 3 divided doses.
Insomnia	Adult	Single dose of 2-4 mg at bedtime
Status Epilepticus	Adult	2.5-10mg/dose IV; may repeat in 15-20 min.
	Child	0.03-0.1mg/kg/dose IV; may repeat in 15-20 min.
Preanesthetic Medication	Adult Child	0.05mg/kg IV 15-20 min or IM 2 hrs prior to the procedure. Max: 4mg.

The initial doses should be reduced by about one-half in elderly and debilitated patients.

PHARMACOKINETICS: Oral Absorption: 2 hours, max.; Elimination Half-Life: 15 hours (range 8-25 hours); Volume of Distribution: 1-1.3 liter/kg. Clearance: 0.7-1.2ml/min/kg. Metabolized to an active derivative; eliminated principally as the inactive glucuronide; cumulative effects are not likely.

ADVERSE EFFECTS: The most common untoward effects of lorazepam are sedation (16%), dizziness (7%), weakness (4%), and ataxia (3%). These reactions abate in over 50% of patients during continued administration; the remainder usually respond to reduction of dose. May cause respiratory depression.

Other adverse effects include disorientation, nausea, headache, agitation, leukopenia and hepatic toxicity.

CONTRAINDICATIONS: Acute narrow-angle glaucoma, lactation, psychosis, depression, pregnancy.

LABORATORY MONITORING: Some patients develop leukopenia and hepatic toxicity; therefore, monitor white cell count and liver function tests before administration of the drug at 2 weeks and then at monthly intervals.

LOVASTATIN

(Mevacor)

USES: Lovastatin has been approved by the FDA for the treatment of **hypercholesterolemia;** it is effective in lowering total cholesterol and low-density lipoprotein (LDL)-cholesterol (Types IIa or IIb). Mean reductions in total cholesterol of 20% to 35% and LDL-choesterol of 25-45% have been obtained in both familial and nonfamilial forms of hypercholesterolemia (Lovastatin Study Group II, JAMA 256, 2829-2834, 1986; Illingworth, D.R., Ann. Int. Med. 101, 598-604, 1984). In addition to lowerng LDL-cholesterol levels, lovastatin produces modest reductions in triglyceride levels.

Lovastatin decreased LDL cholesterol by 28%, triglycerides by 31% and VLDL cholesterol by 42% in non-insulin-dependent diabetes mellitus and mild hypercholesterolemia (Garg, A. and Grundy, S.M., N. Engl. J. Med 318, 81, 1988). Lovastatin is more effective in lowering elevated total and LDL cholesterol than cholestyramine (JAMA 260, 359, July 15, 1988).

The clinical use of lovastatin has been studied for only a few years; its long-term safety and effects on coronary artery disease have not yet been established.The yearly wholesale cost of treatment using lovastatin is approximately $900.

Mechanism of Action: Lovastatin, a HMG CoA reductase inhibitor, has the effects listed in the next Table:

Effects of Lovastatin
Blocks HMG CoA reductase
Increase of LDL receptor activity in the liver
Increase of rate of receptor-mediated removal of LDL
Decrease in production of LDL

Lovastatin inhibits HMG CoA reductase, the enzyme regulating the production of cholesterol as illustrated in the next Figure (Brown, M.S. and Goldstein, J.L., Science 232, 34-47, April 4, 1986):

Inhibition of HMG CoA Reductase by Lovastatin

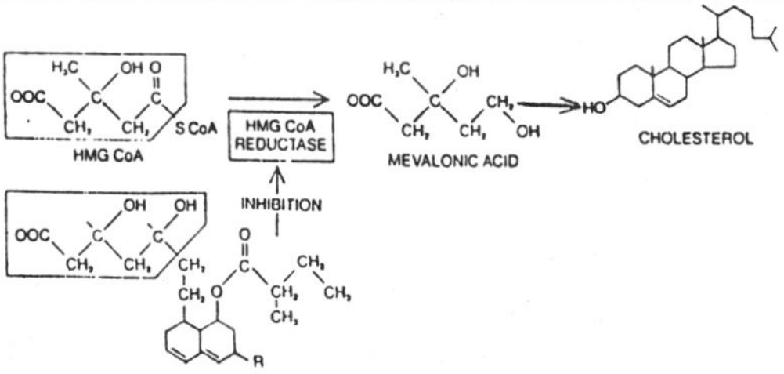

The side chain of lovastatin is so similar to that of HMG CoA that it competitively blocks the synthesis of mevalonic acid, the precursor of cholesterol.

The effect of decreased synthesis of cholesterol by hepatic cells is illustrated in the next Figure (Brown, M.S. and Goldstein, J.L., Science 232, 34-47, April 4, 1986):

Effect of Decreased Synthesis of Cholesterol by Hepatic Cells

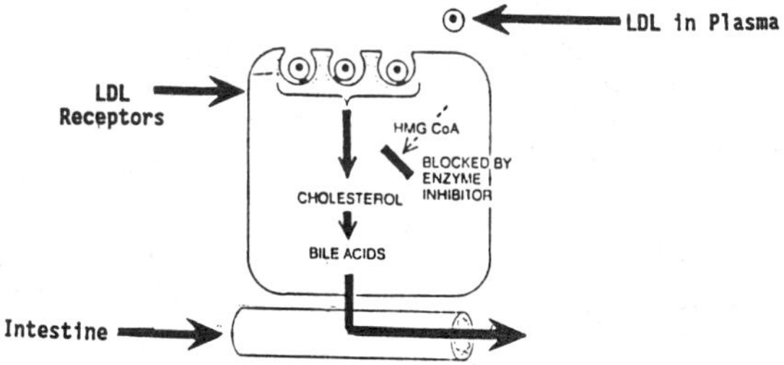

LOVASTATIN (Cont.)

The decrease in synthesis of cholesterol by the liver stimulates an increase of LDL receptors and the liver takes up LDL (low density lipoprotein) and IDL (intermediate density lipoprotein). The cholesterol of these lipoproteins is then converted to bile acids and excreted in the bile. Thus, serum cholesterol levels are decreased.

DOSAGE FORMS: Tabs: 20, 40mg

DOSAGE: Initially, 20mg once daily with the evening meal. Increase, if necessary at 4 week intervals. Maximum dose is 80mg daily in single or divided doses.

Lovastatin is not recommended for children.

ADVERSE EFFECTS: Adverse effects are often transient and collectively have occurred in less than 5% of patients; adverse effects are given in the next Table:

Adverse Effects of Lovastatin

System	Effect
Liver	Hepatotoxicity; approximately 2% of patients have developed persistent increases in transaminases of greater than 3 times normal after 3-16 months of therapy requiring discontinuance of therapy. Monitor liver function.
G.I.	Nausea; change in bowel function
Muscle	Myalgia and myositis reflected by elevated CPK levels
CNS	Headache, insomnia
Lens	No effects detected in humans
Hypersensitivity	Pruritis and skin rash
Other	Fatigue

DRUG INTERACTIONS: Additive effects with cholestyramine.

CONTRAINDICATIONS: Liver disease, pregnancy, lactation.

PRECAUTIONS: Use with caution in alcoholics; discontinue if the patient develops a myositis or elevated CPK levels.

MONITOR: Liver function tests should be performed every 6 weeks because of the possibility of hepatotoxicity due to lovastatin.

Observe for lens opacities.

Monitor CPK levels for possible myositis.

Monitor total cholesterol and LDL-cholesterol just prior to starting therapy, in 4 to 6 weeks, and at 3 months. If LDL-cholesterol goal is achieved, monitor total cholesterol annually.

LUNGS: ABSCESS, PATHOGENS

Pathogens: The pathogens that cause lung abscesses are given in the next Table (Handbook of Antimicrobial Therapy, The Medical Letter, 1990):

Pathogens that Cause Lung Abscesses

1. Anaerobic streptococci
2. Bacteroides
3. Staphylococcus aureus
4. Klebsiella (or other gram-negative bacilli)
5. Streptococcus pneumoniae
6. Fungi
7. Actinomyces, Nocardia

LUPUS ERYTHEMATOSUS, TREATMENT

Treatment of lupus erythematosus are given in the next Table:

Treatment of Lupus Erythematosus

Condition	Treatment
Minor Symptoms without Major Organ Involvement	Nonsteroidal Antiinflammatory Drugs (NSAIDs), e.g., salicylates, ibuprofen and naproxen
Cutaneous Manifestations	Hydroxychloroquine Sulfate (200-600mg Daily) and Topical Corticosteroids
Acute Serologic Changes and Severe Clinical Manifestations	Short Acting Corticosteroids (Prednisone, Prednisolone or Methylprednisolone
Diffuse Proliferative Glomerulonephritis, Myocarditis, CNS involvement	Moderate to High Dose Corticosteroid Therapy Cyclophosphamide or Azathioprine Plasmapheresis

LYPRESSIN

(Diapid)

USE: Lypressin is used to prevent or control polydipsia, polyuria, and dehydration in patients with diabetes insipidus caused by a deficiency of endogenous posterior pituitary antidiuretic hormone(ADH).

The pharmacologic action of lypressin is similar to that of vasopressin

DOSAGE FORMS: (Diapid) Nasal Spray: 185mcg/ml

DOSAGE: Lypressin is applied topically as a spray to the nasal mucosa; do not inhale. Each spray of the nasal solution containing 185mcg/ml delivers approximately 7mcg of lypressin which is equivalent to 2 USP Posterior Pituitary Units. The nasal solution may be sprayed once or twice into one or both nostrils whenever urinary frequency increases or significant thirst develops. The usual dose for children and adults is 1 or 2 sprays in each nostril 4 times daily and at bedtime.

ADVERSE EFFECTS: Coronary vasoconstriction may occur with large doses.

MAGNESIUM CITRATE

(Citrate of Magnesia)

USES: Magnesium citrate is a saline **laxative.**

Mechanism of Action: The action of magnesium citrate may result from the hyperosmotic effect of poorly absorbed magnesium within the small intestine and from the retention of water which indirectly stimulates stretch receptors and increases peristalsis.

DOSAGE FORMS: (Citrate of Magnesia) Sol'n: 15-19mg/ml (0.77-0.94mEq/ml).

DOSAGE: The usual oral dosage of magnesium citrate solution is given in the next Table:

Usual Oral Dose of Magnesium Citrate Solution

Age (Years)	Volume (ml)
Child	4ml/kg/dose
Adults	100-300

Magnesium citrate should be administered at infrequent intervals. Laxatives should be used cautiously.

ADVERSE EFFECTS: Use with caution in renal insufficiency. May cause hypermagnesemia. Up to 20% is absorbed.

MAGNESIUM HYDROXIDE

(Milk of Magnesia)

USES: Laxative; magnesium hydroxide is a saline laxative.

Mechanism of Action: The action of magnesium hydroxide may result from the hyperosmotic effect of poorly absorbed magnesium within the small intestine and from the retention of water which indirectly stimulates stretch receptors and increases peristalsis.

DOSAGE FORMS: (Milk of Magnesia) Susp: 77.5mg/g; Tabs: 300, 600mg

DOSAGE: The usual oral dosage of magnesium hydroxide (milk of magnesia) is given in the next Table:

Usual Oral Dose of Magnesium Hydroxide (Milk of Magnesia)

Age (Years)	Volume (ml)
Child(by wt)	0.5ml/kg/dose (40mg/kg/dose)
2-5	5-15 (0.4g-1.2g of Magnesium Hydroxide)
6-12	15-30 (1.2-2.4g of Magnesium Hydroxide)
Adults	30-60 (2.4-4.8g of Magnesium Hydroxide or 82-164mEq Magnesium)

Magnesium hydroxide (Milk of Magnesia) should be administered at infrequent intervals. Laxatives should be used cautiously.

ADVERSE EFFECTS: Use with caution in renal insufficiency. May cause hypermagnesemia.

MAGNESIUM SULFATE (Oral)

(Epson Salt)

USES: Magnesium sulfate is a saline **laxative.**

Mechanism of Action: The action of magnesium sulfate may result from the hyperosmotic effect of poorly absorbed magnesium within the small intestine and from the retention of water which indirectly stimulates stretch receptors and increases peristalsis.

DOSAGE: The usual oral dosage of magnesium sulfate is given in the next Table:

Usual Oral Dose of Magnesium Sulfate

Age (Years)	Dose (g)
Child	0.25gm/kg/dose
2-5	2.5-5g
6-12	5 - 10g
Adults	10-30g (81-243mEq Magnesium)

Magnesium sulfate should be administered at infrequent intervals. Laxatives should be used cautiously.

MAGNESIUM SULFATE (Parenteral)

USES: Magnesium sulfate acts as an **anticonvulsant** in patients with severe preeclampsia or eclampsia when administered parenterally. Doses sufficient to cause hypermagnesemia depress the CNS and block peripheral neuromuscular transmission. Magnesium is also used to prevent or treat magnesium deficiency. Magnesium deficiency is associated with various conditions, including glomerulonephritis, hypothyroidism, pancreatitis, inadequate intake, or excessive intestinal, renal, or other body fluid losses. The uses of magnesium sulfate are given in the following Table:

Uses of Magnesium Sulfate
Severe Preeclampsia or Eclampsia
Treat Magnesium Deficiency
Prevent Magnesium Deficiency
Asthma (possibly)

DOSAGE FORMS: Injection: 10, 12.5, 50%.

DOSAGE: Magnesium sulfate may be administered IM or IV; the oral form is used as a laxative (see previous section). In adults, IM administration should be in concentrations of 25-50%; in children, the maximum concentration should be 20%. For IV administration, the concentration should not exceed 20%; the rate of infusion should not exceed 150mg/min (1.5ml of 10% solution/min) and children should have the drug administered by slow IV infusion. The dosage of magnesium sulfate in various conditions are given in the next Table:

Use and Dosage of Magnesium Sulfate

Condition	Dosage
Severe Preeclampsia or Eclampsia	Initial: 4g of magnesium sulfate in 250ml of 5% dextrose, IV, 1-2g magnesium sulfate/hour by constant IV infusion. or Initial: 4g of magnesium sulfate in 250ml of 5% dextrose, IV, plus 4-5g IM into each buttock followed by 4-5 g, IM into alternate buttocks at 4-hour intervals as needed. Total dosage of magnesium sulfate should not exceed 30-40g daily. In patients with severe renal insufficiency, monitor serum magnesium concentrations frequently and maximum dosage of magnesium sulfate is 20g per 48 hours. or Initial: 8-15g of magnesium sulfate, depending on weight of patient, i.e., 8g for a 45kg patient to 15g for a 90kg patient, is administered as follows: 4g in 250ml of 5% dextose,IV and the remainder of the initial dose is given IM. Dosage for next 24 hours based on serum conc. and urinary excretion of magnesium following initial dose. Subsequent doses as necessary to replace the magnesium excreted in the urine and will be approx. 65% of the initial dose, administered IM at 6-hour intervals.
Mild Magnesium Deficiency	Adult: One gram, IM, every 6 hours for 4 doses. or 3g, orally, every 6 hours for 4 doses. Child: 25-50mg/kg/dose IV or IM 4 times daily.
Severe Magnesium Deficiency	Max: 250mg/kg, IM, over a 4-hr period or 5g of magnesium sulfate added to one liter of 5% dextrose injection or 5% dextrose in 0.9% NaCl injection and administered by IV infusion over a 3-hr period. Child: 25-100mg/kg/dose every 4-6 hrs for 3-4 doses IV or IM.
Part of Total Parenteral Nutrition	Children: 0.25-0.5mEq/kg daily or 30-60mg/kg daily IV. Usual max: 1gm daily IV. Adults: 0.5-3g of magnesium sulfate (4-24mEq of magnesium) daily.
Hypomagnesemic Seizures associated with Glomerulonephritis or Hypothyroidism	Adult: 1g IV or IM
Asthma	1.2g of magnesium sulfate IV may be beneficial adjunct therapy in adults with moderate to severe asthma who fail to respond to beta-agonists (Skobeloff, E.M. et al., "Intravenous Magnesium Sulfate for the Treatment of Acute Asthma in the Emergency Department," JAMA 262, 1210-1213, 1989).

Reference Values: IV: Onset of action immediate; duration of action, 30 min. IM: Onset of action, 1 hour; duration of action, 3-4 hours. As an anticonvulsant, effective serum concentrations, 2.5-7.5mEq/liter.

MONITOR: Serum level, BP and respirations.

Antidote: Calcium gluconate (IV) should be available as antidote.

MANNITOL

USES: Mannitol is an **osmotic diuretic**. The uses of mannitol are given in the next Table:

Uses of Mannitol
Oliguric Acute Renal Failure
Reduction of Intracranial Pressure
Reduction of Intraocular Pressure
Severe Intoxication by Certain Drugs
Transurethral Prostatic Resection

Mechanism of Action: Mannitol induces diuresis mainly by elevating the osmotic pressure of the glomerular filtrate to such an extent that tubular reabsorption of water and solutes is hindered.

DOSAGE FORMS: Sol'n: 50mg/ml (5%), 100mg/ml (10%), 150mg/ml (15%); 200mg/ml (20%); 250mg/ml (25%)

DOSAGE: Mannitol injections are administered by IV infusion; a filter should be used for infusion of injections containing 20% or more because mannitol crystals may be present. For transurethral prostatic resection, mannitol irrigation solutions are instilled into the bladder via an indwelling urethral catheter.

The use and dosage of mannitol in different conditions are given in the next Table:

Use and Dosage of Mannitol

Condition	Dosage
Prevention and/or Treatment of Oliguric Acute Renal Failure	Test Dose for Children or Adults: 0.2g/kg as a 15% or 20% solution infused over 3-5 min.; a response is at least 30-50ml of urine over the next 2-3 hours. Prevention of Oliguria; mannitol may be given before or immediately following surgery. Give 50-100g of mannitol, initially as a concentrated solution followed by a 5 or 10% solution. Treatment of Oliguria: 100g of mannitol is a 15-20% solution over 90 minutes to several hours. For Children, give 0.5-2g/kg.
Reduction of Intracranial or Intraocular Pressure	Children or Adults: 0.25-1gm/kg as a 15,20, or 25% solution IV push. Use high dose for acute management. May be used in combination with furosemide. Preoperatively, give 1.5-2gm/kg 1-1.5 hours prior to surgery to achieve maximum reduction of pressure before surgery.
Severe Drug Intoxications to Promote Diuresis	Attempt to maintain a urinary output of at least 100 ml/hour, and a positive fluid balance of 1-2 liters. Give loading dose of 25g followed by rate to maintain urinary output of at least 100ml/hour. Barbiturate Poisoning: Initial dose, 0.5g/kg followed by a 5 or 10% solution at a rate to maintain desired urine output. or Give one liter of a 10% solution given during the first hour. Measure urine volume and pH and calculate cumulative fluid balance at end of first hour and subsequent 2-hour periods. If positive fluid balance remains at 1-2 liters, another liter of 10% mannitol may be given over the next 2 hours. If positive fluid balance falls below 1 liter, mannitol should be replaced with 1 liter of 1/6 M sodium lactate over the next 2 hours (if urine pH is less than 7) or 1 liter of 0.9% sodium chloride over 2 hours (if urine pH is greater than 7). If positive fluid balance is more than 2 liter, 10% mannitol may be given at slowest possible rate.
Transurethral Prostatic Resection	Give 2.5-5% mannitol as irrigating solution.

MONITORING: Keep serum osmolality at 310-320mOm/kg during hyperosmolar therapy for increased intracranial pressure.

ADVERSE EFFECTS: Circulatory overload and electrolyte imbalances.

MEBENDAZOLE

(Vermox)

USES: **Mebendazole** is used in the treatment of **helmintics.** Mebendazole causes irreversible inhibition of glucose uptake in susceptible helminths but not in mammals.

DOSAGE FORMS: (Vermox) Tabs: Chewable: 100mg

DOSAGE: Mebendazole is administered orally; dosage in adults and children is the same. The dosage of mebendazole in the treatment of patients with helmintics is given in the next Table:

Anthelmintic Activity of Mebenazole

Anthelmintic Activity	Dosage of Mebenazole
Enterobius Vermicularis (Pinworm)	100mg as a single dose
Trichuris Trichiura (Whipworm) **Ascarsis Lumbricoides (Roundworm)** **Hookworm Infections** **Ancylostoma Duodenale** **Necator Americanus** **Mixed Infections**	200mg daily, given in 2 equally divided doses in the morning and evening for 3 consecutive days. If the patient is not cured (as indicated by the absence of helminth ova in the feces) within 3-4 weeks following initial therapy, a second course may be administered.
Capillaria Philippinensis	400mg daily in 2 equally divided doses in the morning and evening for 20 days
Hydatid Disease: Echinococcus Granulosus	40mg/kg daily for 1-6 months or longer or 1.2-1.8g daily for 21-30 days

Mebendazole is the drug of choice for Trichuris trichiura. Mebendazole has also been used in the treatment of toxocariasis, trichinosis, gnathostomiasis, Mansonella perstans, and Angiostrongylus cantonensis.

PHARMACOKINETICS: Absorption: 2-10%; Peak: 0.5-7 hours; Half-Life: 2.8-9hours

ADVERSE EFFECTS: Use with caution in children <2 years. Diarrhea, abdominal cramps.

MECLIZINE

(Antivert, Bonine, D-Vert, Others)

USES: Meclizine is a piperazine - derivative antihistamine; uses are given in the next Table:

Uses of Meclizine
Prevention and Treatment of Motion Sickness
Antiemetic to Prevent and Treat Nausea and Vomiting associated with:
a. Vertigo of Vestibular Origin, eg, Labyrinthitis and Meniere's Disease.
b. Radiation Sickness

Meclizine has a slower onset and longer duration of action (24 hours) than most other antihistamines used for motion sickness.

DOSAGE FORMS: Caps: 15,25,30mg; Tabs: 12.5, 25, 50mg; Tabs (chewable): 25mg (nonprescription).

DOSAGE: Dosage for children has not been established. Dosage in different conditions is given in the next Table:

Dosage of Meclizine

Condition	Dosage
Motion Sickness	25 to 50mg once daily. The initial dose should be taken at least one hour prior to departure.
Vertigo and Radiation Sickness	25 to 100mg daily depending upon clinical response.

PHARMACOKINETICS: Onset: One hour; Duration of Action: 8-24 hours; Half-Life: 6 hours.

ADVERSE EFFECTS: Drowsiness, blurred vision, dryness of mouth, and fatigue.

PRECAUTIONS: Asthma, glaucoma, prostatic hypertrophy, GI or urinary tract obstruction, pregnancy, lactation.

INTERACTIONS: Alcohol; tranquilizers; sedative-hypnotic potentiate CNS depression.

MECLOFENAMATE

(Meclomen)

USES: **Meclofenamate** is a nonsalicylate, nonsteroidal, **anti-inflammatory** drug(NSAID) with **analgesic** and **antipyretic activity.** Uses are given in the next Table:

Uses of Meclofenamate
Rheumatoid Arthritis
Osteoarthritis

Mechanism of Action: Meclofenamate acts like other NSAIDs by blocking the synthesis of prostaglandins by inhibiting cyclo-oxygenase, which converts arachidonic acid to cyclic endoperoxides, precursors of prostaglandins. It also competes for binding at prostaglandin receptor sites.

DOSAGE FORMS: Caps: 50, 100mg

DOSAGE: For rheumatoid arthritis and osteoarthritis, give 200 to 400mg daily in three or four equal doses. The drug may be taken with meals or milk. Symtomatic improvement may occur after several days; optimum effects may require 2-3 weeks.

PHARMACOKINETICS: Peak after Oral Dose: 0.5-1 hour; when taken with foood, absorption is delayed but the total amount absorbed is the same;' Protein Binding: 99%; Half-Life: 2-3.3 hours; Excretion: 2/3 in urine and 1/3 in feces

ADVERSE EFFECTS: Diarrhea: 10-33% of patients; 4% of patients discontinued drug because of this effect; nausea with or without vomiting, 10%; abdominal patients with a history of ulcers. Central nervous system reactions include confusion. Anemia, jaundice and hepatitis have been observed.

DRUG INTERACTIONS: Oral anticoagulants potentiated.

MEDROXYPROGESTERONE

(Provera, Depo-Provera, Amen, Curretab)

USES: **Medroxyprogesterone,** a synthetic **progestin,** transforms an estrogen-primed proliferative endometrium into a secretory endometrium; Uses are given in the next Table:

Uses of Medroxyprogesterone
Abnormal Uterine Bleeding caused by Hormonal Imbalance
Secondary (Pituitary) Amenorrhea
Endometrial or Renal Carcinoma, Inoperable
Contraceptive Use
Paraphilia in Males

Medroxyprogesterone is used for the treatment of abnormal uterine bleeding caused by hormonal imbalance in patients without underlying organic pathology such as fibroids or uterine cancer.

Medroxyprogesterone has been used parenterally as a long-acting (3 months) contraceptive in females. One IM injection every 3 months provides almost completely effective contraception.

Medroxyprogesterone has been used for the management of paraphilia (homosexual, heterosexual, or bisexual pedophlia, heterosexual voyeurism, sexual sadism, or exhibitionism; transvestism) in males. The frequency of erotic imagery and the intensity of erotic cravings is decreased.

DOSGE FORMS: Tab: 2.5, 5, 10mg Inj: 100, 400mg/ml

DOSAGE: Administered orally or IM; dosage is given in the next Table:

Dosage of Medroxyprogesterone

Condition	Route	Dosage
Abnormal Uterine Bleeding	Oral	5-10mg for 10 days beginning on the assumed or calculated 16th or 21st day of the menstrual cycle. Progestin-induced withdrawal bleeding usually occurs within 3-7 days after discontinuing therapy with the drug. When bleeding is caused by a deficiency of estrogen & progestin, as indicated by a poorly proliferative endometrium, use estrogens in conjunction with medroxyprogesterone. If bleeding is controlled satisfactorily, 2 subsequent cycles of combined therapy should be used.
Secondary Amenorrhea	Oral	5-10mg for 5-10 days beginning on the assumed 16th to 21st day of the menstrual cycle. In patients with a poorly developed endometrium, use estrogen therapy in conjunction with medroxyprogesterone. Progestin-induced withdrawal bleeding usually occurs within 3-7 days after discontinuing therapy with the drug.
Menopausal Replacement Therapy	Oral	10mg for last 10 days of estrogen administration
Endometrial or Renal Carcinoma, Inoperable	Oral	400mg to 1g per wk. initially;then maintenance of 400mg every month.
Contraceptive Use	IM	150mg IM every 3 months. Not FDA approved.
Paraphilia in Males	IM	200mg, 2 or 3 times daily or 500mg wkly.;maintenance dosage, 100mg once wkly.to once a month

PHARMACOKINETICS: Withdrawal bleeding in estrogen-primed endometrium occurs 2-7 days after the last dose; duration of 3 months or longer when given IM for contraception. The drug is metabolized by hydroxylation; 20-40% of dose is excreted as glucuronide and sulfate conjugates in the urine; 10% of dose is excreted in the feces; Half-Life: 15 hrs.

ADVERSE EFFECTS: Menstrual irregularities and breakthrough bleeding, amenorrhea, weight gain; masculinization of female fetus and congenital abnormalities when taken during pregnancy; thromboemboli, edema, rash, depression, decreased glucose tolerance.

MENINGITIS, PATHOGENS, TREATMENT

Pathogens: The bacterial pathogens that usually cause meningitis are given in the next Table:

Bacterial Pathogens Causing Meningitis

Neonates: Escherichia coli (33%); Group B streptococci (29%); Listeria monocytogenes (7%); other streptococci (except Streptococcus pneumoniae) (3.5%); Pseudomonas species (3.3%); Streptococcus pneumoniae (3.3%); Proteus species (2.7%); Staphylococcus aureus (2.7%); Klebsiella species (2.5%). (Report, Brit. Med. J. 290, 778-780, 1985; McCracken, G.H. et al., JAMA 252, 1427-1432, 1984). Other studies suggest that E. coli is much less common and that Group B Streptococci make up more than half of cases of neonatal meningitis (Wenger, J.D. et al., J. Infect. Dis. 162, 1316-1323, 1990).

Children, >2 months: Haemophilus influenzae, type b (67%); N. meningitidis (16%); Str. pneumoniae (9%); group B streptococci (5%); Listeria monocytogenes (4%).

Healthy Adults: Neisseria meningitidis (meningococci); Streptococcus pneumoniae (pneumococci); H. influenzae.

Elderly: Streptococcus pneumoniae (pneumococci); enteric gram-negative bacteria.

Bacterial meningitis may occur as an isolated infection or secondary to pneumonia, endocarditis, osteomyelitis or extension of infections of the sinuses and ears. Bacteremia occurs in 40 percent of patients with meningitis. Neonates: In the first week of life, meningitis is likely to be caused by bacteria colonizing the maternal birth canal, and from organisms transmitted from people looking after the newborn infant (usually via the hands) and from organisms flourishing in the humidification apparatus that is used in neonatal intensive care units.

Other pathogens that may cause meningitis are given in the next Table:

Meningitis, Other Pathogens

Viral agents (enterovirus, coxsackie, echovirus, mumps, herpes simplex, HIV and others)
Mycobacterium tuberculosis
Cryptococcus neoformans and other fungi
Treponema pallidum
Leptospira

Antibiotic Treatment: Antibiotic treatment of bacterial meningitis is given in the next Table (Medical Letter 30, 33-40, Mar 25, 1988; Committee on Infectious Diseases, Pediatrics 81, 904-907, June 1988):

Antibiotic Treatment of Bacterial Meningitis

Age	Bacteria	Treatment
Adults	Pending identification of bacterial pathogen	Penicillin G or Ampicillin, I.V., for meningococcal or pneumococcal or susceptible H. influenzae meningitis or Cephalosporin, eg, cefotaxime or ceftriaxone for beta-lactamase producing H. influenzae. or Chloramphenicol for beta-lactamase-producing H. influenzae.
	Enteric gram-negative bacteria	Cephalosporin, eg, cefotaxime, ceftriaxone or ceftizoxime.
	Pseudomonas aeruginosa or Acinetobacter	Extended-spectrum penicillins, eg, carbenicillin, or ticarcillin or mezlocillin or piperacillin, or azlocillin plus an aminoglycoside or Ceftazidime plus an aminoglycoside
	Listeria monocytogenes	Ampicillin with or without gentamicin
Children	H. influenzae S. pneumoniae N. meningitidis	Cephalosporin, eg, cefotaxime or ceftriaxone or Ampicillin and chloramphenicol
Newborns	Pending identification of bacterial pathogen	Ampicillin plus aminoglycoside or Ampicillin plus cefotaxime or ceftazidime.

MENINGITIS (Cont.)
Penicillin-Allergic Patients: In patients with a history of allergy to penicillin, alternative therapy for treatment of meningitis is given in the next Table:

Penicillin-Allergic Patients	
Drug	Comment
Cephalosporin	Patients may also be allergic to cephalosporins.
Chloramphenicol	May not be effective against enteric gram-negative bacilli. Some H. influenzae are resistant.
Aztreonam	No activity against gram-positive bacteria
Imipenem	Patients may also be allergic to imipenem
Penicillin	Penicillin may be tried if the patient has not had a history of anaphylactic reaction to penicillin and if the physician is prepared to treat anaphylaxis promptly.

Neonates: In the hospitalized low birth weight premature infant in whom nosocomial Pseudomonas infection is a possibility, ceftazidime is preferred over cefotaxime.
Infants and Children: In the first 6 to 8 weeks of life, it is advisable to add ampicillin to the cephalosporin regimen because of the possibility of Listeria or enterococcus as causative agents.

If facilities for monitoring serum concentrations are not immediately available, if pharmacologic interaction of drugs is likely, or if hepatic or renal insufficiency is present, it is advisable to avoid chloramphenicol or the aminoglycosides.
Dexamethasone: Dexamethasone therapy combined with antibiotics helps decrease the neurologic abnormalities (ataxia, hemiparesis, hypertonic extremities and cranial nerve abnormalities) and hearing loss. Dexamethasone decreases the inflammatory response in the CSF; ideally, dexamethasone should be given prior to antibiotic therapy (Odio, C.M. et al., N. Engl. J. Med. 324, 1525-1531, 1991). The antibiotic and dexamethasone schedule is given in the next Table (Lebel, M.H. et al., N. Engl. J. Med. 319, 964-971, 1988; Odio, C.M. et al., N. Engl. J. Med. 324, 1525-1531, 1991):

Antibiotic plus Dexamethasone for Bacterial Meningitis		
Antibiotic	Dosage	Dosage of Dexamethasone
Ceftriaxone	80mg/kg IV at diagnosis, 12 and 24 hours and daily thereafter.	0.15mg/kg IV every 6 hours for the first four days.
Cefotaxime	50mg/kg IV at diagnosis, and every 6 hours thereafter.	

Duration of Therapy: Minimum duration of therapy was 10 days for patients with Haemophilus influenzae, type b or Streptococcus pneumoniae meningitis.

Minimum duration of therapy was 7 days for patients with Neisseria meningitidis infections although many clinicians treat for 10 days.

MEPERIDINE HCl
(Demerol)

USES: Meperidine is a strong **analgesic** used in the relief of **moderate to severe pain;** the uses of meperidine in different conditions are given in the next Table:

Uses of Meperidine
Relieve moderate to severe pain.
Preoperative sedation as a supplement to anesthesia
Analgesia during labor
Reduce anxiety in pulmonary edema

Meperidine has been used to relieve the pain of acute myocardial infarction; however, it is probably not as effective as morphine sulfate. It has been used to relieve the pain associated with renal or biliary colic, malignancy, surgical procedures, burns, trauma and many other causes of acute pain.

Meperidine is useful for preanesthetic medication because of its sedative, antianxiety and analgesic effects.

Meperidine is sometimes used to provide analgesia during labor; however, it crosses the placenta and may depress fetal respiration. If meperidine-induced respiratory depression is suspected in the neonate, naloxone should be given as an adjunct to mechanical ventilatory support.

Mechanism of Action: Meperidine acts like other opioids in that it acts on specific opioid binding sites (receptors) in the central nervous system.

DOSAGE FORMS: Sol'n: 50mg/5ml; Tabs: 50mg, 100mg; Injection: 25mg/ml, 50mg/ml, 75mg/ml, 100mg/ml

DOSAGE: Administered orally, subcutaneously, IM or slow IM injection; or by slow, continuous IV infusion. Morphine equivalent: 75mg IV meperidine equals 10mg IV morphine. The usual dosages of meperidine are given in the next Table:

Dosages of Meperidine

Patient	Dosage
Adult	Oral, IV, IM or subcutaneously: 50-150mg every 3-4 h, as needed. Slow continuous IV infusion: 15-30mg/hour
Children	Oral, IV, IM or subcutaneously: 1-1.5mg/kg every 3-4 h, as needed. Single pediatric doses should not exceed 100mg.
Preoperative	
Adult	50-100mg IM or subcutaneously, 30-90 min. before beginning anesthesia
Children	1-1.5mg/kg (max. up to adult dose) IM or subcutaneously, 30-90 min. before beginning anesthesia
Analgesia during Labor	50-100mg, IM or subcutaneously when labor pains become regular; may repeat at 1-to 3-hour intervals, as necessary.

PHARMACOKINETICS: Peak: Orally, 1 hour; subcutaneously, 40-60 minutes; IM, 30-50 minutes. Analgesic Effect: 2-4 hours. Metabolism: Hydrolyzed and also metabolized in the liver to normeperidine (an active metabolite) which is also hydrolyzed. Half-Life: 3 hours. Normeperidine has a half-life of 14-21 hours in patients with normal renal function; it increases to 35 hours in renal failure. Excretion: Urine.

ADVERSE EFFECTS: The most common adverse effects are dizziness, nausea and vomiting. Other adverse effects include sweating, hypotension, headache, decreased respiration, and constipation. Withdrawal may occur. Accumulation of normeperidine in patients on prolonged or high dose therapy, or in patients with renal or hepatic impairment, may lead to CNS stimulation including nervousness, agitation, myoclonus, seizures, etc.

DRUG INTERACTIONS: Reduce dose of meperidine when used with the following drugs: antipsychotic drugs, sedative-hypnotics, or other CNS depressants. Effects are potentiated by monoamine oxidase inhibitors (MOAI) and isoniazid.

CONTRAINDICATIONS: Use with extreme caution or not at all in patients with cardiac arrhythmias, asthma, increased intracranial pressure, or renal failure.

METAPROTERENOL

(Metaprel, Alupent)

USES: Metaproterenol is used as a bronchodilator in the symptomatic treatment of bronchial asthma and reversible bronchospasm which may occur in association with chronic obstructive pulmonary diseases such as chronic bronchitis, pulmonary emphysema and bronchiectasis.

Mechanism of Action: Metaproterenol is a synthetic sympathomimetic drug that is similar to isoproterenol in chemical structure and in pharmacologic action. Metaproterenol stimulates the beta-2 receptors to relax bronchial smooth muscle and the smooth muscle of peripheral vasculature, metaproterenol has little or no effect on alpha-adrenergic receptors. Metaproterenol has less effect on beta-1 receptors (cardiac stimulation) than isoproterenol.

DOSAGE FORMS: Oral(sol'n): 10mg/5ml; Oral(tabs): 10, 20mg; Inhalation (aerosol): 650mcg/metered spray; Inhalation(sol'n): 0.4% (4mg/ml); 0.6% (6mg/ml); 5% (50mg/ml).

DOSAGE: Metaproterenol is administered by oral inhalation via metered dose inhaler or small volume nebulization and orally.

Dosage of Metaproterenol

Route	Age	Dosage
Inhalation (Aerosol)	Adult Older Children	1.3-2.0mg (2-3 metered sprays) up to every 3-4 hrs (Max. 12 inhalations/day)
Inhalation (Sol'n)	Adult	0.3ml of 5% solution (15mg) diluted to 2.5ml every 4-6 hrs or more often if necessary
	Child	0.1-0.3ml of 5% solution (5-15mg) diluted to 2.5ml every 4-6 hrs or more often if necessary.
Oral	Adult	20mg/dose 3 to 4 times daily
	Child	0.3-0.5mg/kg/dose 3 to 4 times daily. Max: 20mg/dose.

ADVERSE EFFECTS: Cardiovascular effects (tachycardia, arrhythmias) and CNS effects (anxiety, tremor, headache) predominate. Tachyphylaxis may lead to decreased effectiveness; paradoxical bronchoconstriction occurs occasionally.

METHADONE

(Dolophine)

USES: The uses of methadone are given in the next Table:

Uses of Methadone
Relief of Severe Pain
Detoxification and Maintenance of Opiate Dependence

Methadone is used to relieve severe, chronic pain, especially in terminally ill patients.

Methadone is used in detoxification treatment and maintenance treatment as an oral substitute for heroin or other morphine-like drugs to suppress the abstinence syndrome in patients who are dependent on these drugs.

DOSAGE FORMS: Oral: Tabs: 5mg, 10mg; Tabs(Dispersible): 40mg; Sol'n: 5mg/5ml, 10mg/5ml, 10mg/ml; Parenteral: 10mg/ml

DOSAGE: Administered orally, subcutaneously, IV or IM. Morphine equivalent: 8-10mg IM or SC methadone equals 10mg IM or SC morphine. The dosage of methadone is given in the next Table:

Dosage of Methadone

Condition	Dosage
Severe Pain	Adult: Oral, subcutaneous IV or IM: 2.5-10mg every 3-4h as necessary Child: Oral, subcutaneous, IV or IM: 0.7mg/kg daily in divided doses every 4-6hrs as necessary. Titrate to effect.
Severe, Chronic Pain in Terminally Patients	Adult: 5-20mg every 6-8h, orally. Higher doses may be used in patients who become tolerant to analgesic effects. Child: 0.7mg/kg daily in divided doses every 6-8h orally. Titrate to effect.
Detoxification	Administer methadone daily. Single oral dose of 15-20mg will often suppress withdrawal symptoms. Stabilizing dosage: 40mg in single or divided doses, daily. With stabilization for 2 or 3 days, decrease dosage daily or at 2 day intervals.
Maintenance:	See package insert

PHARMACOKINETICS: Onset: rapid, well absorbed from GI tract. Duration (IM,SC): 4-6 hrs in patients on methadone maintenance. Relieves symptoms of withdrawal longer than symptoms of pain.

ADVERSE EFFECTS: Respiratory depression, hypotension, pulmonary edema, constipation, excessive sweating. CNS depression may outlast pain relief.

METHENAMINE MANDELATE

(Mandelamine)

USES: Methenamine is used for **prophylaxis** or **suppression** of recurrent **urinary tract infections**, especially when long-term therapy is considered necessary. Methenamine should be used only after the urinary tract infection has been eradicated by other antibiotics and should not be used alone for acute infections.

Mechanism of Action: Methenamine acts by the release of formaldehyde from the drug in an acid medium. Resistance is unusual since the antibacterial effects of mandelic acid and formaldehyde are nonspecific.

DOSAGE FORMS: Tabs: 500, 1000mg; Susp.: 250mg/5ml, 500mg/5ml

DOSAGE: Dosages are given in the next Table:

Dosages of Methenamine

Patient	Dosage (After Meals and at Bedtime)
Children, <6 years	50-75mg/kg/day divided 4 times daily
Children, 6-12 years	500mg, 4 times daily
Children, >12 years & Adults	1g, 4 times daily

For maximal antibacterial effects, the urine pH should be maintained a pH 5.5 or less. Urinary pH should be monitored during methenamine therapy and, if required, supplementary acidification may be achieved by dietary regulation and/or concommitant administration of acidifying agents such as ammonium chloride.

ADVERSE EFFECTS: GI Disturbances: Nausea, vomiting, diarrhea, abdominal cramps, and anorexia.

Contraindicated in renal insufficiency.

METHICILLIN
(Staphcillin)

USES: Methicillin is a parenteral penicillinase-resistant penicillin; its use is generally limited to the treatment of infections caused by susceptible penicillinase-producing staphylococci.
DOSAGE FORMS: For Injection: 1,4,6,10g. For Injection for IV Infusion: 1g.
DOSAGE: Methicillin sodium is administered by slow IV injection or infusion or by deep IM injection. Dosage is given in the next Table:

Dosage of Methicillin Sodium

Condition	Age	Route	Dosage
Usual (Mild to Moderate infections)	Adults	IM or IV	1g every 4 or 5 h.
	Child. >1 mo. & <40kg	IM or IV	25mg/kg every 6 h.
	Neonates <2kg	IM or IV	25mg/kg every 12 h. during the first week of life; same dose every 8 h. from 1-4 weeks.
	Neonates >2kg	IM or IV	25mg/kg every 8 h. during first week of life; same dose every 6 h. from 1-4 weeks.
Meningitis	Child. Neonates	IV	Same dosage schedule as above, use 50mg/kg/dose.
Endocarditis	Adults	IV	1.5-2g every 4 h.
Acute or Chronic Osteomyelitis	Adults	IV	1.5-2g every 4 h.
Acute Osteomyelitis	Child.	IV	200-400mg/kg daily in divided doses every 4 h.

Dosage must be adjusted in patients with renal impairment.

ADVERSE EFFECTS: Frequent: Allergic reactions, rarely anaphylactic; rash; diarrhea. Occasional: Hemolytic anemia, neutropenia; pseudomembranous colitis; platelet dysfunction. Rare: Acute interstitial nephritis; hepatitis; granulocytopenia or agranulocytosis; bleeding diathesis; thrombocytopenia;hemorrhagic cystitis.
PHARMACOKINETICS: Half-Life: 0.4-0.5 h. (adults); 4-6 h. in anuric patients; 2-4 h. (neonates). Metabolism: Not to any appreciable extent.
CONTRAINDICATIONS: Hypersensitivity to penicillins.
MONITOR: Parameters to monitor are given in the next Table:

Parameters to Monitor, Methicillin Therapy

Parameter	Comment
Leukocyte Count, Total and Differential	Prior to Therapy; 1-3 times weekly during therapy to monitor for neutropenia, granulocytopenia, agranulocytosis and thrombocytopenia; eosinophilia may indicate allergic reaction.
Urinalysis, BUN and Creatinine	Acute interstitial nephritis; hemorrhagic cystitis
AST(SGOT) and ALT(SGPT)	Hepatitis

METHIMAZOLE
(Tapazole)

USES: Uses of methimazole are given in the next Table:

Uses of Methimazole
Palliative treatment of hyperthyroidism
Ameliorate hyperthyroidism in preparation for surgical treatment or radioactive iodine therapy

Methimazole is used to control the symptoms of hyperthyroidism associated with Grave's disease and maintain the patient in a euthyroid state for about 1 to 2 years until a spontaneous remission occurs; however, spontaneous remission may not occur and the patient may require ablative therapy, such as, surgery or radioactive iodine.

Mechanism of Action: Methimazole inhibits the synthesis of thyroid hormones by blocking the incorporation of iodine into tyrosyl residues of thyroglobulin and by inhibiting the coupling of these iodotyrosyl residues to form iodothyronine.

DOSAGE FORMS: (Tapazole) Tabs: 5mg, 10mg

DOSAGE: Methimazole is given orally, daily in 3 equally divided doses at about 8-hour intervals. Dosage in different hyperthyroid conditions are given in the next Table:

Dosage of Methimazole in Adults

Condition	Dosage
Mild Hyperthyroidism	Adult, initial: 15mg daily
Moderately Severe, Hyperthyroidism	Adult, initial: 30-40mg daily
Severe Hyperthyroidism	Adult, initial: 60mg daily

In general, once full control of symptoms has been achieved, therapy is continued at initial dosage levels for about 2 months. Subsequent dosage should be adjusted according to the patient's tolerance and therapeutic response.

Adult maintenance dose ranges from 5 to 30mg daily.

For the treatment of hyperthyroidism in children, the usual initial dosage of methimazole is 0.5-0.7mg/kg daily in 3 divided doses; the usual maintenance dosage is approximately one-half the initial dosage.

PHARMACOKINETICS: Peak, 1 hour; half-life, 5-13 hours; excreted in urine.

ADVERSE EFFECTS: Occur in less than 3% of patients and are listed in the next Table:

Adverse Effects of Methimazole
Agranulocytosis
Pancytopenia
Exfoliative Dermatitis
Hepatitis

Dermatologic effects are most common with rash, uriticaria, pruritis, abnormal hair loss, skin pigmentation.

Inhibition of myelopoiesis with resultant agranulocytosis, granulocytopenia and thrombocytopenia may occur; most cases appear in the first two months of therapy and rarely after 4 months. Furthermore, the risk is increased in patients older than 40 years of age and in patients receiving dosages greater than 40mg daily.

Monitor: Patients should be instructed to contact their physician immediately if the following signs or symptoms develop: sore throat, skin eruptions, fever, chills, headache or general malaise.

Leukocyte and differential counts must be done in patients with fever or sore throat.

METHOCARBAMOL
(Robaxin)

USES: Methocarbamol is used to relieve the pain of local muscle spasm.

Methocarbamol is a CNS depressant; the skeletal muscle relaxant effects are minimal and are probably related to its sedative effects.

DOSAGE FORMS: Tabs: 500, 750mg; take with milk or food. IV: 100mg/ml.

DOSAGE: Adults: Initially, 1.5 to 2g four times daily for 48 to 72 hours; for maintenance, 1g four times daily. IV or IM: 1g every 8hrs; max rate of infusion, 300mg/min.

PHARMACOKINETICS: Absorption: Rapid and almost complete; Onset: 30 min.; Peak: 1-2 hours; Half-Life: 1-2 hours; Metabolism: Liver; Excretion: Urine.

ADVERSE EFFECTS: Drowsiness, dizziness, headache, anorexia, vertigo, and mild nausea occur occasionally. Skin eruptions occur rarely. IV administration may cause thrombophlebitis.

METHOTREXATE
(Folex)

USES: **Methotrexate** is used to treat patients with certain **cancers** and to treat **psoriasis.**

Uses of methotrexate in the treatment of different cancers are given in the next Table:

Uses of Methotrexate in Treatment of Tumors
Prolonged Survival and Probably some Cures:
Choriocarcinoma, Low Risk: Methotrexate alone
Choriocarcinoma, High Risk: Methotrexate + Dactinomycin + Chlorambucil(MAC)
Burkitt's Lymphoma: Cyclophosphamide + Vincristine + Methotrexate + Doxorubicin + Prednisone
Acute Lymphocytic Leukemia of Childhood: Prophylaxis of CNS disease: Intrathecal Methotrexate
Maintenance: Methotrexate + Mercaptopurine
Non-Hodgkin's Lymphomas, Rapidly Growing Types (e.g. Diffuse Histiocytic Lymphoma): Bleomycin + Doxorubicin + Cyclophosphamide + Methotrexate + Dexamethasone(M-BACOD)
or Cyclophosphamide + Vincristine + Methotrexate (High Dose with Leucovorin Rescue) + Cytarabine(COMLA)
Palliation and Probable Prolongation of Life:
Breast Carcinoma, Adjuvant Therapy: Cyclophosphamide + Methotrexate + Fluorouracil(CMF)
Breast Carcinoma, Advanced Disease: Cyclophosphamide + Methotrexate + Fluorouracil(CMF) ± Prednisone(CMFP) ± Vincristine(CMFPP)
Small Cell Carcinoma of Lung: Cyclophosphamide + Lomustine + Methotrexate

Other tumors that may be responsive to methotrexate, in combination with other antitumor drugs, include ovarian carcinomas and osteogenic sarcoma. Head and neck carcinomas have been treated with methotrexate. Other tumors treated with methotrexate are cutaneous T-cell lymphomas (mycoses fungoides) and medulloblastoma.

Methotrexate is used in the treatment of conditions other than cancer; these conditions are listed in the next Table:

Treatment of Conditions Other than Cancer with Methotrexate
Psoriasis
Rheumatoid Arthritis, severe
Asthma (investigational)

Mechanism of Action: Methotrexate is a folic acid analogue. Methotrexate blocks the action of the enzyme, dihydrofolate reductase, as illustrated in the next Figure:

Methotrexate and Folate Metabolism

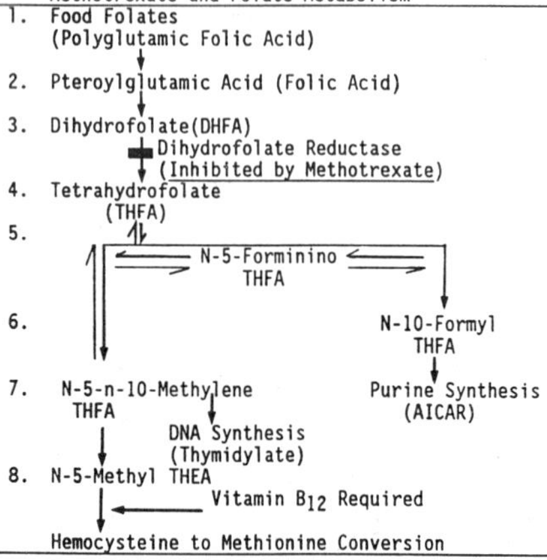

METHOTREXATE (Cont.)

As illustrated in this Figure, methotrexate blocks the synthesis of THFA which is normally converted to various coenzymes required for one-carbon transfer reactions involved in the synthesis of thymidylate, purines, methionine, and glycine. Thus, inhibition of dihydrofolate reductase by methotrexate can lead to inhibition of DNA, RNA, and protein synthesis.

Methotrexate is cell cycle-specific for the S phase.

The **block** of dihydrofolate reductase is **bypassed** by use of **leucovorin** calcium (see Leucovorin); this "rescue" agent allows for recovery of normal tissue and allows use of larger doses of methotrexate.

DOSAGE FORMS: Tabs: 2.5mg; Injection: 20, 50, 100, 250, 1000mg; 2.5, 25mg/ml.

DOSAGE: Methotrexate is administered orally. Methotrexate sodium is administered by IM, IV or intrathecal injection; the drug may also be administered intra-arterially. Dosage is given in the next Table (Alternative dosing schedules may be used):

Dosage of Methotrexate

Condition	Age	Route	Dosage
Trophoblastic Neoplasms	Adults	Oral or IM	15-30mg daily for 5 days; repeat in one or more weeks if toxicity has disappeared; 3-5 courses. Monitor HCG levels during therapy
Meningeal Leukemia		Intrathecal	$12mg/m^2$ or 15mg at 2-5 day intervals until CSF cell counts return to normal; then one additional dose is administered or $12mg/m^2$ once weekly for 2 weeks and then once monthly thereafter. Children: 6mg (<1 yr); 8mg (1-2 yr); 10mg (2-3 yr); 12mg (≥3 yr).
Mycosis Fungoides	Adults	Oral	2.5-10mg daily for several weeks or months
	Adults	IM	50mg once weekly or 25mg twice weekly
Burkitt's Lymphoma Stages I or II		Oral	10-25mg/day for 4-8 days
Psoriasis	Adults		Test for idiosyncratic reactions by giving a single 5mg to 10mg dose of methotrexate 1 week prior to initiation of therapy. There are three dosage schedules suggested by the manufacturers. Optimum dosage has not been established.
Rheumatoid Arthritis	Adults	Oral or IM	7.5mg as a single dose IM or orally or in 3 divided doses orally every 12 hours once a week. Dosage is increased gradually until optimal therapeutic response. Usual max: 20mg weekly. Test dose, as above.
Asthma (investigational)	Adults	Oral	15-50mg weekly may allow reduction of steroid dose in severe steroid dependent asthma (Mullarkey, M.F. et al., Ann. Intern. Med. 112, 577-581, 1990). Another study has shown lack of benefit (Erzurum, S.C. et al., Ann. Intern. Med. 114, 353-360, 1991).

Methotrexate should only be administered by physicians experienced with its use.

PHARMACOKINETICS: Half-Life: After intravenous infusion, methotrexate distributes within the total body water and the initial half-life is about one hour. After this initial distribution, the half-life is about 3 hours.

ADVERSE EFFECTS: With high-dose methotrexate, nephrotoxicity is a common problem. More than 90 percent of methotrexate is excreted by the kidney within 24-48 hours. At acid pH, methotrexate may deposit in the renal cells; one of the major metabolites, 7-OH methotrexate, is relatively soluble at acid pH, Nephrotoxicity is reversible.

Hepatotoxicity may occur and may progress to cirrhosis. Elevated transaminases may occur in 15% of patients on chronic therapy.

METHOTREXATE (Cont.)

Toxicities, other than nephrotoxicity or hepatotoxicity that occur with high-dose methotrexate include B-lymphocyte dysfunction and acute dermatitis, bone marrow depression, leukopenia, thrombocytopenia, anemia, stomatitis, vomiting and diarrhea.

LABORATORY MONITORING: Specimen: Red top tube, separate serum as soon as possible. Stable at 4°C for at least 24 hours and at -20°C for one month. Collect specimens at 24, 48 and 72 hours past high-dose infusion. Keep specimen in the dark.

Excretion: More than 90 percent of methotrexate is excreted by the kidney and renal toxicity is common; determine serum creatinine and creatinine clearance before starting therapy.

High dose methotrexate is usually accompanied by leucovorin rescue depending on the concentration of methotrexate at 24, 48 and 72 hours.

Sampling Times: Sampling times are usually 24, 48 and 72 hours after starting methotrexate infusion, and ideally everyday during leucovorin rescue.

Toxicity: Without leucovorin rescue: >8 x 10^{-8}M for > 42 hours. With leucovorin rescue: 10^{-7}M when leucovorin is discontinued; 10^{-5}M at 24 hours; 10^{-6}M at 48 hours; 10^{-7}M at 72 hours.

Monitor transaminases prior to institution of chronic therapy and periodically thereafter.

METHOXAMINE HYDROCHLORIDE
(Vasoxyl)

USES: Methoxamine hydrochloride is a **sympathomimetic amine** that is similar to phenylephrine in pharmacologic action. Sympathomimetics are drugs that partially or completely mimic the actions of norepinephrine or epinephrine. Methoxamine acts almost exclusively by a direct effect on alpha-adrenergic receptors. Uses of methoxamine are given in the next Table:

Uses of Methoxamine
Hypotension and Shock
Hypotension during Anesthesia
Supraventricular Paroxymsal Tachycardia

In the treatment of hypotension and shock, methoxamine is used to produce vasoconstriction to raise blood pressure.

DOSAGE FORMS: Parenteral: 20mg/ml

DOSAGE: Methoxamine hydrochloride is administered IM or IV. Dosage is given in the next Table:

Dosage of Methoxamine Hydrochloride

Condition	Age	Route	Dosage
Hypotension & Shock	Adults	IM	5-20mg
		IV	3-5mg
	Child	IM	0.25mg/kg
		IV	0.08mg/kg
Prevent Hypotension During Spinal Anesthesia	Adults	IM	Shortly before or at time of administration; 10mg for low spinal; 15-20mg for high spinal
	Child.	IM	0.25mg/kg

ADVERSE EFFECTS: May cause sustained excessive blood pressure elevation, decreased cardiac output and decreased organ perfusion due to vasoconstriction.

METHSUXIMIDE
(Celontin)

USES: Methsuximide is an **anticonvulsant**; uses are given in the next Table:

Uses of Methsuximide
Absence (Petit Mal) Seizures
Combined Absence and Tonic-Clonic Seizures, especially in conjunction with other anticonvulsants, eg, phenytoin or phenobarbital.
Partial Seizures with Complex Symptomatology (Psychomotor Seizures)

Methsuximide is often used for combined absence and tonic-clonic seizures, often in conjunction with other anticonvulsants. Ethosuximide which is the drug of choice for absence seizures, may precipitate tonic-clonic seizures; methsuximide does not usually have this effect.

DOSAGE FORMS: Caps: 150, 300mg

DOSAGE: Give orally, dosage is given in the next Table:

Dosage of Methsuximide

Adults or Children:
- Initial: 300mg daily for the first week.
- As necessary, increase dosage by 300mg daily at weekly intervals thereafter up to a maximum dosage of 1.2g daily in divided doses.
- Usual maintenance dose, 10mg/kg daily

PHARMACOKINETICS: Peak: 1-3 hours; half-life: 3 hours

ADVERSE EFFECTS: GI; CNS; hematologic, eg, leukopenia, pancytopenia, eosinophilia, monocytosis. Use with extreme caution in patients with hepatic or renal disease. Systemic lupus erythematosis has been associated.

LABORATORY MONITORING: Complete blood count (CBC), hepatic function tests and urinalysis at periodic intervals.

METHYLDOPA
(Aldomet)

USES: Methyldopa is a centrally acting alpha-blocker, used in the treatment of **hypertension;** it is often considered to be the drug of choice for treating chronic hypertension during pregnancy.

Methyldopa has been used to reduce the neurogenic vasoconstriction in some patients with Raynaud's phenomenon.

Hypertension: Treatment of hypertension with methyldopa is given in the next Table (The 1988 Report of the Joint National Committee on Detection, Evaluation, and Treatment of High Blood Pressure, Arch.Intern. Med.148, 1023-1038, 1988):

Treatment of Hypertension with Methyldopa

Step 1: Nonpharmacologic Approaches (see **HYPERTENSION**)
↓
Step 2: **Diuretic** or **Beta-Blocker** or **Calcium Antagonist** or **ACE Inhibitor**
Observe up to 6 months; if treatment ineffective
↓
Step 3: Add a second drug of a different class eg, methyldopa
or Increase the dosage of the first drug
or Substitute another drug
↓
Step 4: Add a third drug of a different class
or Substitute a second drug
↓
Step 5: Consider further evaluation and/or referral
or Add a third or fourth drug

Mechanism of Action: The antihypertensive action of methyldopa is thought to be mediated by its metabolism to alpha-methylnorepinephrine; this metabolite lowers blood pressure by activating inhibitory alpha-adrenergic receptors in the brainstem, thereby reducing sympathetic outflow.

DOSAGE FORMS: Oral Preparations: Susp.: 250mg/5ml; Tabs: 125, 250, 500mg; Parenteral (Methyldopate HCl): Injection: 50mg/ml

DOSAGE: Methyldopa is administered orally. Methyldopate hydrochloride, the intravenous preparation, is used mainly to treat postoperative hypertension. Dosage is given in the next Table:

Dosage of Methyldopa

Condition	Age	Route	Dosage
Chronic Hypertension	Adult	Oral	Initially, 250mg at bedtime; this dose increased to 250mg twice daily after one week. Increased gradually until blood pressure controlled (1 or 1.5g/day); max. 3g.
	Child.	Oral	Initially, 10mg/kg daily in two to four doses. The dose is increased or decreased at two-day or longer intervals. Max. 65mg/kg daily
HYPERTENSIVE EMERGENCIES (Use Methyldopate)	Adult	IV	250-500mg every 6-8 h. as required. Max. 1g every 6h
	Child.	IV	20-40mg/kg daily divided into 4 doses

ADVERSE EFFECTS: Drowsiness is a common side which often subsides with continued therapy. Excessive hypotension is the most common side effect in hospitalized patients. Orthostatic hypotension may occur, especially in elderly patients. Sodium and water retention may occur if a diuretic is not given.

Other: Mental depression; fatigue; dryness of the mouth; nasal congestion; nausea; vomiting; diarrhea; sexual dysfunction; hepatitis. Positive Coombs' test in 10-20% with prolonged treatment but hemolytic anemia occurs rarely.

PHARMACOKINETICS: Onset: 6 hours (oral); 2-3 hours (IV); Duration: 6-12 hours Half-Life: 1.8 hours. Excretion: Urine.

CONTRAINDICATIONS: Active hepatic disease.

METHYLDOPA (Cont.)

MONITOR: Monitor parameters as given in the next Table:

Monitor Methylodopa

Parameter	Comments
Complete Blood Count (CBC)	Baseline values then periodically for hemolytic anemia and eosinophilia (hypersensitivity reaction)
Direct Coombs' Test	Baseline values then after 6 and 12 months of therapy
Liver Function Tests	Baseline values and every 2 weeks during first 6-12 weeks of therapy or whenever unexplained fever occurs, to detect hepatitis

LABORATORY TEST INTERFERENCE: Methyldopa may interfere with the determination of urinary catecholamines by the fluorescent technique and thus gives a false positive result in the work-up of a patient for pheochromocytoma. Before treatment is started, it is desirable to do a blood count,(hematocrit, hemoglobin, or red cell count) which should then be repeated at periodic intervals. Do a direct coombs test before therapy and at 6 and 12 months after the start of therapy.

METHYLDOPA AND HYDROCHLOROTHIAZIDE

(Aldoril)

USES: The combination, methyldopa, a centrally acting alpha-blocker, and hydrochlorothiazide, a diuretic, is used in the management of moderate to severe hypertension. Methyldopa is generally most effective when used with a diuretic. Advantages of using the combination of methyldopa and hydrochlorothiazid are given in the next Table:

Advantages of Combination of Methyldopa plus Hydrochlorothiazide
May prevent tolerance to methyldopa.
Permit reduction of methyldopa dosage.
Hydrochlorothiazide may prevent sodium retention.
Hydrochlorothiazide may prevent increased plasma volume which may occur after prolonged methyldopa therapy.
Permits a reduction in the dosage of each drug thus minimizing adverse effects.

Treatment of hypertension with Aldoril is given in the next Table(The 1988 Report of the Joint National Committee on Detection, Evaluation, and Treatment of High Blood Pressure, Arch. Intern. Med. 148, 1023-1038, 1988):

Treatment of Hypertension with Aldoril

Step 1: Nonpharmacologic Approaches (see **HYPERTENSION**)

↓

Step 2: Aldoril should not be used initially. The dosage of hydrochlorothiazide is adjusted first; then, as appropriate, adjust the dosage of methyldopa. If it is determined that the optimum maintenance dosage corresponds to the ratio in the available fixed combination preparation (see **DOSAGE FORMS**)then use one of the available products.

DOSAGE FORMS: Dosage forms of Aldoril are given in the next Table:

Dosage Forms of Aldoril

Drug	Methyldopa (mg)	Hydrochlorothiazide (mg)
Aldoril 15	250	15
Aldoril 25	250	25
Aldoril D 30	500	30
Aldoril D 50	500	50

DOSAGE: Dosage should first be adjusted by administering each drug separately

ADVERSE EFFECTS: When fixed combinaton; hypotensive agents such as Aldoril are used, the cautions, precautions, contraindications, and adverse effects are those associated with each alone.-see methyldopa and hydrochlorothiazide. These effects are as follows: positive Coombs test, hemolytic anemia, fever, jaundice, hepatic necrosis, granulocytopenia, fluid or electrolyte imbalance, sedation, headache, asthenia, orthostatic hypotension, bradycardia, GI upset rash, nasal congestion, hyperprolactinemia, arthralgia.

PARAMETERS TO MONITOR: See methyldopa.

METHYLENE BLUE

USES: The uses of methylene blue are given in the next Table:

Uses of Methylene Blue
Treatment of Idiopathic and Drug-induced Methemoglobinemia
Management of Chronic Urolithiasis

In the treatment of methemoglobinemia, the reactions are as follows:

$$\text{Methylene Blue} \xrightarrow[\text{Reductase in RBC's}]{\text{Methemoglobin}} \text{Leukomethylene Blue}$$

$$\text{Methemoglobin}(Fe^{+3}) \xrightarrow{\text{Leukomethylene Blue}} \text{Hemoglobin}(Fe^{+2})$$

Methylene blue is reduced to leukomethylene blue by methemoglobin reductases in erythrocytes; leukomethylene blue then reduces methemoglobin to hemoglobin.

DOSAGE FORMS: Tabs: 65mg; Injection: 10mg/ml

DOSAGE: Methylene blue may be administered orally or by IV injection. In the treatment of acute methemoglobinemia, the IV route is usually preferred because IV is more rapid in onset than the oral route. The dosages of methylene blue are given in the next Table:

Dosages of Methylene Blue

Condition	Age	Route	Dosage
Acute Methemoglobinemia	Adults and Children	IV	1-2mg/kg injected slowly over several minutes or 25mg/m^2. Repeat after 1 hour as necessary.
	Adults	Oral	65-130mg, 3 times daily, after meals with a full glass of water.
Maintenance Therapy in Chronic Methemoglobinemia	Adults	Oral	100-300mg daily
Chronic Urolithiasis	Adults	Oral	65mg, 3 times daily.

ADVERSE EFFECTS: Oral dose: Bladder irritation: GI: nausea, vomiting, diarrhea; fever. IV: GI, precordial pain, CNS: dizziness, headache, mental confusion; hypertension, profuse. Long-term administration may cause marked anemia; monitor hemoglobin frequently. Hemolysis may occur, especially in infants and patients with G-6-PD deficiency. Causes blue-green discoloration of urine.

CONTRAINDICATIONS: Patients with severe renal impairment or known hypersensitivity, G-6-PD deficiency.

METHYLPHENIDATE
(Ritalin)

USES: **Methylphenidate** is used to treat **attention deficit disorder** with **hyperactivity** (hyperkinetic syndrome of childhood, minimal brain dysfunction) in carefully selected children older than 6 years of age and narcolepsy (a condition characterized by deep sleep).

DOSAGE FORMS: (Ritalin) Tabs: 5, 10, 20mg; Tabs; slow release: 20mg(8 hour duration)

DOSAGE: Administered orally. The dosage is given in the next Table:

Dosage of Methylphenidate

Condition	Dosage
Hyperactivity	Initial Dose: 0.25mg/kg daily. Dosage may be doubled each week. Maximum dosage 60mg daily. Some authors recommend maintenance dose of 0.6mg/kg daily (McBride, M.C., J. Pediatr. 113, 137-145, 1988); manufacturers recommend 1-2mg/kg daily. or Initial Dose: 5mg before breakfast and lunch. Dosage may be increased by 5-10mg daily at weekly intervals. Oral Dosage in children should not exceed 60mg daily. Discontinue if beneficial effect is not attained in one month. If treatment is successful, discontinue periodically to assess patient's condition.
Narcolepsy	Adult: 10mg 2 or 3 times daily, given 30-45 minutes before meals. Range 10-60mg daily.

METHYLPHENIDATE (Cont.)
ADVERSE EFFECTS: Most frequent adverse effects are dose related and include nervousness and insomnia. Prolonged administration at 30-40mg daily may suppress normal weight gain in children. Other adverse effects include: anorexia, nausea, dryness of the throat, dizziness, palpitation, headache, dyskinesia (eg, choreoathetosis) and drowsiness. CV Effects: angina, cardiac arrhythmias, hyper- or hypotension and increase or decrease in pulse rate.
LABORATORY MONITORING: Periodic complete blood cell(CBC) and platelet counts in patients on prolonged therapy are suggested by the manufacturers. Many clinicians follow these parameters only if clinical signs suggest hematologic toxicity.
DRUG INTERACTIONS: MAOI's; Metabolism of coumarin, anticonvulsants, tricyclic antidepressants and other drugs is inhibited.

METHYLPREDNISOLONE
(Medrol, Solu-Medrol, Others)
USES: Uses of **methylprednisolone** are listed in the next Table:

Uses of Methylprednisolone
Anti-Inflammatory
Immunosuppressant
Concomitant Therapy with a Mineralocorticoid for Treatment of Adrenocorticoid Insufficiency

Methylprednisone is used principally as an **anti-inflammatory** or an **immunosuppressant drug.** It has only minimal mineralocorticoid activity and if used in the treatment of adrenocortical insufficiency, a mineralocorticoid is required.
DOSAGE FORMS: Oral(methylprednisolone): 2,4,8,16,24,32mg tabs; IM(methylprednisolone acetate): 20,40,80mg/ml; IV or IM(methylprednisolone sodium succinate): 40,125,500,1000,2000mg.
DOSAGE: Methylprednisolone dosage is given in the next Table:

Dosage of Methylprednisolone

Preparation	Route	Dosage
Methylprednisolone	Oral	Adult: 2-60mg daily in 4 divided doses Child: 0.12-1.7mg/kg daily in 3-4 divided doses. Dose varies, depending on disease being treated.
Methylprednisolone acetate	IM	Adult: 10-80mg; total daily dose or weekly dose may be administered once.
Methylprednisolone sodium succinate	IV or IM	Adult: Usual dosage range 10-250mg up to 6 times daily. Child: Asthma dosage; load with 1-2mg/kg once followed by 2-4mg/kg daily in 4 divided doses. Life-threatening shock: 30mg/kg initially, repeat doses every 4-6hrs for 24-48hrs has been given. Use is controversial; no clear benefit in randomized controlled trials (Sprung, C.L. et al., NEJM 311, 1137-1143, 1984; Bone, R.C. et al., NEJM 317, 653-658, 1987). Adjunct therapy for pneumocystis: 30mg twice daily for 5 days, then once daily for 5 days, then 15mg once daily for 11 days.

Wide dosage ranges exist; dosage must be individualized to the patient and the condition being treated.
ADVERSE EFFECTS: Dermatologic: acne, thin fragile skin, poor wound healing, petechiae, ecchymoses, facial erythema. Endocrine: Cushing's syndrome, growth suppression, pituitary-adrenal axis suppression, menstrual changes, glucose intolerance, negative nitrogen balance, decreased protein anabolism. Fluid and Electrolyte Disturbances: salt and water retention, hypertension, congestive heart failure, potassium depletion, hypokalemic alkalosis. Gastrointestinal: peptic ulcers, pancreatitis, esophageal ulceration. Immunologic Suppression: exacerbation of deep fungal or mycobacterial infection or herpes keratitis; chronic use may predispose to infections caused by unusual organisms. Musculoskeletal: weakness, myopathy, decreased muscle mass, osteoporosis, pathologic fractures. Neurologic: increased intracranial pressure (pseudotumor cerebri), vertigo, headache, euphoria, psychosis, convulsions. Ophthalmic: posterior subcapsular cataracts, increased intraocular pressure, glaucoma.

METHYSERGIDE
(Sansert)

USES: Methysergide is a semisynthetic ergot alkaloid; uses are given in the next Table:

Uses of Methysergide
Prophylaxis for **Severe Disabling Migraine** and **Episodic Cluster Headaches** that do not respond to other prophylactic drugs such as propranolol

Serious adverse reactions occur with prolonged use of methysergide. Methysergide is ineffective in terminating acute migraine or cluster headaches.

DOSAGE FORMS: Tabs: 2mg.

DOSAGE: Methysergide is given orally; dosage is given in the next Table:

Dosage of Methysergide

Condition	Dosage
Prophylaxis of Migraine or Cluster Headaches	Usual adult dosage: 4-8mg daily in divided doses with meals. Should not be administered continously for more than 6 months; a gradual wean should lead to a 3-4 week drug-free interval.

Methysergide has been used to control diarrhea in patients with carcinoid, although it is not approved for this purpose. Initial dose is 2mg 3 times/day, increase to 4-6mg 3 times/day as needed.

ADVERSE EFFECTS: The most serious adverse effects are fibrotic changes in retroperitoneal, pleuropulmonary and cardiac tissues that may occur with long-term uninterrupted use.

Adverse vascular effects include peripheral vascular insufficiency with cold, numb, painful extremities with or without paresthesias and diminished or absent pulse. Angina-like pain has been reported.

Central nervous system effects include insomnia, nervousness, euphoria, dizziness, ataxia, rapid speech, nightmares and hallucinations. Other effects include drowsiness, lethargy, loss of initiative, and mental depression.

Gastrointestinal effects include nausea, vomiting, diarrhea, and abdominal pain.

Other adverse effects include dermatitis, alopecia, peripheral and localized edema, weight gain, and myalgia.

CONTRAINDICTIONS: Hypertension, cerebrovascular disease, coronary artery disease, angina pectoris, severe peripheral vascular disease, thyrotoxicosis, hepatic or renal impairment, sepsis, severe pruritis, malnutrition, pregnancy, (category X).

METOCLOPRAMIDE
(Reglan)

USES: Metoclopramide is a **dopamine receptor antagonist,** an **antiemetic** and a **stimulant** of **upper GI motility.** The uses of metoclopramide are given in the next Table:

Uses of Metoclopramide
Diabetic Gastric Stasis
Prevention of Postoperative Nausea and Vomiting
Prevention of Cancer Chemotherapy-Induced Emesis
Facilitate Intubation Small Intestine
Radiographic Exam of Upper GI Tract in Patients with Delayed Gastric Emptying
Gastroesophageal Reflex

DOSAGE FORMS: (Reglan) Oral: Tabs: 5,10mg; Sol'n: 5mg/5ml; Parenteral: 5mg/ml

DOSAGE: The dosage of metoclopramide in different conditions is given in the next Table:

Uses of Metoclopramide

Condition	Dosage
Diabetic Gastric Stasis	Adults: Oral: 10mg, 4 times daily, 30 min before meals and at bedtime. Same dosage may be given IV or IM if necessary. Continue therapy for 2-8 weeks
Prevention of Post-operative Nausea and Vomiting	Adults: 10-20mg IM near the end of the surgical procedure and every 4-6 hrs as necessary.
Prevention of Cancer Chemotherapy-Induced Emesis	Adults or Children: IV: Initially, 2mg/kg, 30 min. before admission of a known emetrogenic drug,such as, cisplatin, dacarbazine, dactinomycin; repeat twice at 2-hour intervals following initial dose. If vomiting not suppressed, give 2mg/kg at 3-hour intervals for 3 additional doses. If vomiting is suppressed following initial 3 doses, give 1mg/kg at 3-hour intervals for 3 additional doses.
Facilitate Intubation Small Intestine	If tube has not passed through pylorus during 10 min., then give metoclopramide as follows: Adults: 10mg, I.V., single dose Children: <6 years: 0.1mg/kg, IV; 6-14 years: 2.5-5mg, IV
Radiographic Exam of Upper GI Tract in Patients with Delayed Gastric Emptying	Adult: IV, 10mg, single dose Children, <6 years, 0.1mg/kg; 6-14 years, 2.5-5mg
Gastroesophageal Reflex	Adult: Oral, 10-15mg given up to 4 times daily 30 min. before each meal and at bedtime as needed. For treatment of intermittent symptoms, give single, oral dose, up to 20mg prior to provoking situation. Child: 0.1mg/kg/dose 4 times daily IV or orally (Tolia, V. et al., J. Pediatr. **115**, 141-145, 1989).

ADVERSE EFFECTS: CNS effects, eg, restlessness, drowsiness, fatigue and lassitude, occur in about 10% of patients. May cause extrapyramidal reactions, dystonic reactions, tardive dyskinesia, Parkinsonian symptoms, and neuroleptic malignant syndrome (NMS).

METOLAZONE

(Diulo, Mykrox, Zaroxolyn)

USES: Metolazone is a quinazoline-derivative diuretic, structurally similar to the thiazides. Metolazone is used in the treatment of edema and hypertension. Uses of metolazone are given in the next Table:

Uses of Metolazone

Condition	Comment
Hypertension	Step 2 drug; see below
Edema	May be more useful in patients with impaired renal function. May be useful in patients with refractory congestive cardiac failure (Kiyingi, A., et al., Lancet 335, 29-31, 1990).

Hypertension: Diuretics initially lower blood pressure by reducing the plasma volume; during long-term therapy, peripheral resistance also is decreased. Treatment of hypertension with metolazone is given in the next Table (The 1988 Report of the Joint National Committee on Detection, Evaluation, and Treatment of High Blood Pressure, Arch. Intern. Med. 148, 1023-1038, 1988):

Treatment of Hypertension with Metolazone

Step 1: Nonpharmacologic Approaches (see HYPERTENSION)

↓

Step 2: Metolazone (Usual Minimum, 1.25mg/day; Usual Maximum, 10mg/day); Observe up to 6 months; if ineffective then,

↓

Step 3: Add a second drug of a different class
or Increase the dosage of metolazone
or Substitute another drug

↓

Step 4: Add a third drug of a different class
or Substitute a second drug

↓

Step 5: Consider further evaluation and/or referral
or Add a third or fourth drug

"Step-Down": For patients with mild hypertension after 1 year of control, consider decreasing or withdrawing metolazone and other hypotensive drugs.

Mechanism of Action: Metolazone, which is similar to the thiazide diuretics, acts on the cortical thick ascending loop of Henle and the proximal distal tubule where it inhibits sodium chloride reabsorption. The urinary excretion of sodium chloride and water is increased. Unlike the thiazides, metolazone does not decrease the glomerular filtration rate (GFR) and may produce diuresis in patients with a creatinine clearance <20ml/min.

DOSAGE FORMS: Tabs: Mykrox: 0.5mg; Diulo, Zaroxolyn: 2.5, 5, 10mg.

DOSAGE: Metolazone is administered orally; unlike the thiazides, metolazone may produce diuresis when creatinine clearance is <20ml/min. Mykrox tablets are more rapidly and extensively absorbed and are not therapeutically equivalent to other preparations. Dosage is given in the following Table:

Condition	Dosage
Edema	Usual Adult Dose: 5-10mg once daily as Zaroxolyn or Diulo. Some patients may respond to doses as low as 1.25mg/day. Patients with renal disease may require up to 20mg once daily. Child: 0.2-0.4mg/kg/day given in 1 to 2 doses (Arnold, W.C., Pediatrics, 74, 872-875, 1984). Some patients may respond to lower doses: 0.04-0.06mg/kg daily in one dose (Garin, E.H. and Richard, G.A., International J. of Pediatr. Nephrol., 2, 181-184, 1981).
Hypertension	Initial dose: 1.25-2.5mg once daily as Zaroxolyn or Diulo, 0.5mg once daily as Mykrox. Increase dosage gradually to desired effect, usual maximum 5-10mg once daily as Zaroxolyn or Diulo or 1mg once daily as Mykrox.

PHARMACOKINETICS: Peak: 2-4 hours (Mykrox), 8 hours (Zaroxolyn); Volume of Distribution: 113 liters, one-third protein bound; Elimination half-life: 14 hours, excreted unchanged in the urine.

ADVERSE EFFECTS: See HYDROCHLOROTHIAZIDE. Also, abdominal bloating, chest pain.

CONTRAINDICATIONS: Hepatic coma or pre-coma.

MONITOR: Electrolytes should be followed closely, monitor calcium and magnesium periodically.

METOPROLOL TARTRATE
(Lopressor)

USES: **Metoprolol** tartrate is a **beta-1 adrenergic blocking agent;** uses are given in the next Table:

Uses of Metoprolol
Hypertension
Angina
Acute Myocardial Infarction

Treatment of hypertension with metoprolol is given in the next Table (The 1988 Report of the Joint National Committee on Detection, Evaluation, and Treatment of High Blood Pressure, Arch. Intern. Med. 148, 1023-1038, 1988):

Treatment of Hypertension with Metoprolol

Step 1: Nonpharmacologic Approaches (see **Hypertension**)
↓
Step 2: Metoprolol (Usual Minimum, 50 mg/day; Usual Maximum, 200 mg/day)
Observe up to 6 months; if ineffective then,
↓
Step 3: Add a second drug of a different class
or Increase the dosage of metoprolol
or Substitute another drug
↓
Step 4: Add a third drug of a different class
or Substitute a second drug
↓
Step 5: Consider further evaluation and/or referral
or Add a third or fourth drug

"Step-Down": For patients with mild hypertension, after 1 year of control, consider decreasing or withdrawing metoprolol and other hypotensive drugs.

Metoprolol may be used as initial therapy or may be given with a diuretic as Step 2 in the antihypertensive regimen. Beta-1 receptors are found in the heart and are stimulated by norepinephrine. Metoprolol like other beta-1 blockers, produces a fall in blood pressure by decreasing the cardiac output. With continued treatment, the cardiac output returns to normal but the blood pressure remains low because the peripheral vascular resistance is "reset" at a lower level.

Angina: Metoprolol, like other beta-1 blocking agents, reduces heart rate, myocardial contractility, and cardiac output; myocardial oxygen demand is reduced by prolonging the diastolic interval during which coronary flow occurs.

Acute Myocardial Infarction: Metoprolol tartrate may reduce estimated myocardial infarct size when given I.V. in the early stages of acute myocardial infarction and may decrease mortality when used for long term therapy.

DOSAGE FORMS: Tabs: 50, 100mg; I.V. Solution: 1mg/ml in 5ml containers.

METOPROLOL TARTRATE (Cont.)
DOSAGE: Metoprolol by oral route is taken with meals; the drug is not recommended for children. Dosage is given in the next Table:

Dosage of Metoprolol Tartrate

Condition	Route	Dosage
Hypertension	Oral	Initially, 100-150mg daily as a single or divided dose. Dosage may be increased at weekly (or longer) intervals until hypotensive effect is maintained. Maintenance Dose: 100-450mg daily, usually given in one or two doses. If control is not adequate, the drug should be given three times daily.
Angina	Oral	50mg, 2-4 times daily; sublingual and long acting nitrates should be continued as needed.
Acute Myocardial Infarction	IV	Initially, three 5mg rapid IV injections at 2 min. intervals (total, 15mg). Monitor blood pressure, heart rate and ECG.
	Oral	Oral therapy may then be instituted 15 minutes after the last IV dose if IV therapy is tolerated. The oral dosage is 25-50mg every 6 hrs. for 48 hrs. followed by oral maintenance dosage of 100mg twice daily

Metoprolol must be withdrawn gradually; sudden withdrawal is dangerous. Taper over 1-2 weeks.
PHARMACOKINETICS: Bioavailability: 50%; Half-Life: 3-4 hrs. increased in poor hydroxylators; Protein Binding: 10%; Urinary Excretion: 10%; Metabolism: Liver; Active Metabolites: None.
ADVERSE EFFECTS: The most frequent adverse effects dizziness, fatigue, insomnia, and gastric upset.
Cardiovascular Effects: The most common adverse cardiovascular effects are shortness of breath and bradycardia especially with the IV routes. Bradycardia is treated with IV atropine sulfate. If there is inadequate response to atropine, IV isoproterenol may be administered with caution.
Other effects include cold extremities, Raynaud's phenomenon, palpitation, peripheral arterial insufficiency, intermittent claudication, angina pectoris and CHF. Hypotension may occur after IV metoprolol.
Nervous System Effects: Central nervous system effects include dizziness, fatigue, insomnia, headache, nightmares, and increased dreams and reversible mental depression. Rarely, hallucinations, visual disturbances, nervousness and impotence have been reported.
GI Effects: Diarrhea, nausea, gastric pain, constipation, flatulence,heartburn and hiccups have been observed.
Other Effects: Bronchoconstriction and wheezing may occur with dosages greater than 100mg daily, particularly in patients with asthma. Decreased exercise tolerance may be observed. Sexual dysfunction. Hypertriglyceridemia and decreased HDL cholesterol.
CONTRAINDICATIONS: Should not be used in patients with asthma, COPD, congestive heart failure, heart block >first degree, and sick sinus syndrome.
Use with caution in insulin-treated diabetic patients and patients with peripheral vascular disease; should not be discontinued abruptly in patients with ischemia heart disease.
DRUG INTERACTIONS: Drug interactions of metoprolol are given in the next Table:

Drug Interactions of Metoprolol

Drug	Interactions
Cimetidine	Reduces bioavailability of metoprolol
Hydralazine	Increases plasma concentration of metoprolol
Drugs metabolized by liver, (eg, Lidocaine, Chlorpromazine, Coumarin)	Plasma clearance of these drugs may be reduced
Calcium Channel Blockers	May promote negative inotropic effects on the myocardium

METRONIDAZOLE
(Flagyl)

USES: Metronidazole is unique in that it is both an **antiprotozoal** and **antibacterial drug;** uses are given in the next Table (Rosenblatt, J.E. and Edson, R.S., Mayo Clin. Proc. 62, 1013-1017, 1987):

Uses of Metronidazole
Trichomoniasis (T. vaginalis)
Amebiasis (E. histolytica; Dientamoeba fragilis)
Giardiasis (Giardia lamblia)
Anaerobic Bacterial Infections

Metronidazole is the only drug rapidly bactericidal against the Bacteroides fragilis group. It is used for prophylaxis during elective colorectal surgical procedures and the treatment of deep abdominal sepsis (usually in combination with another drug such as an aminoglycoside). Metronidazole is the treatment of choice for bacterial vaginosis and may be as effective as vancomycin for treatment of Clostridium difficile-related diarrhea and colitis. Metronidazole should not be taken during the first trimester of pregnancy (Rosenblatt, J.E. and Edson, R.S., Mayo Clin. Proc. 62, 1013-1017, 1987).

Mechanism of Action: The mechanism of action of metronidazole is based on its reduction by a nitroreductase enzyme to reactive intermediates which disrupt DNA and inhibit nucleic acid synthesis.

DOSAGE FORMS: Tabs: 250, 500mg; Injection: 500mg; 5mg/ml.

DOSAGE: Dosage of metronidazole in different conditions is given in the next Table:

Dosage of Metronidazole

Condition	Dosage
Trichomoniasis	Adults: 7-Day Regimen: 250mg, 3 times daily or 500mg twice daily for 7 days. Single Dose: 2g as single dose or as 2 divided doses on the same day. The single dose is given to sexual contacts and lactating women. If organism reconfirmed by wet smear and/or culture and an interval of 4-6 weeks between courses, retreat with 7 day course. Children: 15mg/kg daily in 3 divided doses for 7-10 days Infants beyond the 4th Week of Life: 10-30mg/kg daily for 5-8 days.
Amebiasis (E. histolytica)	Adults: 750mg, 3 times daily for 5-10 days. Metronidazole is given alone or, preferably, in conjunction with iodoquinol (650mg orally 3 times daily for 20 days) or with diloxanide furoate (500mg orally 3 times daily for 10 days). Children: 35-50mg/kg daily in 3 divided doses for 10 days.
Dientamoeba fragilis	Children: 250mg, 3 times daily for 7 days.
Giardiasis	Adults: 250mg, 3 times daily for 5-7 days or 2g as a single dose for 3 days For adults with coexistent amebiasis, give 750mg, 3 times daily for 5-10 days. Children: 15mg/kg daily in 3 divided doses for 7-10 days.
Anaerobic Bacterial Infections	Adults and Children: IV loading dose of 15mg/kg followed by maintenance doses of 7.5mg/kg, given over 1 hr, every 6 hrs. Max. daily adult IV or oral dose is 4g. Usual duration of therapy is 7-10 days but may require 2-3 weeks of therapy. Neonates: IV loading dose of 15mg/kg followed by maintenance doses of 7.5mg/kg/dose every 12 hours beginning 24 hrs after loading dose for term infants, 48 hrs after loading dose for preterm infants.
Prophylaxis, Perioperative	Adults: 15mg/kg by IV over 30-60 min. 1 hour prior to procedure, and, if necessary, 7.5mg/kg by IV infusion over 30-60 min. at 6 and 12 hours after initial dose. Complete within 12 hours after surgery. or Oral metronidazole with oral neomycin or oral kanamycin; 750mg oral metronidazole 2-3 times daily beginning 2 days prior to surgery
Gardnerella Vaginitis	Adults: 500mg oral doses twice daily for 7 days or single 2g oral dose.

METRONIDAZOLE (Cont.)
ADVERSE EFFECTS: Side effects are infrequent and minimal. In patients with severe hepatic impairment, reduce dosage and monitor drug. GI Effects of Oral Dose: Nausea, headache, anorexia, metallic taste. CNS: Peripheral neuropathy, dizziness and vertigo.
LABORATORY INTERFERENCE: Falsely decreased SGOT (AST) and SGPT (ALT).
MONITOR: Reversible neutropenia occurs in less than 1% of patients; total and differential leukocyte counts are recommended before and after therapy.
PHARMACOKINETICS: Oral Absorption: Well absorbed; not affected by food; Peak: 1-2 hours; Protein-Binding: 20%; Metabolism: Liver; the hydroxy metabolite is 65% as effective as metronidazole and may play a major therapeutic role. Half-Life: 6-8 hours, prolonged with severe hepatic impairment; not increased in renal failure; Distribution: CSF; crosses placenta; appears in breast milk; Excretion: Urine.
DRUG INTERACTIONS: Intolerance to alcohol similar to that produced by disulfiram (Antabuse); avoid alcohol for 48 hours after taking metronidazole. Potentiates anticoagulant effect of warfarin and other coumarins; avoid concomitant use or reduce dosage of anticoagulant.
CONTRAINDICATIONS: Alcohol.

MEXILETINE
(Mexitil)
USES: Mexiletine is an orally active lidocaine congener that "appears to be about as effective as quinidine for treatment of some symptomatic ventricular arrhythmias but may be ineffective for patients with sustained ventricular tachycardia." (The Medical Letter 28, 65-66, 1986).
Mechanism of Action: Mexiletine decreases the duration of the action potential and the rate of rise of phase 0. The drug has little effect on sinus rate or atrial refractoriness. Mexiletine (like lidocaine and tocainide; unlike quinidine, procainamide, and disopyramide) does not prolong the PR, QRS or QT intervals. It is classified as a class 1B antiarrhythmic agent.
DOSAGE FORMS: Caps: 150, 200 and 250mg.
DOSAGE: 150-400mg every 6-12 hrs. Begin with low dose and titrate to effect. Maximum dose: 1200mg/day. Minimum of 2-3 days between dosage adjustments, increase by 50-100mg increments. Should be taken with food or antacids.
ADVERSE EFFECTS: Adverse effects of mexiletine occur in 50% of patients causing 30% to discontinue the drug; adverse effects are given in the next Table(Kreeger, R.W. and Hammill, S.C., Mayo Clin. Proc. 62, 1033-1050, 1987):

Adverse Effects of Mexiletine

Adverse Effects	Percent (%)
Cardiac Toxicity	
Proarrhythmia	10
Congestive heart failure	<3
Heart block	1
Noncardiac Toxicity	
Light-headedness, paresthesias tremor, ataxia, confusion, loss of memory	20
Nausea	39

PHARMACOKINETICS: Absorption: 80% to 90% bioavailability; Onset: 0.5-2 hours; Peak: 1-3 hours; Half-Life: 12-13 hours; Therapeutic Range: 1-2 microgram/ml; Metabolism: 100% hepatic.

MEZLOCILLIN
(Mezlin)

USES: **Mezlocillin** is an **extended-spectrum penicillin** with a spectrum of activity similar to that of **carbenicillin** and **ticarcillin.** **Mezlocillin** is used primarily for the treatment of suspected or proven infections caused by **P. aeruginosa;** its activity against P. aeruginosa is about equal to that of ticarcillin but less than that of piperacillin and azlocillin. However, some ticarcillin and carbenicillin resistant organisms are susceptable to mezlocillin; activities of mezlocillin are given in the next Table (Parry, M.F., Med. Clin. No. Am. 71, 1093-1112, Nov. 1987):

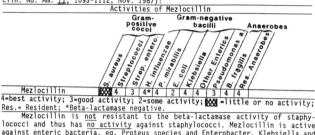

Activities of Mezlocillin

	Gram-positive cocci			Gram-negative bacilli						Anaerobes	
	S. aureus	Streptococci	Strep. entero.	H. influenzae	P. mirabilis	E. coli	Klebsiella	Other Enterics	Pseudomonas a.	B. fragilis	Res. Anaerobes
Mezlocillin	▩	4	3	4*	4	2	4	4	3	4	4

4=best activity; 3=good activity; 2=some activity; ▩ =little or no activity; Res.= Resident; *Beta-lactamase negative.

Mezlocillin is not resistant to the beta-lactamase activity of staphylococci and thus has no activity against staphylococci. Mezlocillin is active against enteric bacteria, eg, Proteus species and Enterobacter, Klebsiella and anaerobes. However, beta-lactamase producing Bacteroides species are not predictably susceptible.

DOSAGE FORMS: Inj: 1, 2, 3, 4g vials

DOSAGE: Mezlocillin sodium is administered by slow IV injection or infusion or by deep IM injection. Give IV for treatment of life-threatening infections. Dosage is given in the next Table:

Dosage of Mezlocillin Sodium

Condition	Age	Route	Dosage
Uncomplicated Urinary Tract Infections	Adults	IV or IM	100-125mg/kg daily in divided doses every 6 hrs. or 1.5-2g every 6 hrs.
Complicated Urinary Tract Infections	Adults	IV	150-200mg/kg daily in divided doses every 6 hrs. or 3g every 6 hrs.
Lower Respiratory Tract Infections, Intra-Abdominal Infections, Gynecologic Infections, Skin and Skin Structure Infections, and Septicemia	Adults	IV	225-300mg/kg daily in divided doses every 6 hrs. or 3g every 4 hrs. or 4g every 6 hrs.
Life-Threatening Infections	Adults	IV	Max. 350mg/kg daily or 4g every 4 hrs.
Pediatric	1 month to 12 yrs.	IV or IM	50-75mg/kg every 4-6 hrs.
	<7 days	IV or IM	75mg/kg every 12 hrs.
	>7 days <2kg	IV or IM	75mg/kg every 8 hrs.
	>7 days >2kg	IV or IM	75mg/kg every 6-8 hrs.

Duration of Therapy: Continue for at least 48 hrs. after all evidence of infection has disappeared, usual duration is 10-14 days.

MEZLOCILLIN (Cont.)
Dosage in Renal and Hepatic Impairment: Dosage in adults with renal failure is given in the next Table:

Dosage of Mezlocillin Sodium in Renal Failure in Adults

Infection	Creatinine Clearance 10-30ml/min	Creatinine Clearance <10ml/min
Uncomplicated Urinary Tract	1.5g every 8 hr.	1.5g every 8 hr.
Complicated Urinary Tract	1.5g every 6 hr.	1.5g every 8 hr.
Serious Systemic	3g every 8 hr.	2g every 8 hr.
Life-Threatening	3g every 6 hr.	2g every 6 hr.

Hepatic Impairment: Decrease dose by 50% or double dosing time.
PHARMACOKINETICS: Half-Life: 1 hr., dose dependent; Plasma Protein-Binding: 16% to 42%; Excretion: 60% in urine; probenecid delays excretion;
ADVERSE EFFECTS: Adverse reactions to mezlocillin are given in the next Table (Parry, M.F., Med. Clin. No. Am. 71, 1093-1112, Nov. 1987):

Adverse Reactions to Mezlocillin

Reaction	Expected Frequency(%)
Cutaneous reactions	2-4
Drug fever	1-2
Diarrhea	2-3
Leukopenia	1-2
Abnormal transaminase	1-2
Hypokalemia	1-2

Most common side effects are skin rashes and minor GI disturbances. Other adverse effects are as follows: hypersensitivity reactions; thrombophlebitis; leukopenia; eosinophilia; platelet dysfunction; hepatic dysfunction with elevated hepatic enzyme levels; hypokalemia and central nervous system irritation.

Each gram of mezlocillin contains 1.85mEq (42.6mg) of sodium; large doses may add to sodium load.

MICONAZOLE

(Monistat, Micatin)

USES: Miconazole is an antifungal agent; uses are given in the next Table:

Uses of Miconazole

Vulvovaginal Candidiasis
- Note: Miconazole is not effective in treating vulvovaginitis caused by Trichomonas or Gardnerella vaginalis (formerly Haemophilus vaginalis)

Dermatophytoses, Superficial Mycoses and Cutaneous Candidiasis
- Trichophyton mentagrophytes: Tinea pedis
- Trichophyton rubrum: Tinea cruris
- Epidermophyton floccosum: Tinea corporis
- Malassezia furfur: Tinea versicolor
- Moniliasis: Cutaneous candidiasis

Severe Systemic Fungal Infections and Fungal Meningitis
- Coccidoidomycosis
- Cryptococcosis
- Paracoccidoidomycosis
- Petrieltidrosis
- Candidiasis
- P. boydii
- Sporotrichosis

Vulvovaginal Candidiasis: Miconazole vaginal preparation (Monistat) is used to treat vulvovaginal candidiasis (moniliasis) which has been confirmed by potassium hydroxide microscopic mounts and/or culture.
Dermatophytoses: Miconazole topical cream is used for the treatment of tinea pedis, tinea cruris, and tinea corporis caused by T. mentagrophytes, T. rubrum, or Epidermophyton floccosum and for the treatment of cutaneous candidiasis (moniliasis).
DOSAGE FORMS: Dosage forms of Monistat for treatment of vulvovaginal candidiasis are given in the next Table:

Dosage Forms of Monistat

Product	Miconazole Nitrate
Monistat 7 Vaginal Cream	2%
Monistat 7 Vaginal Suppository	100mg
Monistat 3 Vaginal Suppository	200mg
Monistat Dual Pak, Suppository and Topical Cream	200mg 2%

Topical: Aerosol, 2%; Cream, 2%; Lotion, 2%; Powder, 2%. Injection: 10mg/ml.

MICONAZOLE (Cont.)

DOSAGE: Dosage of Monistat is given in the next Table:

Miconazole Vaginal Preparations

Preparation	Dosage
Monistat 7 Vaginal Cream	One applicatorful vaginally at bedtime for 7 days.
Monistat 7 Suppository	One suppository, vaginally at bedtime for 7 days.
Monistat 3 Suppository	One suppository, vaginally at bedtime for 3 days.
Monistat Dual Pak, Suppository and Topical Cream	One suppository, vaginally at bedtime for 3 days. Apply topical cream twice daily for 2 weeks

Topical: apply twice a day for 2-4 weeks.
IV: >1 yr: 20-40mg/kg/day, every 8h, max. of 15mg/kg/dose; Adults: 200-1200mg/dose every 8h.
ADVERSE EFFECTS: Side Effects of Vaginal Preparations: Vulvovaginal burning, itching or irritation, cramps, headache, rash, urticaria.

Side Effects of IV Therapy: Phlebitis, pruritus, rash, nausea, vomiting, fever, drowsiness, diarrhea, anorexia and flushes. Decrease in hematocrit and platelets has been reported.
DRUG INTERACTIONS: Enhances anticoagulant effect of coumarin. Limited data suggests that amphotericin B and miconazole may be antagonistic. Enhances hypoglycemic effects of sulfonylurea antidiabetic agents.

MIDAZOLAM
(Versed)

USES: Midazolam is a benzodiazepine; uses are given in the next Table:

Uses of Midazolam
Preoperative Sedation
Conscious Sedation
Anesthesia: Induction and Maintenance

Midazolam provides sedation, relieves anxiety and has good amnestic properties. Midazolam has a rapid onset and short duration of effect making it a good choice for short surgical procedures.
DOSAGE FORMS: Parenteral: 1,5mg/ml.
DOSAGE: Midazolam is administered IM or IV. Dosage is given in the next Table:

Dosage of Midazolam

Condition	Age	Dosage
Preoperative Sedation	Adult or Children	70-80micrograms/kg IM 30-60 minutes prior to surgery (usual adult dose: 5mg)
Conscious Sedation	Adult <60 years	1-2.5mg IV over at least 2 minutes. Usual total dose: 5mg for conscious sedation.
	Adult >60 years	1-1.5mg IV over at least 2 minutes. Usual total dose: 3.5mg for conscious sedation.
	Children	0.035-0.2mg/kg IV over at least 2 minutes. Start with low dose and titrate to effect.
Anesthesia	Adults <55	Induction dose 300-600micrograms/kg. Premedicated patients should receive 250micrograms/kg
	Adults ≥55	Induction dose 200-300micrograms/kg. Debilitated patients should receive 150micrograms/kg. Premedicated patients should receive 150-200micrograms/kg.

Midazolam has been used to maintain sedation in intubated intensive care patients. Dose range for continuous infusion: 0.1-10micrograms/kg/minute, titrate to effect (Shapiro, J.M. et al., Anesthesiology 64, 394-398, 1986).
PHARMACOKINETICS: Oral Administration: rapidly absorbed, extensive first-pass metabolism in the liver (50-60% metabolized); Maximal Effect: 1 hr; IM Administration: rapidly and completely (>90%) absorbed. Onset: 5-15 min; Maximal Effect: 20-60 min; Duration: 2 hrs (range: 1-6 hrs); IV Administration: Onset: 1-5 min; Duration: <2 hrs. Elimination Half-Life: 1-4 hrs; Volume of Distribution: 0.8-2.5 liters/kg; Clearance: Midazolam is extensively metabolized in the liver.
ADVERSE EFFECTS: May cause respiratory depression. Facilities for oxygen and controlled respiration must be available. Hypotension occurs rarely. Central nervous systems effects include excessive sedation, headache, combativeness, dizziness, weakness and slurred speech may occur. Effects potentiated by concomitant administration of narcotics or other sedatives. Paradoxical agitation may occur, unresponsive to increasing dosage. Withdrawal may occur with prolonged or high doses.
CONTRAINDICATIONS: Acute narrow-angle glaucoma, known hypersensitivity.

MINOCYCLINE
(Minocin)

USES: Minocycline is a synthetic **tetracycline** antibiotic derived from tetracycline; uses are given in the next Table:

Uses of Minocycline
Asymptomatic meningococcus carriers
Mycobacterial infections
Gonococcal and spirochetal infections
Chlamydial and mycoplasmal infections

DOSAGE FORMS: (Minocin) Oral: Caps: 50, 100mg; Susp: 50mg/5ml; Tabs: 50, 100mg; Parenteral: 100mg

DOSAGE: Minocycline is usually administered orally and should not be taken with milk or dairy products. When oral therapy is not feasible, the drug may be given IV. Dosages are given in the next Table:

Dosages of Minocycline

Condition	Dosage
Usual	Adult: Oral or IV, 200mg initially; then 100mg every 12 hours or 100-200mg initially; then 50mg every 6 hours. Children, 8 years of age or older: 4mg/kg initially; then 2mg/kg every 12 hours.
Asymptomatic Meningococcus Carriers	Use rifampin when drug susceptibility unknown or organism known to be sulfa-resistant. Minocycline, orally, 5 days is used when rifampin is contraindicated.
Mycobacterial Infection Granulomas of the Skin	100mg, orally, twice daily for 6-8 weeks
Gonococcal Infections	Usual oral dose for a minimum of 4 days. However, tetracycline and doxycycline are the tetracycline derivatives currently recommended by the CDC for treatment of gonorrhea.
Syphilis	Usual oral dose for 10-15 days. However, doxycycline or tetracycline are the tetracycline derivatives currently included in the CDC recommended treatment schedule for syphilis.
Uncomplicated Urethral, Endocervical, or Rectal Infection caused by Chlamydia Trachomatis or Ureaplasma Urealyticum	Adults: Oral minocylcine, 100mg, twice daily for at least 7 days.
Nongonococcal Urethritis caused by C. Trachomatis or Mycoplasma	Adults: Oral minocycline, 100mg daily, in one or two divided doses for 1-3 weeks.

ADVERSE EFFECTS: Vestibular dysfunction occurs more frequently with minocycline than with other currently available tetracyclines. Symptoms may occur in 30-90% of patients receiving the usual dose of minocycline. Photosensitivity may occur.

CONTRAINDICATIONS: Tetracyclines may cause permanent discoloration of the teeth if given during development. Therefore, tetracyclines are contraindicated in children <8 years.

MINOXIDIL

(Loniten; Rogaine (topical))

USES: Uses of minoxidil are given in the next Table:

Uses of Minoxidil
Stimulates Hair Growth
Hypertension

Stimulates Hair Growth: Minoxidil, applied topically, causes elongation of follicles in the area of alopecia; new follicles are not formed. Minoxidil, applied topically as a 1%-3% preparation twice daily for months, has given good responses in about one-third of subjects (Weiss, V.C. and West, D.P., Arch. Dermatol. 121, 191-192, 1985).

Hypertension: Minoxidil is a **vasodilator,** used in the management of moderate to severe hypertension. Treatment of hypertension with minoxidil is given in the next Table (The 1988 Report of the Joint National Committee on Detection, Evaluation, and Treatment of High Blood Pressure, Arch. Intern. Med. 148, 1023-1038, 1988):

Treatment of Hypertension with Minoxidil

Step 1: Nonpharmacologic Approaches (see **HYPERTENSION**)

↓

Step 2: **Diuretic** or **Beta-Blocker** or **Calcium Antagonist** or **ACE Inhibitor**
Observe up to 6 months; if ineffective then,

↓

Step 3: Add a second drug of a different class, usually one of the group of four listed above .
or Increase dosage of the first drug
or Substitute another drug

↓

Step 4: Add a third drug of a different class, such as minoxidil
or Substitute a second drug, such as minoxidil

↓

Step 5: Consider further evaluation and/or referral
or Add a third or fourth drug

A combination of hypotensive drugs that is used is a diuretic plus a beta-blocker plus minoxidil. Minoxidil may be substituted for hydralazine if a more potent vasodilator is needed. If fluid retention occurs, substitute furosemide for a thiazide and those already receiving furosemide should receive a larger dose. Consider using combined therapy of furosemide with the thiazide, metolazone.

Mechanism of Action: Minoxidil is an antihypertensive drug which reduces peripheral resistance and blood pressure as a result of a direct vasodilatory effect on vascular smooth muscle; the effect on arterioles is greater than on veins. The minoxidil-induced decrease in blood pressure is accompanied by increased heart rate, cardiac output, and stroke volume, probably because of a reflex response to decreased peripheral resistance. Minoxidil has no direct effect on the heart.

DOSAGE FORMS: Tabs: 2.5mg, 10mg. Topical: 2% solution (20mg/ml metered dose)

DOSAGE: Minoxidil is usually given with a diuretic and a beta-blocker. Dosage for treatment of hypertension is given in the next Table:

Dosage of Minoxidil for Treatment of Hypertension

Age	Dosage
Adults and Children >12 years	Initially: 5mg once daily. As necessary, increase dosage at intervals of three days or longer to 10,20 and then 40mg daily. The usual dosage range is 10-40mg; max. 100mg, in single or divided doses
Children <12 years	Initially, 0.1-0.2mg/kg daily as a single dose. As necessary, increase dosage in increments of 0.1 to 0.2mg/kg until control is achieved (usual, 0.25 to 1mg/kg daily; max. 50mg daily). (Balfe, J.W., et al., "Hypertension in Childhood," Adv. Pediatr. 36, 201-246, 1989).

MINOXIDIL (Cont.)

ADVERSE EFFECTS: Adverse effects are given in the next Table:

Adverse Effects of Minoxidil

Effect	Comment
Fluid Retention	Fluid retention is common and is characterized by edema and weight gain. If fluid retention occurs, furosemide should be substituted for a thiazide and those already receiving furosemide should receive a larger dose. Consider using combined therapy of furosemide with the thiazide, metolazone. Manifestations of fluid retention, other than edema and weight gain, include congestive heart failure, pericardial effusion and pulmonary hypertension.
Anginal Attacks	Anginal attacks may occur secondary to reflex cardiac stimulation combined with reduced coronary perfusion; this may occur because beta-blockage may be inadequate.
Orthostatic Hypotension	Orthostatic hypotension may develop especially when minoxidil is administered with guanethidine.
Hypertrichosis	Inappropriate hair growth occurs in 80% of patients and is particularly a concern in women and children.
Other: Nausea, Headache, Fatigue, Dermatologic Reactions, Stevens-Johnson Syndrome, Breast Tenderness	Some of these reactions occur occasionally.

PHARMACOKINETICS: Bioavailability: 90%; Onset: 30 min.; Peak Activity: 2-8 hours; Half-Life: 4.2 hours; Therapeutic Effect: 24 hours; Metabolism: 90%; Protein-Binding: none; Excretion: Kidney; Dialyzable: yes.

DRUG INTERACTIONS: Profound orthostatic hypotension frequently occurs when minoxidil is administered to patients receiving guanethidine. Guanethidine should be discontinued 1 to 3 weeks before starting minoxidil therapy.

MISOPROSTOL
(Cytotec)

USES: Misoprostol is used in patients at high risk for developing stomach ulcers while on arthritis drugs. Ulcers that develop in these patients may not cause pain and may go undetected until they have caused bleeding.

According to the FDA, there are about 200,000 cases of gastrointestinal bleeding each year, resulting in 10,000 to 20,000 deaths due to the 68 million prescriptions of non-steroidal anti-inflammatory drugs (NSAIDs).

Gastric ulcers occurred over 3 months in 22% of users of NSAIDs with abdominal pain. 5.6% and 1.4% of similar groups receiving misoprostol 400 micrograms daily or 800 micrograms daily respectively, had gastric ulcers (Graham, D.Y. et al., Lancet 2, 1277-1280, Dec. 31, 1988; Editorial, Lancet 2, 1293-1294, Dec. 3, 1988).

Duodenal ulcer is as prevalent as gastric ulcer in patients receiving NSAIDs (2-month prevalence in the placebo group was 8% for duodenal and 6% for gastric ulcers)(Ehsanullah, R.S.B. et al., Br. Med. J. 297, 1017-1021, 1988). Duodenal ulcers are less effectively treated with misoprostol than with H_2 receptor antagonists. However, ranitidine significantly reduces the frequency of duodenal ulcer but has no effect on gastric ulceration in patients receiving NSAIDs (Ehsanullah, R.S.B. et al., Br. Med. J. 297, 1017-1021, 1988). It is suggested that patients taking NSAIDs should receive both misoprostol (to prevent gastric ulcer) and ranitidine (to prevent duodenal ulcer)(Editorial, Lancet 2, 1293-1294, Dec. 3, 1988).

Mechanism of Action: Misoprostol is a synthetic prostaglandin E_1 analogue; it has gastric antisecretory and cryoprotective properties. Prostaglandins appear to protect the mucosal layers below the epithelial layers, facilitating recovery of the mucosa after exposure to an NSAID.

DOSAGE FORMS: 100, 200 micrograms.

DOSAGE: 200 microgram misoprostol four times daily with meals and at bedtime, concurrently with the NSAID. Dosage may be reduced to 100micrograms four times daily in patients who do not tolerate the usual dosage.

MISOPROSTOL (Cont.)

ADVERSE EFFECTS: Adverse effects of misoprostol are given in the next Table (Graham, D.Y. et al., Lancet 2, 1277-1280, Dec. 3, 1988):

Adverse Effects of Misoprostol(200 microgram, 4x daily)

Effect	% of Group
Diarrhea	39
Dyspepsia	16
Flatulence	18
Abdominal Pain	18
Nausea	16

Mild to moderate, self-limiting diarrhea is the most frequently reported adverse effect.

CONTRAINDICATIONS: Misoprostol may cause miscarriages in pregnant women. Misoprostol is contraindicated in women of childbearing potential unless the patient must receive NSAIDs and is at high risk of development of gastric ulcers. In these women, the physician must obtain a negative pregnancy test before prescribing misoprostol and be sure that the patient has been informed of the need to avoid getting pregnant while taking the drug.

MORPHINE SULFATE

(Roxanol, Generic)

USES: Morphine is an **opiate;** uses are given in the next Table:

Uses of Morphine
Relief of Pain: Drug of choice for relief of pain of myocardial infarction
Preoperative Sedation: as a supplement to anesthesia
Analgesia during labor

DOSAGE FORMS: Sol'n: 10mg/5ml, 20mg/5ml; 20mg/ml; Tabs: 15mg, 30mg; Tabs, Soluble: 10mg, 15mg, 30mg; Tabs, Extended Release: 15, 30, 60, 100mg; Injection: 0.5, 1, 2, 4, 5, 8, 10, 15mg/ml; Rectal(supp): 5,10,20,30mg.

DOSAGE: The dosage is given in the next Table:

Dosage of Morphine Sulfate

Subject	Dosage
Oral: Adult	Oral: 10-30mg every 4 hours as necessary; or extended-release tablets, 30mg every 12 hours
Parenteral:	
Adult	Subcutaneous or IM: 10mg every 4 hours as necessary; range 5-20mg every 4 hours. IV: 2.5-15mg diluted in 4-5ml water and injected slowly over 4-5 minutes
Children	Subcutaneous: 0.1-0.2mg/kg every 4 hours as necessary; single dose should not exceed 15mg IV: 0.1-0.2mg/kg/dose (max: 15mg/dose) every 2-4 hours as needed.
Pain of Myocardial Infarction	8-15mg; very severe pain, give smaller doses every 3-4 h.
Analgesia during Labor	10mg, subcutaneous or IM
Severe Chronic Pain	Continuous IV; Initial; Adult: 1-10mg/h & then increased to effective dosage; maintenance dosages of 20-150mg/h Children: 0.025-2mg/kg/hr; begin at low dose and titrate to effect.
Rectal	Adult: 10-20mg every 4 hours as necessary

ADVERSE EFFECTS: Addicting. The most serious adverse effect is respiratory depression. Naloxone may be used to reverse respiratory depression. Urinary retention, pruritis, nausea, vomiting may occur.

Use with caution in infants less than 6 months of age; pharmacokinetics are unpredictable in the very young.

MOUNTAIN SICKNESS, PREVENTION, TREATMENT

Mountain (high-altitude) sickness varies from person to person; it depends on altitude and rate of climb. Mild symptoms may occur at 8,000 feet; severe symptoms may occur at 15,000 feet.

Management of acute mountain sickness is given in the next Table (Johnson, T.S. and Rock, P.B., N. Engl. J. Med. 319, 841-845, Sept. 29, 1988):

Management of Acute Mountain Sickness

Prevention

- Staging: spend two to five days at an intermediate altitude (2000m)
- Slow ascent: above 3000m, ascend only 300m per day
- Acetazolamide (Diamox): 250mg every eight hours, begun the day before the ascent and continued for at least five days at the higher altitude.
- Dexamethasone: 4mg every six hours, begun the day of the ascent, continued for three days at the higher altitude, then tapered over five days. Potential side effects should be considered.

Treatment

- Primary: Descent (increasingly important as the severity of acute mountain sickness increases)
- Secondary:
  - Mild cases: Rest; acetaminophen or ibuprofen; acetazolamide*
  - Moderate cases: Rest; dexamethasone: 4mg every six hours by mouth for one to three days, then tapered over five days; acetazolamide
  - Severe cases: Oxygen*; dexamethasone: 4-8mg initially, then 4mg every six hours orally or intramuscularly (Levine, B.D. et al., NEJM 321, 1707-1713, 1989); acetazolamide.

*A recommended but not clearly beneficial treatment.

Acetazolamide (Diamox) is used to increase altitude tolerance in the prevention or amelioration of symptoms associated with acute high-altitude sickness. The dosage of acetazolamide is as follows: 250mg every 8-12 hours or 500mg every 12-24 hours as extended-release caps; begin 24-48 hours before and continue during ascent; continue at high altitude as necessary.

MOUTH, PATHOGENS

Pathogens: The pathogens that cause infection of the mouth are given in the next Table (Handbook of Antimicrobial Therapy, The Medical Letter, 1990):

Infection of the Mouth
Herpes viruses
Candida albicans
Leptotrichia buccalis (Vincent's infection)
Bacteroides
Mixed anaerobes
Treponema pallidum
Actinomyces

MYOCARDIAL INFARCTION, TREATMENT

General recommendations for treatment of acute myocardial infarction among patients who have no specific contraindications is as follows: Give a thrombolytic drug within the first six hours of the onset of symptoms (up to 24 hours). Add aspirin to streptokinase regimen. Intravenous beta blockers reduce mortality. Continue aspirin and beta-blocker therapy for at least two years. Intravenous nitroglycerin may benefit patients with moderate and large-sized infarcts expecially if they have pulmonary congestion (Yusuf, S. et al., Circulation 82, Suppl. II, II117-II134, September, 1990; Gunnar, R.M. et al., ACC/AHA Task Force Report, JACC 16, 249-292, August, 1990).

Neither a antiarrhythmic drug nor a calcium channel blocker should be routinely recommended to patients who have had an acute myocardial infarction.

The therapeutic objective in early treatment of myocardial infarction is to reduce "infarct size" or prevent fatal arrhythmias. The drugs that reduce infarct size are those that increase oxygen or nutrient supply (eg, thrombolytic agents) or those that reduce the need for nutrients and oxygen by the ischemic myocardium (eg, beta-blockers, nitrates, and calcium channel blockers).

Drugs that may help to prevent arrhythmias are beta-blockers, other antiarrhythmic drugs, antiplatelet drugs, anticoagulants and other strategies to decrease the risk of atherosclerosis.

The effects of treatment of patients with myocardial infarction are given in the next Table (Yusuf, S. et al., JAMA 260, 2088-2093, Oct. 14, 1988):

Treatment of Patients with Myocardial Infarction

Disease/Drug	Risk Reductions Mortality (%)
Short-Term Acute Interventions	
Reduction of Infarct Size-Thrombolytic Drugs-Reperfusion:	
Streptokinase	
Intracoronary	-18
Intravenous	-24
Intravenous, given <6 hr.	-26
Intravenous, given >6 hr.	-17
Tissue Plasminogen Activator (alteplase, t-PA) IV given <6 hr.	-26
Anisolyated Plasminogen-Streptokinase Activator Complex (APSAC) anistreplase, IV given <6 hr.	-52*
Reduction in Need for Nutrients and Oxygen:	
Beta-Blockers	-13
Nitrates, IV	-35
Calcium Channel Blockers	+10
Antiarrhythmic Drugs:	
Lidocaine	+11
Anticoagulants	-22
Aspirin	-21
Combined Therapy:	
Streptokinase plus Aspirin	-42
Long-Term Chronic Interventions	
Beta-Blockers	-22
Antiplatelets	-11
Calcium Channel Blockers	+6

*APSAC has not been definitively shown to be more efficacious than streptokinase in direct comparison, but data are limited.

Reperfusion: Thrombolytic treatment should be routine in acute myocardial infarction and be given as early as possible. There are four currently available thrombolytic drugs: urokinase, streptokinase, tissue plasminogen activator (t-PA) and anisolyated plasminogen-streptokinase activator complex (APSAC) (anistreplase) reduce the risk of death following acute myocardial infarction. The reduction in mortality varied from 18% to 52%; these data should not be taken as definitive considering variations in parameters in the studies. In a 12,490 patient comparison of streptokinase with t-PA, each given with or without heparin, showed no specific difference between the two agents with regard to the end-point (severe left ventricular damage or death). Heparin therapy did not show additional benefit; all patients received atenolol and

MYOCARDIAL INFARCTION, TREATMENT (Cont.)
aspirin (GISSI-2, Lancet 336, 65-71, 1990). For review of streptokinase vs t-PA literature, see Sherry, S. and Marder, V.J., Ann. Intern. Med. 114, 417-423, 1991.

Absolute contraindications to thrombolytic therapy include active internal bleeding, suspected aortic dissection, prolonged CPR, recent head trauma, intracranial neoplasm, hemorrhagic ophthalmic condition (eg, diabetic hemorrhagic retinopathy, pregnancy, previous allergy to thrombolytic agent, BP>200/120, history of hemorrhagic cerebrovascular accident, or recent trauma or surgery (<2 weeks). Relative contraindications include recent trauma or surgery (>2 weeks), history of chronic severe hypertension, active peptic ulcer, history of cerebrovascular accident, known bleeding diathesis or anticoagulant therapy, significant liver dysfunction, or prior use of streptokinase or APSAC, especially within 6-9 months (does not apply to t-PA)(Gunnar, R.M. et al., ACC/AHA Task Force Report, JACC 16, 249-292, August 1990).

Reduction in Need for Nutrients and Oxygen:

Beta-Adrenergic Blocking Agents: Beta-blockers reduce oxygen demand by lowering heart rate and blood pressure; they block the adverse effects of catecholamines and have antiarrhythmic effects. Beta-adrenergic blocking agents reduced mortality by 13%. The data indicate that starting treatment early with intravenous beta-blockers and then continuing treatment orally for at least two years is a reasonable approach. Contraindications include bradycardia (HR<60), hypotension (systolic BP<100), moderate to severe left ventricular failure, peripheral hypoperfusion, AV conduction abnormalities or severe COPD; relative contraindications include asthma, concurrent use of calcium channel blockers, severe peripheral vascular disease, or difficult to control insulin-dependent diabetes (Yusuf, S. et al., Circulation 82, Suppl. II, II117-II134, September, 1990; Gunnar, R.M. et al., ACC/AHA Task Force Report, JACC 16, 249-292, August, 1990).

Nitrates: IV nitrates, nitroglycerin and sodium nitroprusside reduce oxygen demand and myocardial wall stress by reducing afterload and preload. Nitrates reduced the risk of mortality by 35%(Yusef et al., Lancet 1, 1088-1092, 1988).

Calcium Channel Blockers: Calcium channel blockers reduce oxygen demand by lowering blood pressure and reducing contractility; diltiazem and verapamil also reduce heart rate. There is no data to indicate that calcium channel blockers are useful after myocardial infarction with the exception of diltiazem which is recommended in patients with non-Q wave infarction (The Diltiazem Reinfarction Study Group, NEJM 319, 385-392, 1988; Gunnar, R.M. et al., ACC/AHA Task Force Report, JACC 16, 249-292, August, 1990).

Antiarrhythmic Drugs; Lidocaine: Ventricular fibrillation may occur within hours following acute myocardial infarction. The current data do not support the routine use of antiarrhythmic drugs in asymptomatic patients. Lidocaine is indicated for patients with myocardial ischemia or infarction who have documented arrhythmias including ventricular tachycardia, ventricular fibrillation or ventricular premature beats that are frequent (>6/min), closely coupled (R on T), multiform configuration, or short bursts of three or more (Gunnar, R.M. et al., ACC/AHA Task Force Report, JACC 16, 249-292, August, 1990).

Anticoagulants: Anticoagulants reduce mortality by about 22%; combined use of a thrombolytic drug and anticoagulants may lead to an increased risk of bleeding and stroke (Timmis, G.C. et al., Arch. Intern. Med 146, 667-672, 1986). Heparin: Low dose subcutaneous heparin is indicated for prevention of deep venous thrombosis and pulmonary embolism. High dose heparin is indicated for patients with large anterior transmural myocardial infarct; heparin should be continued for at least 3 months in patients with ventricular mural thrombosis or a large akinetic region at the apex of the left ventricle, and indefinitely in patients with dilated and poorly contracting left ventricle (Gunnar, R.M. et al., JACC 16, 249-292, August, 1990).

Combined Therapy: Combined therapy is done to assess whether drugs that reduce mortality and myocardial infarction are additive.

Streptokinase plus Aspirin: Thrombolytic treatment with streptokinase and aspirin are equally beneficial in treating acute myocardial infarction but their effects are additive (42% reduction in mortality). (ISIS-2 [Second International Study of Infarct Survival] Collaborative Group. Randomised trial of intravenous streptokinase, oral aspirin, both, or neither among 17,187 cases of suspected acute myocardial infarction: ISIS-2. Lancet 2, 349-360, 1988).

MYOCARDIAL INFARCTION, TREATMENT (Cont.)

UNSTABLE ANGINA: Unstable angina may lead to an increased risk of myocardial infarction and death; occlusive or nonocclusive thrombi are thought to be a precipitating factor for unstable angina.

The effects of treatment of patients with unstable angina are given in the next Table (Yusuf, S. et al., JAMA 260, 2259-2263, Oct. 21, 1988):

Treatment of Unstable Angina

Treatment	Risk Reductions: Mortality (%)	Risk Reductions: Myocardial Infarction (%)
Aspirin	-42	-40
Intravenous Heparin	Inadequate data	-44
Beta-Blockers	Inadequate data	-13
Calcium Channel Blockers	Inadequate data	- 4

Aspirin and Heparin: Aspirin reduces the risk of death and myocardial infarction; apparently, intravenous heparin also prevents myocardial infarction. More recent data from the RISC Group again confirms reduction of the risk of MI and death in patients with unstable angina treated with low dose aspirin (75mg/ day) but fails to confirm benefits of intravenous heparin. It should be noted, however, that heparin was administered by intermittent (rather than continuous) infusion, and that 81% of patients began treatment more than 24 hrs after admission (median 33 hrs)(RISC Group, Lancet 336, 827-830, October, 1990).

Beta-Blockers: Initial treatment with IV beta-blockers followed by oral treatment for a week leads to a 13% reduction in the risk of developing a myocardial infarction (Yusuf, S. et al., Prog. Cardiovasc. Dis. 27, 335-371, 1985). Beta-blockers are useful in relieving symptoms.

Calcium Channel Blockers: Routine use of calcium channel blockers do not appear to be useful in preventing death or myocardial infarction in patients with unstable angina.

CONGESTIVE HEART FAILURE: The mainstays of therapy of congestive heart failure are diuretics, inotropic agents and vasodilators [especially the angiotensin converting enzyme (ACE) inhibitors]. Although therapy must be individualized, a general approach to therapy for heart failure is given in the following Table (Parmley, W.W. "An Overview of Integration of Therapy for Congestive Heart Failure", J. of Cardiovasc. Pharm. 14 (Suppl. 5), S73-S77, 1989):

Therapy for Mild Heart Failure

Consider diuretic, inotropic agent, or vasocilator as first-line therapy.

Special Considerations:

For:	Consider:
Edema	Diuretic
CAD with angina	Nitrates or (?) Beta-blocker
LV dysfunction only	ACE inhibitor (?)
Dilated heart, Decreased ejection fraction	Digitalis, Xamoterol or ACE inhibitor

Therapy for Moderate-Severe Heart Failure

Combination therapy with ACE inhibitors, diuretics, and inotropic agents.

Special Considerations:

For:	Consider:
Refractory edema	Add metolazone to loop diuretic
Low cardiac output	Add hydralazine or PDE inhibitor to ACE inhibitor
Cardiomyopathy with tachycardia	Low dose metoprolol (?)
Persistent elevation of LV pressure	Add nitrate to ACE inhib. and diuretic
Renal Insufficiency	Hydralazine plus isosorbide dinitrate in place of ACE inhibitor
Severe arrhythmias	Amiodarone (?)
Refractory CHF	PDE inhibitor, intermittent dobutamine (?), transplant (?)

CAD = coronary artery disease; PDE inhibitor = phosphodiesterase inhibitor (eg, amrinone); LV = left ventricle.

MYOCARDIAL INFARCTION, TREATMENT (Cont.)

The effects of treatment of patients with congestive heart failure with angiotensin converting enzyme inhibitors and hydralazine/nitrates are given in the next Table (Yusuf, S. et al., JAMA 260, 2259-2263, Oct. 21, 1988):

Treatment of Congestive Heart Failure	
Treatment	Risk Reductions, Mortality (%)
Angiotensin Converting Enzyme Inhibitors	-37
Hydralazine/Nitrates	-12

Angiotensin Converting Enzyme (ACE) Inhibitors: The angiotensin-converting enzyme (ACE) inhibitors, captopril and enalapril are now widely used to treat chronic congestive heart failure (Medical Letter 30, 13 Jan. 29, 1988). Enalapril maleate, given for an average of six months, reduced mortality by 27% (N. Engl. J. Med. 316, 1429-1435, 1987). Large-scale studies are in progress to determine if early treatment with ACE inhibitors of patients with acute myocardial infarction can prevent the development of heart failure and decrease mortality in these patients.
Hydralazine/Nitrates: Results on these drugs are suggestive of benefit in patients with mild to moderate congestive heart failure (Cohn, J.N. et al., NEJM 314, 1547-1552, 1986).
Diuretics: Patients with edema may benefit from diuretic therapy. Therapy is usually begun with a thiazide diuretic, however, patients with moderate to severe symptoms will usually require addition of a loop diuretic (eg, furosemide). Serum potassium must be monitored closely with supplementation as needed; concomittant use of a potassium-sparing diuretic (spironolactone, amiloride or triamterene) should be considered (Parmley, W.W., JACC 13, 771-785, 1989).
Inotropic Agents: The most widely used agent is digitalis. Sicker patients, especially those with a dilated heart and reduced ejection fraction, seem to respond most to digoxin (Review: Kulick, D.L. and Rahimtoola, S.H., "Current Role of Digitalis Therapy in Patients with Congestive Heart Failure," JAMA 265, 2995-2997, June 12, 1991). Toxicity occurs frequently and overall effect on mortality is questionable. Other inotropic agents including phosphodiesterase inhibitors (eg, amrinone) and dobutamine improve cardiac output on a short-term basis, but must be given intravenously making chronic use impractical (Parmley, W.W., JACC 13, 771-785, 1989; Dickstein, K. and Smith, T.W., J. of Cardiovasc. Pharmacol. 14 (Suppl. 5), S48-S56, 1989).

NADOLOL

(Corgard)

USES: Nadolol is a long-acting **beta-adrenergic blocking agent,** acting on both beta-1 and beta-2 receptors, that is structurally and pharmacologically similar to propranolol. Uses of nadolol are given in the next Table:

Uses of Nadolol
Hypertension
Angina Pectoris
Cardiac Arrhythmias

Hypertension: Nadolol is as effective as propranolol in hypertensive patients. Treatment of hypertension with nadolol is given in the next table (The 1988 Report of the Joint National Committee on Detection, Evaluation, and Treatment of High Blood Pressure, Arch. Intern Med. 148, 1023-1038, 1988):

Treatment of Hypertension with Atenolol

Step 1: Nonpharmacologic Approaches (see **HYPERTENSION**)

↓

Step 2: **Diuretic** or **Beta-Blocker** (eg, Nadolol) or **Calcium Antagonists** or **ACE Inhibitor**

Observe up to 6 months; if treatment ineffective then,

↓

Step 3: If nadolol choosen as first drug, increase the dosage.
or Add a second drug of a different class
or Substitute another drug

↓

Step 4: If nadolol choosen as first drug, add a second drug
or Add a third drug of a different class
or Substitute

↓

Step 5: Consider further evaluation and/or referral
or Add a third or fourth drug

"Step-Down": For patients with mild hypertension, after 1 year of control, consider decreasing or withdrawing nadolol and other hypotensive drugs.

NADOLOL (Cont.)
Mechanism of Action: The mechanism for nadolol's hypotensive action is not known; it is thought that nadolol, like other beta-adrenergic blocking drugs, reduces blood pressure by blocking peripheral, (especially cardiac) adrenergic receptors resulting in decreasing cardiac output by decreasing sympathetic outflow from the CNS and/or by suppressing renin release. Nadolol decreases heart rate and decreases cardiac output.
Angina Pectoris: Nadolol is thought to block catecholamine-induced increases in heart rate, velocity and extent of myocardial contraction and blood pressure which result in net decrease in myocardial oxygen consumption.
Cardiac Arrhythmias: Nadolol decreases conduction velocity through the atrioventricular (AV) node and decreases myocardial automaticity via beta-1 blockage.
DOSAGE FORMS: Tabs: 20, 40, 80, 120, 160mg.
DOSAGE: Nadolol is administered orally once daily. If long-term therapy is to be discontinued, dosage of the drug should be gradually reduced over a period of 1-2 weeks. Dosage is given in the next Table:

Dosage of Nadolol

Condition	Dosage
Hypertension	Initially: 40mg once daily, alone or in combination with a diuretic. Dosage may be gradually increased at 2 to 14 day intervals until the desired blood pressure response is obtained. The usual maintenance dosage is 40 or 80mg once daily. Doses up to 640mg may be required rarely.
Angina	Initially: 40mg once daily; the amount may be increased gradually by 40 to 80mg increments at 3 to 7 day intervals until the desired response is obtained. The usual maintenance dose is 40 or 80mg once daily. Doses up to 240mg may be required. Sublingual and long-acting nitrates should be continued.
Cardiac Arrhythmias	Initially: 40mg once daily. The dose may be increased gradually at weekly intervals as needed. The usual maintenance dose is 60-160mg daily.

Dosage in Renal Impairment: Dosage in renal impairment is given in the next Table:

Dosage in Renal Impairment

Creatinine Clearance ($ml/min/1.73M^2$)	Dosage Interval (Hours)
>50	24
31-50	24-36
10-30	24-48
<10	40-60

PHARMACOKINETICS: Half-Life: 10-24 hours (increased in uremia); Protein Binding:30%; Urinary Excretion of Unchanged Drug:76%; Active Metabolites:None.
ADVERSE EFFECTS: Most adverse effects are mild and transient and occur more frequently at the onset of therapy. Bradycardia if severe, can be treated with IM or IV atropine sulfate or if necessary, IV isoproterenol. Cardiac failure, postural hypotension, palpitation, and cardiac arrhythmias may occur. CNS effects are dizziness and fatigue. Paresthesias, sedation, malaise and change in behavoir may occur. GI effects may include nausea, diarrhea, abdominal discomfort, constipation, vomiting, indigestion, nausea, bloating and flatulence.

Bronchospasm, peripheral arterial insufficiency, fatique, insomnia, sexual dysfunction. Exacerbation of congestive heart failure; masking of symptoms of hypoglycemia; hypertriglyceridemia, decreased HDL cholesterol.
PRECAUTIONS: Should not be used in patients with asthma, COPD, CHF, heart block > first degree and sick sinus syndrome. Use with caution in insulin-treated diabetic patients and patients with peripheral vascular disease.
DRUG INTERACTIONS: Drug interactions are given in the next Table:

Drug Interactions of Nadolol

Drug	Comment
Lidocaine, Chlorpromazine, Coumarin	Clearance of these drugs, which are metabolized by the liver, may be reduced.
Calcium Channel Blockers	May promote negative inotropic effects on the failing myocardium.
Reserpine	May cause marked bradycardia and syncope.

NAFCILLIN

(Unipen, Nafcil)

USES: Nafcillin is a penicillin which is used only in the treatment of infections caused by, or suspected of being caused by, **penicillinase-producing Staphylococci**. Some strains of Staphylococcus aureus and many strains of Staphylococcus epidermidis are resistant (Parry, M.F., Med. Clin. No. Am. 71, 1093-1112, Nov. 1987).

DOSAGE FORMS: Oral; Caps: 250mg; Sol'n: 250mg/5ml; Tabs: 500mg; Parenteral: Injection: 500mg, 1, 2g; Injection; IV infusion: 1, 1.5, 2g.

DOSAGE: Nafcillin is adminstered orally, by slow IV injection or infusion or by deep IM injection.

Orally administered nafcillin is used as follow-up after parenteral therapy. However, when an oral pencillinase-resistant penicillin, cloxacillin or dicloxacillin is generally preferred because of greater and more predictable GI absorption. Dosage is given in the next Table:

Dosage of Nafcillin

Age	Route	Dosage
Adults	Oral	2-4g daily divided every 6 h.
	Parenteral	2-12g daily divided every 4-6 h.
Children	Oral	50-100mg/kg daily; divided every 6 h.
	Parenteral	100-200mg/kg daily; IV every 6 h, IM every 12 h, max. 12g
Neonate <2kg; < 1 wk.	Parenteral	50mg/kg/day; divided every 12 h.
Neonate <2kg; >1 wk.	Parenteral	75mg/kg/day; divided every 8 h.
Neonate >2kg; < 1 wk.	Parenteral	50mg/kg/day; divided every 8 h.
Neonate >2kg; > 1 wk.	Parenteral	75mg/kg/day; divided every 6 h.

Modification of dosage may be necessary in patients with both severe renal impairment and hepatic impairment.

Duration of Therapy: For severe staphylococcal infections, therapy should be continued for at least 2 weeks.

ADVERSE EFFECTS: As with other penicillins, hypersensitivity reactions are the most frequent adverse reactions. Other adverse effects include hemolytic anemia; agranulocytosis; acute interstitial nephritis (rarely); hypokalemia; and toxic hepatitis. Sodium concentration 2.9mEq/gm.

PHARMACOKINETICS: Absorption: Erratic (oral); rapid (IM); Peak: 30 min.-2 hr. (oral); 30-60 min (IM); Protein-Binding: 70-90%; Half-Life: 0.5-1.5 h.; half-life mildly prolonged with renal failure.

MONITOR: Monitor parameters as given in the next Table:

Monitor, Nafcillin

Parameter	Monitor for Complications
Complete Blood Count(CBC) including Differential	Monitor for hemolytic anemia, agranulocytosis and hypersensitivity (eosinophil count)
Renal Function Tests: Urinalysis, BUN, Creatinine & Serum Electrolytes	Interstitial nephritis and hypokalemia
Liver Function Tests: AST(SGOT); ALT(SGPT)	Toxic hepatitis

NALOXONE

(Narcan)

USES: Naloxone is an **opiate antagonist**, which is used to treat **respiratory depression** caused by **opiate overdose**; uses are given in the next Table:

Uses of Naloxone
Neonatal Opiate Depression: Treatment of asphyxia resulting from opiates administered to the mother during labor and delivery.
Postoperative Opiate Depression
Known or Suspected **Opiate Overdose** or as an **Aid** in the **Diagnosis** of Suspected Opiate Overdose

Naloxone, accompanied by other resuscitative measures such as oxygen, and mechanical ventilation is used for the treatment of respiratory depression caused by opiates.

Mechanism of Action: Naloxone is a specific antagonist at opiate receptors in the central nervous system.

DOSAGE FORMS: Injections: 0.02mg/ml, 0.4mg/ml, 1.0mg/ml

DOSAGE: Naloxone is rapidly inactivated following oral administration; it is given parenterally, IV, IM or subcutaneously. Doses are given in the next Table:

Dosages of Naloxone

Condition	Dosage
Neonatal Opiate Depression	0.1mg/kg, administered into the umbilical or other vein of neonate at 2-or 3-minute intervals until desired response is obtained. Additional doses may be necessary at 1-to 2-hour intervals. The drug may also be given by IM, subcutaneous or intratracheal injection.
Postoperative Opiate Depression	Adults: 0.1-0.2mg, IV, given at 2-to 3-minute intervals until desired response is obtained; additional doses may be necessary at 1- to 2-hour intervals. or 0.005mg/kg, IV, repeated every 15 minutes as needed. Children: 0.005-0.1mg/kg IV, given at 2-to 3-minute intervals until desired response is obtained; additional doses may be necessary at 1-to 2-hr intervals (Max. 2.0mg/dose)
Known or Suspected Opiate Overdose(or Aid in Diagnosis of Suspected Opiate Overdose)	Adult: 0.4-2mg, IV, given at 2-to 3-minute intervals until desired response is obtained, up to a max. of 10mg. IM, subcutaneous or intratracheal if necessary. Children: 0.1mg/kg, IV, IM, subcutaneous or intratracheal up to 5 yrs of age or 20kg. Beyond 5 yrs or for patients weighing more than 20kg, naloxone 2.0mg should be given. Continuous Infusion: Recommendations vary; adults and children: 0.4mg/hr or children: 0.005-0.16mg/kg/hr.

The currently recommended dose of naloxone for complete opiate reversal is 0.1mg/kg for infants and children from birth to 5 years of age or 20kg of body weight; children older than 5 years or weighing more than 20kg should receive 2.0mg (Committee on Drugs, American Academy of Pediatrics, Pediatrics 86, 484-485, September, 1990). Smaller doses may be used and titrated to effect in cases of postoperative opiate depression in which the patient's respiratory status is stable and only partial reversal of opiate effect is desirable.

PHARMACOKINETICS: Onset: 2-3 minutes; Metabolized in liver; Plasma half-life in adults, 60-90 minutes; in neonates, 3 hours. Excreted in urine.

ADVERSE EFFECTS: Use with caution in patients with cardiovascular disease. No adverse effects in doses used to reverse respiratory depression. Will cause narcotic withdrawal in chronically dependent patients.

NAPROXEN

(Anaprox, Naprosyn)

USES: Naproxen is a **nonsteroidal anti-inflammatory drug (NSAID)** structurally and pharmacologically related to fenoprofen and ibuprofen. It has pharmacologic activites similar to NSAID's, that is, **anti-inflammatory, analgesic** and **antipyretic activity.** Uses of naproxen are given in the next Table:

Uses of Naproxen
Rheumatoid Arthritis
Osteoarthritis
Juvenile Rheumatoid Arthritis
Ankylosing Spondylitis
Acute Gouty Arthritis
Acute Painful Shoulder, Tendinitis, Bursitis
Dysmenorrhea

In patients with rheumatoid arthritis or osteoarthritis, naproxen therapy is reserved for treatment of active disease unresponsive to an adequate trial with salicylates.

DOSAGE FORMS: Tabs: 250, 375. 500mg; Susp: 125mg/5ml; Sodium Salt: Tabs: 275mg (equal to 250mg naproxen); 550mg (equal to 500mg naproxen).

DOSAGE: Naproxen and naproxen sodium are administered orally. Adverse GI effects may be minimized by administering the drugs with meals, milk or a magnesium and aluminum hydroxide antacid. Dosage is given in the next Table:

Dosage of Naproxen

Condition	Age	Dosage
Inflammatory Diseases: Acute or Chronic (Excluding Acute Gouty Arthritis)	Adults	250-500mg of naproxen twice daily, morning and evening; or 275mg of naproxen sodium in the morning and 550mg in the evening. Adjust dosage according to response and tolerance. Max. 1.5g naproxen or 1.65g of naproxen sodium. Symptomatic improvement usually begins within 2 weeks;if no improvement, continue for another 2 weeks
Juvenile Rheumatoid Arthritis	Child.	10mg/kg daily in 2 divided doses
Acute Gouty Arthritis	Adults	750mg of naproxen followed by 250mg every 8 hrs. or 825mg of naproxen sodium followed by 275mg every 8 hrs. Continue therapy until attack subsides; expect relief in 24-48 hrs.
Pain & Dysmenorrhea	Adults	500mg of naproxen followed by 250mg every 6-8 hrs. as necessary.Max 1.25g of naproxen. or 550mg of naproxen sodium followed by 275mg every 6-8 hrs. as necessary. Max. 1.375g of naproxen sodium.

PHARMACOKINETICS: Onset: 1 hr; Duration: 7 hrs; Peak effect: 2-4 weeks; Half-Life: 12-15 hrs. Absorption: Readily and complete; more rapid with sodium form. Protein Binding: 99.6%. Excretion: 95% in urine.

ADVERSE EFFECTS: GI: Indigestion, abdominal discomfort, nausea, vomiting, heartburn; these effects are less frequent than with aspirin and indomethacin. GI bleeding. CNS: headache, drowsiness, vertigo, tinnitus.

Rare: Visual disturbances, thrombocytopenia, agranulocytosis, jaundice, interstitial nephritis and nephrotic syndrome.

CONTRAINDICATIONS: Patients exhibiting syndrome of nasal polyps, angioedema and bronchospasm induced by aspirin or other nonsteroidal anti-inflammatory agents.

PRECAUTIONS: Pregnancy. Pre-existing ulcer disease or history of GI bleeding.

NEOMYCIN SULFATE
(Mycifradin, Neo-Tabs, Neo-IM)

USES: Neomycin is an **aminoglycoside** antibiotic; uses are given in the next Table:

Uses of Neomycin
Hepatic Encephalopathy
Preoperative Intestinal Antisepsis
Diarrhea caused by Enteropathogenic E. Coli
Bacteriuria and Bacteremia Assoc. with Indwelling Catheters
Ophthalmic Infections
Otic Infections
Skin Infections

Neomycin sulfate is used orally in the treatment of GI bacteria, hepatic encephalopathy -(see below), preoperative intestinal antisepsis and diarrhea caused by E. coli; approximately 3% of an oral dose of neomycin is absorbed from the normal GI tract.

Hepatic Encephalopathy: Neomycin is used orally or as a retention enema to inhibit ammonia-forming bacteria in the GI tract as an adjunct to protein restriction and supportive therapy in patients with hepatic encephalopathy. Note that other aminoglycosides, kanamycin or paromomycin can be used orally for hepatic encephalopathy.

DOSAGE FORMS: Oral: 125mg/5ml; Tabs: 500mg; Injection: 500mg; Ophthalmic, Otic, and Skin preparations: Many available.

DOSAGE: The dosages of neomycin sulfate are given in the next Table:

Dosages of Neomycin Sulfate

Condition	Dosages
Hepatic Encephalopathy	Adult: 4-12g, oral, in 4 divided doses for 5-6 days; patients with chronic hepatic insufficiency may need up to 4g daily for an indefinite period. Children: 2.5-7g/M^2 daily in 4 divided doses for 5-7 days; chronic therapy, 2.5g/M^2 daily in 4 divided doses.
Preoperative Intestinal Antisepsis for Colorectal Surgery	Low residue diet; saline cathartic immediately preceding neomycin therapy. 24 Hour Regimen: Adult: 1g every hour for 4 doses, then 1g every 4 hours for the balance of the 24 h. 2-to 3-Day Regimen: Adults and Children: daily dose, 90mg/kg in 6 equally divided doses at 4-hour intervals. 19-Hour Regimen for Preparation for 8 A.M. Surgery: 1g neomycin and 1g of erythromycin base at 1 P.M., 2 P.M., 11 P.M. on day preceding surgery
Diarrhea Caused by Enteropathogenic E. Coli	Adults: 3g/day in 4 divided doses for 2-3 days; Premature and Newborn: 50mg/kg/day in 4 divided doses; Infants and Children: 50-100mg/kg/day in 4 divided doses.
Ophthalmic Infections	Combined with other drugs; place ointment into conjunctival sac every 3-4 hours. When solutions or suspensions are used, 1 or 2 drops into affected eye 2-4 times daily.
Otic Infections	Combined with other drugs; 3-4 times daily. Limit, 7-10 days.
Skin Infections	Alone or Combined with other drugs; some experts question the efficacy of topical antibiotics
Bacteriuria and Bacteremia Assoc. with Indwelling Catheters	Neomycin sulfate in combination polymyxin B sulfate is used for irrigation of the urinary bladder to prevent bacteriuria and bacteremia assoc. with indwelling catheters when open drainage urinary catheters are used.

Reduce dosage in renal impairment.

ADVERSE EFFECTS: Renal and ototoxicity. Contraindicated in ulcerative bowel disease or intestinal obstruction.

NEONATE, TOXIC DRUG REACTIONS

Toxic reactions in the neonate are given in the next Table (Warner, A., Clin. Chem. 32, 721-727, 1986):

Toxic Reactions in the Neonate

Drug/Chemical	Toxic Manifestation	Mechanism of Toxicity
Chloramphenicol	Gray Baby Syndrome	Slowed Clearance with Accumulation to Toxic Concentrations
Diazepam	Floppy Infant Syndrome	Reduced Clearance
Benzyl Alcohol	Gasping Syndrome	Large Amount of Dose Related to Size and Decreased Clearance
Tetracycline	Delayed Bone Growth	Interference with Ca Metabolism
Methyl Parabens	Kernicterus	Bilirubin Displacement
Sulfisoxazole	Kernicterus	Bilirubin Displacement
Boric Acid Powder	Diarrhea, Skin Changes, Death	Inc. Percutaneous Absorption --> Systemic Toxicity
Corticosteroids	Risk of Growth Retardation	Inc. Percutaneous Absorption --> Systemic Toxicity
Hexachlorophene	Vacuolar Encephalopathy of the Reticular Formation	Inc. Percutaneous Absorption --> Systemic Toxicity
Vitamin K (Water Soluble)	Kernicterus and Hemolytic Anemia	Unknown
E-Ferol	Hepatic Toxicity	Unknown

NEOSTIGMINE
(Prostigmin)

USES: Neostigmine is a **parasympathomimetic (cholinergic) drug** which mediates its effects by its anticholinesterase activity; uses of neostigmine are given in the next Table:

Uses of Neostigmine
Differential **Diagnosis** of **Myasthenia Gravis**
Treatment of Myasthenia Gravis
Postoperative Distention and Urinary Retention
Reversal of Nondepolarizing Neuromuscular Blocking Agents

Myasthenia Gravis: Myasthenia gravis is manifested clinically by weakness of skeletal muscle. Neostigmine is used to diagnose myasthenia gravis; patients with myasthenia gravis show a dramatic increase in muscle strength in response to neostigmine methylsulfate. Neostigmine is used to improve muscle strength in the symptomatic treatment of myasthenia gravis.

Mechanism of Action: The reaction catalyzed by acetylcholinesterase is as follows:

$$\text{Acetylcholine} + H_2O \xrightarrow[\text{Cholinesterase}]{\text{Acetyl-}} \text{Acetate} + \text{Choline}$$

Skeletal Muscle: Muscular contraction is mediated by release of acetylcholine from motor nerve terminals and its binding to receptor proteins on muscle; contraction is terminated by the enzyme acetylcholinesterase which catalyzes the hydrolysis of acetylcholine to choline plus acetate.

Acetylcholine mediates parasympathomimetic (cholinergic) effects.

Neostigmine inhibits the hydrolysis of acetylcholine by competing with acetylcholine for attachment to acetylcholinesterase. Acetylcholine accumulates at cholinergic synapses and its effects are prolonged and exaggerated; cholinergic responses of neostigmine are listed in the next Table:

Cholinergic Responses of Neostigmine
Increased Tonus of Skeletal and Intestinal Musculature
Miosis
Constriction of Bronchi and Ureters
Bradycardia
Stimulation of Secretion of Salivary and Sweat Glands

DOSAGE FORMS: Tabs: 15mg (Bromide); Injection: 0.25mg/ml, 0.5mg/ml, 1mg/ml.

DOSAGE: The dosages of neostigmine are given in the next Table:

Dosages of Neostigmine

Condition	Dosage
Diagnosis of Myasthenia Gravis	Discontinue all anticholinestase medications for at least 8 hours. Give atropine sulfate, 0.01mg/kg IV with, or IM or subcutaneously 30 minutes before, neostigmine methylsulfate, to prevent adverse muscarinic (sweating, vasodilation, salivary and bronchial secretion, miosis, bradycardia, stim. of smooth muscle) effects. Children: Atropine sulfate, 0.01mg/kg subcutaneously, IV or IM followed by neostigmine methylsulfate, 0.025-0.04mg/kg IM. Adults: Atropine sulfate, 0.01mg/kg IV with, or IM or subcutaneously before, neostigmine methylsulfate 0.022 mg/kg by IM injection. If a cholinergic reaction occurs, the test should be discontinued and 0.4-0.6 mg or more of atropine sulfate administered IV.
Treatment of Myasthenia Gravis Oral	Neonate: 1-4mg orally, neostigmine bromide every 2-3 hrs. Children: 7.5-15mg orally, neostigmine bromide, 3-4 times daily or 0.333mg/kg, orally, 6 times daily. Adults: 15mg, orally, neostigmine bromide, 3 times daily, the daily dose is gradually increased at intervals of one or more days(range: 15-375mg/day; average: 150mg/day)
Treatment of Myasthenia Gravis Parenteral	Neonate: 0.1-0.2mg neostigmine methylsulfate subcutaneously or 0.03mg/kg IM every 2-4 hrs. Children: 0.01-0.04mg/kg/dose IV, IM, or SC every 2-3 hrs. Adults: 0.5-2.5mg of neostigmine methylsulfate, IV, IM or SC as needed.

NEOSTIGMINE (Cont.)

Dosage of Neostigmine	
Condition	Dosage
Prevention of Postoperative Distention and Urinary Retention	Adults: 0.25mg neostigmine methylsulfate, subcutaneously or IM, every 4-6 hours for 2-3 days.
Treatment of Postoperative Urinary Retention	0.5-1mg, neostigmine methylsulfate, subcutaneously or IM. If in the treatment of urinary of urinary retention, there has been no response within an hour of the first dose, patient should be catheterized Doses repeated every 3 hours for 5 doses after bladder emptied. Mechanical obstruction must be excluded.
Reversal of Nondepolarizing Neuromuscular Blockade	Neonates and Infants: 0.02mg/kg of atropine sulfate with 0.025-0.1mg/kg neostigmine methylsulfate, IV. Adults: 0.6-1.2mg atropine sulfate or 0.2-0.6mg of glycopyrrolate (about 0.2mg of glycopyrrolate for each 1mg of neostigmine methylsulfate) with 0.5-2.5mg neostigmine methylsulfate, slowly, IV. Neuromuscular blockade may return, especially if longer acting agents are given just prior to reversal.

Neostigmine is not the drug of choice for diagnosis, or therapy of myasthenia gravis or postoperative urinary retention; **drugs of choice for these conditions** are given in the next Table:

Drugs of Choice for Myasthenia Gravis and Urinary Retention	
Condition	Drug of Choice
Differential Diagnosis of Myasthenia Gravis	**Edrophonium**
Oral Therapy of Myasthenia Gravis	**Pyridostigmine**
Therapy of Severe Myasthenia Gravis	**Pyridostigmine or Ambenonium plus Neostigmine**
Postoperative Distention and Urinary Retention	**Bethanechol Chloride**

ADVERSE EFFECTS: Exaggerated response to parasympathetic stimulation: nausea, vomiting, diarrhea, miosis, excessive salivation and sweating, increased bronchial secretions, abdominal cramps, bradycardia, and bronchospasm. Weakness, muscle cramps, and hypotension may occur. Contraindicated in intestinal and urinary obstruction.

Atropine sulfate injection should always be readily available as an antagonist for the muscurinic effects of neostigmine.

CONTRAINDICATIONS: Asthma.

NETILMICIN
(Netromycin)

USES: **Netilmicin** is a **aminoglycoside** antibiotic; because of its potential ototoxic and nephrotoxic effects, netilmicin is only used in **serious complicated aerobic gram-negative infections** principally the **Enterobacteriaceae** and **Pseudomonas aeruginosa.**

DOSAGE FORMS: Injection: 100mg/ml

DOSAGE: Netilmicin sulfate is administered by IM injection or IV infusion; dosage is identical for IM or IV administration and is given in the next Table:

Dosage of Netilmicin

Age	Route	Dosage
Adults	IM or IV	4-6.5mg/kg daily, divided every 8 h.
Children	IM or IV	5.5-8mg/kg daily, divided every 8 h.
Neonate <1 wk.	IM or IV	5mg/kg/day, divided every 12 h.
Neonate 1-4 wks.	IM or IV	7.5mg/kg/day, divided every 8 h.

Renal failure: load with 1.3-3.25mg/kg, then dosage as given in the next Table:

Dosage of Netilmicin in Renal Failure

Dose	Creatinine Clearance(ml/min) 80-50	50-10	<10
1.3-2.2mg/kg	Every 8-12 h.	Every 12-24 h.	Every 24-48 h.

See GENTAMICIN for more specific method of adjustment for renal failure.

ADVERSE EFFECTS: Toxicity and untoward effects are listed in the next Table; (Edson, R.S. and Keys, R.F., Mayo Clin. 58, 99-102, 1983):

Toxicity of Aminoglycosides

Major:
- **Renal Toxicity**
- **Vestibular Toxicity**
- **Auditory Toxicity**
- **Neuromuscular Blockade**

Minor: Skin Rash, Drug-Induced Fever

Hypomagnesemia (less than 1.6ml/dl in almost 40% of patients) is a frequent early occurrence in patients receiving aminoglycoside therapy; aminoglycosides may produce hypocalcemia and hypokalemia; it may be advisable to monitor serum magnesium for patients receiving aminoglycoside therapy, with use of magnesium replacement therapy when low levels are found (Zaloga, G.P. et al., Surg. Gynecol. Obstet. 158, 561-565, 1984).

Permanent hearing losses are due to destruction of sensory hair cells of the inner ear.

Aminoglycosides are eliminated by the kidney and cause nephrotoxicity; therefore, serum creatinine should be measured.

PHARMACOKINETICS: The pharmacokinetics of the parenterally administered aminoglycosides are similar.

Absorption: Poorly absorbed (oral); 100%(IM); Peak: 30-90 min.(IM); Protein Binding: <10%; Volume of Distribution: 0.2-0.3 liter/kg; Half-Life: 2-3 hr. (adults and children >6 months); 8-11 hr. (premature); 5 hr. (neonate).

MONITOR: Peak and trough levels (Peak: 6-12mcg/ml; Trough: 0.5-2mcg/ml), magnesium, calcium, potassium, creatinine or BUN, and audiograms. See GENTAMICIN for recommendations.

NIACIN (NICOTINIC ACID)
(Nicobid, Nicolar)

USES: Niacin, a **B vitamin,** may be effective in **lowering cholesterol** and **triglyceride** in all types of hyperlipoproteinemias except type I. Administration of niacin is associated with a reduction in recurrent myocardial infarctions and in long-term total mortality (Canner, P.L. et al., J. Am. Coll. Cardiol. 8, 1245-1255, 1986).

Niacin lowers total and LDL-cholesterol and triglycerides and raises HDL-cholesterol levels. Total cholesterol is decreased 25% and LDL-cholesterol is decreased 15-30%. It may be useful in treating type II hyperlipoproteinemias when the bile acid sequestrants, cholestyramine or colestipol, alone are ineffective. Lipids are reduced to normal in type III hyperlipoproteinemia; however, the apoprotein E-III defect is not affected. It is often highly successful in lowering triglyceride in type V hyperlipoproteinemia.

Mechanism of Action: Niacin reduces the rate of synthesis of LDL and apolipoprotein B by depressing the synthesis of VLDL. As a result, VLDL and LDL cholesterol decrease and HDL cholesterol increases.

DOSAGE FORMS: Caps(timed release): 125, 250, 300, 400, and 500mg; Elixir: 50mg/5ml; Tabs: 25, 50, 100, 250, 500mg; Tabs(timed release): 150, 250, 500, 750mg.

DOSAGE: Niacin is initiated with a single dose of 100-250mg daily. This initial dose is usually given after dinner to minimize problems with flushing during normal daily activities. The frequency of dose and total daily dose are slowly increased every 4-7 days until the first level therapeutic dose of 1.5-2 gram daily is reached. If the LDL-cholesterol is not lowered sufficiently, the dose should be increased to 3g daily (1.0g three times daily). In patients with marked elevations of plasma cholesterol, consider dosage up to 6g daily.

ADVERSE EFFECTS: Adverse effects of niacin is given in the next Table:

Adverse Effects of Niacin

System	Effect
Prostaglandin Release	Flushing mediated through release of prostaglandins occurs initially in almost all patients and persists in 10% to 15%; flushing can be ameliorated by concomitant use of aspirin 300mg daily or nonsteroidal anti-inflammatory drugs (NSAIDS). Tolerance to flushing develops rapidly over several weeks. Flushing is reduced by slowly increasing nicotinic acid to full dose, by avoiding administration on an empty stomach, and by use of sustained-release preparations (Knopp, R.H. et. al., Metabolism 34, 642-647, 1985). Flushing will return if doses are omitted from the prescribed schedule.
Gastro-intestinal	Nausea, vomiting, flatulence and diarrhea may subside with continual therapy. Also activation of peptic ulcer may occur.
Metabolism	Impaired glucose tolerance and hyperuricemia; these effects are usually reversible when niacin is discontinued; niacin is contraindicated in diabetics mellitus and gouty arthritis.
Liver	Hepatotoxicity including cholestatic jaundice.
Integument	Pruritis, dry skin with scaling, acanthosis nigricans.

CONTRAINDICATIONS: Hepatic disease, peptic ulcer, gouty arthritis, or diabetes mellitus; pregnancy, Category C.

MONITOR: Uric acid, liver function tests and blood glucose. Monitor total cholesterol, total triglycerides, LDL-cholesterol, VLDL and HDL, as appropriate, just prior to starting therapy, in 4 to 6 weeks, and at 3 months. If the "goal" is achieved, monitor total cholesterol or triglyceride (as appropriate) at 4 month intervals and lipoproteins annually.

DRUG INTERACTIONS: Niacin potentiates the effects of ganglionic blocking agents; when niacin is used with these drugs in hypertensive patients, it may cause orthostatic hypotension.

PHARMACOKINETICS: Absorption: Rapid and almost complete; Peak: 45 minutes; Excretion: Urine; Metabolism: Niacin concentrates mainly in the liver but also appears in adipose tissue and kidneys; plasma clearance is reduced in patients with hepatic impairment. Effective in 2 weeks-2 months.

NICARDIPINE

(Cardene)

USES: Nicardipine is a calcium-entry blocker; uses are given in the next Table:

Uses of Nicardipine
Chronic Stable Angina Pectoris
Hypertension

Chronic Stable Angina Pectoris: Nicardipine causes an increase in ejection fraction and cardiac output with minimal change in LVEDP. Coronary blood flow is increased. Although most patients experience fewer episodes of angina and increased exercise tolerance, some patients (7%) experience increased frequency, duration or severity of angina.

Hypertension: Nicardipine may be used in the stepped-approach to treatment of hypertension (see HYPERTENSION, TREATMENT). Nicardipine has also been used successfully for IV treatment of severe hypertension (Wallin, J.D. et al., Arch. Intern. Med. 149, 2662-2669, 1989). Nicardipine reduces systemic vascular resistance, leading to decreased systolic and diastolic blood pressure.

Mechanism of Action: Nicardipine inhibits calcium influx, thus inhibiting the contractile processes of cardiac and vascular smooth muscles; nicardipine is more selective to vascular smooth muscle than cardiac muscle and has less negative inotropic effect than nifedipine (Rousseau, M.F. and Pouleur, H., Abstract 1217, Circulation, 70(suppl. 2), 304, 1984).

DOSAGE FORMS: Caps: 20, 30mg; IV(tentative): 1.0, 2.5mg/ml.

DOSAGE: Nicardipine is administered orally: parenteral preparation is currently under investigation. Dosage of nicardipine is given in the next Table:

Uses of Nicardipine

Condition	Dosage
Stable Angina Hypertension	Initially: 20mg orally three times daily, may be increased gradually to 40mg orally three times daily to achieve desired effects.
Severe Hypertension	Use is investigational; initially: 1mg/hr IV; increase as needed until desired effect is achieved or a maximum dose of 15mg/hr is reached. Usual range: 2-4mg/hr. Peak effect occurs at 8-12 hrs (Wallin, J.D., Amer. Heart J., 119, 434-437, 1990).

PHARMACOKINETICS: Absorption: 100%; Peak: 0.5-2 hrs; Protein Binding: >95%; Metabolism: Liver.

ADVERSE EFFECTS: Headache, nausea, vomiting, dizziness, flushing, hypotension, pedal edema, and palpitations. Some patients with angina experience worsening of symptoms (7%).

Nicardipine is more likely to cause edema but less likely to cause constipation or AV block than verapamil (Medical Letter 31, 27, 1989).

Nicardipine is less likely to cause side effects such as dizziness, flushing, headache, pedal edema, and palpitations than nifedipine when used to treat angina pectoris (DeWood, M.A. et al., Amer. Heart J. 119, 468-478, 1990).

DRUG INTERACTIONS: Experience with this drug is limited; drug interactions are probably similar to other calcium-entry blockers. Drug interactions are shown in the next Table:

Drug Interactions of Nicardipine

Drug(s)	Interactions
Beta-Blockers	Combination is generally well tolerated.
Cimetidine	Increases nicardipine levels.
Fentanyl	Severe hypotension.
Digoxin	Nicardipine usually does not alter digoxin levels, however, drug levels should be evaluated.
Cyclosporine	Nicardipine elevates cyclosporine levels.

NICLOSAMIDE
(Niclocide)

USES: **Niclosamide** is used in the treatment of **helminthics.**

DOSAGE FORMS: Tabs: 0.5gm

DOSAGE: Niclosamide is administered orally; tablets should be chewed or crushed. The dosage of niclosamide in the treatment of patients with helminthics is given in the next Table:

Antihelmintic Activity of Niclosamide

Antihelmintic Activity	Dosage of Niclosamide
Hymenolepsis Nana (Dwarf Tapeworm)	Adults: 2g daily, given as single doses for 7 days. Children: >34kg: 1.5g as a single dose on the first day, followed by 1g daily, given as single daily doses for 6 days. 11-34kg: 1g as a single dose on the first day, followed by 500mg daily, given as single daily doses for 6 days.
Diphyllobothrium Latum (Fish Tapeworm); Dipylidium Caninum (Dog and Cat Tapeworm); Taenia Saginata (Beef Tapeworm); Hymenolepis diminuta (Rat tapeworm); Taenia Sodium (Pork Tapeworm). Drug of choice for all except Taenia Solium.	Adults: Single 2g dose Children: >34kg: 1.5g as a single dose 11-34kg: 1g as a single dose

Proglottids and/or eggs may be present in stools for up to 3 days after effective therapy; persistence in stool for 7 days or longer after therapy indicated failure and a repeat course of therapy may be given at that time. Absence of proglottids and eggs in stools for a minimum of 3 months after therapy with the drug is considered indicative of a cure.

ADVERSE EFFECTS: Nausea, vomiting, abdominal discomfort.

NICOTINE POLACRILEX
(Nicorette)

USES: **Nicorette** is a **chewing gum** that is used as an adjunct to a **behavoir modification** program for **smokers** who want to **quit smoking;** it is effective as a smoking cessation aid for people who are physically addicted to nicotine.

Mechanism of Action: Nicorette is a complex of nicotine and the cation exchange resin, polacrilin. Nicotine is released from the complex when the gum is chewed; the nicotine is then absorbed through the buccal mucosa. The trough blood nicotine concentrations produced by smoking one cigarette per hour are approxomately 1.5 times those achieved by chewing one piece of Nicorette every hour.

DOSAGE FORMS: Each piece of the chewing gum contains 2mg of nicotine.

DOSAGE: One piece of gum is chewed whenever the urge to smoke occurs and each piece should be chewed slowly and intermittently for 30 minutes. Most patients require approximately 10 pieces of gum per day during the first month of treatment. Patients should not exceed 30 pieces of gum per day. The use of nicotine resin complex for more than six months is not recommended.

PHARMACOKINETICS: One piece of gum containing 2mg of nicotine hourly produces a mean steady-state plasma nicotine level of 12ng/ml compared to a mean plasma nicotine trough concentration during usual cigarette smoking of 16ng/ml.

ADVERSE EFFECTS: Adverse effects are usually mild and transient; these include non-specific gastrointestinal distress (10%), eructation (6%), nausea and/or vomiting (19%), lightheadedness, insomnia, irritability and headache, (1%-2%), mouth and throat soreness (37%), muscle ache of the jaw (18%), hiccups (15%) and excessive salivation (2%).

PRECAUTIONS: Coronary heart disease, serious arrhythmias, hypertension, vasospastic disease, hyperthyroidism, pheochromocytoma, insulin dependent diabetes, peptic ulcer.

NIFEDIPINE
(Adalat, Procardia)

USES: **Nifedipine** is a **calcium-entry blocker** used for its **vasodilating** properties; uses are given in the next Table:

Uses of Nifedipine
Prinzmetal Variant Angina
Chronic Stable Angina Pectoris
Hypertension Acute or Chronic

Prinzmetal Variant Angina (Vasospastic Angina): Nifedipine inhibits spontaneous coronary artery spasm resulting in increased myocardial oxygen delivery.

Chronic Stable Angina Pectoris: Nifedipine has the following effects: dilation of systemic arteries resulting in decrease in total peripheral resistance; decrease in systemic b.p. (5-10mm Hg); decrease in afterload of the heart; small reflex increase in heart rate. The reduction in afterload and its resultant decrease in myocardial oxygen consumption is probably responsible for the effects of nifedipine in patients with angina.

Hypertension Acute or Chronic: Nifedipine may be used in the stepped-approach to treatment of hypertension as suggested by the 1988 Report of the Joint National Committee on Detection, Evaluation, and Treatment of High Blood Pressure (Arch. Intern. Med. 148, 1023-1038, 1988)(see HYPERTENSION, TREATMENT). Nifedipine has a rapid onset and may be given orally or sublingually for emergency treatment of hypertension.

Mechanism of Action: Nifedipine inhibits calcium influx, thus inhibiting the contractile processes of cardiac and vascular smooth muscles; coronary arteries and systemic arteries dilate.

DOSAGE FORMS: Caps: 10, 20mg; Tabs(extended release): 30, 60, 90mg.

DOSAGE: Nifedipine is administered orally or sublingually. Capsule must be punctured for sublingual administration. Dosage is given in the next Table:

Dosage of Nifedipine

Condition	Dosage
Prinzmetal Variant Angina or Chronic Stable Angina Pectoris Hypertension-Adults	Initial: 10mg, 3 times daily; then increase dosage gradually at 7-to 14-day intervals until optimal control is obtained. Maintenance: Usually, 30-60mg daily in 3 divided doses; Usual max. 180mg daily in 3-4 divided doses. or if symptoms warrant, increase dosage to 90mg daily in increments of 30mg/day over a over a 3-day period. Alternatively, initiate therapy with extended release tablets at dosage of 30-60mg once daily. Usual max. 120mg daily. Hospitalized Patients, Closely Monitored: Dosage may be increased in 10mg increments at 4- to 6-hour intervals, as necessary; single dose should not exceed 30mg.
Hypertension-Severe	Adult: 10mg orally or sublingual. Repeat 10-20mg oral dose at 30-45 min or sublingual dose at 15 min. if needed. Children: 0.2-0.5mg/kg (max. 10mg) orally or sublingual.
Hypertension-Child	Initial: 0.25mg/kg daily in 3-4 divided doses. Max. 1mg/kg daily; 5mg equals approx. 0.175ml

PHARMACOKINETICS: Absorption: 90%; Peak: 0.5-2 hrs.; Plasma Protein Binding: 92-98%; Half-Life: 2-5 hrs.; Metabolism: Liver; Excretion: Urine, 70-80%; Feces, 15%.

ADVERSE EFFECTS: Headache, tachycardia, dizziness, weakness, nausea, flushing, transient hypotension, severe muscle cramps, dermatologic reactions. Leg edema is relatively common and may be caused by local vasodilation. Worsening of myocardial ischemia may occur, and is more common in patients with angina of effort.

NIFEDIPINE (Cont.)

DRUG INTERACTIONS: Drug interactions of nifedipine are shown in the next Table:

Drug Interactions of Nifedipine

Drug(s)	Interactions
Beta-Adrenergic Blocking Agents, e.g., Propranolol, Atenolol, Timolol	Increases risk of severe hypotension, congestive heart failure (CHF) and arrhythmias; exacerbation of anginal pain has been noted when beta-blocker therapy is being withdrawn concurrently with initiation of nifedipine therapy.
Fentanyl (Opiate Agonist)	Severe hypotension
Digoxin	May increase digoxin concentration but data are controversial.
Cimetidine	Concomittant, administration increases peak nifedipine concentration by 80-90% and decreases clearance by 40%.
Phenytoin	Phenytoin toxicity may occur 4 weeks after initiating nifedipine therapy.

NITROFURANTOIN

(Macrodantin, Furadantin)

USES: **Nitrofurantoin** is an antibiotic that is used in the **treatment** of **uncomplicated urinary tract infections.**

DOSAGE FORMS: (Macrodantin, Furadantin) Tabs: 50, 100mg; Susp: 25mg/5ml; Caps: 25, 50, 100mg

DOSAGE: The drug is given orally; dosages are given in the next Table:

Dosages of Nitrofurantoin

Patient	Dosage
Adults	50-100mg, 4 times daily; continue for at least 1 week and for at least 3 days after sterility of the urine is attained.
Infants older than 1 month and Children	5-7mg/kg daily in 4 divided doses; continue for at least 1 week and for at least 3 days after sterility of the urine is attained.
Long-Term Therapy:	
Adults	50-100mg as a single evening dose.
Children	1-2mg/kg daily as a single evening dose or in 2 divided doses.

ADVERSE EFFECTS: The toxic effects of greatest importance are hypersensitivity pneumonitis, pulmonary fibrosis, and hepatotoxic reactions.

Other side effects include gastrointestinal intolerance, peripheral neuropathy, and anemia. May cause urine to be dark yellow or brown colored. Causes false positive urine glucose by clinitest (Benedicts reagent) but not by glucose oxidase reaction (Tes-Tape).

Careful monitoring for the presence of pulmonary, hepatic, and neurologic toxicity is necessary with long-term administration.

CONTRAINDICATIONS: Severe renal disease, G6PD deficiency; infants less than one month of age.

DRUG INTERACTIONS: Probenicid and sulfinpyrazone result in decreased efficacy and increased toxicity of nitrofurantoin. Nitrofurantoin may antagonize the effects of Quinolone antibiotics.

NITROGLYCERIN

[Tridil (IV), Nitrostat (Sublingual), Nitro-Bid (Oral)]

USES:Nitroglycerin, like other nitrates, acts as a **direct-acting vasodilator** resulting in **relaxation** of **vascular smooth muscle;** the venous system is affected to a greater degree than the arterial system. Nitroglycerin is used primarily for treatment of **angina pectoris.** The uses of nitroglycerin are given in the next Table:

Uses of Nitroglycerin
Treatment of **Angina Pectoris:**
Acute Relief of **Angina Pectoris** (Sublingual Nitroglycerin is Drug Choice)
Prophylactic Management in **Situations** likely to Provoke Angina Attacks
Long-Term Prophylactic Management of Angina Pectoris
IV Nitroglycerin:
Perioperative Hypertension especially Associated with Cardiovascular Procedures
Congestive Heart Failure Associated with Acute Myocardial Infarction
Produces Controlled Hypotension During Surgical Procedures.
Angina Pectoris Refractory to Nitrates and/or a Beta-Adrenergic Blocking Agent
IV or Topical Nitroglycerin:(alone or in combination with cardiac glycosides and diuretics or with hydralazine).
Refractory Congestive Heart Failure or other Low Cardiac Output States.
IV, Sublingual or Topical Nitroglycerin:
May Reduce Myocardial Ischemia and Possibly Decrease the Extent of Infarction During Acute Myocardial Infarction.

Nitroglycerin is administered lingually, sublingually, intrabuccally, orally, topically, or by IV infusion. **Sublingual nitroglycerin is the drug of choice for the acute relief of an attack of angina pectoris because it has a rapid onset, is inexpensive, and is effective.**

In long-term prophylaxis of angina pectoris, oral or topical nitroglycerin are administered.

Nitroglycerin dilates normal coronary arteries but may have little or no effect on atherosclerotic coronary arteries. Nitroglycerin increases subendocardial blood flow resulting in decreased myocardial ischemia.

IV nitroglycerin is used to control blood pressure in perioperative hypertension, expecially hypertension associated with cardiovascular procedures; for the treatment of congestive heart failure associated with acute myocardial infarction; and to produce controlled hypotension during surgical procedures.

Mechanism of Action: Nitroglycerin acts both peripherally and centrally. Nitroglycerin relaxes vascular smooth muscle, resulting in generalized vasodilation, decreased peripheral venous resistance, venous "pooling" of blood, decreased venous return to the heart, decreased left ventricular end-diastolic pressure and volume and decreased ventricular size and ventricular wall tension, resulting in decrease in myocardial oxygen consumption.

DOSAGE FORMS: Sublingual Tab (Nitrostat) : 0.15, 0.3, 0.4, 0.6 mg; **Topical Ointment:** 2%; Transdermal Systems: 2.5, 5, 7.5, 10, 15mg/24 hours; the most popular are the 5 and 10mg/24 hours. **Buccal** (Transmucosal) (Nitrogard): 1, 2, 3mg; **Lingual Aerosol** (Nitrolingual): 0.4mg/metered spray; **Oral:** Caps(extended release): 2.5, 6.5, 9mg; Tabs(extended release): 2.6, 6.5mg; **Parenteral:** 0.5, 0.8, 5, 10mg/ml.

NITROGLYCERIN (Cont.)

DOSAGE: Nitroglycerin is administered lingually, sublingually, intrabuccally, orally, topically, or by IV infusion. Dosage is given in the next Table:

Dosage of Nitroglycerin

Condition	Route	Dosage
Acute Anginal Attack	Sublingual(Under Tongue or in Buccal Pouch	0.15-0.6mg;if necessary, additional doses at 5 min. intervals; max. is 3 doses in 15 minutes.
	Lingual (Spray)	0.4mg per metered spray (1 or 2 sprays); if necessary, repeat in 3-5 minutes; max. 3 sprays (1.2mg) in 15 minutes.
Long-Term Prophylactic Management of Angina Pectoris	Buccal (Transmucosal) Tabs. (between lip and gum).	Extended-release tabs: 1mg 3 times daily, every 5 hrs. during waking hrs. Assess over 4-5 days.Titrate dosage upward until angina controlled or adverse effects occur. Usual dosage interval, 3-5 hours; Usual maintenance dosage,2mg, 3 times daily.
	Topical Dosage: Transdermal Sys.: Apply at same time each day to areas of hairless skin of the upper arm or body; rotate to avoid skin irritation. Ointment: See package insert.	Initially, use smallest dose of transdermal unit applied every 24 hours. Nitroglycerin may be applied as an ointment: initially 0.5inch of 2% conc. (approx. 7.5 mg) every 8 h.
	Oral	Extended-release: 1.3-9mg every 8 or 12 hours.
	Lingual (Spray)	Prophylactically, 5-10 minutes before situations that may provoke attack.
Control b.p. in perioperative hypertension; treatment of congestive heart failure (CHF) associated with acute myocardial infarction; produce controlled hypotension	IV: Dilute in 5% dextrose or 0.9% sodium chloride. Use glass or polypropylene because nitroglycerin migrates into polyvinyl chloride (PVC)	Non-polyvinyl chloride: Initially, 5mcg/min. with increases of 5mcg/min. every 3-5 min. until a b.p. response is obtained or until infusion rate is 20mcg/min. If no effect, increase dosage by 10mcg/min. and if necessary, by 20mcg/min. When partial b.p.response is obtained, reduce increases in dosage and lengthen interval. Monitor: b.p., heart rate, pulmonary, capillary wedge pressure. Polyvinyl Chloride: Higher doses required; initial dosage is usually 25mcg/min.
Children	IV	Initially: 1mcg/kg/min by IV infusion. Increase by 1mcg/kg/min every 20 minutes, titrate to effect. Max dose: 5mcg/kg/min.

PHARMACOKINETICS; Onset and duration are given in the next Table:

Onset and Duration

Dosage Form	Onset	Duration
Antianginal Effects		
Sublingual	Within 2 min.	Up to 30 min.
Buccal (Transmucosal) Extended-Release	Within 2-3 min.	3-5 hours
Ointment	30 min.	3 hours
Hemodynamic Effects		
Sublingual	2 min.	Up to 30 min.
Buccal (Transmucosal) Extended-Release	Within 2 min.	Up to at least 3 hours
Ointment	Within 1 hour	3-6 hours

NITROGLYCERIN (Cont.)
Metabolized in the liver; Half-life: 1-4 min; Plasma Protein-Binding: 60%.
ADVERSE EFFECTS: Serious adverse effects are uncommon; adverse effects are mainly cardiovascular, e.g., hypotension and tachycardia; bradycardia is occasionally associated with hypotension and responds to atropine; transient cerebral ischemia may occur. Other adverse effects include headache which occurs most frequently, dizziness, weakness, nausea and vomiting. Methemoglobinemia may occur in infants and patients on high doses of nitrates. The IV preparation contains alcohol and propylene glycol which may lead to toxicity (Curry, S.C. and Arnold-Capell, P., Crit. Care Clin. 1991, In Press).
PRECAUTIONS: Remove nitroglycerin patches before cardioversion; avoid use in patients with cardiomyopathy.
PARAMETERS TO MONITOR: Headache and other side effects. In patients with congestive heart failure, monitor hemodynamic and functional measurements. During IV use, monitor b.p., heart rate and capillary wedge pressure.
CONTRAINDICATIONS: Increased intracranial pressure, cerebral hemorrhage. Nitroglycerin IV is contraindicated in patients on disulfiram (Antabuse) due to the alcohol content of this preparation.

NITROPRUSSIDE
(Nipride, Nitropress)
USES: **Nitroprusside** is indicated for **immediate reduction** of **blood pressure** of patients in **hypertensive emergencies.** Nitroprusside is also used to produce controlled hypotension during anesthesia in order to reduce bleeding resulting from surgical procedures Nitroprusside is contraindicated in compensatory hypertension, such as arteriovenous shunt or coarctation of the aorta.
IV infusion of nitroprusside produces an almost immediate reduction in blood pressure. Blood pressure begins to rise immediately when the infusion is slowed or stopped and returns to pretreatment levels within 1-10 minutes.
Mechanism of Action: Nitroprusside is a potent vasodilator that acts directly on vascular smooth muscle to produce a peripheral vasodilation.
DOSAGE FORMS: IV: 50mg
DOSAGE: Nitroprusside is administered only by IV infusion using a controlled-infusion device, micro-drip regulator, or similar device that will allow precise measurement of the flow rate. Dilute in D5W and protect from light. The rate of administration should be adjusted to maintain the desired hypotensive effect as monitored with arterial line. Dosage is given in the next Table:

Dosage of Nitroprusside

Patients	Dosage
Adults and Children	0.5-10mcg/kg/minute Do not exceed 10mcg/kg/minute

Maintain diastolic blood pressure about 30-40% below pretreatment levels; systolic blood pressure should not be decreased to less than 60mmHg. Oral hypotensive agents should replace IV infusion of nitroprusside.
Nitroprusside should never be infused at the maximum rate of 10mcg/kg/min for more than 10 minutes. Cyanide toxicity may occur even at approved rates for as little as 35 minutes. Nitroprusside has a low risk of toxicity if used only briefly or at infusion rates less than 2mcg/kg/min.
ADVERSE EFFECTS: Nitroprusside administration may lead to two clinically distinct forms of toxicity. Cyanide toxicity occurs early and is manifest by metabolic acidosis with elevated blood lactate, increased mixed venous oxygen, tachycardia and lethargy leading to coma. Cyanide metabolism in the liver is limited by the availability of sulfur-containing co-factors (mainly thiosulfate). **Cyanide toxicity can be prevented by co-administration of sodium thiosulfate with nitroprusside in a 10:1 weight ratio (i.e. one gram of sodium thiosulfate per 100mg nitroprusside).** Thiocyanate toxicity occurs late and is manifest by nausea, vomiting, cramps, agitation, psychosis, hypothyroidism and seizures. Thiocyanate-toxicity is rare. Treatment is dialysis (Curry, S.L. and Arnold-Capell, P., Crit. Care Clin. 1991, In Press).
MONITOR: Monitor serum thiocyanate concentrations daily when therapy with nitroprusside is extended (>48 hours); especially in patients with impaired renal function. Nitroprusside is metabolized as follows:

Nitroprusside ⟶ Cyanide

Cyanide + Thiosulfate $\xrightarrow[\text{Rhodanase}]{\text{Liver}}$ Thiocyanate + Sulfate ⟶ Renal Excretion

Levels of serum thiocyanate should not exceed 0.1mg/ml.
Levels of red cell cyanide are toxic at >1mg/liter.

NIZATIDINE
(Axid)

USES: Nizatidine is an H_2-receptor antagonist. Uses of nizatidine are given in the next Table (The Medical Letter 30, 77-78, Aug. 12, 1988):

Uses of Nizatidine
Active Duodenal Ulcers
Prophylaxis to Prevent Recurrence of Duodenal Ulcers
Active Gastric Ulcers
Probably useful in Treatment of Zollinger-Ellison Syndrome

Nizatidine healed duodenal ulcers in about 68% of patients compared to 30% with placebo (Dyck, W.P. et al., Scand. J. Gastroenterol 22, Suppl. 136, 47, 1987). Nizatidine is as effective as ranitidine (Zantac) for treatment of duodenal ulcer (Simon, B., et al., Scand. J. Gastroenterol. 22, Suppl. 136, 61, 1987; Bovero. E. et al., Hepatogastroenterology 34, 269, 1987).

During maintenance therapy, patients on nizatidine had a cumulative one-year recurrence rate of 34%, compared to 64% in controls who took placebo (Cerulli, M.A. et al., Scand. J. Gastroenterol. 22, Suppl. 136, 79, 1987). The recurrence rate with nizatidine was 19%, compared to 13% in patients who took ranitidine (Zantac) (Hentschel, E., Scand. J. Gastroenterol. 22, Suppl. 136: 84, 1987).

Mechanism of Action: Nizatidine competitively inhibits the action of histamine on H_2 receptors of parietal cell, thus reducing acid secretion by parietal cells of the stomach; it acts like the other H_2 receptor antagonists, i.e., cimetidine (Tagamet), ranitidine (Zantac), and famotidine (Pepcid).

DOSAGE FORMS: Caps: 150mg, 300mg.

DOSAGE: Dosage of nizatidine is given in the next Table:

Dosage of Nizatidine

Condition	Dosage
Active Ulcer	300mg daily at bedtime
or	150mg twice daily both for up to 8 weeks.
Maintenance	150mg daily at bedtime for at least one year.

Dosage in renal insufficiency is given in the next Table:

Dosage in Renal Insufficiency

Condition	Creatinine Clearance	Dosage
Active Duodenal Ulcer	20 to 50ml/min	150mg daily.
Maintenance		150mg every other day.
Active Duodenal Ulcer	<20ml/min	150mg every other day.
Maintenance		150mg every three days.

Adverse Effects: Sweating, urticaria, somnolence and hepatic toxicity (Black, M., Am. J. Med. 83, Suppl 6A, 68, 1987).

Cimetidine (Tagamet), and to a lesser extent, ranitidine (Zantac) interfere with the hepatic metabolism of various drugs, such as oral anticoagulants and theophyllines which can accumulate in toxic amounts; nizatidine and famotidine apparently do not interfere with hepatic metabolism.

Nizatidine does not increase prolactin concentrations; however, gynecomastia occurs rarely.

PHARMACOKINETICS: Absorption: >90%; increased by about 10% with food; antacids may decrease absorption (Knadler, M.P. et al., Clin. Pharmacol. Ther. 42, 514, 1987); Acid Suppression: Prompt after oral dose of 300mg at bedtime, persists all night but not during the next day. Half-Life: 1-2 hours with normal renal function; Excretion: 65% excreted unchanged in urine.

NONSTEROIDAL ANTI-INFLAMMATORY DRUGS (NSAIDs)

The nonsteroidal anti-inflammatory drugs (NSAIDs) have anti-inflammatory, antipyretic and analgesic effects. The rheumatic diseases are the most common inflammatory conditions for which they are employed. Currently available nonsteroidal anti-inflammatory drugs are given in the next Table:

Nonsteroidal Anti-Inflammatory Drugs (NSAIDs)

Class, Generic and Trade Name
Salicylates
Acetylsalicylic Acid (Aspirin)
Diflunisal (Dolobid)
Propionic Acids
Naproxen (Naprosyn)
Naproxen Sodium (Anaprox)
Ibuprofen (Motrin, Rufen, Advil, Haltran, Medipren, Nuprin)
Fenoprofen (Nalfon)
Indoles
Indomethacin (Indocin)
Sulindac (Clinoril)
Oxicams
Piroxicam (Feldene)
Pyrroles
Tolmetin (Tolectin)
Fenamates
Meclofenamate Sodium (Meclomen)
Mefenamic Acid (Ponstel)
Pyrazoles
Phenylbutazone (Butazolidin)

The clinical usefulness of NSAIDs resides in their ability to counteract prostaglandin-mediated pain and inflammation. The biosynthetic pathway of prostaglandins is illustrated in the next Figure:

Biosynthetic Pathway of Prostaglandins

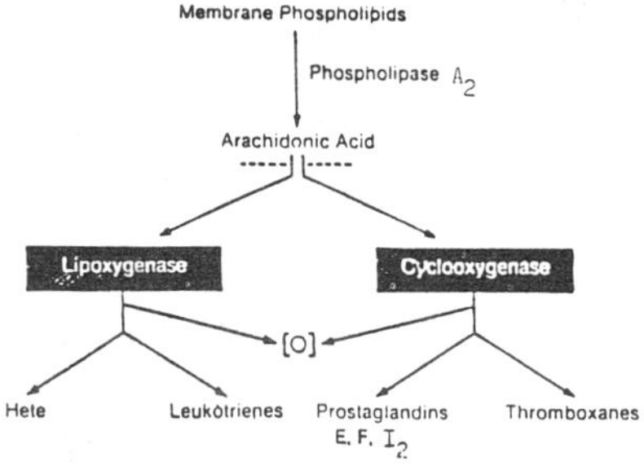

NSAIDs mediate their effects by inhibiting the enzyme cyclooxygenase, which catalyzes the reaction transforming arachidonic acid to the endoperoxide compounds.

NONSTEROIDAL ANTI-INFLAMMATORY DRUGS (NSAIDs) (Cont.)

The site and mechanism of action of aspirin, acetaminophen, and the nonsteroidal anti-inflammatory drugs (NSAIDs), including mefenamic acid and diflunisal are given in the next Table (Amadio, P., Am. J. Med. 77(3A), 17-26, 1984):

Site and Mechanism of Action of Aspirin, Acetaminophen, and the Nonsteroidal Anti-Inflammatory Drugs, Including Mefenamic Acid and Diflunisal

Compound	Prostaglandin Cyclo-Oxygenase Inhibition	Stimulation of $PGG_2 \to PGH_2$	Free [0]* Scavenger	Prostaglandin Receptor Site Inhibition
Acetylsalicylic acid	+	0	0	0
Acetaminophen	0	+++	+	0
NSAIDs	+++	0	0	0
Diflunisal	++	++	+	0
Mefenamic acid	++	0	0	+

*Free radical oxidation products; PGG_2=prostaglandin G_2; PGH_2=prostaglandin H_2; 0=free oxygen radicals.

Pharmacokinetic profiles of NSAIDs are given in the next Table (Amadio, P., Am. J. Med. 77(3A), 17-26, 1984):

Pharmacokinetic Profiles of Analgesic Nonsteroidal Anti-Inflammatory Drugs

Drug	Time of Peak (hours)	Half-Life	Protein Binding (percent)	Major Metabolic Pathway and (Excretion)
Diflunisal	2-3	8-12	99	Hepatic (Renal)
Mefenamic acid	2-4	2	Extensive	Hepatic (Renal [6%]) (Fecal [20-25%])
Fenoprofen	2	2.5-3	99	Hepatic (Renal)(Fecal)
Ibuprofen	1-2	1.8-2	90-99	Hepatic (Renal) (Biliary/fecal)
Naproxen	2-4	13	99	Hepatic (30%) (Renal 90%) (Fecal 5%)
Naproxen sodium	1-2	13	99	Hepatic (30%) (Renal 90%) (Fecal 5%)

ADVERSE REACTIONS: Adverse reactions common to all nonsteroidal anti-inflammatory drugs are given in the next Table (Amadio, P., Am. J. Med. 77(3A), 17-26, 1984):

Adverse Reactions Common to All Nonsteroidal Anti-Inflammatory Drugs

Gastrointestinal upset: nausea, vomiting, dyspepsia, diarrhea, constipation
Major gastrointestinal bleeding, ulcer, or perforation (Review: Soll, A.H. moderator, "Nonsteroidal Anti-Inflammatory Drugs and Peptic Ulcer Disease," Ann. Intern. Med. 114, 307-319, 1991).
Toxic Hepatitis
Skin rash: pruritus, urticaria, alopecia
Ocular: reversible blurring of vision
Central nervous system toxicity: headache, tinnitus, drowsiness, dizziness, light-headedness, agitation, confusion, lethargy, weakness, depression
Cardiovascular toxicity, palpitations, arrhythmias
Renal toxicity: Sodium and water retention, hyperkalemia, decreased renal blood flow and glomerular filtration, parenchymal disease (Review: Scharschmidt, L.A. and Feinfeld, D.A., Hosp. Physician, 29-33, August 1989)

The relative side effects of analgesic nonsteroidal anti-inflammatory drugs (NSAIDs) are given in the next Table (Amadio, P., Am. J. Med. 77(3A), 17-26, 1984):

Relative Side Effects of Analgesic Nonsteroidal Anti-Inflammatory Drugs

Drug	GI Irrita.	Peptic Ulcer	CNS Effects	Tinnitus	Hepatic Toxi.	Renal Toxi.	Bone Marrow Toxi.	Hypersensi.
Aspirin	+++*	++*	+	+++	++	+	+	+
Diflunisal	+	+	+	+	+	+	...	...
Mefenamic acid	+(++)	+	+	...	...	++	+	...
Fenoprofen	++	+	++	+++	+	+	+	...
Ibuprofen	++	+	+	+	+	+	+	+
Naproxen	++++	++++	++	++	+	+	+	+

*For aspirin in anti-inflammatory doses, these side effects would be present at a +++++ level.

NORFLOXACIN

(Noroxin)

USES: **Norfloxacin**, an **oral fluoroquinolone**, offers an alternative to parenteral therapy for serious infections; activities of norfloxacin are given in the next Table (Neu, H.C., Med. Clin. No. Am. 72, 623-636, 1988; Wolfson, J.S. and Hooper, D.C., Ann. Intern. Med. 108, 238-251, 1988; Adams, H.G., Personal Comm.):

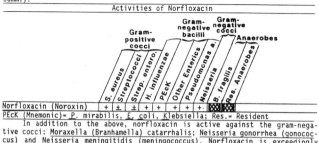

Activities of Norfloxacin

	Gram-positive cocci: S. aureus	Gram-positive cocci: Streptococci	Gram-positive cocci: Strep. entero.	H. influenzae	Gram-negative bacilli: PEcK	Gram-negative bacilli: Other Enterics	Gram-negative bacilli: Pseudomonas a.	Gram-negative cocci: Neisseria	Anaerobes: B. fragilis	Anaerobes: Res. Anaerobes
Norfloxacin (Noroxin)	+	±	±	+	+	+	+	+		

PEcK (Mnemonic)= P. mirabilis, E. coli, Klebsiella; Res.= Resident

In addition to the above, norfloxacin is active against the gram-negative cocci: Moraxella (Branhamella) catarrhalis; Neisseria gonorrhea (gonococcus) and Neisseria meningitidis (meningococcus). Norfloxacin is exceedingly potent in-vitro against enteric gram-negative bacilli, Neisseria species, and Haemophilus species. It is potent against Pseudomonas aeruginosa and some gram-positive bacteria. It has minimal activity against anaerobes.

Norfloxacin is approved by the FDA for the treatment in adults of complicated and uncomplicated **urinary tract infections** caused by susceptible organisms. Other potential uses include the treatment of bacterial gastroenteritis, prophylaxis of traveler's diarrhea, gonorrhea and bacterial prostatitis and prevention of infection with gram-negative bacilli in neutropenic patients.

Mechanism of Action: Norfloxacin, like ciprofloxacin, apparently acts to block DNA gyrase (topoisomerase II). DNA gyrase is responsible for proper coiling of DNA, for DNA replication, transcription of certain genes, and aspects of DNA repair and recombination. (Wolfson, J.S. and Hooper, D.C., Antimicrob. Agents Chemother. 28, 581-586, 1985).

DOSAGE FORMS: Tabs: 400mg. Norfloxacin is not recommended for children less than 18 years of age or during pregnancy.

DOSAGE: Norfloxacin is administered orally. The tablets should be taken one hour before or 2 hours after meals with a glass of water. Dosage is given in the next Table:

Dosage of Norfloxacin

Condition	Dosage
Urinary Tract Infection, Uncomplicated	400mg twice daily for 7-10 days.
Urinary Tract Infection, Complicated	400mg twice daily for 10-21 days, max. 800mg daily.

Continue treatment for 2 days after symptoms improve. For creatinine clearances of less than 30ml/min, the dosing interval should be doubled, or the dose should be halved (Arrigo, G. et. al., Int. J. Clin. Pharmacol. Ther. Toxicol. 23, 491-496, 1985). No dosage alterations are recommended in the elderly or in patients with hepatic dysfunction.

PHARMACOKINETICS: Oral Bioavailability: Excellent; Peak Serum Concentration: 1-2 hours; Protein-Binding: 15%; Metabolism: Metabolized to at least six metabolites, some of which are active. Excretion: Excreted in part by the kidneys; the concentration of norfloxacin in the urine exceeds the minimal inhibitory concentrations for virtually all urinary bacterial pathogens. Secreted in the urine by glomerular filtration rate and by renal tubular secretion. Half-Life: 3 to 4 hours.

NORFLOXACIN (Cont.)
ADVERSE EFFECTS: The incidence of adverse effects is 12.5% (Wang, C. et al., Scand. J. Infect. Dis. 48 (suppl.), 81-89, 1986). Adverse effects are dose related. In almost all patients, adverse effects are mild and do not require cessation of therapy. Adverse effects are given in the next Table:

Adverse Effects of Norfloxacin

System	Effects
Gastrointestinal Tract	Incidence, 4%; nausea
Central Nervous System	Incidence, 3%; headache and lightheadedness. Seizures occur rarely.
Rashes	Incidence, 0.3%
Cartilage Deterioration	Norfloxacin is not recommended for use in children and during pregnancy because of reports of cartilage deterioration in animals.

CONTRAINDICATIONS: Children or during pregnancy.
DRUG INTERACTIONS: Avoid nitrofurantoin; avoid concomitant antacids; excretion reduced by probenecid. Sucralfate, iron, calcium, magnesium, aluminum, and bismuth all interfere with absorption.

NYSTATIN

(Mycostatin, Nilstat)

USE: **Nystatin** is an **antifungal antibiotic** that is used for the treatment of cutaneous and mucocutaneous **candidal infections.** The infections caused by candida that are treated with nystatin are listed in the next Table:

Candidal Infections
Oral Cavity (Thrush)
Cutaneous Candidiasis
Candidal Diaper Rash
Vulvovaginal Candidiasis
Intestinal Candidiasis

DOSAGE FORMS: (Mycostatin, Nilstat) Tabs: 500,000 Units; Susp.: 100,000 U/ml; Vaginal Tab: 100,000 U; Powder: 100,000 Units/g; Powder(for susp): 50 million-5 billion units. Cream or Ointment: 100,000 U/g with Triamcinolone Acetonide (0.1%)

DOSAGE: Nystatin may be applied topically as a cream, ointment, powder, vaginal tablet or oral suspension; dosages are given in the next Table:

Dosages of Nystatin

Candidal Infections	Dosages
Oral Candidiasis (Thrush)	Adults and Children: 400,000 to 600,000 units as an oral suspension, 4 times daily. Infants: 200,000 units as an oral suspension, 4 times daily. Premature and Low-Birth Weight Infants: 100,000 units as an oral suspension, 4 times daily. Divide so that one-half is placed in each side of the mouth. Suspension should be retained in the mouth for several minutes before swallowing. Treatment should be continued for 48-72 hours after oral symptoms have subsided and/or cultures have returned to normal.
Cutaneous Candidiasis	A cream or ointment of nystatin, containing 100,000units/g in fixed combination with or without triamcinolone acetonide, 0.1% (a glucocorticoid) is applied to affected area in the morning and evening, gently and thoroughly massaging the preparation into the skin after application. Candidal Infection of Feet: Dust powder in shoes, stockings and on feet. Keep area dry and exposed to air. Candidal Diaper Rash: Apply cream or ointment to diaper area 2-4 times daily. As an adjunct to topical nystatin therapy, use oral suspension, 100,000 units, 4 times daily.
Vulvovaginal Candidiasis	Vaginal tablets, 100,000 units, inserted high in vagina, once or twice daily, even during menstruation, usually for 2 weeks; cleansing douches may be used by nonpregnant patients.
Intestinal Candidiasis	Therapy as above plus oral tablets, 500,000 to 1 million units, 3 times daily; continue for 48 h after clinical cure to prevent relapse.
Prevent Thrush in Neonate	Vaginal tablets, 100,000 to 200,000 units daily for 3-6 weeks prior to delivery

Treatment of cutaneous or mucocutaneous candidal infections produces symptomatic improvement within 1-3 days. Treatment of cutaneous candidal infections should be continued for at least 2 weeks and discontinued only after 2 successive negative tests for Candida. Topical therapy for cutaneous candidiasis using nystatin in combination with triamcinolone acetonide should be discontinued if signs and symptoms persist after 25 days of therapy.

Infections by candida of skin surrounding the fingernails (paronychia) may require months of therapy.

ADVERSE EFFECTS: When the glucosteroid, triamcinolone acetonide is used with nystatin for long-term therapy, corticosteroid-induced hypothalamic-pituitary-adrenal axis may occur with development of Cushing's syndrome; children are more susceptible than adults.

GI symptoms with diarrhea may occur.

OMEPRAZOLE

(Prilosec; formerly Losec)

USES: Uses of **omeprazole** are given in the following Table:

Uses of Omeprazole
Active Duodenal Ulcers
Active Gastric Ulcers
Reflux Esphagitis
Pathologic Hypersecretory Conditions, eg, Zollinger-Ellison Syndrome

Omeprazole is the most effective inhibitor of acid secretion available. Omeprazole is superior to H_2 blockers in the treatment of gastric ulcers (Walan, A. et al., N. Engl. J. Med. 320, 69-75, 1989), duodenal ulcers (Lauritsen, K., et al., N. Engl. J. Med. 312, 958-961, 1985), and reflux esophagitis (Klinkenberg-Knol, E.C., et al., Lancet, 349-351, 1987). Omeprazole is also very effective in Zollinger-Ellison syndrome and is likely to become the drug of choice for this condition (Wolfe, M.M. and Jensen, R.T., N. Engl. J. Med. 317, 1200-1209, 1987).

Mechanism of Action: Omeprazole is an inhibitor of H^+, K^+-ATPase or "proton pump" on the secretory surface of the parietal cell. Acid secretion from the parietal cell is inhibited at the final step.

DOSAGE FORMS: Caps: 20mg. Capsules should not be chewed or crushed since omeprazole is acid labile and granules are enteric coated.

DOSAGE: Omeprazole is administered orally. Dosage is given in the following Table:

Dosage of Omeprazole

Condition	Dosage
Gastric Ulcers, Duodenal Ulcers, Reflux Esophagitis	20-40mg once daily for 4-8 weeks.
Zollinger-Ellison Syndrome	60-360mg daily; Doses greater than 80mg daily should be divided.

No dosage adjustment necessary in renal failure or geriatrics.

PHARMACOKINETICS: Oral Absorption: 70%; Metabolized: Liver; Excretion: Urine; Half-Life: 30-90 minutes; Plasma Protein Binding: 95%; Duration of Effect: Gastric acid secretion is inhibited for 4-5 days after discontinuation of the drug; new enzyme must be synthesized.

ADVERSE EFFECTS: Side effects are infrequent and usually minor. Gastrointestinal (3%): nausea, diarrhea, abdominal pain; CNS: Headache; skin, rash, leukopenia, and elevated transaminases occur rarely. Potential risk of bacterial overgrowth and nosocomial pneumonia. Animal studies have demonstrated an increased rate of gastric carcinoid tumors; no increased incidence of tumors has been shown in humans to date.

DRUG INTERACTIONS: Omeprazole is metabolized in the liver by cytochrome P-450; other drugs with hepatic metabolism (diazepam, warfarin, phenytoin, etc.) may have delayed metabolism.

ONDANSETRON

(Zofran)

USES: **Ondansetron** is the first of a new class of **serotonin ($5\text{-}HT_3$) antagonists;** uses are given in the following Table:

Uses of Ondansetron
Chemotherapy Induced Nausea and Vomiting
Schizophrenia(?)

Ondansetron has been shown to be effective for treatment of cisplatin-induced nausea and vomiting (Cubeddu, L. et al., N. Engl. J. Med. 322, 810-816, 1990).

Mechanism of Action: Ondansetron is a selective $5\text{-}HT_3$ receptor antagonist; it has no effect on dopamine receptors.

DOSAGE FORMS: Injection: 2mg/ml.

DOSAGE: Manufacturer's (Glaxo) suggested dosing regimen is 0.15mg/kg IV 30 min. before chemotherapy with additional doses 4 and 8 hours later. Oral formulation is in Phase III trials.

PHARMACOKINETICS: Onset: Within 30 minutes; Duration: unknown; Metabolism: liver.

ADVERSE EFFECTS: Headache, constipation, transaminase elevation. Experience is limited overall, especially in children.

ORPHAN DRUGS

There are more than 300 experimental drugs that have been designated as orphan drugs (Orphan Drug Act, Jan. 3, 1983), 54 have been approved for marketing as of April 1991. These are drugs that could not otherwise become commercially available because the targetted patient populations are too small for normal commercialization. The marketed drugs are given in the next Table:

Orphan Drugs

Generic (Product)	Use
Alglucerase Inj. (Ceredase) (Genzyme)	Replacement therapy in patients with Gaucher's disease type I (4/5/91).
Alpha-1-Proteinase Inhibitor (Prolastin) (Cutter)	Chronic replacement therapy in individuals who have congenital deficiency of alpha-1-proteinase deficiency (12/23/87).
Altretamine (Hexalen) (US Bioscience)	Treatment of advanced ovarian adenocarcinoma (12/26/90).
Antithrombin III - human (Antithrombin)(Kabi Vitrum Inc.)	Treatment of hereditary antithrombin III deficiency in connection with surgical or obstetric procedures, or when they have thromboemboli (12/13/89).
Benzoate and Phenylacetate (Ucephan)(Kendall McGaw)	Management of hyperammonemia in patients with urea cycle enzymopathies (UCE)(12/23/87).
Botulinum toxin type A (Oculinum)(Oculinum, Inc)	Treatment of blepharospasm or strabismus (12/19/89).
Calcitonin (human)(Ciba-Geigy)	Symptomatic Paget's disease of bone (osteitis deformans) (10/31/86).
Calcium acetate (PhosLo) (Braintree Labs)	Treatment of hyperphosphatemia in end stage renal disease (12/10/90).
Chenodiol (Rowell Laboratories)	Dissolution of radiolucent gallstones in patients who are poor surgical risks (7/28/83).
Citric Acid, Glucono-delta-lactone and mag carbonate (Renacidin Solution) (United-Guardian)	Renal or bladder calculi (apatite or struvite variety)(10/2/90).
Clofazimine (Ciba-Geigy)	Lepromatous leprosy, including Dapsone-resistant lepromatous leprosy and lepromatous complicated by erythema nodosum leprosum (12/15/86).
Coagulation factor IX-human (AlphaNine)(Alpha Therapeutic)	Hemophilia B - replacement therapy for prevention and control of bleeding (12/31/90).
Colfosceril palmitate (Exosurf)(Burroughs Wellcome)	Prevention and treatment of hyaline membrane disease (8/2/90).
Cromolyn Sodium (Gastrocrom) (Fisons)	Mastocytosis (12/22/89).
Cromolyn sodium 4% ophthalmic solution (Fisons)	Vernal keratoconjunctivitis (10/30/84).
Cytomegalovirus Immune Globulin (human)(Mass. Pub. Health Bio. Labs)	Prevention and attenuation of primary CMV disease in immunosuppressed organ transplant patients (4/17/90).
Digoxin-specific antibody fragments (Burroughs Wellcome)	Potentially life-threatening digitalis intoxication (4/21/86).
Eflornithine HCl (Ornidyl)(Merrell Dow)	Treatment of *Trypanosoma brucei gambiense* infection (sleeping sickness) (11/28/90).
Epoetin alfa (Epogen) (Amgen)	Anemia due to end stage renal disease (6/1/89).
Ethanolamine oleate (Ethamolin)(Glaxo)	Bleeding esophageal varices (12/12/88).
Etidronate disodium (Norwich Eaton)	Hypercalcemia of malignancy not responding to dietary modification, oral hydration or both (4/21/87).
Fludarabine phosphate (Fludara)(Triton Bioscience)	Treatment of refractory B-cell chronic lymphocytic leukemia (4/18/91).

ORPHAN DRUGS (Cont.)
Table Continued

Orphan Drugs	
Generic (Product)	Use
Gallium nitrate (Ganite) (Fujisawa)	Treatment of hypercalcemia of malignancy (1/17/91).
Ganciclovir sodium (Cytovene)(Syntex)	CMV retinitis in AIDS patients (6/23/89).
Gonadorelin acetate (Lutrepulse)(R.W. Johnson Research Institute)	Induction of ovulation in women with hypothalamic amenorrhea due to Gn-RH deficiency (10/10/89).
Hemin (Abbott Laboratories)	Hepatic porphyria (7/20/83).
Idarubicin (Idamycin)(Adria)	Acute nonlymphocytic leukemia (9/27/90).
Ifosfamide (Ifex)(Bristol-Myers)	Testicular cancer, bone and soft tissue sarcomas (12/30/88).
Interferon alfa-2a (Roferon-A)(Hoffmann LaRoche)	Treatment of AIDS related Kaposis sarcoma (11/21/88).
Interferon alfa-2b (Intron A)(Schering)	Treatment of AIDS related Kaposis sarcoma (11/21/88).
Interferon gamma-1b (Actimmune)(Genentech)	Treatment of chronic granulomatous disease (12/20/90).
Leucovorin (Lederle)	Rescue therapy following high dose methotrexate for osteosarcoma (8/31/88).
L-carnitine enteral liquid (Kendal McGaw Laboratories)	Primary systemic carnitine deficiency (4/10/86).
L-carnitine tablets (Sigma-Tau, Inc.)	Primary systemic carnitine deficiency (12/27/85).
Mefloquine HCl (Lariam) (Hoffmann LaRoche)	Treatment of plasmodium falciparum and vivax malaria, prophylaxis of resistant plasmodium falciparum malaria (5/2/89).
Mesna (Mesnex)(Degussa Corp; Adria)	Prophylaxis for ifosfamide-induced hemorhagic cystitis or inhibition of urotoxic effects of cyclophosphamide (12/30/88).
Metronidazole (topical) gel (Flagyl)(Searle)	Decubitus ulcers, Grade III and IV, anaerobically infected (11/22/88).
Mitoxantrone (Novantrone) Lederle Larboratories	Initial therapy of acute nonlymphocytic leukemia (ANLL) in adults (12/23/87).
Monooctanoin (Moctanin) (Ethitek Pharmaceuticals)	Dissolution of cholesterol gallstones retained in the biliary tract after cholecystectomy, for use when other means of stone removal are unsuccessful or contraindicated (10/31/85).
Naltrexone (DuPont)	Narcotic addition (11/30/84).
PEG-adenosine deaminase (PEG-ADA)(Adagen)(Enzon)	Enzyme replacement for ADA deficiency in severe combined immunodeficiency (3/21/90).
Pentamidine isethionate (Nebupent)(Fujisawa)	Prevention of Pneumocystis carinii pneumonia in high risk patients (6/15/89).
Pentamidine isethionate (Pentam 300)(Fujisawa)	Treatment of Pneumocystis carinii pneumonia (10/16/84).
Pentastarch (Pentaspan) (DuPont Critical Care)	Adjunct in leukapheresis, to improve harvest and increase yield of leukocytes by centrifugal means (5/19/87).
Potassium citrate (Urocit K) (University of Texas)	Management or renal tubular acidosis with calcium stones, hypocitraturic calcium oxalate nephrolithiasis of any etiology, and uric acid lithiasis with or without calcium stones. (8/30/85).
Rifampin (Rifadin IV) (Merrell Dow)	Antituberculosis treatment when oral therapy is not feasible (5/25/89).
Sargramostim (Leukine) (Immunex Corp)	Treatment of neutropenia following bone marrow transplant following non-Hodgkin's and Hodgkin's lymphoma and acute lymphoblastic leukemia (3/5/91).
Selegiline HCl (Deprenyl) (Somerset)	Adjunct to levodopa/carbidopa in Parkinson's Disease and Parkinsonism (6/5/89).

ORPHAN DRUGS (Cont.)
Table Continued

Orphan Drugs	
Generic (Product)	Use
Somatrem (Protropin) (Genentech, Inc)	Long-term therapy for children with growth failure due to insufficient endogenous growth-hormone secretion (10/17/85).
Somatropin (Humatrope) (Eli Lilly)	Long-term treatment of growth failure in growth hormone deficient children (3/8/87).
Succimer (Chemer) (Johnson and Johnson)	Treatment of lead poisoning in children (1/30/91).
Teriparatide (Parathar) (Rorer Pharmaceuticals)	Distinguish between hypoparathyroidism and pseudohypoparathyroidism (12/23/87).
Tiopronin (Thiola)(Charles Y.C. Pak, MD)	Cystinuria-prevention of cystine nephrolithiasis (8/11/88).
Tranexamic acid (Kabi Vitrum)	Short-term treatment of hemophilia (2-8 days) (12/30/86).
Trientine HCl (Merck Sharp & Dohme)	Wilson's disease in patients intolerant of or inadequately responsive to penicill-amine (11/8/85).
Urofollitropin (Serono laboratories, Inc.)	Induction of ovulation in women with poly-cystic ovarian disease with elevated LH/FSH ratio who have failed to respond to clomiphene citrate (9/18/86).
Zidovudine (Burroughs Wellcome Co.)	Certain cases of AIDS and ARC (3/19/87).

Inquiries can be made to:

National Information Center for Orphan Drugs
and Rare Diseases (NICODARD)
P.O. Box 1133
Washington, DC 20013-1133
(800) 456-3505 or (202) 565-4167

or Office of Orphan Products Development
5600 Fishers Lane
Rockville, MD 20857
(301) 443-4903

OTITIS EXTERNA; PATHOGENS, TREATMENT

Pathogens: The pathogens that cause otitis externa are given in the next Table (Handbook of Antimicrobial Therapy, The Medical Letter, 1990):

Pathogens Causing Otitis Externa
1. Pseudomonas aeruginosa (or other gram-negative bacilli)
2. Staphylococcus aureus
3. Streptococcus pyogenes (Group A)
4. Streptococcus pneumoniae
5. Haemophilus influenzae (in children)
6. Aspergillus and other fungi

Clinical forms of otitis externa are given in the next Table (Pelton, S.I. and Klein, J.O., Infect. Dis. Clin. North Am. 2, 117-129, 1988; Hawke, M. et al., J. Otolaryngol. 13, 289-295, 1984):

Clinical Forms of Otitis Externa

Clinical Form	Pathogens
Acute Otitis Media with Perforation	Streptococcus pneumoniae Haemophilus influenzae Streptococcus pyogenes (Group A) Moraxella (Branhamella) catarrhalis
Otitis Externa (Swimmer's Ear, Diffuse External Otitis)	Pseudomonas aeruginosa Staphylococcus aureus Enterobacter species Escherichia coli Proteus mirabilis Klebsiella species Streptococcus viridans Enterococcus species
Otomycosis	Aspergillus
Necrotizing External Otitis (Malignant Otitis Externa, Invasive Otitis Externa)	Pseudomonas aeruginosa

Treatment: Treatment of the three different clinical forms of otitis externa is given in the next Table (Pelton, S.I. and Klein, J.O., Infect. Dis. Clin. North Am. 2, 117-129, 1988):

Treatment of Otitis Externa

Clinical Form	Treatment
Acute Otitis Media with Perforation	Oral antibiotics are the primary therapy: Amoxicillin; Amoxicillin-clavulanic acid (Augmentin); Erythromycin-sulfamethoxazole; Trimethoprim-sulfamethoxazole; Cefaclor. Ototopical therapy is used when otitis externa is also present. Use is controversial (Bluestone, C.D., Pediatr. Infect. Dis. 4, 507-612, 1985).
Otitis Externa	Suction and irrigation of external canal; irrigate with saline, warm water or acetic acid. Ototopical therapy for 1 week. Packing with antibiotic-steroid medication. Oral antibiotics: Used when cellulitis is present. Amoxicillin; Tetracycline(8 yrs. of age or older); Erythromycin-sulfamethoxazole; Trimethoprim-sulfamethoxazole; amoxicillin-clavulanic acid (Augmentin), Cefaclor. Relief for pain if necessary.
Otomycosis	M-cresyl acetate (25%) or Tolnaftate (Tinactin), 4 drops applied 4 times a day for 3 weeks (Liston, S.L. and Siegel, L.G., Laryngoscope 96, 699, 1986).
Necrotizing External Otitis	Prolonged medical therapy in conjunction with local debridement of granulation tissue and infected cartilage. Antibiotics: Tobramycin plus anti-pseudomonal penicillin, eg, carbenicillin, ticarcillin, mezlocillin, azlocillin, piperacillin.

OTITIS EXTERNA; PATHOGENS, TREATMENT (Cont.)

Ototopical agents which may be appropriate for treatment of otitis externa are given in the following Table (Pelton, S.I. and Klein, J.O., Infect. Dis. Clin. North Am. 2, 117-129, 1988):

Ototopical Agents for Otitis Externa

Product	Generic
Cortisporin Otic Susp Pediotic Susp Lazersporin-C soln	Polymyxin B, Neomycin sulfate, Hydrocortisone
Coly-Mycin S Otic	Colistin sulfate, Neomycin sulfate, Thonzonium bromide, Hydrocortisone
Pyocidin-otic	Polymyxin B, Hydrocortisone

OTITIS MEDIA, PATHOGENS, TREATMENT

Pathogens: The pathogens that cause otitis media are given in the next Table (Giebink, G.S., Pediatr. Infect. Dis. 8, S18-S20, 1989):

Causative Organisms in Otitis Media

Organism	Percent
Acute:	
Streptococcus pneumoniae (pneumococci)	29
Hemophilus influenzae	20
Moraxella (Branhamella) catarrhalis	6
Staphylococcus aureus	2
Streptococcus pyogenes (Group A)	2
Others	6
Mixed	6
No Growth	27
*Chronic:(Bluestone, C.D.,Pediatr. Infect. Dis. J. 7, S137-140, Nov. 1988)	
Pseudomonas aeruginosa	88
Staphlococcus aureus	27
Diphtheroids	24
Staphylococcus epidermidis	11
Streptococcus pneumoniae	11
Haemophilus influenzae	11
Streptococcus pyogenes	6
Proteus mirabilis	5
Candida albicans	5
Escherichia coli	3
Moraxella (Branhamella) catarrhalis	3
"Other"	44

***Note:** Many cases of chronic, suppurative otitis media are mixed infections thus, the percents add up to more than 100%.

Treatment: Efficacy of selected antibiotics for the common pathogens in acute otitis media is given in the next Table (Bluestone, C.D., Pediatr. Infect. Dis. J. 7, No. 11, S129-S136, Nov. 1988):

Efficacy of Selected Antibiotics for Common Pathogens in Acute Otitis Media

Antibiotics	Streptococcus pneumoniae	Haemophilus influenzae	Moraxella catarrhalis	Streptococcus pyogenes	Staphylococcus aureus
Amoxicillin	(+)	(+,-)	(+,-)	(+)	(+,-)
Amoxicillin-clavulanate (Augmentin)	(+)	(+)	(+)	(+)	(+)
Erythromycin and sulfisoxazole(Pediazole)	(+)	(+)	(+)	(+)	(+)
Trimethoprim-sulfamethoxazole	(+)	(+)	(+)	(-)	(+)
Cefaclor (Ceclor)	(+)	(+)	(+,-)	(+)	(+)
Cefuroxime axetil	(+)	(+)	(+)	(+)	(+)

(+), effective; (+,-), effective for strains not producing bata-lactamase; (-), not effective.

OTITIS MEDIA, PATHOGENS, TREATMENT (Cont.)

Oral antibiotic treatment of acute otitis media is given in the next Table:

Antibiotic Treatment of Acute Otitis Media

Antibiotics	Dose
Amoxicillin	20-40mg/kg daily in three divided doses for 10-14 days. Adults: 250-500mg every 8 hours for 10-14 days
Erythromycin Ethylsuccinate (200mg/5ml) and Sulfisoxazole (600mg/5ml)(Pediazole)	50mg/kg daily (as erythro) and 150mg/kg daily (as sulfa) in 4 divided doses for 10-14 days. Adults: Max. dose: 6gm sulfisoxazole daily in 4 divided doses for 10-14 days.
Cefaclor (Ceclor)	40mg/kg daily in 3 divided doses for 10-14 days Adults: 250-500mg every 8 hours for 10-14 days.
Trimethoprim-sulfamethoxazole (Bactrim, Septra)	8-10mg/kg daily (as trimethoprim) in two divided doses for 10-14 days. Adults: 160mg (as trimethoprim) every 12 hours for 10-14 days.
Amoxicillin-Clavulanic acid (Augmentin)	20-40mg/kg daily (as amoxicillin) in three divided doses for 10-14 days. Adults: 250-500mg (as amoxicillin) every eight hours for 10-14 days.
Cefuroxime (Ceftin)	30mg/kg daily in 2 divided doses for 10-14 days Adults: 250mg every 12 hours for 10-14 days.
Cefixime (Suprax)	8mg/kg daily as a single dose or in 2 divided doses for 10-14 days. Adults: 400mg daily in 1-2 doses for 10-14 days

OXACILLIN

(Bactocill, Prostaphlin)

USES: Oxacillin is a **penicillinase-resistant penicillin** (cloxacillin, dicloxacillin, methicillin, nafcillin and oxacillin) which is generally limited to the treatment of infections caused by susceptible **penicillinase-producing staphylococci**. Some strains of staphylococcus aureus and many strains of staphylococcus epidermidis are resistant (Parry, M.S., Med. Clin. No. Am. 71, 1093-1112, November, 1987).

Oxacillin (or nafcillin) usually is preferred to methicillin in adults and older children because of the association of interstitial nephritis with methicillin.

DOSAGE FORMS: Oral; Caps: 250, 500mg; Sol'n: 250mg/5ml; Parenteral; Injection: 250, 500mg, 1, 2, 4g; For Injection, for IV Infusion: 1, 2, 4g.

DOSAGE: Oxacillin sodium is administered orally, by slow IV injection or infusion or by deep IM injection. Orally administered oxacillin should not be used for the initial treatment of severe, life-threatening infections. Children weighing 40kg or more may receive the usual adult dosage of oxacillin. Dosage is given in the next Table:

Dosage of Oxacillin

Condition	Age	Route	Dosage
Mild to Moderate Infections of Upper Resp. Tract or Skin or Skin Structures	Adults	Oral	500mg every 4-6 h.
Follow-Up to Parenteral Penicillinase-Resistant Penicillin Therapy	Adults	Oral	1g every 4-6 h.
Mild to Moderate Infections of Upper Resp. Tract or Skin or Skin Structures	Adults	IM or IV	250-500mg every 4-6h.
Severe Infections	Adults	IM or IV	1-1.5g every 4-6 h.
Endocarditis or Acute and Chronic Osteomyelitis	Adults	IV	1.5-2g every 4 h. Max: 12g daily.
Usual	Child.	Oral	50-100mg/kg daily div. every 6 h.
		IM or IV	100-200mg/kg daily div. every 6 h.
	Newborn < 2 kg < 1 wk	IM or IV	50mg/kg daily div. every 12 h.
	Newborn > 2 kg < 1 wk	IM or IV	75mg/kg daily div. every 8 h.
	Newborn < 2 kg > 1 wk	IM or IV	100mg/kg daily div. every 8 h.
	Newborn > 2 kg > 1 wk	IM or IV	150mg/kg daily div. every 6 h.

Duration of Therapy: In serious infections, therapy should be continued for 1-2 weeks; for endocarditis or acute and chronic osteomyelitis, therapy is generally continued for 4-8 weeks.

ADVERSE EFFECTS: Adverse reactions are usually mild and most commonly consist of allergic reactions that are typical of penicillins. Abnormal liver function tests occur more frequently than with other antistaphylococcal penicillins; abnormal test results are reversible when the drug is discontinued.

PHARMACOKINETICS: Absorption: 33% (oral); Protein-Binding: 90%; Half-Life: 0.3-0.8 hour.; 0.5-1 hour (anuric); Percent Unchanged in Urine: 55%.

MONITOR: Liver function tests, renal function tests, complete blood count. See NAFCILLIN.

OXAZEPAM
(Serax)
USES: **Oxazepam** is a **benzodiazepine;** uses are given in the next Table:

Uses of Oxazepam
Situational Anxiety and Generalized Anxiety Disorder
Management of Agitation associated with Acute Alcohol Withdrawal
Insomnia

DOSAGE FORMS: Caps: 10, 15 and 30mg; Tabs: 15mg
DOSAGE: Serax is not recommended for children. Dosage of oxazepam is given in the next Table:

Condition	Dosage
Anxiety	30 to 60mg daily divided into three or four doses. Elderly Patients: Initially, 30mg daily divided into three doses; if necessary, the dose may be increased cautiously to 45 to 60 mg daily divided into three or four doses.

PHARMACOKINETICS: Half-Life: 5 to 15 hours; short half-life because it is metabolized to inactive glucuronide metabolites which are excreted by the kidney. Liver disease does not alter the pharmacokinetics.
ADVERSE EFFECTS: The incidence of adverse effects is low. The most common is drowsiness. Other adverse effects that occur occasionally include rash, nausea, dizziness, syncope, hypotension, tachycardia, edema, nightmares, lethargy, slurred speech, excitement, confusion and ataxia. Other adverse effects that occur rarely include leukopenia, eosinophilia, and hepatic dysfunction. The long-term use of larger than usual doses may result in psychological and physical dependence. Abrupt discontinuation may precipitate withdrawal.

OXYTOCIN
(Pitocin, Syntocinon)
USES: Oxytocin is a peptide hormone primarily used to stimulate uterine contraction. The uses of oxytocin are given in the following Table:

Uses of Oxytocin
Induction of Labor when continuation of pregnancy is a greater risk to mother or fetus than risk of oxytocin therapy
Augmentation of Labor during first and second stages in dysfunctional labor
Control Uterine Bleeding during the third stage of labor
Oxytocin Challenge Test in high-risk pregnancies tests for uteroplacental insufficiency

Oxytocin therapy carries inherent risks to both mother and fetus. In all cases in which oxytocin is considered, benefits must outweigh the risks.

Oxytocin is the drug of choice for induction of labor. Termination of pregnancy may be desirable in certain circumstances, including hypertension (preeclampsia or eclampsia), diabetes mellitus, erythroblastosis fetalis, bleeding, or prolonged pregnancy with placental insufficiency. Fetal lung maturity and fetopelvic disproportion should be considered prior to induction. Other contraindications include unfavorable fetal position, fetal distress, placental abnormalities (eg, placenta previa), previous major uterine surgery, prolapsed cord, and active genital herpes.

Oxytocin is used for augmentation of labor during the first and second stages when labor is dysfunctional. Use of oxytocin when labor is progressing slowly is controversial; potential hazards of oxytocin include uterine rupture, cervical or soft tissue laceration, trauma to the infant, or impaired placental blood flow with compromised fetal oxygenation.

Oxytocin has been used during the third stage of labor and puerperium to control uterine bleeding. Routine use of oxytocin following normal vaginal deliveries is not usually necessary.

Oxytocin challenge test is used to test for uteroplacental insufficiency in high risk pregnancies. This test involves infusion of oxytocin with concurrent monitoring of fetal heart rate. Oxytocin produces uterine contraction with transient reduction in uteroplacental blood flow and fetal oxygenation. A positive (abnormal) test is the occurence of late deceleration of the fetal heart rate with uterine contraction.

Oxytocin has been used as an adjunct therapy in incomplete spontaneous or therapeutic abortion. Oxytocin has also been used intranasally to promote breast milk ejection.

OXYTOCIN (Cont.)

Mechanism of Action: Oxytocin is a nine amino acid hormone produced in the supraoptic and paraventricular nuclei of the hypothalamus and stored in the posterior pituitary. Commercially available preparations are synthetic. Oxytocin stimulates the frequency and force of contraction of the uterus; high estrogen concentrations during the third trimester of pregnancy markedly increases the uterine responsiveness to oxytocin. Oxytocin promotes milk ejection in the mammary glands. Large doses of oxytocin produces a transient relaxation of vascular smooth muscle with transient hypotension.

DOSAGE FORMS: Injection: 10 units/ml; Intranasal: 40 units/ml.

DOSAGE: Oxytocin is given by IV infusion; intranasal administration is used to promote milk ejection. Dosage of oxytocin is given in the following Table:

Dosage of Oxytocin

Condition	Route	Dosage
Induction of Labor	IV	1 milliunit/minute; increase by 1 milliunit/min every 15 minutes (usual maximum: 9-10 milliunits/min).
Augmentation of Labor	IV	2 milliunits/minute; increase slowly to a maximum of 20 milliunits/min. Decrease dosage when labor is established.
Postpartum Bleeding	IV	20-40 milliunits/min to a total of 10 units.
Oxytocin Challenge Test	IV	0.5 milliunits/min; increase rate slowly until contractions occur every 3-4 minutes. Usual maximum: 20 milliunits/min.
Breast Milk Ejection	Intra-nasal	1 spray into one or both nostrils immediately prior to nursing.

PHARMACOKINETICS: Onset: almost immediate; Half-Life: 3-5 minutes; Elimination: Liver, kidney metabolism.

ADVERSE EFFECTS: Hyperstimulation of the uterus with hypertonic and/or tetanic contractions, uterine rupture, cervical or vaginal lacerations, placental abruption, impaired uterine blood flow with fetal hypoxia, fetal trauma. Potential benefits to the fetus and mother must outweight the risks.

CONTRAINDICATIONS: Oxytocin is contraindicated in any condition in which vaginal delivery is contraindicated (eg, placenta previa, vasa previa, prolapsed cord, active genital herpes). Other contraindications include cephalopelvic disproportion, unfavorable fetal position, fetal distress, and previous major cervical or uterine surgery.

PAIN, TREATMENT

Drugs used for the treatment of pain are given in the next Table:

Drugs Used for the Treatment of Pain

Non-Narcotic Analgesics
- Acetaminophen
- Nonsteroidal Anti-Inflammatory Drugs (NSAIDs)
- Combinations of Two or More Analgesics, eg, Aspirin, Acetaminophen and Caffeine

Narcotic-Type Analgesics (Opioids)

Combinations: Non-Narcotic Analgesics plus Narcotic-Type Analgesics

Acetaminophen or codeine may be adequate for mild pain but morphine is needed for more severe pain.

NON-NARCOTIC ANALGESICS:

Acetaminophen: Acetaminophen is an effective analgesic; it is not associated with the numerous side effects of aspirin, and the other non-steroidal anti-inflammatory drugs(NSAIDs). If a rare sensitivity reaction occurs, the patient should stop the drug.

Nonsteroidal Anti-Inflammatory Drugs (NSAIDs): NSAIDs are all effective analgesics; they are useful for the treatment of pain associated with inflammation. Select NSAIDs that are used for analgesia are given in the next Table (Amadio, P., Am.J. Med. 77(3A), 17-26, 1984):

Nonsteroidal Anti-Inflammatory Drugs for Analgesia

Class and Generic Name	Trade Name
Salicylates	
Acetylsalicylic acid	Aspirin
Diflunisal	Dolobid
Fenamates	
Mefenamic acid	Ponstel
Propionic acid	
Fenoprofen	Nalfon
Ibuprofen	Motrin
Naproxen	Naprosyn
Naproxen sodium	Anaprox

Combination of Two or More Analgesics: Formerly, the combination of aspirin, phenacetin and caffeine (APC) was the most popular analgesic combination. However, concern about the safety of long-term, high-dose consumption of phenacetin-containing analgesics has led to the removal of phenacetin from these preparations or its replacement with acetaminophen. Aspirin and acetaminophen in combinations offers no advantage in inducing analgesia instead of one of these drugs alone. (Beaver, W.T., Am.J. Med. 77(3A), 38-53, 1984). Caffeine enhances the analgesic effect of antipyretic-analgesics (Laska, E.M. et al., JAMA 251, 1711-1718, 1984; Beaver, W.T., JAMA 251, 1732-1733, 1984).

PAIN, TREATMENT (Cont.)

NARCOTIC-TYPE ANALGESICS: The narcotic-type analgesics used for pain are given in the next Table (Inturrisi, C.E., Am. J. Med. 77(3A), 27-37, 1984; Fernandez, F., AIDS Medical Report 1, 25-31, Nov. 1988):

Narcotic Type Analgesics Commonly Used for Pain

Name (Oral Efficacy)	Route (Duration, hrs)	Comments	Precautions
Hydromorphone* (Dilaudid) (Very Good)	Oral, IM (4-5)	Very potent; like heroin	Impaired ventilation, bronchial asthma, incr. intracranial pres., liver failure
Methadone* (Dolophine) (Good)	Oral, IM (3-20)	Good oral potency, long plasma half-life	Like morphine, may accumulate with repetitive dosing causing excessive sedation.
Levorphanol* (Good)	Oral, IM (4-6)	Like methadone	Like hydromorphone.
Morphine* (Fair-Good)	Oral, IM (4-6)	Standard of comparison for narcotic type analgesics	Same
Heroin*	Oral, IM	Biotransformed to morphine; not legally available in U.S.	Same
Oxymorphone*	IM	Like morphine	Same
Oxycodone* (Fair-Good)	Oral (3-4)	Available in combination with acetaminophen (Percocet) or aspirin (Percodan)	Same
Codeine* (Fair)	Oral, IM (4-6)	"Weak" morphine; often used in combination with non-narcotic analgesics; biotransformed, in part to morphine	Impaired ventilation, bronchial asthma, increased intracranial pressure.
Propoxyphene* (Darvon) Propoxyphene Napsylate (Fair)	Like codeine	"Weak" narcotic; often used in combination with non-narcotic analgesics; long half-life.	Biotransformed to potentially toxic metabolite (norpropoxyphene); accumulates with repetitive dosing; overdose complicated by convulsions.
Meperidine* (Demerol) (Poor)	Oral, IM (4-5)	Biotransformed to normeperidine, a toxic metabolite.	Normeperidine accumulates with repetitive dosing causing CNS excitation; not for patients with impaired renal function or receiving monoamine oxidase inhibitor
Mixed agonist-antagonist			
Pentazocine** (Talwin) (Poor-Fair)	Oral IM (2-3)	Less abuse liability than morphine; in combination with non-narcotics; in combination with naloxone to discourage parenteral abuse.	May cause psychotomimetic effects; may precipitate withdrawal in narcotic-dependent patients; not used in patients with myocardial infarction.
Nalbuphine**	IM	Like pentazocine but not scheduled.	Incidence of psychotomimetic effects lower than with pentazocine.
Butorphanol**	IM	Like nalbuphine.	Like pentazocine.
Partial agonist			
Buprenorphine***	IM Sublingual	Less abuse liability than morphine; does not produce psychotomimetic effects; not yet available in U.S.	May precipitate withdrawal in narcotic-dependent patients.

*Morphine-like agonists; **Mixed agonist-antagonist; ***Partial agonist

PAIN, TREATMENT (Cont.)
Morphine-Like Agonists: The morphine-like agonists are all morphine surrogates that qualitatively mimic the pharmacologic profile of morphine, that is, both desirable and adverse effects.
Mixed Agonist-Antagonists: The mixed agonist-antagonists produce analgesia and other narcotic effects characteristic of morphine but do not have the capacity to produce the degree of respiratory depression as does morphine.
Partial Agonists: The partial agonist has less abuse liability as compared to the morphine-like drugs.
COMBINATIONS: NON-NARCOTIC ANALGESICS PLUS NARCOTIC-TYPE ANALGESICS:
Aspirin and acetaminophen are the mainstays of oral analgesic combinations. There is evidence that combining an optimal dose of acetaminophen or aspirin with an oral opioid such as codeine, propoxyphene, oxycodone or hydrocodone produces an additive analgesic effect greater than that obtained by doubling the dose of either constituent administered alone.
Representative combinations of antipyretic-analgesic with narcotics or narcotic antagonist analgesics are given in the next Table (Beaver, W.T., Am. J. Med. 77(3A), 38-53, 1984):

Representative Combinations of Antipyretic-Analgesic Agents with Narcotics or Narcotic Antagonist Analgesics

Codeine Combinations:		
Tylenol with Codeine	Empirin with Codeine	Codalan
Acetaminophen, 300mg plus codeine phosphate, either No. 1, 7.5 mg No. 2, 15 mg No. 3, 30 mg No. 4, 60 mg	Aspirin, 325mg plus codeine phosphate, either No. 2, 15 mg No. 3, 30 mg No. 4, 60 mg	Acetaminophen 500mg and caffeine 30mg plus codeine phosphate, either No. 1, 8 mg No. 2, 15 mg No. 3, 30 mg
Propoxyphene Combinations:		
Darvocet-N 50(or Darvocet-N 100) Propoxyphene napsylate, 50mg(or 100mg) Acetaminophen, 325mg(or 650mg)		
Darvon Compound(or Darvon Compound-65) Propoxyphene hydrochloride,32mg(or 65mg) Aspirin, 389mg Caffeine, 32.4mg		
Oxycodone Combinations:		
Percodan(or Percodan-Demi)	Percocet	Tylox
Oxycodone hydrochloride, 4.5mg (or 2.25mg) Oxycodone terephthalate, 0.38mg (or 0.19mg) Aspirin, 325mg	Oxycodone hydrochloride, 5mg Acetaminophen, 325mg	Oxycodone hydrochloride, 5mg Acetaminophen, 500mg
Hydrocodone Combinations:	**Pentazocine Combinations:**	
Vicodin, Others	Talwin Compound	Talacen
Hydrocodone bitartrate, 5mg Acetaminophen, 500mg	Pentazocine (as the hydrochloride), 12.5mg Aspirin, 325mg	Pentazocine (as the hydrochloride), 25mg Acetaminophen, 650mg

PANCREATIN
(Creon)
USES: **Pancreatin** is used as **replacement therapy** in the symptomatic treatment of malabsorption syndrome caused by **pancreatic insufficiency**; the causes of pancreatic insuffiency are given in the next Table:

Causes of Pancreatic Insufficiency
Cystic Fibrosis
Chronic Pancreatitis
Pancreatectomy
Cancer of the Pancreas

Pancreatin contains enzymes, principally amylase, lipase, and protease.
DOSAGE FORMS: Tabs and Enteric-Coated Tabs. Pancreatin preparations are given in the next Table:

Pancreatin Preparations

	USP Units		
Source	Lipase	Amylase	Protease
Creon, Reid-Rowell	8,000	30,000	13,000
Pancreatin 5x Tabs, Vitaline	12,000	60,000	60,000
Pancreatin 8x Tabs, Vitaline	22,500	180,000	180,000

DOSAGE: The usual initial dosage of pancreatin is 8,000-24,000 USP units of lipase activity before or with each meal or snack; occasionally up to 36,000 USP units of lipase activity may be required with meals.

As an alternative, the total daily dose may also be given in divided doses at 1-to 2-hour intervals throughout the day.
ADVERSE EFFECTS: Diarrhea, hyperuricemia; retention in the mouth before swallowing may cause irritation of the mucosa with irritation. Hypersensitivity reactions have been reported.

PANCRELIPASE
(Cotazyme, Entolase, Ilozyme, Pancrease, Viokase, Zymase)
USES: See Pancreatin.
DOSAGE FORMS: Delayed release preparations are used to minimize inactivation by gastric juices. Pancrelipase preparations are given in the next Table:

Pancreatic Preparations

	USP Units		
Source	Lipase	Amylase	Protease
Capsules:			
Cotazyme, Organon	8,000	30,000	30,000
Capsules, Delayed Release:			
Pancrease, MT4, McNeil	4,000	12,000	12,000
Pancrease, Enteric-Coated, McNeil	4,000	20,000	25,000
Cotazyme-S, Enteric-Coated, Organon	5,000	20,000	20,000
Entolase-HP, Robins	8,000	40,000	50,000
Pancrease MT10, McNeil	10,000	30,000	30,000
Zymase, Organon	12,000	24,000	24,000
Pancrease MT16, McNeil	16,000	48,000	48,000
Powder:			
Viokase, Robins	16,800	70,000	70,000
Tablets:			
Viokase, Robins	8,000	30,000	30,000
Ilozyme, Adria	11,000	30,000	30,000

DOSAGE: The usual initial dosage of pancrelipase is 4,000-33,000 USPunits of lipase activity (1-3 capsules or tablets) before or with each meal or snack. For the treatment of severe deficiency, the dose may be increased to 88,000 USP units of lipase activity with each meal or the dosing interval may be increased to hourly if necessary and if nausea, cramping, and/or diarrhea do not occur. Titrate to eliminate diarrhea and minimize steatorrhea. Approximately 8000 USP units of lipase activity is required for each 17g of dietary fat.
ADVERSE EFFECTS: Nausea, cramping, and/or diarrhea with excessive dosage; extremely high doses of enzymes have been associated with hyperuricemia.

PANCURONIUM BROMIDE
(Pavulon)

USES: **Pancuronium** bromide is a competitive, nondepolarizing neuromuscular blocking agent used mainly to produce **skeletal muscle relaxation** in conditions listed in the next Table:

Uses of Pancuronium Bromide as Skeletal Muscle Relaxant
During **Surgery** after **General Anesthesia** has been Induced
Increase Pulmonary Compliance during Assisted or **Controlled Respiration**
Faciliate Mechanical Respiration in Patients with **Status Asthmaticus**
Facilitate **Endotracheal Intubation**

DOSAGE FORMS: Injection: 1mg/ml, 2mg/ml

DOSAGE: Pancuronium bromide is given IV; dosages are given in the next Table:

Dosages of Pancuronium Bromide

Patient	Dosage
Neonate (up to 1 month)	Initial Dose: 0.02mg/kg/dose Maintenance: 0.03-0.09mg/kg/dose every 30 min. to 4 hours, as needed
1 Month to Adult Adjunct to General Anesthesia Skeletal Muscle Relaxation Endotracheal Intubation	Initial: 0.04-0.1mg/kg/dose Maintenance: 0.01-0.1mg/kg/dose, every 30-60 minutes.
Defasciculating dose during Intubation	0.005-0.01mg/kg/dose

ADVERSE EFFECTS: Respiratory paralysis may occur; thus, be prepared to intubate within minutes of induction. Tachycardia occurs frequently. Use with caution in patients with renal, hepatic, pulmonary impairment, respiratory depression and in geriatric or debilitated patients. Reduce dosage in patients receiving magnesium sulfate since magnesium salts enhance neuromuscular blockade. Effects are reversed by neostigmine (with atropine or glycopyrrolate).

PANIC DISORDER, TREATMENT

Anxiety can occur in the form of spontaneous panic attacks; these are characterized by sudden, inexplicable feelings of **terror** or **impending doom**, accompanied by prominent autonomic symptoms. Drugs used to treat panic disorder are given in the next Table (Katon, W. et al., Patient Care, pgs. 148-173, March 30, 1988):

Drug Treatment of Panic Disorder
Tricyclic Antidepressants:
Imipramine HCl (Janimine, Tofranil)
Desipramine HCl (Norpramin, Pertofrane)
Amitriptyline HCl (Amitril, Elavil, Endep, etc.)
Benzodiazepines:
Alprazolam (Xanax)
Clonazepam (Klonopin)
Monoamine Oxidase (MAO) Inhibitors

Tricyclic Antidepressants: A protocol for initiating imipramine HCl or desipramine therapy for panic disorder is given in the next Table (Katon, W. et al., Patient Care, pgs. 148-173, March 30, 1988):

Imipramine or Desipramine Therapy for Panic Disorder

	Number of 25mg Tablets			
Day	Breakfast	Lunch	Dinner	Bedtime
1-3	0	0	0	1
4-7	1	0	0	1
8-12	1	0	0	2
13-19	1	0	1	2
20-26	1	1	1	2
27-33	2	1	1	2
34-40	2	1	2	2
41-47	2	2	2	2

If side effects are tolerable, the dosage is increased by one tablet every three days to a maximum of 150-300mg daily. Suppression of panic attacks usually requires a minimum dose of 150mg daily.

Amitriptyline HCl may be used if panic episodes disturb the patient's sleep.

Clinical benefit may be obtained after 2-6 weeks of tricyclic antidepressant therapy.

If a patient fails to respond to dosages of 150 to 200mg/day of imipramine, obtain a blood level 9-12 hours after the last dose. A blood level of less than 150ng/ml is an indication to continue increasing the dosage until a blood level of 150-200ng/ml is obtained.

PANIC DISORDER, TREATMENT (Cont.)
Benzodiazepines: The benzodiazepine, **alprazolam,** may be advisable for a patient with severe, incapacitating panic anxiety who requires rapid relief of symptoms, that is, hours instead of weeks. A protocol for use of alprazolam (Xanax) for panic disorders is given in the next Table (Katon, W. et al., Patient Care, pgs. 148-173, March 30, 1988):

Alprazolam Therapy for Panic Disorder

	Mg Alprazolam		
Day	Breakfast	Lunch	Dinner
1-2	0.5	0.5	0.5
3-4	1.0	0.5	0.5
5-6	1.0	0.5	1.0
7-8	1.0	1.0	1.0
9-10	1.5	1.0	1.0
11-12	1.5	1.0	1.5
13-14	1.5	1.5	1.5
15-16	2.0	1.5	1.5
17-18	2.0	1.5	2.0
19-20	2.0	2.0	2.0

The dosage of alprazolam is increased by 0.5mg every two days to a maximum of 6mg daily.
Monoamine Oxidase (MAO) Inhibitors: MAO inhibitors provide excellent control of panic anxiety. However, MAO inhibitors have potential for serious side effects; furthermore, there are restrictions for the intake of certain foods and medications. Therefore, use of MAO inhibitors is reserved for those patients in whom benzodiazepines and tricyclics are ineffective.

PARALDEHYDE
USES: Uses of paraldehyde are given in the next Table:

Uses of Paraldehyde
Sedative, Hypnotic
Management of Seizures due to Tetanus
Treatment of Status Epilepticus
Alcohol Withdrawal Syndromes
Basal Anesthetic in Children

DOSAGE FORMS: Oral or Rectal: 1gm/ml.
DOSAGE: Paraldehyde may be administered orally or rectally. Do not administer subcutaneously because of tissue irritation. IV preparation was used in the past, but paraldehyde is no longer available in parenteral form. Rectal doses similar to oral doses may be given; the drug should be dissolved in 200ml of 0.9% sodium chloride or at least 2 volumes of olive or cottonseed to prevent rectal irritation. Avoid plastic equipment since paraldehyde reacts with plastic; use glass or rubber.

The dosage of paraldehyde in different conditions is given in the next Table:

Dosage of Paraldehyde

Condition	Dosage
Hypnotic	Adults: 10-30ml orally Children: 0.30ml/kg orally
Sedative	Adult: 5-10ml orally Children: 0.15ml/kg (150mg/kg) orally
Management of Seizures due to Tetanus	Adult: Up to 12ml (diluted 1:10) via gastric tube every 4 hours as needed.
Seizures due to Poisons	Adult: 5-15ml via gastric tube or rectally
Status Epilepticus	Adult: 5-15ml via gastric tube or rectally Children: 0.3ml (300mg)/kg/dose, max 5ml/dose
Alcohol Withdrawal Syndromes	Adults; Orally: 5-10ml orally every 4-6 hours for the first 24 hours, then every 6 hours on the following days with a maximum dose of 60ml orally on the first day and 40ml orally on following days.
Basal Anesthetic for Children	Children: 0.5ml/kg rectally with a maximum dose of 30ml as a 10% solution in 0.9% sodium chloride.

ADVERSE EFFECTS: The most frequent adverse effects are gastric irritation and erythematous rash. Contraindicated in hepatic or pulmonary disease; overdose may cause cardiorespiratory depression. **Do not use discolored solution.**

PAREGORIC

(Camphorated opium Tincture)

USES: Paregoric contains morphine; its uses are given in the next Table:

Uses of Paregoric
Diarrhea
Withdrawal Symptoms in Neonates Born to Women Addicted Opiates

Paregoric, because of its morphine content, increases smooth muscle tone of the GI tract, inhibits GI motility and delays the passage of intestinal contents. Paregoric should not be used in patients with diarrhea caused by poisoning until the toxic material is eliminated from the GI tract.

Paregoric preparations are often used in combination with kaolin and pectin or bismuth salts which have adsorbent and protective properties.

Although paregoric has been used to treat severe withdrawal symptoms in neonates born to women addicted to opiates, some clinicians recommend diluted opium tincture since paregoric contains camphor and benzoic acid which may cause adverse effects.

DOSAGE FORMS: (Camphorated opium Tincture) Tincture: 2mg of morphine/5ml; Contents: 2mg of morphine (0.4mg morphine/ml), 0.02ml of anise oil, 20mg of benzoic acid, 20mg of camphor, 0.2ml of glycerin, and diluted with alcohol to make 5ml

DOSAGE: The usual dosages of paregoric are given in the next Table:

Dosage of Paregoric

Patient	Dosage
Treatment of Diarrhea	Adult: 5-10ml, 1-4 times daily Children: 0.25-0.5ml/kg, 1-4 times daily
Withdrawal Symptoms in Neonates Born to Women Addicted to Opiates	Neonates: 0.2-0.3ml every 3 hours; dosage increased 0.05ml every 3 hours until symptoms are controlled; it is rarely necessary to exceed 0.7ml. Max. dose: 2ml/kg/day or 0.7ml/kg/dose. After withdrawal symptoms have been stabilized for 3-5 days, dosage should be decreased gradually (eg, 10% every 2-3 days) over a 2- to 4-week period.

Note: Opium Tincture contains 25 times more morphine than paregoric.

ADVERSE EFFECTS: Same side effects as morphine; nausea and other GI disturbances. Use with caution in patients with asthma or hepatic disease. Acute Toxicity: Depression of the CNS; reversed by opiate antagonist, naloxone hydrochloride.

PARKINSONISM, TREATMENT

Parkinsonism is a disorder of the **extrapyramidal system** located in the basal ganglia, caudate nucleus, putamen, globus pallidus, characterized by degeneration and loss of the pigment cells of the substantia nigra, with resultant **deficiency** of the neurotransmitter, **dopamine** in the nigrostriatial pathway. **Dopamine** is believed to act principally as an **inhibitory neurotransmitter**; acetycholine is an excitatory neurotransmitter (Review: Agid, Y., Lancet 337, 1321-1324, 1991).

The classic features of the disease are resting tremor, lead-pipe rigidity, bradykinesia, loss of normal postural reflexes and impaired gait.

The neural pathway and drugs used in treatment are given in the next Figure:

Neural Pathway and Drugs Used in Treatment of Parkinsonism

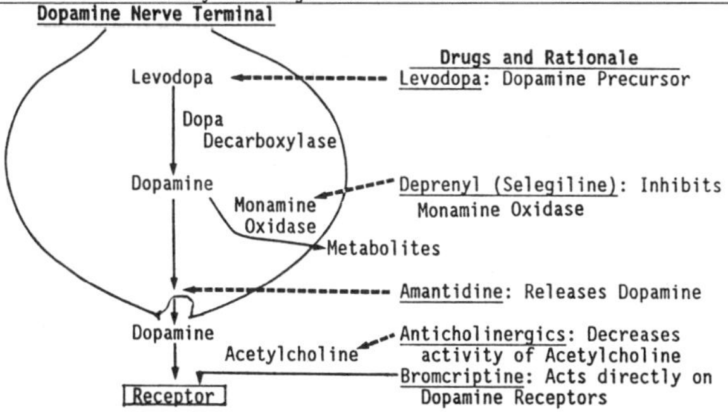

The choice of drug is related to the severity of the disease and is given in the next Table:

Choice of Drug in Treatment of Parkinson's Disease

Stage	Comment
Early Stages Selegiline (Deprenyl)	Selegiline may block the production of toxic metabolites by inhibiting monoamine oxidase. Selegiline slows disease progression in the first few years (The Parkinson Study Group, N. Engl. J. Med. 321, 1364-1371, 1989). Dosage: 10mg daily.
Anticholinergic Drugs	In Parkinson's disease, the decreased activity of dopamine in the caudate nucleus makes the excitatory effects of acetylcholine more prominent. Anticholinergic drugs may be useful early in the disease. These drugs can decrease tremor, rigidity, and akinesia and may have an additive therapeutic effect at any stage of the disease when taken concurrently with levodopa or bromocriptine
Amantadine (Symmetrel)	Amantadine may increase release of dopamine in the brain. Dosage: 100mg, twice daily. When amantadine and anticholinergics are used together, their adverse effects on mental function may be additive.
Fully Developed Disease **Levodopa and Carbidopa** (Sinemet) **Levodopa** (Dopar, Larodopa)	Sinemet (levodopa and carbidopa) is the most effective drug for the treatment of Parkinsonism. Carbidopa, a peripheral decarboxylase inhibitor, prevents peripheral decarboxylation of levodopa. Preparations of Sinemet are as follows: 10mg carbidopa, 100mg levodopa; 25mg carbidopa, 100mg levodopa; 25mg carbidopa, 250mg levodopa. The usual daily dosage range is 300 to 1250mg levodopa; relatively complete inhibition of peripheral decarboxylase requires at least 75 mg daily of carbidopa. Amantadine, bromocriptine and/ or anticholinergics may be given concurrently.

PARKINSONISM, TREATMENT (Cont.)

Stage	Comment
Late Stages of Parkinson's Disease **Levodopa** (Dopar, Larodopa) **Levodopa and Carbidopa** (Sinemet)	Levodopa may lose its effectiveness with time. More frequent administration of levodopa may be helpful.
Bromocriptine (Parlodel)	The best results with bromcriptine are obtained when bromocriptine and levodopa are given concurrently.
Amantadine (Symmetrel)	see above

PEMOLINE

(Cylert)

USES: Pemoline is a **stimulant** that is used to treat **attention deficit disorders.**

Attention Deficit Disorder: Pemoline is used in the treatment of attention deficit disorder with hyperactivity (hyperkinetic syndrome of childhood, minimal brain dysfunction) in carefully selected children older than 6 years of age.

Pemoline is a CNS and respiratory stimulant; neither the mechanism nor site of action are known. It may be that the CNS stimulatory action of pemoline may be mediated by brain dopamine. Functionally, pemoline is similar to amphetamines and to methylphenidate (Ritalin).

DOSAGE FORMS: Tabs: 18.75, 37.5, 75mg; Tabs, Chewable: 37.5mg

DOSAGE: Pemoline is given orally. Give drug in the morning to provide maximal effects during waking hours and to avoid insomnia. Dosages are given in the next Table:

Dosage of Pemoline

Patient	Dosage
6 Years of Age and Older	37.5mg daily; may be increased by 18.75mg at weekly intervals until desired clinical response is achieved. Usual effective dosage, 56.25-75mg daily. Dosage in children should not exceed 150mg daily. Beneficial results may not be evident for 3-4 weeks.
Dosage by Weight	Maintenance: 0.5-3mg/kg daily; Max. dose: 150mg/day

In children who have responded to pemoline, the drug should be discontinued periodically to assess the patient's condition. Improvement may be maintained temporarily or permanently after the drug is discontinued. The drug can usually be discontinued when the child reaches adolescence.

ADVERSE EFFECTS: Most frequently, adverse effects are dose related and include insomnia and anorexia. Adverse effects: GI: anorexia; Nervous System: insomnia, usually transient and repsonds to reduction in dosage; Hepatic: elevated liver enzymes, usually after several months of therapy; hepatitis may occur. May cause choreoathetosis. Decreases seizure threshold.

PENICILLAMINE

(Cuprimine, Depen)

USES: The uses of penicillamine are given in the next Table:

Uses of Penicillamine

Condition	Mechanism
Wilson's Disease	Chelates copper
Lead Poisoning	Chelates lead
Arsenic Poisoning	Chelates arsenic
Cystinuria	Combines chemically with cystine to form soluble complex, penicillamine-cysteine disulfide; penicillamine reduces the concentration of cystine in urine to less than that believed to be critical for the formation of cystine stones; existing stones may be dissolved.
Rheumatoid Arthritis	Penicillamine may inhibit the collagen formation. Penicillamine decreases immunoglobulin M rheumatoid factor levels; in-vitro, penicillamine depolymerizes rheumatoid factor.

Mechanism of Action: Penicillamine is a **chelating agent.** It is a degradation product of all penicillins but has no antibiotic activity. Penicillamine chelates **copper**, **lead**, **mercury** and **other heavy metals.**

PENICILLAMINE (Cont.)
DOSAGE FORMS: Caps: 125, 250mg; Tabs: 250mg
DOSAGE: The dosage of penicillamine is given in the next Table:

Dosage of Penicillamine

Condition	Dosage
Wilson's Disease	Adults and Older Children: 250mg, 4 times daily preferably 30-60 minutes before meals and at least 2 hours after the evening meal. Infants <6 months: 250mg/dose once daily. Children <12 years: 250mg/dose 2-3 times daily. or Children: 20mg/kg daily in 1-4 divided doses. After dosage has been established, 24-hour urinary copper analyses should be performed at 3-month intervals and adjusted accordingly; the patient will probably be in negative copper balance if the 24-hour urinary copper excretion is 0.5-1mg. Usual max. dosage: 2g/day. Pyridoxine 25mg daily should be administered to minimize toxicity of penicillamine.
Lead Poisoning	CaEDTA and BAL (Dimercaprol) are the mainstays of therapy for lead poisoning, and must be given parenterally. Penicillamine has been given orally as follow-up therapy in moderate to severe cases. Adults: 0.5-1.5g daily in 2-4 divided doses. Children: 25-40mg/kg daily in 2-4 divided doses or 500-750mg/m^2 daily in 2-4 divided doses. Pyridoxine 25mg daily should be administered to minimize toxicity of penicillamine.
Arsenic Poisoning	100mg/kg daily in 4 divided doses for 5 days. Maximum dose: 1g/day.
Cystinuria	Dosage should be based on urinary cystine excretion which should be maintained less than 100mg daily in patients with renal calculi and/or pain or at 100-200mg daily in patients without a history of renal calculi. While receiving penicillamine, patients should drink 500ml of water at bedtime and again during the night. Penicillamine should be given in 4 equal doses daily. Children: 30mg/kg daily Adult: 2g daily (range 1-4g daily). Initiating therapy with 250mg daily and then gradually increasing dosage will reduce adverse effects. Pyridoxine 25mg daily should be administered to minimize toxicity of penicillamine.
Rheumatoid Arthritis	Give penicillamine at least 1 hour before a meal and at least 1 hour apart from any other drug, food or milk. Adult: 125-250mg daily; dosage may be increased by 125-250mg/day at 1- to 3-month intervals. Remission of symptoms is attained and maintained in many patients with 500-750mg daily. In patients who respond to penicillamine but in whom disease suppression is incomplete after the first 6-9 months of therapy, daily penicillamine dosage may be increased by 125-250mg at 3-month intervals. Maximum dose: 1-1.5g daily.

ADVERSE EFFECTS: Allergic reactions occur in about one-third of patients; skin reactions, occurring early in treatment, may be controlled by concomitant use of an antihistamine. Renal effects: Proteinuria (less than 2g/24 hours) commonly occurs and may improve spontaneously with continued therapy or if dosage is reduced. Hematologic Effects: Leukopenia, thrombocytopenia, bone marrow depression, thrombotic thrombocytopenia purpura, and other hematologic abnormalities have been reported. Mucocutaneous Effects: Increased fragility of the skin may occur at pressure or trauma sites.
MONITOR: Complete blood count, liver function tests, urinalysis.

PENICILLIN

The important activities of penicillins are given in the next Table (Adams, H.G., Personal Communication):

Activities of Penicillins

Classification	Gram-positive cocci: S. aureus	Strep	Enterococci	Gram-negative bacilli: H. influenzae	E. coli	Klebsiella	P. mirabilis	Other enterics	Pseudomonas a.	Anaerobes: B. fragilis	Others
Natural Penicillins, eg, Penicillin G		4	3	3*						2	3
Aminopenicillins, eg, Ampicillin, Amoxicillin		4	4	4*	2		4			2	3
Amoxicillin/Clavulanate (Augmentin)	4	4	4	4	3	4	4	3			4
Ampicillin/Sulbactam (Unasyn)	4	4	4	4	3	4	4	3		3	4
Penicillinase-Resistant, eg, Nafcillin, Oxacillin	4	4									
Extended-Spectrum, eg, Ticarcillin		4		4*	3		4	3	3	3	4
Ticarcillin/Clavulanate (Timentin)	4	4		4	4	4	4	4	3	4	4
Extended-Spectrum, eg, Piperacillin		4	3	4*	3	4	4	4	4	4	4

4 = best activity; 3 = good activity; 2 = some activity

* = beta-lactamase negative

Classification: Classification of penicillins is given in the next Table:

Classification of the Penicillins

Type and Generic Name	Trade Names
Natural Penicillins	
Penicillin G	Many
Benzathine penicillin G	Bicillin, Permapen
Procaine penicillin G	Crysticillin, Wycillin
Penicillin V	V-Cillin, Pen-Vee K
Penicillinase-Resistant: Antistaphylococcal Penicillins	
Methicillin	Staphcillin
Oxacillin	Prostaphlin
Nafcillin	Unipen
Cloxacillin	Tegopen
Dicloxacillin	Dynapen, Dycill
Aminopenicillins(extended spectrum)	
Ampicillin	Polycillin, Omnipen
Amoxicillin	Amoxil, Larotid
Bacampicillin	Spectrobid
Cyclacillin	Cyclapen-W
Extended-Spectrum Penicillins	
Carboxypenicillins	
Carbenicillin	Geopen, Geocillin
Ticarcillin	Ticar
Acylaminopenicillins	
Mezlocillin	Mezlin
Azlocillin	Azlin
Piperacillin	Pipracil
Amidinopenicillins	
Amidinocillin (mecillinam)	Coactin (Not available)
Combinations with Beta-lactamase inhibitors	
Amoxicillin plus potassium clavulanate	Augumentin
Ticarcillin plus potassium clavulanate	Timentin
Ampicillin plus sulbactam	Unasyn

Penicillins can be divided into 5 groups **(natural, penicillinase-resistant, aminopenicillins, extended-spectrum and amidinopenicillins)** based principally on their spectra of activity. The spectra of activity is induced by changes in the structure of penicillins as described in the next section.

PENICILLIN (Cont.)

Structure of Penicillins: The basic structure of the penicillins is given in the next Figure:

Basic Structure of the Penicillins

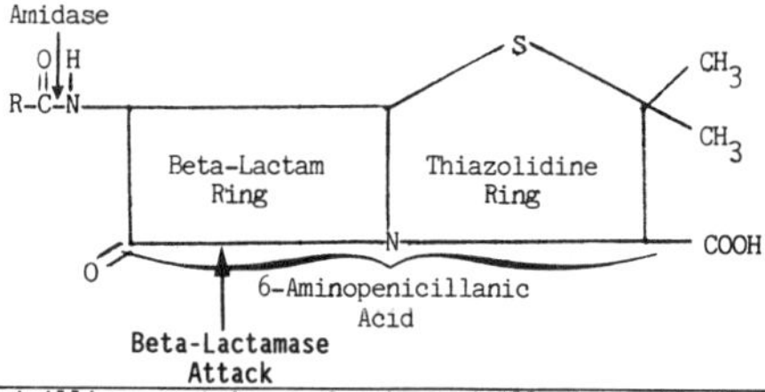

All penicillins contain a 6-aminopenicillanic acid (6-APA) nucleus, which is composed of a beta-lactam ring fused to a 5-membered thiazolidine ring. A free carboxyl group on the thiazolidine ring and one or more substituted amino side chains at R are also essential for antibacterial activity. Cleavage at any bond in the 6-APA nuclear ring results in complete loss of antibacterial activity.

Addition of various side chains at R on the penicillin nucleus results in penicillin derivatives with differences in activity, stability against hydrolysis by beta-lactamases, acid stability, GI absorption, and protein-binding.

Beta-lactamases are enzymes that hydrolyze the cyclic amide bond of the beta-lactam ring and render it inactive.

Mechanism of Action of the Penicillins: Like most other beta-lactam antibiotics, penicillins are bactericidal because they inhibit bacterial cell-wall synthesis and may increase breakdown of the cell wall; the exact mechanism is not completely understood. Penicillins are believed to inhibit bacterial cell-wall synthesis by inhibiting cross-linking of the linear polysaccharide chains by peptide bonds.

In gram-positive bacteria, there is an inhibitor of a cell wall autolytic enzyme. Penicillins decrease the availability of the inhibitor and thus enzymatic breakdown of the cell wall may occur.

Penicillins bind to penicillin-binding proteins (PBPs). These proteins are believed to be enzymes that are involved in bacterial cell wall division, wall elongation, septum formation and the maintenance of cell shape. Penicillins bind to PBP2 and/or PBP3, which cause bacterial cell lysis and the production of long filamentous forms, respectively.

Mechanisms of Bacterial Resistance to Beta-Lactam Antibiotics: The most important mechanism of bacterial resistance to the beta-lactam antibiotics is bacterial production of beta-lactamases, enzymes that hydrolyze the cyclic amide bond of the beta-lactam ring and render it inactive; the action of beta-lactamase on penicillins is illustrated in the next Figure:

Action of Beta-Lactamase on Penicillins and Cephalosporins

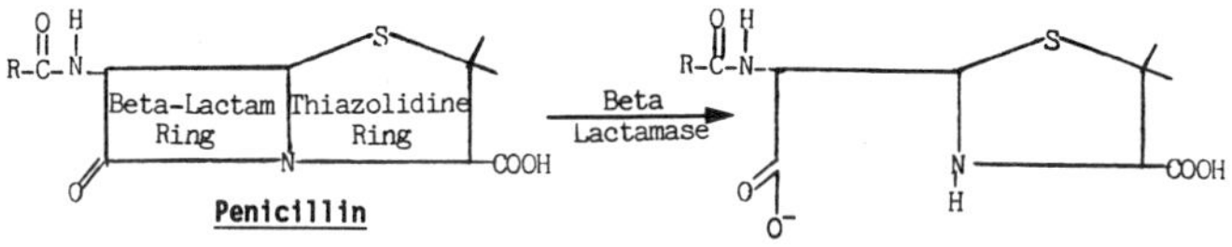

PENICILLIN (Cont.)

Incidence of Beta-Lactamase Production in Bacterial Isolates: The incidence of beta-lactamase production in bacterial isolates is given in the next Table (Neu, H.C., Am. J. Med. 79 (suppl.5B), 2-12, 1985; Doern, G.V. et al., Antimicrob. Agents Chemother. 32, 180-185, 1988; Yogev, R., Adv. Pediatr. Infect. Dis. 3, 181-206, 1988):

Incidence of Beta-Lactamase Production in Bacterial Isolates

Organism	Beta-Lactamase-Producing (%) Hospital Isolates	Community Isolates
Staphylococcus aureus	85	85
Staphylococcus epidermis	80-95	
Moraxella catarrhalis	75	75
Neisseria gonorrhoeae	5-10	
Hemophilus influenzae	20	20
Escherichia coli	20	21
Klebsiella pneumoniae	90	88
Bacteroides fragilis	90	
Pseudomonas aeruginosa	90-100	

NATURAL PENICILLINS: The main uses of the natural penicillins are given in the next Table (Wilkowske, C.J. and Hermans, P.E., Mayo Clin. Proc. 62, 789-798, 1987):

Natural Penicillins and Their Main Uses

Drug	Main Indications
Penicillin G (Parenteral)	Streptococci: Severe infections due to beta-hemolytic streptococci (A, B, C, G, and H), Streptococcus pneumoniae (Pneumonoccus). Also in viridans streptococcal and S. bovis endocarditis. In combination with an aminoglycoside for severe enterococcal infection. Neisseria meningitidis (Meningococcus) Susceptible anaerobes. Lyme Disease (spirochete: Borrelia burgdorferi)
Penicillin G (Oral)	Group A streptococcal pharyngitis and pyoderma. Prophylaxis and treatment of rheumatic fever. Simple urinary tract infections due to enterococci.
Penicillin V (Oral)	Same as for penicillin G; GI absorption is better than Pen G.
Benzathine penicillin G (Parenteral)	Prophylaxis of rheumatic fever. Treatment of group A streptococcal infections. Primary, secondary, and latent syphilis (normal findings on cerebrospinal fluid examination).
Procaine penicillin G (Parenteral)	Pneumococcal pneumonia. Syphilis

Penicillin V: Penicillin V is preferred over penicillin G for oral treatment caused by gram-positive cocci other than penicillinase-producing staphylococc because it is more reliably absorbed and can be administered with food.

Penicillin G: For initial therapy of severe infections, penicillin G administered parenterally, is first choice.

Procaine Penicillin G: For somewhat longer action in less severe infections due to Group A streptococci, pneumococci, or Treponema pallidum, procaine penicillin G, an intramuscular formulation, is given once or twice daily.

Benzathine Penicillin G: Benzathine penicillin G, a slowly absorbed intramuscular preparation, is usually given in a single monthly injection for prophylaxis of rheumatic fever, once for treatment of Group A streptococcal pharyngitis, and once or more for treatment of syphilis.

PENICILLIN (Cont.)

Recommendations by consultants of the Medical Letter for use of the natural penicillins as first-choice or alternative antimicrobial therapy are given in the next Table (The Medical Letter 30, 33-40, Mar. 25, 1988):

Antimicrobial Therapy with Natural Penicillins

Bacterial Pathogen	Penicillin
GRAM-POSITIVE COCCI	
Staph. aureus or epidermidis, non-penicillinase	G or V
Streptococci	
Strep. pyogenes (Group A) and Groups C and G	G or V
Strep., Group B	G
Strep., viridans group	G with or without gentamicin
Strep., bovis	G
Strep., enterococcus group, endocarditis or other severe infection	G or ampicillin, with gentamicin
Strep., anaerobic or Peptostreptococcus	G
Strep. pneumoniae (pneumococcus)	G or V
GRAM-POSITIVE BACILLI	
Bacillus anthracis (anthrax)	G
Clostridium perfringens	G
Clostridium tetani	G
Corynebacterium diphtheriae	G (as alternative drug)
ACTINOMYCETES	
Actinomycetes israelii (actinomycosis)	G
GRAM-NEGATIVE COCCI	
N. meningitidis (Meningococcus)	G
N. gonorrhoeae (Gonococcus)	G (for sensitive strains)
ENTERIC GRAM-NEGATIVE BACILLI	
Bacteroides, Oropharyngeal strains	G
OTHER GRAM-NEGATIVE BACILLI	
Fusobacterium	G
Leptotrichia buccalis	G
P. multocida	G
Spirillum minus (rat bite fever)	G
Streptobaccillus moniliformis (rat bite fever; Haverhill fever)	G
SPIROCHETES	
Borrelia burgdorferi (Lyme disease)	G or V(as alternative drug)
Borrelia recurrentis (relapsing fever)	G (as alternative drug)
Leptospira	G
Treponema pallidum	G
Treponema pertenue (yaws)	G

PENICILLINASE-RESISTANT ANTISTAPHYLOCOCCAL PENICILLINS: The main uses of the penicillinase-resistant antistaphylococcal penicillins are given in the next Table (Wilkowske, C.J. and Hermans, P.E., Mayo Clin. Pro. 62, 789-798, 1987):

Penicillinase-Resistant Antistaphylococcal Penicillins and Their Main Uses

Drug (Route)	Main Indications
Oxacillin (Parenteral)	Severe Staphylococcus aureus infections
Nafcillin (Parenteral)	
Dicloxacillin (Oral)	Mild S. aureus infections, such as pyodermal infections.
Cloxacillin (Oral)	

The penicillinase-resistant penicillins are drugs of choice for staphylococcal infections.

Methicillin has been associated with interstitial nephritis more frequently than oxacillin or nafcillin; thus, these latter drugs are preferred for parenteral use in patients with severe Staphylococcal aureus infections.

Oral dicloxacillin or cloxacillin may be used for mild to moderate infections.

When penicillin-resistant strains of Staphylococcus aureus or S. epidermidis are known or suspected to be present, vancomycin is required.

PENICILLIN (Cont.)

AMINOPENICILLINS: The main uses of the aminopenicillins are given in the next Table(Wilkowske, C.J. and Hermans, P.E., Mayo Clin. Proc. 62, 789-798, 1987):

Aminopenicillins and Their Main Uses

Drug	Main Indications
Ampicillin (Parenteral)	Complicated urinary tract infections and systemic infections caused by susceptible microorganisms. Endocarditis prophylaxis (IV), combined with gentamicin.
Ampicillin (Oral)	Simple urinary tract infections, if causative microorganism is susceptible (many hospital strains are resistant). Shigellosis and severe salmonellosis.
Amoxicillin (Oral)	Bacterial sinusitis, otitis, and bronchitis caused by susceptible microorganisms; also, ampicillin indications. Endocarditis prophylaxis (oral).

Recommendations by consultants of the Medical Letter for use of the aminopenicillins as first-choice or alternative antimicrobial therapy are given in the next Table (The Medical Letter 30, 33-40, Mar. 25, 1988):

Aminopenicillins as First-Choice or Alternative Antimicrobial Therapy

Bacterial Pathogen	Penicillin
GRAM-POSITIVE COCCI	
Strep faecalis enterococcus group:	
Endocarditis or other severe infection	G or ampicillin with gentamicin.
Uncomplicated urinary tract infection	Ampicillin or amoxicillin
GRAM-POSITIVE BACILLI	
Listeria monocytogenes	Ampicillin with or without gentamicin
ENTERIC GRAM-NEGATIVE BACILLI	
Escherichia coli	Ampicillin with or without gentamicin, tobramycin, or amikacin
Proteus mirabilis	Ampicillin
Salmonella typhi	Ampicillin or amoxicillin (as alternatives)
Salmonella other than S. typhi	Ampicillin or amoxicillin
Shigella	Ampicillin as alternate therapy
OTHER GRAM-NEGATIVE BACILLI	
Eikenella corrodens	Ampicillin
H. influenzae other than meningitis, epiglottis, arthritis and other serious infections.	Ampicillin or amoxicillin

Amoxicillin is closely related to ampicillin in chemical structure and in antibacterial activity. Amoxicillin is more completely absorbed orally in comparison with ampicillin with resultant blood levels about twice those obtained with similar oral doses of ampicillin.

EXTENDED-SPECTRUM PENICILLINS: The extended-spectrum penicillins are listed in the next Table:

Extended-Spectrum Penicillins
CARBOXYPENICILLINS
Carbenicillin
Ticarcillin
ACYLAMINOPENICILLINS
Mezlocillin
Azlocillin
Piperacillin

The main uses of the extended-spectrum penicillins are given in the next Table (Wilkowske, C.J. and Hermans, P.E., Mayo Clin. Proc. 62, 789-798, 1987):

Extended-Spectrum Penicillins and Their Main Uses

Drug (Route)	Main Indications
Ticarcillin (parenteral)	Severe infections due to Enterbacteriaceae or Pseudomonas aeruginosa (with an aminoglycoside), but resistant strains are common.
Piperacillin (parenteral) **Azlocillin** (parenteral) **Mezlocillin** (parenteral)	Severe infections due to Enterobacteriaceae. May be used as initial (empiric) therapy. Severe infections due to P. aeruginosa in combination with an aminoglycoside (amikacin, tobramycin, or gentamicin).

PENICILLIN (Cont.)

Recommendations by consultants of the Medical Letter for use of extended-spectrum penicillins as first or alternative choice antimicrobial therapy are given in the next Table (The Medical Letter 30, 33-40, Mar. 25, 1988):

Extended-Spectrum Penicillins as First Choice or Alternative Antimicrobial Therapy

Bacterial Pathogen	Extended-Spectrum Penicillin
GRAM-POSITIVE COCCI	None
GRAM-POSITIVE BACILLI	None
GRAM-NEGATIVE COCCI	None
ENTERIC GRAM-NEGATIVE BACILLI	
Bacteroides, Gastrointestinal Strains	Alternative
Enterobacter	Alternative
E. Coli	Alternative
P. Mirabilis	Alternative
Proteus, Indole-Positive	Alternative
Providencia Rettgeri	Alternative
Morganella Morganii	Alternative
Proteus Vulgaris	Alternative
Providencia Stuartii	Alternative
Serratia	Alternative
OTHER GRAM-NEGATIVE BACILLI	
Acinetobacter	Alternative
Pseudomonas Aeruginosa	First Choice, with aminoglycoside

The extended-spectrum penicillins have an antibacterial range similar to that of aminopenicillins with added activity against certain strains of P. aeruginosa, the indole-positive Proteus species and Enterobacter species.

COMBINATIONS OF PENICILLINS WITH BETA-LACTAMASE INHIBITORS: The addition of a beta-lactamase inhibitor (clavulanate or sulbactam) restores amoxicillin, ampicillin and ticarcillin to its original spectra of activity. Beta-lactamase inhibitors resemble penicillin structurally and enhance the in-vitro activity of certain beta-lactam antibiotics by protecting them from hydrolysis by beta-lactamases. They are termed "suicide inhibitors" because they bind to and inactivate beta-lactamases but are destroyed in the process. Examples are given in the next Table:

Combinations of Penicillins with Beta-Lactamase Inhibitors

Combination	Additional Susceptible Bacteria
Ampicillin and Sulbactam (Unasyn)	S. aureus, H. influenzae, Moraxella catarrhalis, Klebsiella species, and Bacteroides fragilis.
Amoxicillin and Clavulanate (Augmentin)	H. influenzae, E. coli, Proteus, K. pneumoniae; S. aureus and S. epidermidis (but not methicillin-resistant strains); M. catarrhalis, N. gonorrhoeae, and Legionella pneumophila.
Ticarcillin and Clavulanate (Timentin)	S. aureus, H. influenzae, N. gonorrhoeae, E. coli, Klebsiella, Providencia and B. fragilis.

Augmentin is an oral clavulanate

ADVERSE REACTIONS TO PENICILLINS: Adverse reactions to penicillins are given in the next Table (Wright, A.J. and Wilkowske, C.J., Mayo Clin. Proc. 62, 806-820, 1987):

Adverse Reactions to Penicillins

Shared by all penicillins
- Allergic reactions (rarely anaphylactic)
- Skin rashes
- Diarrhea
- Neuromuscular irritability, including seizures associated with large doses or renal failure
- Hematologic changes such as neutropenia and anemia (at times hemolytic)
- Drug-induced fever
- Nephropathy (as component of serum sickness-type reaction) or interstitial nephritis (especially methicillin)

(Cont.)

PENICILLIN (Cont.)

Table Continued

Adverse Reactions to Penicillins
Commonly associated with the following individual drugs
Ampicillin/Amoxicillin
Skin rashes
Diarrhea
Pseudomembranous colitis
Carbenicillin and ticarcillin
Hypokalemic alkalosis, sodium overload
Platelet dysfunction
Methicillin
Interstitial nephritis
Anemia, neutropenia, granulocytopenia
Nafcillin
Thrombophlebitis
Elevated AST (SGOT)
Oxacillin
Elevated AST (SGOT)
Granulocytopenia
Potassium penicillin G
Hyperkalemia and arrhythmias associated with intravenous doses given rapidly when renal failure is present
Procaine penicillin G
Neurologic reaction and abnormal behavior associated with high doses

From 5% to 20% of patients have a history of a rash or some other reaction while taking a penicillin.

Cross-Reactions with Other Beta-Lactams: Patients allergic to penicillin occasionally have allergic reactions to cephalosporins and imipenem, a parenteral beta-lactam. However, aztreonam (Azactam), which is also a parenteral beta-lactam, is not associated with allergic reactions. (Saxon, A. et al., Ann. Intern. Med. 107, 204, 1987).

Alternative Drugs to Penicillin: Drugs used as an alternative to penicillin in penicillin-allergic patients are given in the next Table (Medical Letter 30, 79, Aug. 12, 1988):

Alternative to Penicillin in Penicillin-Allergic Patients

Condition	Drug-Alternative
Gram-Positive Organisms	Vancomycin
Meningitis	Chloroamphenicol (may not be effective for enteric-gram-negative bacilli)
Bacteremia (unknown organism)	Vancomycin or clindamycin and aztreonam (active against aerobic gram-negative bacilli; inactive against anaerobes or gram-positive organisms).

Other alternatives include erythromycin, trimethoprim/sulfamethoxazole, the aminoglycosides and the fluoroquinolones, eg, ciprofloxacin.

PENICILLIN G

(Pentids, Bicillin, and others)

USES: **Penicillin G** is a **first generation penicillin** (natural penicillin); it is preferred in serious infections, especially when parenteral administration of large doses is required. Activities of penicillin G are given in the next Table (Parry, M.F., Med. Clin. No. Am. 71, 1093-1112, Nov. 1987; Adams, H.G., Personal Comm.):

Activities of Penicillin G

	Gram-positive cocci: S. aureus	Gram-positive cocci: Streptococci	Gram-positive cocci: Strep. entero.	Gram-negative bacilli: H. influenzae	Gram-negative bacilli: PEcK	Gram-negative bacilli: Other Enterics	Gram-negative bacilli: Pseudomonas a.	Anaerobes: B. fragilis	Anaerobes: Res. Anaerobes
Penicillin G	▩	4	3	3*	▩	▩	▩	2	3

4=best activity; 3=good activity; 2=some activity; ▩=little or no activity;
*Beta-lactamase negative.
PEcK (Mnemonic)= P. mirabilis, E. coli, Klebsiella; Res.= Resident

Infectious organisms for which penicillin G may be the **antibiotic of choice** are given in the next Table (The Medical Letter, 30, 33-40, March 25, 1988; Wilkowske, C.J. and Hermans, P.E., Mayo Clin. Proc. 62, 789-798, 1987; Wright, A.J. and Wilkowske, C.J., Mayo Clin. Proc. 62, 806-820, 1987):

Infectious Organisms for which Penicillin G may be Antibiotic of Choice

Gram-Positive: Cocci	Gram-Positive: Bacilli	Gram-Negative
Staphylococcus Aureus or Epidermidis	Bacillus Anthracis (Anthrax)	**Enteric Bacilli**
Non-Penicillinase Producing	Clostridium Perfringens or Tetani	Bacteroides, Oropharyngeal Strains
Streptococcus		**Other Bacilli**
Pyogenes (Group A)		Fusobacterium
Groups B,C, and G		Leptotrichia Buccalis
Viridans		Pasteurella Multocida
Bovis		Spirillum Minus (Rat Bite Fever)
Enterococcus Group Endocarditis or other Severe Infections		Streptobacillus Moniliforms (Rat Bite Fever)
Anaerobic or Peptostreptococcus		**Cocci**
Pneumoniae (Pneumococcus)		Neisseria Meningitidis (Meningococcus)
Actinomycetes	**Spirochetes**	
Actinomyces Israelii (Actinomycosis)	Leptospira	
	Treponema Pallidum	
	Treponema Pertenus (Yaws)	
	Borrelia Burgdorferi (Lyme Dis.)	

PENICILLIN G (Cont.)

The main indications for the use of penicillin G are given in the next Table (Wilkowske, C.J. and Hermans, P.E., Mayo Clin. Proc. 62, 789-798, 1987):

Main Indications for Use of Penicillin G

Form and Route	Main Indications
Penicillin G, Parenteral	Severe infections due to B-hemolytic streptococci (A,B,C,G,and H), Streptococcus pneumoniae (pneumococcus), Neisseria meningitidis (meningococcus), and susceptible anaerobes. Viridans streptococcal and S. bovis endocarditis. In combination with an aminoglycoside for severe enterococcal infection. Lyme disease (late) - persistent arthritis, severe carditis, meningitis or encephalitis (Rahn, D.W. and Malawista, S.E., Ann. Intern. Med. 114, 472-481, 1991).
Penicillin G, Oral	Group A streptococcal pharyngitis and pyoderma. Prophylaxis and treatment of rheumatic fever. Simple urinary tract infections due to enterococci.
Benzathine Penicillin G, Parenteral	Prophylaxis of rheumatic fever. Treatment of group A streptococcal infections. Primary, secondary and latent lues (normal findings on cerebrospinal fluid examination)
Procaine Penicillin G, Parenteral	Pneumococcal pneumonia. Syphilis

The disadvantages of penicillin G are that it is (1) degraded by gastric acid (2) destroyed by the enzyme penicillinase, and (3) its use is associated with an allergic reaction in approximately 10% of patients.

Mechanism of Action: The antibacterial activity of penicillin G results from inhibition of mucopeptide synthesis in the bacterial cell wall. The rigid structure of the bacterial cell wall is due to peptidoglycan, a mucopeptide made up of linear polysaccharide chains cross-linked by peptide bonds.

DOSAGE FORMS: The dosage forms of penicillin G are given in the next Table:

Dosage Forms of Penicillin G

Preparation	Route	Forms
Penicillin G Potassium	Oral	Powder(for solution):200,000 and 400,000 units/5ml Powder(for suspension):250,000 and 400,000units/5ml Tabs:200,000; 250,000; 400,000; 500,000; 800,000 units.
Penicillin G (Aqueous) Potassium	IM or IV	Powder:200,000; 500,000 and 1,5,10 and 20 million units Powder(buffered): 1 and 5 million units
Penicillin G (Aqueous) Sodium	IM or IV	Powder: 5 million units
Procaine Penicillin G	IM	300,000; 500,000; 600,000 units/ml.
Benzathine Penicillin G	IM	Bicillin L-A:300,000units/ml in 10ml containers. 600,000units/ml in 1,2 and 4ml containers. Permapen:600,000units/ml in 2ml containers.
	Oral	Bicillin, Tabs: 200,000 units

PENICILLIN G (Cont.)

DOSAGE: The oral form is taken one hour before or two hours after meals. The dosage of penicillin G in different conditions is given in the next Table:

Dosage of Penicillin G

Condition	Route and Dosage Form	Age	Dosage
Usual	Oral; G Potassium	Adults, Child.>12yrs.	0.8-3.2 million units daily in divided doses 4 times daily.
		Child.<12yrs.	40,000 to 80,000 units/kg daily in divided doses every 6 hours.
High-Dose IV Penicillin G is used in **Meningitis eg, Pneumococcal Meningitis)** **Some forms of Endocarditis, eg, Enterococcal and Severe Clostridial Infections**	IM or IV; G Potassium or G Sodium	Adults	20-30 million units daily; daily dosage in 2-6 hour intervals or by constant IV infusion. Large doses should be given IV
		Children	100,000 to 300,000 units/kg daily in divided doses every 4-6 hours.
Meningitis,eg, (Pneumococcal Meningococcal Gonococcal)	IM or IV, G Potassium or G Sodium	>7 days and >2kg	200,000 units/kg daily in divided doses every 6 hours.
		>7 days and <2kg	150,000 units/kg daily in divided doses every 8 hours.
		<7 days and >2kg	150,000 units/kg daily in divided doses every 8 hours.
		<7 days and <2kg	100,000 units/kg daily in divided doses every 12 hours.
Gonococcal Infection Disseminated*	IV, Aqueous	Adults	10 million units daily for at least 3 days, complete 7-10d course with oral therapy, eg, Amoxicillin. **Penicillin sensitive strains only.**
Gonococcal Ophthalmia*	IV, Aqueous	Adults	10 million units daily for 5 days. **Pen. sensitive strains only.**
Neonatal Gonococcal Infections (No apparent) Infection but born to mother with Gonococcal Infection*	IV, IM Aqueous	Full-Term	50,000 units as a single injection
		Low-Birth Weight	20,000 units as a single injection
			Pen. sensitive strains only.
Neonatal Gonococcal Ophthalmia*	IV, Aqueous	Neonates	100,000 units/kg daily in four divided doses (two doses if <7d) for seven days. **Pen. sensitive strains only.**
Neonatal Gonococcal Bacteremia and Arthritis*	IV, Aqueous	Neonates	100,000 units/kg daily in four divided doses (two doses if <7d) for at least seven days. **Pen. sensitive strains only.**
Gonococcal Meningitis*	IV, Aqueous	Neonates	See Meningitis listing in this chart (above). **Pen. sensitive strains only.**
Syphilis, Early; Primary, Secondary or Latent of less than one years duration.	IM, Benzathine Penicillin G	Adults	2.4 million units in a single dose
Syphilis, > one year (except Neurosyphilis)	IM, Benzathine, Penicillin G	Adults	2.4 million units weekly for three successive weeks (7.2 million units total.

PENICILLIN G (Cont.)

Neurosyphilis	IV, Aqueous and IM Benzathine, Penicillin G	Adults	2-4 million units every 4 hours for 10-14 days followed by IM benzathine penicillin G, 2.4 million units weekly for 3 successive weeks.
or	IM, Aqueous Procaine Penicillin G	Adults	2.4 million units daily plus probenecid 500mg orally four times daily; both drugs for 10 days followed by benzathine penicillin G, IM 2.4 million units for 3 successive weeks.
Syphilis in Pregnancy			Treat as for nonpregnant patients.
Congenital Syphilis	IM or IV Aqueous Penicillin G	Neonates Symptomatic or Asymptomatic	50,000 units/kg 2-3 times daily for 10-14 days.
or	IM, Aqueous Procaine Penicillin G	Neonates Symptomatic or Asymptomatic	50,000 units/kg once IM daily for 10-14 days. If more than 1 day of therapy is missed, restart course.
Lyme Disease Arthritis, Carditis, Meningitis	IV, Penicillin G	Adults	20 million units daily in divided doses; Arthritis 14-21d, carditis 14d, meningitis 10-21d. Ceftriaxone also effective (Rahn, D.W. and Malawista, S.E., Ann. Intern. Med. 114, 472-481, 1991).
		Children	300,000 units/kg/day in divided doses for 14-21 days. Ceftriaxone also effective (Amer. Acad. Pediatr. Policy Statement, AAP News, May 1991).

*Penicillin G is not the drug of choice for empirical therapy of presumed gonococcal disease due to the emergence of penicillinase-producing N. Gonorrhoeae (PPNG). See GONORRHEA or SEXUALLY TRANSMITTED DISEASES sections.

Combination of benzathine penicillin G and procaine penicillin G is often used to treat Group A streptococcal pharyngotonsillitis. This combination provides early peak levels as well as prolonged levels of penicillin in the blood. The dosage of benzathine penicillin G for treatment of streptococcal sore throat is given in the following Table (Barkin, R.M. and Rosen, P., Emergency Pediatrics, 3rd ed., 1990):

Treatment of Streptococcal Pharyngitis

Weight, kg (lb)	Benzathine Pen G (Bicillin LA)	Benzathine/Procaine Pen G (Bicillin C-R 900/300)
<14 (30)	300,000 units	300,000:100,000
14-27 (31-60)	600,000 units	600,000:200,000
27-41 (61-90)	900,000 units	900,000:300,000
>41 (90)	1,200,000 units	Not available

Penicillin dosage is adjusted downward in renal impairment.

PHARMACOKINETICS: Oral Absorption: Partially destroyed by gastric acid; absorption in neonates and the elderly is higher because gastric pH is higher; absorption erratic and incomplete; usually 20-30% of an oral dose is absorbed, primarily in the duodenum. Food in G.I. tract decreases absorption; give penicillin G one hour before or 2-3 hours after a meal. Peak: Oral: 30-60 min.; IM: 15-30 min. after aqueous penicillin G; IV: Immediately after aqueous penicillin G. Protein-Binding: 60% bound to albumin; Elimination: 60%-90% in urine within one hour. Half-Life: 0.5 hours; 6-10 hours in renal impairment.

Penicillin G Procaine: Penicillin G procaine is relatively insoluble. IM administration of the drug provides a tissue depot from which the drug is slowly absorbed and hydrolyzed to penicillin G. After IM injection, serum penicillin G procaine peaks in 1-4 hours and falls slowly over 15-20 hours.

PENICILLIN G (Cont.)

Penicillin G Benzathine: Penicillin G benzathine is relatively insoluble. IM administration of penicillin G benzathine results in serum concentrations of penicillin G that are generally more prolonged, but much lower, than those attained with an equivalent IM dose of penicillin G procaine or penicillin G potassium or sodium. Peak serum concentration is attained in 13-24 hours are usually detectable for 1-4 weeks depending on the dose.

ADVERSE EFFECTS: The major adverse effects of penicillin are hypersensitivity reactions; the incidence is between 1% and 10%. Also, 5% to 10% of penicillin-allergic patients are sensitive to cephalosporins; patients who have experienced an immediate-type hypersensitivity reaction to penicillins should not receive cephalosporins.

Some adverse effects are due to the dosage form of penicillin G and are given in the next Table:

Adverse Effects and Dosage Form of Penicillin G

Dosage Form	Adverse Effects
Procaine Penicillin G	Immediate-type reactions to the procaine component particularly with a large single dose. IM Injection: Pain and sterile inflammation at the site of IM injection. IV Injection: Phlebitis or thrombophlebitis.
Penicillin G Potassium	Massive IV doses (1.7mEq of potassium/million units) may produce hyperkalemia, arrhythmias, and cardiac arrest, particularly in patients with impaired renal function.

Other adverse effects are given in the next Table:

Other Adverse Effects of Penicillin G

System	Effect
CNS	Damage to a peripheral nerve following accidental IM injection; usually reversible. High concentrations of penicillin may cause convulsions or fatal encephalopathy, especially in epileptics and infants.
Kidney	Allergic reaction manifested as interstitial nephritis.
Hematologic	Reversible neutropenia; Coomb's positive hemolytic anemia is rare.

MONITOR: Initial renal function tests when using high doses.

PENICILLIN V

(Beepen VK, Betapen-VK, Ledercillin VK, Pen-Vee K, V-Cillin K)

USES: Penicillin V is preferred over penicillin G for **oral treatment** of infections caused by **gram-positive cocci** because it is more reliably absorbed and can be administered with food. Activities of penicillin V are given in the next Table (Parry, M.F., Med. Clin. No. Am. 71, 1093-1112, Nov. 1987; Adams, H.G., Personal Comm.):

Activities of Penicillin V

	Gram-positive cocci			Gram-negative bacilli				Anaerobes	
	S. aureus	Streptococci	Strep. entero.	H. influenzae	PEcK	Other Enterics	Pseudomonas a.	B. fragilis	Res. Anaerobes
Penicillin V	▩	4	3	3*	▩	▩	▩	2	3

4=best activity; 3=good activity; 2=some activity; ▩ =little or no activity; *Beta-lactamase negative.

PEcK (Mnemonic)= P. mirabilis, E. coli, Klebsiella; Res.= Resident

Major uses of penicillin V are given in the next Table:

Major Uses of Penicillin V

- Group A Beta-Hemolytic Streptococcal Pharyngitis (10 Day Course)
- Mild Streptococcal Pyoderms (Impetigo) (10 Day Course)
- Mild Respiratory Tract Infections caused by Streptococcus Pneumoniae (Pneumococcus)
- Lyme Borreliosis: Children <9 yrs with early disease, isolated Bell's palsy, arthritis or mild carditis (Amer. Acad. Pediatr. Policy Statement, AAP News, May, 1991).

Penicillin V is the **drug of first choice** for the treatment of infections caused by the **gram-positive cocci,** Staphylococcus aureus or epidermidis, non-penicillinase producing and Streptococcus pyogenes(Group A) and Groups C and G

Penicillin V is sensitive to beta-lactamases and beta-lactamase producing strains of bacteria, eg, most staphylococci, are resistant.

DOSAGE FORMS: Dosage forms of penicillin and potassium penicillin V are given in the next Table:

Dosage Forms of Penicillin V and Potassium Penicillin V

Product	Solution(mg/5ml)	Tablets(mg)
Potassium Penicillin V		
Generic; Beepen VK; Pen-Vee K	125, 250	125, 250, 500

The potassium salt of penicillin V is better absorbed than other penicillin salts.

DOSAGE: Dosage of penicillin V potassium is given in the next Table:

Dosage of Penicillin V Potassium

Condition	Age	Dosage
Usual	Adults	125-500mg four times daily
	Children	25-50mg/kg daily in divided doses every six hours. Max: 3g/day.
Lyme Borreliosis: Early disease, Isolated Bell's Palsy, Arthritis, or Mild Carditis	Children <9 years	25-50mg/kg daily in 3 divided doses for 10-30 days. Amoxicillin, same dose, is also effective. Use tetracycline in older patients (Amer. Acad. Pediatr., Policy Statement, AAP News, May, 1991).
Prophylaxis of Rheumatic Fever or **Pneumococcal Infection**	Adults and Children >5 yrs	250 mg twice daily.
	Children <5 yrs	125mg twice daily.

PHARMACOKINETICS: Absorption: 60% primarily from duodenum. Peak: 30-60 min. Protein Binding: 80%. Half-Life: 30-60 min. Probenecid delays elimination. Excretion: Urine.

ADVERSE EFFECTS: Anaphylaxis, urticaria, GI upset, superinfection.

PRECAUTIONS: Continue therapy for 2 days after symptoms improve. Allergy, pregnancy, lactation. May need dosage adjustment in renal failure.

PENTAMIDINE ISETHIONATE
(Pentam, NebuPent)

USES: **Pentamidine** isethionate is used to treat **protozoal infections** as listed in the next Table:

Uses of Pentamidine Isethionate
Pneumocystis Carinii Pneumonia(PCP)
African Trypanosomiasis
Leishmaniasis

Pneumocystis carinii pneumonia(PCP) occurs in a high percent of patients with acquired immunodeficiency syndrome(AIDS). Trimethoprim-sulfamethoxazole, which is less toxic than pentamidine isethionate, is the initial drug of choice for most AIDS patients with PCP. Pentamidine via inhalation is effective for both primary and secondary prophylaxis of PCP in patients with AIDS (Hirschel, B. et al., N. Engl. J. Med. 324, 1079-1083, 1991; Leoung, G.S. et al., N. Engl. J. Med. 323, 769-775, 1990). Trimethoprim-sulfamethoxazole is also effective prophylaxis, and may be preferable because, as a systemic agent, it may prevent other infections (eg, Salmonellosis, Shigellosis, Haemophilus and Pneumococcal otitis media, sinusitis and pneumonia, Isospora, Toxoplasmosis, Nocardia, Listeria and extrapulmonary pneumocystosis). In addition, trimethoprim-sulfamethoxazole is cheaper and more convenient (Wormser, G.P. et al., Arch. Intern. Med. 151, 688-692, 1991).

DOSAGE FORMS: Injection(Pentam): 300mg; Inhalation(NebuPent): 300mg.

DOSAGE: Pentamidine isethionate is administered by deep IM injection, slow IV infusion, or inhalation. The dosage of pentamidine isethionate is given in the next Table:

Dosage of Pentamidine Isethionate	
Protozoal Infection	Dosage
Pneumocystis Carinii Pneumonia(PCP)	Adults and Children:4mg/kg once daily for 14 days. Inhalation: Pneumocystis prophylaxis (5 years and older): 300mg in 6ml water via Respirgard II jet nebulizer once every month or 60mg in 3ml water via Fisoneb hand-held ultrasonic nebulizer, load with 5 doses, one dose every 24-72 hrs during the first 2 weeks followed by one dose every 2 weeks (Murphy, R.L. et al., Amer. J. Med. 90, 418-426, 1991). Other regimens have been used.
African Trypanosomiasis	4mg/kg once daily for 10 days
Leishmania Donovani	Adults and Children: 2-4mg/kg once daily or every other day for up to 15 doses

ADVERSE EFFECTS: Renal Effects: Nephrotoxicity is the most common adverse effect of pentamidine, occurring in at least 25% of patients with PCP receiving the drug. Pentamidine-induced nephrotoxicity is recognized by an increase in serum creatinine and/or BUN, developing gradually and appearing during the second week of therapy. Renal insufficiency is usually mild to moderate in severity and reversible following discontinuance of pentamidine. Development of acute renal failure (serum creatinine >6mg/dl) or severe renal insufficiency may require discontinuation of the drug.

BUN and serum creatinine should be determined prior to starting pentamidine therapy and daily during and several times after therapy with the drug.

Hypoglycemia and Diabetogenic Effects: Hypoglycemia with blood glucose concentration less than 25mg/dl ocurs in 5 to 10% of patients receiving pentamidine. Hyperglycemia and insulin-dependent diabetes mellitus have also occurred, sometimes months after discontinuance of therapy.

Blood glucose concentration should be determined prior to starting pentamidine therapy and daily during and several times after therapy with the drug.

Hematologic Effects: Leukopenia (leukocyte count less than 1000/mm^3) and thrombocytopenia (platelet count less than 20,000/mm^3) occur occasionally.

Complete blood count(CBC) and platelet counts should be determined prior to starting pentamidine therapy and several times during and after therapy with the drug.

Liver: Increased serum AST(SGOT) and ALT(SGPT) activity occurs occasionally. Liver function tests should be performed before, during and after drug therapy.

Cardiovascular Effects: Pronounced local effects may follow IM injection including sterile abscesses. Phlebitis may occur following IV injection; infuse over 1 hr. to reduce risk of hypotension.

Hypocalcemia: Hypocalcemia has been reported to occur occasionally.

PENTAZOCINE
(Talwin)

USES: Pentazocine is a synthetic opiate partial agonist used as an analgesic for moderate to severe pain. Pentazocine is used primarily for treatment of post-operative pain and to provide analgesia during labor.

DOSAGE FORMS: Pentazocine lactate (IV or IM): 30mg/ml; Pentazocine hydrochloride is used for oral administration and is available in the following combinations:

Pentazocine Hydrochloride Combinations for Oral Use

Trade Name	Pentazocine	Other Drugs
Talwin Nx Caplets	50mg	Naloxone 0.5mg
Talwin Compound Caplets	12.5mg	Aspirin 325mg
Talacen Caplets	25mg	Acetaminophen 650mg

DOSAGE: The dosage of pentazocine in different conditions is given in the next Table:

Dosage of Pentazocine

Condition	Route	Dosage
Usual	Oral	50mg every 3-4 hrs.; increase to 100mg/dose when needed. Max.: 600mg daily.
	IV	30mg/dose every 3-4 hrs.
	IM	30-60mg/dose every 3-4 hrs.
Obstetrics	IV	20mg/dose when contractions are regular; repeat every 2-3 hrs. for 2-3 doses as needed.
	IM	30mg/dose when contractions are regular.

Adjust dosage in patients with hepatic impairment.

PHARMACOKINETICS: Onset: oral: 15-30 min; IM: 15-20 min; IV: 2-3 min; Peak analgesia: oral: 1-3 hrs; IM: 1 hr; IV: 15 min; Duration: oral: 3 hrs or longer; IM: 2 hrs; IV: 1 hr.

ADVERSE EFFECTS: The most serious effect is respiratory depression. Naloxone may be used to reverse this effect. Nausea, vomiting, dizziness, and sedation may occur.

May cause respiratory depression of neonates when given during labor and delivery. Addicting. Pentazocine has significant abuse potential; the oral form has been crushed and administered IV in combination with the antihistamine tripelennamine ("blue velvet"); this combination is known as "T's and blues." The addition of naloxone to the tablets has no effect when administered orally, but will precipitate withdrawal symptoms in opiate dependent persons if given IV, eliminating the IV abuse potential. Oral abuse is still possible.

PENTOBARBITAL
(Nembutal)

USES: Pentobarbital is a **barbiturate;** uses are given in the next Table:

Uses of Pentobarbital
Hypnotic in short-term treatment of **insomnia** for 2 weeks
Preoperatively to relieve **anxiety** and provide **sedation**
Routine **sedation**
Status epilepticus
Acute seizure disorders resulting from meningitis, poison, eclampsia, alcohol withdrawal, tetanus or chorea
Basal hypnosis for general, spinal or regional anesthesia
Facilitate **intubation** procedures
Control acute episodes of **agitated behavior** in **psychoses**
Used to **withdraw barbiturates** or **nonbarbiturate hypnotics** in patients who are physically dependent on these drugs
Induce **coma** in management of **cerebral ischemia** and increased intracranial pressure.

DOSAGE FORMS: Elixir: 18.2mg/5ml; Caps: 50, 100mg; Injection: 50mg/ml; Suppositories: 30, 60, 120, 200mg.

DOSAGE: Pentobarbital is administered orally; pentobarbital sodium may be administered orally, rectally, or by deep IM or slow IV injection. The dosage of pentobarbital is given in the next Table:

Dosage of Pentobarbital

Condition	Age	Route	Dosage
Hypnotic	(Give drug at bedtime; do not give drug for more than 2 weeks.)		
	Adult	Oral	100-200mg at bedtime
	Adult	Rectal	120-200mg at bedtime
	Adult	IM	150-200mg
	Children	IM	2-6mg/kg, max. 100mg
	2mos.-1yr	Rectal,Oral	30mg
	1-4 yrs	Rectal,Oral	30-60mg
	5-12 yrs	Rectal,Oral	60mg
	12-14 yrs	Rectal,Oral	60-120mg
Sedation	Adults	Oral,Rectal	20-40mg, 2-4 times daily
	Children	Oral Rectal	2-6mg/kg, daily, max. 100mg daily 3 divided doses
Preanesthetic Medication	Adults	IM	150-200mg
	Children	IM	Pentobarbital sodium may be administered IM to children as a preanesthetic medication, although rectal or oral administration is preferred. Dose: 2-6mg/kg
		Rectal,Oral	2-6mg/kg; max 100mg.
Seizures	Adults	IV Slowly	100mg initially; one min. is required for effect of drug; additional small doses may be administered up to a total of 200-500mg for adults.
	Children	IV Slowly	50mg initially
Barbiturate Coma	Adults Children	IV	Initially: 3-5mg/kg IV once; Maintenance: 2-3.5mg/kg/hr by continuous infusion or as intermittent bolus on an hourly basis Maintain levels 25-40 micrograms/ml.

Dosage should be reduced in geriatrics, debilitated patients and patients with hepatic dysfunction.

Withdrawal of Barbituates or Nonbarbituates: A stabilizing dose is established and then reduced by no more than 100mg/day. If withdrawal symptoms reappear, maintain or increase dosage. Severely dependent patients can usually be withdrawn from barbiturates in 14-21 days.

PHARMACOKINETICS: Onset: oral, rectal: 15-60 min; IM: 10-25 min; IV: 1 min; Duration: oral, rectal: 1-4 hrs; IV: 15 min.

ADVERSE EFFECTS: Acute Toxicity: CNS depression; respiratory depression; shock syndrome; congestive heart failure; cardiac arrhythmias.

PENTOXIFYLLINE
(Trental)

USES: Pentoxifylline is used for the treatment of **intermittent claudication** associated with chronic occlusive peripheral arterial disease; it is thought that pentoxifylline improves oxygenation of ischemic tissues by decreasing blood viscosity.

Pentoxifylline is not recommended for treatment of severe arterial obstructive disease manifested by pain at rest, ischemic skin ulcers, and/or gangrene.

Mechanism of Action: Pentoxifylline causes an increase in erythrocyte flexibility, inhibition of platelet aggregation, a reduction in plasma fibrinogen levels and an increase in the concentraton of cyclic adenosine monophosphate (cAMP) and adenosine triphosphate (ATP) in erythrocytes. Pentoxifylline decreases blood viscosity and thus apparently improves oxygenation of ischemic tissues.

DOSAGE FORMS: Tablets (timed-release) 400mg.

DOSAGE: Adults, 400mg three times daily with food; continue for at least 8 weeks if a beneficial effect is not apparent during the first few weeks of treatment. If GI or CNS side effects develop, dosage should be reduced to 400mg twice daily.

ADVERSE EFFECTS: Adverse effects usually involve the GI tract. Nausea and dyspepsia are the most common side effects; their incidence is reduced by giving the drug with food. Other GI effects include flatulence, anorexia and vomiting.

Adverse effects also involve the CNS and the cardiovascular system. CNS effects include dizziness, headache, flushing, nervousness, insomnia, drowsiness, anxiety and confusion. Cardiovascular symptoms include palpitations, angina, arrhythmias, hypotension, dyspnea and edema. Overdose is associated with loss of consciousness, fever, agitation, and convulsions.

Other adverse effects include blurred vision, rash, pruritis, urticaria, dry mouth and nasal congestion.

PEPTIC ULCER, THERAPY

Guidelines: Guidelines for therapeutic management of uncomplicated peptic ulcers are illustrated in the next Figure (Drug Evaluations, AMA, Chicago, ILL., 6th ed., 1986, pgs. 937-940):

Guidelines for Therapeutic Management of Uncomplicated Peptic Ulcers

Discontinue All Ulcerogenic Drugs and Cigarette Smoking

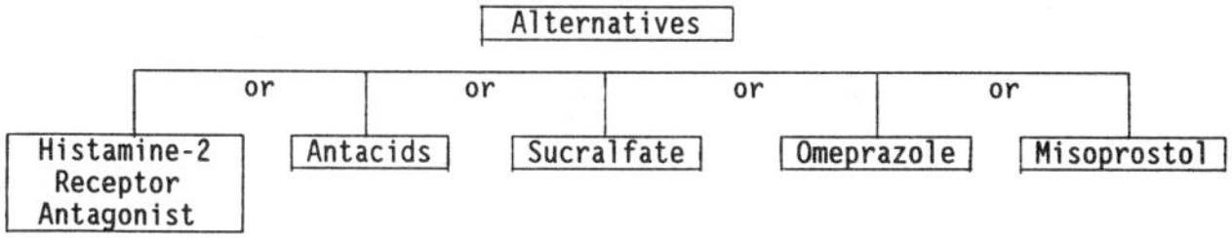

Cimetidine (Tagamet)
or Ranitidine (Zantac)
or Famotidine (Pepcid)
or Nizatidine (Axid)

Treat for 4-6 weeks in patients with duodenal ulcer.
Treat for 8-12 weeks in patients with gastric ulcer.

Nonsteroidal anti-inflammatory drugs are frequently implicated as ulcerogenic drugs (Review: Soll, A.H. moderator, "Nonsteroidal Anti-inflammatory Drugs and Peptic Ulcer Disease," Ann. Intern. Med. 114, 307-319, 1991).

HISTAMINE H_2 RECEPTOR ANTAGONISTS: Some of the uses of histamine-2 receptor antagonists are given in the next Table:

Uses of Histamine-2 Receptor Antagonists

- Active Gastric and Duodenal Ulcers
- Prophylaxis against Recurrence of Duodenal Ulcers
- Stress Ulcer Prophylaxis
- Esophageal Reflux

The H_2 receptor antagonists are used to treat active duodenal ulcer and for maintenance therapy after healing. The H_2 receptor antagonists block the production of acid by the parietal cell and produce gastric luminal anacidity for varying periods throughout 24 hours. The H_2 receptor antagonists are given in the next Table (Medical Letter 30, 77-78, Aug. 12, 1988):

H_2 Receptor Antagonists (Once Daily at Bedtime)

Drug (Trade) Name	Treatment Dosage (mg)	Maintenance Dosage (mg)
Cimetidine (Tagamet)	800	400
Ranitidine (Zantac)	300	150
Famotidine (Pepcid)	40	20
Nizatidine (Axid)	300	150

Cost: The range of the cost to the pharmacist for 30 days treatment varies from $54 (for cimetidine) to $59 for famotidine; the range of the cost to the pharmacist for 30 days maintenance therapy varies from $28 (for cimetidine) to $33 for ranitidine.

Efficacy: The H_2 receptor antagonists have similar healing rates for treatment of duodenal ulcers and for maintenance therapy.

PEPTIC ULCER, THERAPY (Cont.)
Pharmacokinetics: Famotidine has the longest elimination half-life; extended dosing may be possible as compared to the other H_2 receptor antagonists. All of the antagonists are excreted primarily unchanged by the kidneys, necessitating dosing alteration in patients with renal impairment.
Adverse Effects: Overall, the incidence for adverse effects of the H_2 receptor antagonists is 2 to 3% (see individual drugs).
Drug Interactions: Cimetidine interferes with the hepatic metabolism of theophylline, warfarin, phenytoin, lidocaine and certain benzodiazepines (Worden, J., personal communication); these substances can accumulate in toxic amounts. Cimetidine binds to and thus inhibits the P-450 hepatic microsomal oxidase system. This is especially important in the cases of drugs with narrow therapeutic ranges, such as theophylline.

Cimetidine delays the clearance of lidocaine via reduction of hepatic blood flow.

Cimetidine can elevate procainamide concentrations via reduction in renal tubular secretion.

Ranitidine, with only one tenth the affinity of cimetidine for the P-450 enzymes, is much less likely to interfere with the hepatic metabolism of drugs. However, there is a report of three elderly patients who had been receiving theophylline for a prolonged time for treatment of chronic obstructive pulmonary disease and subsequently developed symptoms of peptic ulcers treated with ranitidine; all three developed symptoms of theophylline toxicity with nausea, vomiting, anorexia, abdominal pain and tremulousness (Roy, A. et al., Am. J. Med. 85, 525, 1988).

Famitidine and nizatidine apparently do not interfere with hepatic metabolism of drugs.
Dosing: For active peptic ulcers, ranitidine, famotidine and nizatidine may be taken twice daily while cimetidine is taken four times daily.
Mechanism of Action: The basolateral surface of the gastric parietal cell contains receptors for histamine, muscarine, and possibly gastrin that stimulate the cell to produce acid. These agents, histamine, muscarine, and possibly gastrin, are blocked by the H_2 antagonists (cimetidine, ranitidine, famotidine and nizatidine)and antimuscarinic agents(atropine and pirenzepine). The apical mucosal surface of the parietal secretes acid.
ANTACIDS: The antacids are aluminum, calcium and magnesium salts that neutralize hydrochloric acid. Adequate doses increase gastric pH to 5.0 or more; at this pH, pepsin activity is decreased. Antacids given in sufficient quantity heal duodenal ulcers at a rate comparable to that obtained with H_2 antagonist drugs (Lauritsen, K. et al., Scand. J. Gastroenterol. 20, 123-128, 1985); gastric ulcers may be more resistant.

A neutralizing capacity of 200mmol hydrochloric acid daily is effective in treating most patients with peptic ulceration. However, adverse effects that reduce compliance may occur at dosages required for effective treatment.

Antacids that are commonly used to treat peptic ulcers are given in the next Table:

Antacids Used to Treat Peptic Ulcer

Antacid	Acid Neutralizing Capacity mmol/Tablet	mmol/5ml
Aluminum Hydroxide		
Alterna Gel		12
Amphojel	9.0(300mg tablet)	
Aluminum Hydroxide with Magnesium Hydroxide		
Maalox	8.5 (#1 tablet)	13.5
Maalox Therapeutic conc.(TC)		28.3
Aluminum Hydroxide with Magnesium Hydroxide and Simethicone		
Di-Gel		12.3
Gelusil	11.0	12.0
Gelusil II	21.0	24.0
Maalox Plus	8.5	13.5
Mylanta	11.5	12.7
Mylanta II	23.0	25.4
Calcium Carbonate with Glycine		
Titralac	7.5	19.0
Magaldrate (A Comlex of Aluminum and Magnesium Hydroxides)		
Riopan and Riopan Plus	13.5	15

PEPTIC ULCER, THERAPY (Cont.)

Simethicone is a combination of dimethylpolysiloxanes and silica gel; it has an antifoaming action.

The acid neutralizing capacity of tablets vary from 7.5 to 23mmol/tablet and would require 9 tablets to 27 tablets daily to attain a level of 200mmol neutralizing capacity. The liquid formulation is preferred in patients with duodenal ulcer who would require a large number of tablets daily. The acid neutralizing capacity varies from 12 to 28.3mmol/5ml or about 40 to 85ml daily to attain a level of 200mmol neutralizing capacity.

Adverse effects of magnesium-containing antacids include diarrhea and hypermagnesemia in renal failure patients. Adverse effects of aluminum-containing antacids include constipation, osteomalacia, hypophosphatemia, and aluminum intoxication.

SUCRALFATE: Sucralfate is an amionic sulfated disaccharide that binds to the surface of gastric and duodenal ulcers; sucralfate inhibits the action of pepsin, acid and bile, which allows the ulcer to heal. Sucralfate is not absorbed and provides local protection at the ulcer site. Although data is limited, sucralfate is effective for acute therapy of gastric and duodenal ulcers, prophylaxis of duodenal ulcers, and possibly prophylaxis of gastric ulcers and stress ulceration. The dosage is 1g 4 times daily. See also **SUCRALFATE** section.

OMEPRAZOLE: Omeprazole (Prilosec) is an inhibitor of H^+, K^+-ATPase or "proton pump" on the secretory surface of the parietal cell. Acid secretion is inhibited in its final step. Omeprazole is the most effective inhibitor of acid secretion available. Omeprazole is effective therapy for gastric and duodenal ulcers, reflux esophagitis, and pathologic hypersecretory conditions. Dosage in peptic ulcer therapy is 20-40mg once daily. Adverse effects include multiple drug interactions, since omeprazole interacts with cytochrome P-450. See also **OMEPRAZOLE** section.

MISOPROSTOL: Misoprostol (Cytotec) is a synthetic prostaglandin E_1 analogue with gastric antisecretory effects. Misoprostol is used for acute treatment of gastric ulcers, particularly in patients on NSAID's. Misoprostol appears to be less effective than H_2 receptor antagonists in the treatment of duodenal ulcers. Dosage is 200 micrograms 4 times daily. Adverse effects are primarily gastrointestinal. See also **MISOPROSTOL** section.

PERITONEUM, PATHOGENS, TREATMENT

PATHOGENS: The pathogens that cause spontaneous bacterial peritonitis are given in the next Table (Runyon, B.A., Emergency Med. Reports 9, No. 3, 17-24, Feb. 1, 1988; Hoefs, J.C. and Runyon, B.A., Disease-a-Month 31,(9) 1, 1985):

Pathogens that Cause Infection of the Peritoneum

Pathogen	Percent
Escherichia coli	43%
Klebsiella pneumoniae	8%
Streptococcus pneumoniae	8%
Alpha-hemolytic streptococcus	5%
Group D streptococcus	5%
Unclassified streptococcus	4%
Beta-hemolytic streptococcus	4%
Enterobacteriaceae	3%
Pseudomonas	2%
Staphylococcus aureus	2%
Miscellaneous, including Haemphilus and Pasturella, and Neisseria	16%
Single organism	90%
Multiple organism	10%

Spontaneous bacterial peritonitis is usually caused by a single organism that is derived from the intestines. *E. coli* is the most common bacteria; enteric bacteria are two-thirds of hospital acquired spontaneous bacterial peritonitis (Pinzetto, G.et al., Hepatology 3, 545, 1983) Streptococci account for 26% of the cases. Anaerobes account for 6% of cases.

TREATMENT: The drug of choice is cefotaxime, a third generation cephalosporin with activity against both gram-negative enteric bacteria and gram-positive bacteria; the dosage of cefotaxime is 2g IV every 6-8 hours(Felisart, J.et al.,Hepatology 5, 457, 1985).

If the patient is allergic to cephalosporins, use an aminoglycoside, such as gentamicin or tobramycin. The loading dose is 1.5-1.75mg/kg; the dose and frequency of subsequent treatment depends on patient's renal function and serum levels (Felisart, J. et al, Hepatology 5, 457, 1985).

PHARYNGITIS, PATHOGENS, TREATMENT

Pathogens: The pathogens that cause pharyngitis are given in the next Table (Edson, R.S., Diagnosis, pgs. 85-89, Feb. 1986; Todd, J.K., Infect. Dis. Clin. North Am. 2, 149-162, 1988):

Causative Organisms in Acute Pharyngitis
Bacteria:
Streptococcus pyogenes (Group A)
Neisseria gonorrhoeae
Mixed anaerobes (Vincent's angina)
Mycoplasma pneumoniae
Chlamydia trachomatis
Francisella tularensis (cause of Tularemia)
Corynebacterium diphtheriae
Yeast:
Candida albicans
Viral:
Epstein-Barr virus (EBV)
Rhinovirus; Adenovirus; Coronavirus; Herpes simplex, Coxsackievirus A, Influenza; Parainfluenza

For most patients, pharyngitis is likely to be caused by the group A streptococcus or by viruses.

Streptococcus Pyogenes (Group A): The most common cause of acute bacterial pharyngitis is Streptococcus pyogenes, group A; sequalae of Group A streptococcal infections are acute rheumatic fever and acute glomerulonephritis. There has been a marked decline in morbidity and mortality from rheumatic fever in the United States due to early diagnosis and treatment of Group A streptococcal pharyngitis with penicillin (Massell, B.F. et al., N. Engl. J. Med. 318, 280-286, 1988). However, there has been a resurgence of rheumatic fever in several areas of the United States (Veasy, L.G. et al., N. Engl. J. Med. 316, 421-427, 1987).

Neisseria Gonorrhoeae: Neisseria gonorrhoeae can be found in the throats of patients known to participate in oral-genital sexual practices (Hutt, D.M., Judson, F.N., Ann. Int. Med. 104, 655-658, 1986). Patients with known genital gonococcal infection may have infection of the pharynx but are asymptomatic.

Mixed Anaerobes (Vincent's Angina): Angina is derived from Latin (angere means to strangle). Anaerobes can cause pharyngitis.

Mycoplasma Pneumoniae: Mycoplasma pneumoniae can be isolated from patients with pharyngitis but usually is associated with more prominent lower respiratory tract signs.

Chlamydia Trachomatis: Chlamydia trachomatis has been isolated from some patients with pharyngitis. However, chlamydia trachomatis may be found in asymptomatic patients.

Francisella Tularensis: Francisella tularensis causes tularemia; it may present as pharyngitis associated with pharyngeal ulcers and cervical lymph mode inflammation. It is very rare. Infection is usually transmitted from wild animals or exposure in a laboratory.

Corynebacteria: Corynebacterium diphtheriae rarely occurs in the United States because of our immunization program. It causes membranous pharyngitis that can lead to clinical diphtheria.

Candida Albicans: Candida albicans is a yeast that can cause a sore throat and esophagitis usually in immunosuppressed patients, e g., patients with AIDS, or those on steroids or antibiotics.; thrush refers to an infection of the mucous membranes of the mouth caused by Candida albicans.

Viruses: Epstein-Barr virus (EBV) is the cause of the infectious mononucleosis syndrome characterized by pharyngitis, symmetrical cervical lymphadenopathy and malaise. Many other viruses may cause pharyngitis, including rhinovirus, adenovirus, coronavirus, herpes simplex, coxsackie virus A, influenza, and parainfluenza.

PHARYNGITIS, PATHOGENS, TREATMENT (Cont.)

Treatment of Acute Streptococcal Pharyngitis: Treatment of acute streptococcal pharyngitis is given in the next Table(Bass, J.W., JAMA 256, 740-743, 1986; Todd, J.K., Infect. Dis. Clin. North Am. 2, 149-162, 1988; Dajani, A.S. et al., Pediatr. Infect. Dis. J. 8, 263-266, 1989):

Treatment of Acute Streptococcal Pharyngitis

Antibiotic	Route	Dosage
Penicillin V	Oral	250mg, 3 times daily for ten days
Erythromycin estolate	Oral	20-40mg/kg daily in 2-4 divided doses Adults: 1 gram daily for 10 days.
Erythromycin ethylsuccinate	Oral	40-50mg/kg daily in 2-4 divided doses for 10 days. Adults: 1 gram daily for 10 days.
Penicillin G benzathine	IM (1 dose)	<14kg, 300,000 units; 14-27kg, 600,000 units; 27-41kg, 900,000 units; >41kg, 1,200,000 units.
Combination: 900,000 units of pen G benzathine and 300,000 units of pen G procaine in 2 ml.	IM (1 dose)	<14kg, 0.66ml; 14-27kg, 1.33ml; >27kg, 2ml.

Erythromycin is used in those patients who are allergic to penicillin.

The antibiotics, tetracycline and trimethoprim-sulfamethoxazole are not effective treatments for acute streptococcal disease.

Treatment of Acute Viral Pharyngitis: Of the viral infections, only infection with herpes simplex is amenable to therapy. Acyclovir is the recommended antibiotic.

Prophylaxis for Rheumatic Fever: Prevention regimens for rheumatic fever are given in the next Table (Todd, J.K., Infect. Dis. Clin. North America 2, 149-162, 1988):

Prophylaxis for Rheumatic Fever

Antibiotic	Route	Duration	Dosage
Penicillin G benzathine	IM	3-4wks	Children: 1,200,000 units Adults: 1,200,000 units
Penicillin V	Oral	Daily	Children: <60lb (27kg), 125mg twice daily. Adults: 250mg twice daily.
Sulfadiazine	Oral	Daily	Children: 500mg <60lbs. 1g. >60lbs. once daily Adults: 500mg once daily.

PHENAZOPYRIDINE

(Geridium, Pyridiate, Pyridium, Urodine)

USES: Phenazopyridine is used for the symptomatic relief of pain, burning, urgency, frequency, and other discomforts resulting from irritation of the lower urinary tract mucosa caused by infection, trauma, surgery, endoscopic procedures or the passage of sounds or catheters.

DOSAGE FORMS: Tabs: 100, 200mg

DOSAGE: Phenazopyridine is administered orally after meals; dosage is given in the next Table:

Dosage of Phenazopyridine

Patient	Dosage
Adult	200mg, 3 times daily
Children(6-12 yrs)	12mg/kg daily, given in 3 divided doses

The drug is discontinued when pain and discomfort are relieved, usually after 3-15 days.

ADVERSE EFFECTS: Headache, vertigo, mild GI disturbances; rarely, methemoglobinemia, hemolytic anemia, skin pigmentation, and transient acute renal failure have occurred. Colors urine orange; stains clothing.

PHENOBARBITAL
(Barbita, Luminal, Solfoton)

USES: Phenobarbital is a barbiturate; uses are given in the next Table:

Uses of Phenobarbital
Anticonvulsant - Generalized tonic-clonic seizures and partial seizures
Sedation
Preanesthetic medication - relieves anxiety and provides sedation
Barbiturate and other nonbenzodiazepine withdrawal syndromes in dependent individuals
Hyperbilirubinemia: neonates, congenital nonhemolytic unconjugated hyperbilirubinemia (Gilbert's Syndrome) chronic intrahepatic cholestasis

Anticonvulsant: Phenobarbital is effective for the treatment of generalized tonic-clonic and simple partial (with motor or somatosensory symptoms) seizures. Ease of absorption has made phenobarbital the drug of choice for seizures in infants but effects on cognitive functions have led to decreased use for older children and adults.

Sedation: Phenobarbital is used occasionally as a daytime sedative or for mild anxiety.

Hyperbilirubinemia: Phenobarbital decreases serum bilirubin and is used to lower bilirubin levels in hyperbilirubinemia states.

Mechanism of Action: Phenobarbital, like other barbiturates, is believed to facilitate inhibitory neurotransmission in the central nervous system; it presumably interacts with proteins of the gamma-aminobutyric acid (GABA) chloride ionophore complex to open chloride ion channels and hyperpolarize neuronal membranes.

DOSAGE FORMS: Tabs: 8, 15, 16, 30, 32, 60, 65, 100mg; Elixir: 15mg/5ml, 20mg/5ml; Vials: 30, 60, 65, 130mg/ml; Caps: 16mg.

DOSAGE: Phenobarbital is administered orally; phenobarbital sodium is administered by subcutaneous, IM, or slow IV; IV should be used only for emergency situations such as acute seizures. Dosage of phenobarbital is given in the next Table:

Dosage of Phenobarbital

Condition	Age	Route	Dosage
Sedation		Oral, IM, IV	2-3mg/kg/dose, every 8 hours as needed
Anticonvulsant Maintenance	Neonate	Oral, IM, IV	Initially, 2-4mg/kg daily in 1 or 2 doses for 2 weeks then 5mg/kg daily in 1 or 2 doses
	Infant	Oral, IM, IV	5-8mg/kg daily in 1 or 2 doses
	Children	Oral, IM, IV	3-5mg/kg daily in 1 or 2 doses
	Adults	Oral, IM, IV	100-300mg/day in 1 or 2 doses (1-3mg/kg/day)
Status Epilepticus	Adults	IM, Slow IV	300-800mg initially, then 120-240mg every 20 minutes; max. rate of IV infusion: 60mg/min usual max. dose: 1-2gm.
	Children	IM, Slow IV	10-20mg initially, then 5-10mg/kg/dose every 20 min.; max. rate of IV infusion: 1mg/kg/min; usual max. dose: 40mg/kg.

ADVERSE EFFECTS: At serum levels greater than 30 microgram/ml, side effects may be observed; at serum levels greater than 60 microgram/ml, toxicity is observed.

May cause respiratory depression, especially with rapid IV administration or with concomitant administration of other anticonvulsants.

Sedation and behavior disturbances including hyperactivity, loss of concentration, and depression are the principal adverse effects (Brent, D.A. et al., Pediatrics 80, 909, 1987). Paradoxical excitement and hyperactivity are more common in children and the elderly. Occasionally, skin rashes, disturbances in motor function (ataxia) and megaloblastic anemia may occur.

PHENOBARBITAL (Cont.)
With acute toxicity, CNS depression, respiratory depression, shock syndrome, congestive heart failure and cardiac arrhythmias may develop.
Rarely, Stevens-Johnson syndrome, exfoliative dermatitis, photosensitivity, hepatitis and jaundice have been reported.
PHARMACOKINETICS: Absorption (Oral): 80%; Peak: 6-18 hours; Therapeutic: 15-40mcg/ml (Adults); 15-30mcg/ml (Infants and Children); Toxic: >60mcg/ml; Onset: IV: 5 min; Max. effect (IV): 30 min.; Half-Life: 50-120 hours (Adults); 40-70 hours (Children); Metabolism: Hepatic metabolism to inactive metabolites; Excretion: Approximately 25% of the dose is excreted unchanged in the urine.
CONTRAINDICATIONS: Acute intermittent porphyria; abrupt withdrawal of therapy may exacerbate seizures; respiratory disease when dyspnea or obstruction is present; marked renal impairment.
DRUG INTERACTIONS: Drug interactions are given in the next Table:

Drug Interactions of Phenobarbital

Drug	Comment
Phenytoin	Phenobarbital may either increase or decrease the serum concentration of phenytoin; phenytoin's effect on phenobarbital is variable.
Valproic Acid	Valproic acid increases the serum conc. of phenobarbital
Folic Acid and Carbamazepine	These drugs decrease the serum conc. of phenobarbital
Oral Anticoagulants, Oral Contraceptives, Griseofulvin, Quinidine, Chloramphenicol, Rifampin, Tetracycline	Phenobarbital induces cytochrome P-450 enzymes.
Other Sedative Drugs	Additive Effect.

PARAMETERS TO MONITOR: Plasma levels should be monitored after steady state is achieved. Plasma levels should be obtained any time toxicity is suspected.
When patients receive a loading dose, level may be checked the following day or sooner if necessary.
Blood specimen monitoring schedule is given in the next Table:

Blood Specimen Monitoring for Phenobarbital

Age	Blood Monitoring
Newborns	Frequent because the liver of the neonate metabolizes phenobarbital slowly during the first 4 weeks of life.
Children	Monitor in 10-15 days after starting therapy; then monitor every 3 to 4 months.
Adults:	Monitor in 15-25 days.

Therapeutic monitoring should be done just prior to the next dose; a random specimen will also yield useful information since this drug has a long half-life. Monitoring should be for the following patients: poorly controlled, toxic symptoms, change of medication or dosage allowing 2 to 3 weeks for new steady state and when drugs, such as primidone and mephobarbital, are given. These latter drugs are metabolized to phenobarbital.
Specimen: Red top tube, separate serum; or green (heparin) top tube, separate plasma.

PHENYLEPHRINE

(Neo-Synephrine, Others)

USES: **Phenylephrine** is a **sympathomimetic agent** with primarily **alpha-adrenergic (vasoconstrictor) properties;** uses are given in the next Table:

Uses of Phenylephrine

Hypotension Due to Shock or Spinal Anesthesia
Paroxysmal Supraventricular Tachycardia
Topical Decongestant
Ophthalmic Uses: Causes Mydriasis, Treats Conjunctival Erythema

Phenylephrine causes vasoconstriction directly by stimulation of alpha-adrenergic receptors and indirectly by release of endogenous norepinephrine. Total peripheral resistance is increased resulting in increased systolic and diastolic blood pressure. Vasoconstriction occurs in multiple sites, including coronary, pulmonary, renal and cerebral blood vessels; increased blood pressure may overcome these effects and result in improved organ perfusion. Phenylephrine is particularly useful when treating hypotension during anesthesia; many anesthetic agents sensitize the myocardium to arrhythmias and phenylephrine does not stimulate the myocardium.

Phenylephrine has minimal effects on beta 1-adrenergic receptors in the heart, however, alpha-adrenergic stimulation leads to reflex bradycardia due to increased vagal activity. Reflex bradycardia may terminate episodes of paroxysmal supraventricular tachycardia in some patients.

Phenylephrine is effective as a topical decongestant due to local vasoconstriction. Phenylephrine may be useful in acute situations, but it has a short duration of action and rebound congestion occurs frequently.

Phenylephrine applied to the conjunctiva results in pupillary dilatation (mydriasis) due to contraction of the dilator muscle of the pupil. Phenylephrine causes constriction of the arterioles in the conjunctiva and is used to treat conjunctival erythema secondary to mild irritation.

DOSAGE FORMS: Injection: 10mg/ml (1%); Nasal Solution: 0.125, 0.16, 0.2, 0.25, 0.5, 1%; Ophthalmic Solution: 0.12, 2.5, 10%.

DOSAGE: Dosage of phenylephrine is given in the following Table:

Dosage of Phenylephrine

Condition	Age	Route	Dosage
Mild-Mod Hypotension	Adult	Subcut., IM	Usual: 2-5mg; Range: 1-10mg; repeat every 1-2 hours as needed.
		Slow IV	Usual: 0.2mg; Range: 0.1-0.5mg, repeat every 10-15 minutes as needed.
	Children	Subcut., IM	Usual: 0.1mg/kg; repeat every 1-2 hrs. as needed.
		Slow IV	5-20 micrograms/kg; repeat every 10-15 minutes as needed.
Severe Hypotension	Adult	IV drip	Initially, 0.1-0.18mg/min (1-3micrograms/kg/min); After b.p. stabilizes, 0.04-0.06mg/min (0.5-1.0micrograms/kg/min); Titrate to effect.
	Children	IV drip	Usual range: 0.1-0.5micrograms/kg/min; Titrate to effect.
Paroxysmal Supraventricular Tachycardia	Adult	IV over 20-30 sec.	0.25-1.0mg; repeat dose in 5 min. if no effect; max. single dose: 2mg.
	Children	IV over 20-30 sec.	5-10micrograms/kg/dose; repeat dose in 5 minutes if no effect.
Nasal Decongestant	Adult	Topical Nasal	0.25-1% sol'n 2-3 drops or sprays every 3-4 hours; Max. 3 days.
	Children	Topical Nasal	0.25% sol'n 2-3 drops or sprays every 3-4 hours; Max. 3 days.
	Infants	Topical Nasal	0.125% sol'n 2-3 drops or sprays every 3-4 hours; Max. 3 days.
Pupillary Dilatation	Adult Children	Topical Eye	2.5% sol'n 1-2 drops in each eye 15 min. prior to exam.

PHARMACOKINETICS: Onset: Subcutaneous or IM, 10-15 min.; IV, immediate; Duration of Action: Subcutaneous, 50-60 min.; IM, 1-2 hrs.; IV, 15-20 min.; Metabolism: Liver and intestine by monoamine oxidase (MAO).

ADVERSE EFFECTS: Cardiovascular: Hypertension, severe reflex bradycardia leading to decreased cardiac output, increased cardiac work, increased pulmonary artery pressure; CNS: restlessness, anxiety, nervousness, dizziness; Renal: decreased perfusion and urine output.

PRECAUTIONS: Myocardial or coronary artery disease, bradycardia or heart block, hypertension, geriatric patients, hyperthyroidism.

PHENYLPROPANOLAMINE

(Acutrim, Control, Dexatrim, Others; Many Combination Preparations)

USES: **Phenylpropanolamine** hydrochloride is a **sympathomimetic agent**; uses are given in the following Table:

Uses of Phenylpropanolamine
Relieves Nasal Congestion
Treatment of Obesity

Phenylpropanolamine is used to treat nasal congestion associated with upper respiratory tract infections, allergic rhinitis, and other causes of acute and chronic rhinitis. Prolonged use may lead to tachyphylaxis. Multiple preparations available over-the-counter combine phenylpropanolamine with antitussive, expectorant, analgesic-antipyretic, or antihistamines.

Phenylpropanolamine is also used as an adjunct to diet in patients who wish to lose weight. Phenylpropanolamine is related to amphetamine and has some anorexigenic effects; beneficial effects tend to be minimal and tolerance develops.

DOSAGE FORMS: Caps(extended release): 37.5, 50, 75mg; Tabs: 25, 37.5, 50mg; Tabs(extended release): 75mg; Gum: 8.33mg; Combination preparations: numerous.

DOSAGE: Phenylpropanolamine is administered orally; dosage is given in the next Table:

Dosage of Phenylpropanolamine

Condition	Age	Dosage
Nasal Congestion	Adult	20-25mg every 4 hours or 75mg of extended release preparation every 12 hours; Maximum 150mg daily.
	Children	
	6-12 yrs	10-12.5mg every 4 hours; Max. 75mg daily.
	2-6 yrs	6.25mg every 4 hours; Max. 37.5mg daily.
Obesity	Adult	25mg 3 times daily or 37.5mg twice daily or 50-75mg of extended release preparation once daily.

ADVERSE EFFECTS: CNS: Stimulation with nervousness, restlessness, insomnia, headache; Cardiovascular: severe hypertension, arrhythmias (PAC's or PVC's).

PRECAUTIONS: Hyperthyroidism, cardiovascular disease, hypertension, diabetes mellitus, glaucoma, prostatic hypertrophy.

PHENYLPROPANOLAMINE, CLEMASTINE

(Tavist-D)

USES: Tavist-D is commonly used for rhinitis or the common cold. Tavist-D has two components, **phenylpropanolamine**, a **decongestant** and **clemastine**, an **antihistamine**.

DOSAGE FORMS: Each tablet contains phenylpropanolamine, 75mg and clemastine, 1.34mg.

DOSAGE: One tablet every 12 hours; not recommended for children.

ADVERSE EFFECTS: Drowsiness, sedation, anticholinergic effects, eg, dry mouth, blurred vision, urinary retention, GI upset, dizziness, anxiety, weakness, lightheadedness, insomnia, thickening of bronchial secretions, hypotension, arrhythmias, respiratory depression or difficulty, palpitations, blood dyscrasias.

CONTRAINDICATIONS: Severe hypertension, coronary artery disease, bronchospasm, glaucoma, GI or urinary obstruction, lactation.

PRECAUTIONS: Hypertension, angina, urinary retention, thyroid disease, diabetes, history of bronchospasm, pregnancy.

PHENYTOIN

(Dilantin)

USES: Phenytoin is an **anticovulsant;** uses are given in the next Table:

Uses of Phenytoin

Seizures:
- Tonic-Clonic (Grand Mal) Seizures
- Partial Seizures with Complex Symptomatology (Psychomotor Seizures)
- Prevention and Treatment of Seizures Occurring During Neurosurgery
- Status Epilepticus

Cardiac Arrhythmias:
- Arrhythmias caused by Digitalis Intoxication
- Ventricular Tachycardia
- Paroxysmal Atrial Tachycardia

Phenytoin is used mainly in the prophylactic management of tonic-clonic (grand mal) seizures and partial seizures with complex symptomatology (psychomotor seizures).

Phenytoin is not recommended for the treatment of pure absence (petit mal) seizures since the drug may increase the frequency of these seizures; however, phenytoin may be useful in conjunction with succinimide or oxazolidinedione anticonvulsants in the management of combined absence and tonic-clonic seizures.

The usefulness of phenytoin in the treatment of status epilepticus is limited by the need for slow administration and its slow onset of action. Diazepam is the drug of choice for termination of status epilepticus; however, concurrent IV phenytoin and diazepam is considered the treatment of choice for status epilepticus by some clinicans.

Most clinicians consider IV phenytoin sodium to be the **drug of choice** in the treatment of **arrhythmias** caused by **digitalis intoxication.**

DOSAGE FORMS: Caps: 30, 100mg; Caps(extended) 30, 100mg; Tabs(chewable): 50mg; Susp.: 30mg/5ml, 125mg/5ml; Parenteral: 50mg/ml

DOSAGE: Phenytoin and its sodium salt are administered orally; the sodium salt may also be administered by direct IV injection. IV preparation of phenytoin has a pH of 12 - it is extremely caustic to veins. Extravasation may cause ischemia or gangrene. Phenytoin should be given in a large vein (eg, antecubital) and well diluted. It should not be given intramuscularly. The dosage of phenytoin in different conditions is given in the next Table:

Dosage of Phenytoin

Condition	Age	Route	Dosage
Anticonvulsant Maintenance	Adult	Oral	100mg, 3 times daily; once-daily dosing with 300mg as extended phenytoin sodium capsules; 5-10 days to achieve full anticonvulsant effects. Daily dosage may be gradually increased in increments of 100mg every 2-4 wks Max. dose is 300-600mg daily.
	Children	Oral	5mg/kg daily in 2 or 3 divided doses. Max. dose is 300mg daily. Range: 4-8mg/kg daily.
Prophylaxis Seizures During Neurosurgery	Adult	IV	100-200mg, at 4-hour intervals during surgery and the immediate post-op period.
Status Epilepticus	Adult	IV	15-18mg/kg rate not exceeding 50mg/min; in geriatric patients with heart disease, rate 50mg over 2-3 min. Max. dose: 1.5gm/day.
	Children		15-20mg/kg: Rate: 0.5-1.5mg/kg/min.
Arrhythmias caused by Digitalis Intox.; Ventricular Tachycardia; Paroxysmal Atrial Tachycardia	Adult	IV	100mg, phenytoin sodium, at 5-minute intervals until arrhythmia is abolished or adverse effects appear or until total dose of 1g is given.
		Oral	100mg, 2-4 times daily.
	Children	IV	2-4mg/kg/dose over 5-10 min.
		Oral	2-5mg/kg/day in 1-4 divided doses.

PHENYTOIN (Cont.)

ADVERSE EFFECTS: Adverse effects are as follows: The most common side effect of phenytoin therapy is gingival hyperplasia (overgrowth of the gums over the teeth;) this occurs in about 20 percent of all patients receiving the drug; rash, coarsening of facial features, nausea, vomiting, ataxia; ocular signs and symptoms, such as nystagmus and diplopia; peripheral neuropathy after years of use; hypertrichosis and hirsutism. Phenytoin interferes with vitamin D metabolism and may cause osteomalacia. Folic acid deficiency may cause megaloblastic anemia; however, folic acid replacement therapy may increase the rate of phenytoin's metabolism and excretion.

Rare reactions include hepatitis, bone marrow depression, systemic lupus erythematosus, Stevens-Johnson syndrome, and lymphadenopathy.

Toxicity: Correlation of serum level of Phenytoin and symptoms are given in the next Table:

Serum Level of Phenytoin and Symptoms

Serum Level (mcg/ml)	Symptoms
20mcg/ml	Nystagmus
30mcg/ml	Drowsiness, Ataxia, Diplopia
40mcg/ml	Disorientation and Somnolence

Patients with low serum albumin have a higher percentage of free to bound drug ratio (protein binding, 90 percent) and thus therapeutic or toxic reactions occur at a lower serum level. Hypoalbuminemia in liver disease and renal disease is associated with increased percentage of free phenytoin. In addition, elevated metabolic waste products, bilirubin and urea, can displace phenytoin from albumin binding sites. Free phenytoin level may be measured and may be particularly useful in patients with renal disease and liver disease.

Serum free testosterone is decreased in patients on phenytoin although total testosterone is elevated; these patients have decreased libido. Phenytoin induces the synthesis of sex hormone binding protein; the increase in the circulating level of sex hormone binding globulin elevates total serum testosterone but depresses free testosterone (Toone, B.K. et al., J. Neurol. Neurosurg. and Psych. 46, 824-826, 1983).

Other adverse effects include a lupus-like syndrome, hepatic granulomas, lymphadenopathy, pseudolymphoma, and acute pulmonary infiltrates.

DRUG INTERACTIONS: Drug interactions of phenytoin are given in the next Table: (Drugs of Choice from The Medical Letter, The Medical Letter, Inc, N.Y., 1987, pg. 50 and other sources):

Drug Interactions of Phenytoin

Drug	Effect
Carbamazepine	Serum concentration of carbamazepine is reduced due to increased metabolism; altered phenytoin effect, both increased and decreased. Serum concentration of both drugs should be monitored.
Valproic Acid	Increased phenytoin toxicity due to displacement from binding by valproic acid; monitor phenytoin concentration and clinical status.
Primidone	Serum concentration of primidone is reduced due to increased metabolism; increased phenobarbital due to increased conversion of primidone to phenobarbital. Monitor primidone and phenobarbital concentration.
Ethosuximide	Serum concentration of ethosuximide is reduced due to increased metabolism.
Clonazepam	Decreased clonazepam effect due to increased metabolism; variable effect on phenytoin concentration. Monitor clonazepam and phenytoin concentration.
Chloramphenicol, Cimetidine, Dicumarol, Disulfiram, Isoniazid, Phenylbutazone, Sulfonamides, Trimethoprim	These drugs significantly increase the serum concentration of phenytoin.
Folic Acid, Prolonged Ingestion of Alcohol, Carbamazepine, and possibly Phenobarbital	Serum concentration of phenytoin is decreased.

PHENYTOIN (Cont.)

Drug Interactions of Phenytoin

Drug	Effect
Oral Anticoagulants, Certain Antibiotics (Tetracyline, Rifampin, and Chloramphenicol) Oral Contraceptives, Quinidine	Phenytoin induces enzymes that metabolize these drugs, thereby decreasing their effectiveness.

CONTRAINDICATIONS: Pregnancy, liver disease.

PHARMACOKINETICS: Absorption: Variable (30%-95%). Half-Life, adults: 18-30 hours; children, 12-22 hours; neonates 30-60 hours; Time to Steady State, adults, 4-6 days; children, 2-5 days; Time to Peak Plasma Level, 4-8 hours. Phenytoin exhibits nonlinear pharmacokinetics, resulting in highly variable time to steady state. The effectiveness of phenytoin is increased at higher plasma levels within the "therapeutic range." Metabolism: Phenytoin is oxidized in the liver by cytochrome P-450; about 60 to 70 percent of phenytoin is metabolized to an inactive, hydroxylated derivative (5-p-hydroxyphenyl-5-phenylhydantoin, HPPH) which is conjugated and excreted in the urine. Phenytoin potentiates the metabolism of other drugs, eg, phenobarbital, by this same system (P-450). Five percent of phenytoin appears in the urine unchanged.

The enzymatically mediated reaction utilized for the metabolism of phenytoin is nearly saturated at therapeutic plasma concentrations of the drug. The metabolism of phenytoin is thus said to be saturable, or capacity-limited. When the steady-state serum phenytoin level is within the therapeutic range of 10 to 20 mcg/ml, a very small increase in dose may result in clinical evidence of toxicity and serum levels well above the 20 mcg/ml (Raebel, M.A., N. Engl. J. Med. 309, 925, 1983).

THERAPEUTIC MONITORING: Therapeutic monitoring is done for the reasons listed in the next Table: (Baer, M., "Interpretation of Drug Concentration", Am. Soc. Clin. Path., 1981):

Monitoring Phenytoin Levels for Patients
Seizures Poorly Controlled
Toxic Symptoms
Change of Medication or Dosage; Allow One Week to Reach Steady State
Children 10 to 13 years old every Three to Four Months until Dose-Serum Relationship has Stabilized.

Free phenytoin levels may be measured, and are particularly useful in patients with renal disease and liver disease. Therapeutic levels are 1-2mcg/ml.

PHYSOSTIGMINE SALICYLATE
(Antilirium)

USES: Physostigmine is a reversible acetylcholinesterase inhibitor. Uses of physostigmine are given in the next Table:

Uses of Physostigmine
Antidote for Anticholinergic Poisoning, eg, belladonna alkaloids
Antihistamine Overdose

DOSAGE FORMS: Parenteral: 1mg/ml

DOSAGE: The dosage of physostigmine is given in the next Table:

Dosage of Physostigmine

Patient	Dosage
Children	0.01-.03mg/kg/dose, repeat one time after 15-30 min.
Adult	0.5-2mg/dose

The infusion rate should not exceed 0.01mg/kg/min., 0.5mg/min. in children, or 1mg/min. in adults, whichever is slower. Use of physostigmine should be reserved for severe, symptomatic anticholinergic poisoning.

ADVERSE EFFECTS: Atropine, the antidote for physostigmine, should always be available. Contraindicated in asthma and GI and GU obstruction.

PIPERACILLIN

(Pipracil)

USES: **Piperacillin** is classified as an **extended spectrum penicillin**; activities of piperacillin are given in the next Table (Parry, M.F., Med. Clin. No. Am. 71, 1093-1112, Nov. 1987; Wilkowske, C.J. and Hermans, P.E., Mayo Clin. Proc. 62, 789-798, 1987; Adams, H.G., Personal Comm.):

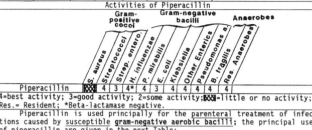

Activities of Piperacillin

	Gram-positive cocci			Gram-negative bacilli						Anaerobes	
	S. aureus	Streptococci	Strep. entero.	H. influenzae	P. mirabilis	E. coli	Klebsiella	Other Enterics	Pseudomonas a.	B. fragilis	Res. Anaerobes
Piperacillin	▩	4	3	4*	4	3	4	4	4	4	4

4=best activity; 3=good activity; 2=some activity; ▩=little or no activity; Res.= Resident; *Beta-lactamase negative.

Piperacillin is used principally for the parenteral treatment of infections caused by susceptible **gram-negative aerobic bacilli**; the principal uses of piperacillin are given in the next Table:

Principal Uses of Piperacillin

Pseudomonas Aeruginosa
Klebsiella Pneumoniae
Bacteroides Fragilis
Proteus Vulgaris
Providencia Rettgeri (formerly Proteus Rettgeni)
Morganella Morganii (formerly Proteus Morganii)
Proteus Mirabilis
Escherichia Coli
Enterobacter
Serratia

Piperacillin should generally be used in combination with an aminoglycoside when it is used for treatment of **serious gram-negative infections.**

DOSAGE FORMS: Parenteral: 2, 3, 4gm.

DOSAGE: Piperacillin sodium is administered by slow IV injection or infusion or by deep IM injection. Give IV rather than IM for treatment of serious infections; give IM for uncomplicated infections and follow-up therapy after IV administration of piperacillin.

If an aminoglycoside is administered concomitantly with piperacillin, the drugs should be administered separately. Dosage labeling for children under 12 years has not been approved. Dosage is given in the next Table:

Dosage of Piperacillin

Condition	Age	Route	Dosage
Uncomplicated Urinary Tract Infect.; or Community-Acquired Pneumonia	Adults	IV or IM	100-125mg/kg daily or 6-8g daily in divided doses every 6-12 hrs.
Complicated Urinary Tract Infections	Adults	IV	125-200mg/kg daily or 8-16g daily in divided doses every 6-8 hrs.
Serious Infections	Adults Children	IV	200-300mg/kg daily or 12-18g daily in divided doses every 4-6 hrs. max. 24g daily
	Neonates	IV	200mg/kg daily in divided doses every 12 hrs.
Febrile Granulocytopenic Patients	Adults	IV	250-300mg/kg daily in 4 or 6 divided doses
Pseudomonas Aeruginosa in Cystic Fibrosis Patients	Adults	IV	300-600mg/kg daily in divided doses every 4-6 hrs.

Duration of Therapy: Usual duration, 10-14 days.

PIPERACILLIN (Cont.)
Dosage in Renal Impairment: Dosage must be adjusted in renal impairment as given in the next Table:

Dosage of Piperacillin in Renal Impairments

Condition	Creatinine Clearance 20-40ml/min	<20ml/min
Uncomplicated Urinary Tract Infections	No Adjustment	3g every 12 hr.
Complicated Urinary Tract Infections	3g every 8 hr.	3g every 12 hr.
Serious Infections	4g every 8 hr.	4g every 12 hr.

PHARMACOKINETICS: Half-Life: 0.7-1 hr. (dose-dependent); greater in renal impairment; Protein-Binding: 16%-22%; Elimination: Renal tubular secretion.
ADVERSE EFFECTS: Most common: Thrombophlebitis, 4%; diarrhea, 3%; skin rashes, 2%. Other adverse reactions include: hypersensitivity reactions, leukopenia and eosinophilia, platelet dysfunction, elevated hepatic enzyme levels, central nervous system irritation, hypokalemia.

PIPERAZINE
(Vermizine)
USES: Piperazine is an **anthelmintic drug;** uses are given in the next Table:

Uses of Piperazine
Enterobius Vermicularis (Pinworm Infection)
Ascaris Lumbricoides (Roundworm Infection)

Piperazine is generally considered an alternative choice to mebendazole or pyrantel pamoate for the treatment of pinworm and roundworm infection.
DOSAGE FORMS: Tabs: 250mg; Syrup: 500mg/5ml.
DOSAGE: The dosage of piperazine is given in the next Table:

Dosage of Piperazine

Condition	Dosage
Enterobiasis	Adults and Children: Single daily dose, 65mg/kg (maximum daily dose, 2.5g), 7 consecutive days. or Adults: Single daily dose, 2g, 7 consecutive days. In severe enterobiasis, treatment may be repeated after a 1-week interval.
Ascariasis	Adults: Single daily dose, 3.5g, 2 consecutive days. Children: Single daily dose, 75mg/kg (max. daily dose, 3.5g), 2 consecutive days.

ADVERSE EFFECTS: Nausea, vomiting, mild diarrhea, abdominal cramps, headache and dizziness.

Contraindicated in patients with impaired renal or hepatic function or seizure disorders. Pyrantel pamoate and piperazine should not be administered concomitantly; these drugs have antagonistic modes of action.

PIROXICAM
(Feldene)

USES: Piroxicam is a nonsteroidal anti-inflammatory drug (NSAID), structurally unrelated to other NSAIDs. It has pharmacologic activities similar to other NSAIDs, that is, anti-inflammatory, analgesic, and antipyretic activity. Uses are given in the next Table:

Uses of Piroxicam
Rheumatoid Arthritis
Osteoarthritis
Juvenile Rheumatoid Arthritis
Ankylosing Spondylitis
Acute Gouty Arthritis
Acute Painful Shoulder, Tendinitis, Bursitis
Dysmenorrhea

Because of its long serum half-life, piroxicam has the advantage of single-daily dose administration.

Mechanism of Action: Anti-inflammatory, analgesic and antipyretic activity may be mediated in part through inhibition of prostaglandin synthesis and release.

DOSAGE FORMS: Caps: 10,20mg

DOSAGE: Piroxicam is administered orally. The drug is usually administered as a single daily dose but may be administered in divided doses. Dosage is given in the next Table:

Dosage of Piroxicam

Condition	Age	Dosage
Usual	Adults	Initial: 20mg daily Maintenance: 20mg daily 30-40mg daily may be required but >20mg daily have been associated with increased frequency of adverse effects.
Juvenile Rheumatoid Arthritis	15-30kg	5mg daily
	31-45kg	10mg daily
	46-55kg	15mg daily

Symptomatic relief usually begins early in therapy and a progressive increase in response may occur over several weeks since the drug has a relatively long half-life.

PHARMACOKINETICS: Half-Life: 41 hrs. (Long half-life allows for single daily dosage regimen); Steady-State: 7-12 days; Protein-Binding: 98%; Peak:3-5 hrs.
Apparent Volume of Distribution: 0.12-0.14 liter/kg.
Excretion: Urine and feces

ADVERSE EFFECTS: G.I.: Gastrointestinal reactions occur in 20% of patients. Epigastric distress and nausea are noted most frequently; abdominal discomfort, constipation, diarrhea and flatulence also occur. Peptic ulcer develops in about 1% of patients; the incidence of gastric irritation and ulcer increases with doses greater than 20mg daily.

Piroxicam, like aspirin, inhibits platelet aggregation and prolongs bleeding time.

Peripheral edema occurs in about 2% of patients.

PLEURA; PATHOGENS

Pathogens: The pathogens that cause infection involving the pleura are given in the next Table (Handbook of Antimicrobial Therapy, The Medical Letter, 1990):

Pathogens that Cause Infection of the Pleura
1. Streptococcus pneumoniae
2. Staphylococcus aureus
3. Haemophilus influenzae
4. Gram-negative bacilli
5. Anaerobic streptococci
6. Bacteroides
7. Streptococcus pyogenes (Group A)
8. Mycobacterium tuberculosis
9. Actinomyces, Nocardia
10. Fungi
11. Fusobacterium necrophorum

PLICAMYCIN

(Formerly known as Mithramycin; Mithracin)

USES: **Plicamycin** is an **antineoplastic** antibiotic; uses are given in the next Table:

Uses of Plicamycin
Testicular Tumors with metastases beyond regional lymphatics
Hypercalcemia and Hypercaliuria associated with advanced cancer

Testicular Tumors: Vinblastine, cisplatin and bleomycin is the treatment of choice for advanced nonseminomatous testicular carcinoma.

Hypercalcemia: Plicamycin is not usually initial therapy. See **HYPERCALCEMIA, TREATMENT** section.

DOSAGE FORMS: Mithracin; Injection: 2.5mg

DOSAGE: Plicamycin is given IV.

Reconstitute as follows: Add 4.9ml of sterile water to vial containing 2.5mg of plicamycin; thus each ml contains 500mcg of drug. Dose is based on ideal body weight. Calculated dose is added to one liter of 5% dextrose or 0.9% NaCl and infused over 4-6 hours. Dosages are given in the next Table:

Dosages of Plicamycin (Mithramycin)

Condition	Dosage
Testicular Tumors	25-30mcg/kg once daily for 8-10 days or until toxicity; do not exceed 30mcg/kg/day or 10 days. Response within 3-4 weeks after initial therapy.
Hypercalcemia and Hypercalciuria of Malignancy	25mcg/kg daily for 3 or 4 days; additional courses may be given at intervals of 1 week or more if initial therapy unsuccessful. Reduction of elevated serum calcium, usually to normal concentrations, is evident within 24-48 hours and lasts 3-15 days following single IV dose. Possible to maintain normal calcium balance with single weekly doses or with 2 or 3 doses per week.

ADVERSE EFFECTS: Bone marrow depression, hemorrhagic diathesis with coagulopathy, cellulitis on extravasation, nausea, vomiting, hypocalcemia, hepatotoxicity, renal toxicity.

PNEUMONIA, PATHOGENS, TREATMENT

Incidence: Pneumonia is the most common infectious cause of death in the United States and the fifth leading cause of death overall.

The incidence of pneumonia is relatively low in children less than six months of age, has a broad incidence peak between six months and five years of age (40/1000) and then gradually declines (9/1000) in nine to 15 year olds (Murphy, T.F. et al., Am. J. Epidemiol. 113, 12-21, 1981):

Pathogens:

Children: The causes of acute pneumonia, by age, are given in the next Table; (Long, S.S., Pediatr. Clin. North Am. 30, 297-321, 1983):

Relative Causes of Acute Pneumonia

Organism	<2 Wk	2 Wk-3 Mo	4 Mo-5 Yr	6-18 Yr
Bacteria	++++	++	++	+
Virus	++	++++	++++	++
Mycoplasma	–	–	+	++++
Chlamydia	–	+++	–	–
Pneumocystis	–	++	–	–
Tuberculosis	–	–	+	+
Fungus	+	–	–	–

*Key to Table: ++++ Most Frequent Cause; +++ Frequent Cause; ++ Less Frequent Cause; + Occasional Cause; — Rare, Warrants Consideration Only in Unusual Circumstances.

Bacteria are the major cause of pneumonia only in the perinatal and nursery period; beyond infancy, bacteria account for less than ten percent of lower respiratory infection (Long, S.S., Pediatr. Clin. North Am. 30, 297-321, 1983).

The pathogens that cause pneumonia in childhood are given in the next Table (Editorial, The Lancet 1, 741-743, 1988; Long, S.S., Ped. Clin. North Am. 30, 297-321, 1983):

Pneumonia in Childhood

Newborn	One Month to Four Years	>4 Years
Chlamydia trachomatis	Viruses	Strep. pneumoniae (pneumococcus)
Group B streptococci	Respiratory syncytial virus (RSV)	Mycoplasma pneumoniae
Gram-negative bacteria (Escherichia coli, Klebsiella pneumoniae)	Parainfluenza	H. influenzae
Listeria monocytogenes	Influenza	Group A strep.
Cytomegalovirus (CMV)	Adenoviruses 3 and 7	S. aureus
Herpes simplex	Streptococcus pneumoniae (pneumococcus)	Tuberculosis
Pneumocystis carinii	Hemophilus influenzae B (HiB)	
Staph. aureus	S. aureus	
	Tuberculosis	

Newborns: Pneumonia in newborns is usually caused by organisms acquired from the mother's vagina during or before delivery. C. trachomatis, group B streptococci and gram-negative bacteria (E. coli, K. pneumoniae) are the most important pathogens.

The incidence of group B streptococcal disease [includes asymptomatic bacteremia to fulminant septicemia, congenital pneumonia, or meningitis (30%)] is 2 cases per 1000 live births and 1,200 neonates in the United States. Early-onset neonatal group B streptococcal disease can be prevented by intrapartum ampicillin prophylaxis (2g of ampicillin intravenously followed by 1g every four hours until delivery) given to women who have prenatal group B streptococcal colonization (positive vaginal or rectal cultures) and various perinatal risk factors (premature labor, prolonged membrane rupture, or intrapartum fever) (Boyer, K.M. and Gotoff, S.P., N. Engl. J. Med 314, 1665-1669. 1986)

Staphyloccal aureus pneumonia in the newborn is usually a complication of hospitalization, another infection or debility; S. aureus pneumonia is associated with influenza and measles infections.

Cytomegalovirus (CMV) can be acquired at or soon after birth from the mother or from other neonates.

PNEUMONIA, PATHOGENS, TREATMENT (Cont.)

One Month to Four Years: Between 1 month and 4 years of age, most pneumonias are viral in origin. Respiratory syncytial virus is the most common pathogen and is the major cause of serious acute lower respiratory tract infection in infants and young children; bronchiolitis and pneumonia are the two common clinical presentations and frequently lead to hospitalization.

Adenoviruses are important pathogens in childhood and in early adult life.

Streptococcus (pneumococcal) pneumoniae is the most frequent cause of bacterial pneumonia in all ages beyond the neonatal period accounting for more than 90% of uncomplicated bacterial pneumonias. S. pneumoniae was classified anatomically as the main cause of lobar pneumonia; however, lobar presentation is less common than in past. Patients often experience an explosive onset, high fever, chills, rust colored sputum, pleuritic pain. A vaccine has been developed to immunize children who are at particularly high risk including children with reticuloendothelial disease, following splenectomy, and children with sickle cell anemia who develop functional asplenia. Blood culture is positive in 20-30% of patients.

H. influenzae is a common cause of both mild and severe pneumonia in preschool children; the majority of patients have clinical and radiographic findings indistinguishable from acute streptococcal pneumonia. Infection is associated with viral pneumonia.

>Four Years: Above the age of 4, Strep. pneumoniae (pneumococcus) and Mycoplasma pneumoniae are the most frequently identified organisms and viruses are of lesser importance.

Mycoplasma Pneumonia: Mycoplasma (primary atypical pneumonia) accounts for 50% of all pneumonias in the age range of 5-10 years. It has a prolonged incubation period and household contacts are often affected; the onset of symptoms in contacts is delayed.

Community-Acquired and Nosocomial (Hospital-Acquired) Pneumonia: The causes of community-acquired and nosocomial (hospital acquired) pneumonia are given in the next Table: (MacFarlane, J.T., Lancet 2, 1446-1449, Dec. 19, 1987):

Community-Acquired and Nosocomial Pneumonia

Pathogen	Community-Acquired	Nosocomial
Bacteria:	70-80%	>90%
Strep. pneumoniae	65-75%	3-9%
H. influenzae	4-5%	?
Legionella species	2-5%	0-25%
Staph. aureus	1-5%	10-20%
Gram-negative bacilli, eg, Klebsiella	Rare	>50%
Anaerobes	Rare	10%(?)
Atypicals	10-20%	Rare
Mycoplasma pneumoniae	5-18%	
Chlamydia psittaci	2-3%	
Coxiella burneti	1%	
Viruses	10-20%	Rare
Influenza	8%	
Other viruses	2-8%	

Community Acquired: The bacteria most often causing community-acquired bacterial pneumonia in the adult are Streptococcus pneumoniae (pneumococcus), Haemophilus influenzae, Legionella pneumophila and the atypicals, Mycoplasma pneumoniae and chlamydia psittaci.

Nosocomial Infection: Pneumonia is the third most common nosocomial infection but it carries the highest mortality rate, 20-50% (Pennington, J.E., Current Pulmonology 7, 1, 1986). Most cases of hospital-acquired pneumonia are caused by aerobic gram-negative bacilli aspirated from a colonized oropharynx. Retrograde pharyngeal colonization by organisms from the stomach may contribute to the pathogenesis of nosocomial pneumonia. Use of antacids or histamine type 2 blockers (cimetidine, ranitidine, famotidine and nizatidine) leading to elevation of gastric pH may favor gastric colonization with gram negative bacilli and increase the risk of nosocomial pneumonia (Driks, M.R. et al., "Nosocomial Pneumonia in Intubated Patients Given Sucralfate as Compared with Antacids or Histamine Type 2 Blockers," NEJM 317, 1376-1382, 1987).

PNEUMONIA, PATHOGENS, TREATMENT (Cont.)

Aspiration Pneumonia: The usual reason for aspiration is loss of consciousness or difficulty in swallowing. Gastric secretions with pH<2.4 cause pulmonary edema. The bacterial pathogens in community-acquired or hospital-acquired aspiration pneumonia are given in the next Table (Mac Farlane, J.T., Lancet 2, 1446-1449, Dec. 10, 1987):

Community-Acquired or Hospital-Acquired Aspiration Pneumonia

Community-Acquired	Hospital-Acquired
Oropharyngeal Anaerobes, eg.,	Gram-negative bacilli
Fusobacterium species	Staph. aureus
B. melaninogenicus	Anaerobes, eg., Bacteroides fragilis
Peptostreptococci	
Peptococci	
Microaerophilic streptococci	

Treatment: The choice of antibiotics will often depend on the likelihood of certain infectious agents since specific etiologies are frequently elusive. If empiric therapy is necessary, provide antibacterial coverage for the most likely etiologic agents and select an antibiotic that will avoid drug toxicity, superinfection, and excessive costs (Griffith, D.E. and Wallace, R.J., Hospital Medicine, pgs. 188-203, Jan. 1988).

Suggested antibiotic therapy for acute bacterial pneumonia based on "likely" pathogens is given in the next Table:

Suggested Antibiotic Therapy for Acute Bacterial Pneumonia

Status	Age	Antibiotic	"Likely" Pathogens
Inpatient	<1 Mo.	Ampicillin plus gentamicin or Ampicillin plus 3rd generation cephalosporin.	Grp. D Streptococci; gram-neg. bacteria (E. coli, K. pneumoniae)
		Nafcillin	Staph. aureus
		Erythromycin	Chlamydial infection
	1 Mo. to 4 yrs.	Penicillin G	Strep. pneumoniae (positive culture)
		Cefuroxime or 3rd generation cephalosporin or ampicillin plus chloramphenicol	H. influenzae
		Nafcillin	S. aureus
	>4 yrs.	Penicillin G	Strep. pneumoniae
		Erythromycin	Mycoplasma, Legionella, Chlamydiae
		Nafcillin	S. aureus
		Cefuroxime or 3rd generation cephalosporin or Ampicillin plus Chloramphenicol.	H. influenzae
Outpatient	1 Mo. to 4 yrs.	Amoxicillin	Strep. pneumoniae(pneumococcus) H. influenzae.
		Erythromycin	Strep. pneumoniae, Mycoplasma
		Amoxicillin/Clavulanate or Sulfamethoxazole(SMX)/Trimethoprim (TMP)	Amoxicillin resistant, H. influenzae
		Cefaclor	Alternative to amoxicillin
	5 yrs. to 19 yrs.	Penicillin V	Strep. pneumoniae
		Erythromycin	Mycoplasma pneumoniae
Nosocomial (Hospital Acquired) Pneumonia	Adults	Nafcillin plus gentamicin	Gram-negative bacilli Staph. aureus
		Cefoxitin alone or substitute clindamycin for nafcillin	

PNEUMONIA, PATHOGENS, TREATMENT (Cont.)

(Table Cont.)

Status	Age	Antibiotic	"Likely Pathogens"
Community-Acquired Aspiration Pneumonia	Adults	Penicillin, parenteral	Anaerobes
		Alternative: Clindamycin	Anaerobes esp. B. fragilis
		Oral amoxicillin (high dose) plus oral metronidazole	
Hospital-Acquired Aspiration Pneumonia	Adults	Gentamicin plus clindamycin or cephalosporin, eg., cefoxitin cefoperazone	Gram-negative bacilli Staph. aureus Anaerobes
Intensive-Care Unit	Children or Adults	Aminoglycoside plus antipseudomonal cephalosporin, eg., ceftazidime	Pseudomonas aeruginosa
		or Aminoglycoside plus Antipseudomonal penicillin, eg, ticarcillin, or azlocillin or piperacillin	

The initial therapy for uncomplicated streptococcus pneumoniae is oral amoxicillin. Cefuroxime or a 3rd generation cephalosporin, eg, cefotaxime or ceftriaxone is substituted for more severely ill in-patients and for possible ampicillin-resistant H. influenzae.

Therapy according to bacterial agent causing pneumonia is given in the next Table:

Therapy According to Bacterial Agent Causing Pneumonia

Etiologic Agent	Therapy
Infants Less than Three Months:	
Group B and D Streptococci	Ampicillin plus Aminoglycoside or Ampicillin plus 3rd Generation Cephalosporin
Enteric Bacilli	Ampicillin plus Aminoglycoside or Ampicillin plus 3rd Generation Cephalosporin
Staphyloccus Aureus	Penicillinase-Resistant Penicillin
Child Three Months to Five Years:	
Streptococcus Pneumonia	Penicillin; Alternatives: Erythromycin (for patients allergic to penicillin); clindamycin; rifampicin; vancomycin, cephalosporin (use with caution in patients allergic to penicillin).
H. Influenzae	Cefuroxime or 3rd generation cephalosporin or ampicillin plus chloramphenicol
S. Aureus	Nafcillin
Children Over Five Years:	
S. Pneumoniae	Penicillin
Mycoplasma	Erythromycin
S. Aureus	Penicillinase-Resistant Penicillin
H. Influenzae	Cefuroxime or 3rd generation cephalosporin or ampicillin plus chloramphenicol
Legionella	Erythromycin; alternative: rifampin
Chlamydial infection	Erythromycin
Respiratory syncytial virus (RSV)	Ribavirin for high risk patients.

PNEUMONIA, PATHOGENS, TREATMENT (Cont.)

Suggested antimicrobial dosages for treatment of pneumonia in infants and children older than one month of age are given in the next Table; (Modified from: Long, S.S., Pediatr. Clin. North Am. 30, 297-321, Apr. 1983):

Suggested Antimicrobial Dosages for Treatment of Pneumonia in Infants and Children Older than One Month of Age

Drug	Route++	Dosage Dose/KG/24 hrs	Adult Daily Dosage##	Dosage Interval
Penicillin G for anaerobic infection	IM,IV	100,000-300,000 U	2-6 million U	4-6 h
Penicillin G (procaine)	IM	25,000-50,000 U	1 million U	12 h
Penicillin V	PO	50 mg	2 gm	6 h
Ampicillin	IM,IV	100-150 mg	4 gm	4-6 h
Amoxicillin	PO	40-50 mg	1.5 gm	8 h
Carbenicillin	IV	400-600 mg	30 gm	4-6 h
Ticarcillin	IV	200-300 mg	18 gm	4-6 h
Methicillin	IM,IV	100-400 mg	8 gm	4-6 h
Nafcillin	IM,IV	100-200 mg	6 gm	4-6 h
Erythromycin	PO	30-50 mg	2 gm	6 h
Erythromycin	IV	20-50 mg	4 gm	6 h
Clindamycin	PO	10-25 mg	2 gm	6 h
Clindamycin	IM,IV	25-40 mg	2 gm	6 h
Vancomycin	IV	30-50 mg	2 gm	6-8 h
Cefazolin	IM,IV	50-100 mg	4 gm	6-8 h
Cefaclor	PO	40 mg	1.5 gm	8 h
Cefoxitin	IM,IV	80-160 mg	8 gm	4-6 h
Cefamandole	IM,IV	50-150 mg	8 gm	4-6 h
Cefuroxime	IM,IV	50-100 mg	4.5 gm	6-8 h
Cefotaxime	IM,IV	50-200 mg	4 gm	6 h
Ceftriaxone	IM,IV	50-75 mg	2 gm	12-24 h
Ceftazidime	IM,IV	90-150mg	4 gm	8 h
Erythromycin-sulfa +	PO	50 mg as erythromycin	2gm as erythromycin	8 h
Trimethoprim-sulfa #	PO	10 mg dosed as TMP	320 mg TMP	8-12 h
for P. carinii	PO	20 mg dosed as TMP	640 mg TMP	6 h
Chloramphenicol	IV	50-100 mg	4 gm	6 h
Gentamicin	IM,IV	6-7.5 mg	3-5 mg/kg	6-8 h

++Intravenous doses administered over 30 to 60 minutes.
##Usual adult dosage for treatment of pneumonia. Higher doses may be used for severe infections in some situations.
+Fixed combination erythromycin 200mg-sulfisoxazole 600mg
#Fixed combination trimethoprim 40mg-sulfamethoxazole 200mg.

POLYETHYLENE GLYCOL ELECTROLYTE PREPARATIONS

(Colyte, GoLYTELY)

USES: This preparation is used for bowel cleansing before colonoscopy and barium enema x-ray examination. Administration should begin 4-5 hours before a diagnostic procedure. Up to one liter of the fluid may be retained in the colon but can be removed by suctioning during colonoscopy. However, when administered on the same day as a barium enema, polyethylene glycol preparations can interfere with barium coating of the bowel wall; addition of bisacodyl to the regimen evacuates residual fluid and may significantly improve coating with barium (Girard, C.M., Am. J. Roentgenol. 142, 1147-1149, 1984).

Mechanism of Action: This preparation is an osmotic agent. The solutions cleanse the bowel rapidly by producing a voluminous liquid stool without significant changes in water and electrolyte balance or mucosal histology (Michael, K.A. et al., Clin. Pharmacy 4, 414-424, 1985).

DOSAGE FORMS: Disposable jug containing polyethylene glycol (PEG) 236g, sodium sulfate 22.74g, sodium bicarbonate 6.74g, sodium chloride 5.86g, potassium chloride 2.97g; water is added to jug until a 4 liter volume is reached. In patients who are to receive a barium enema, the solution can be given the evening before the examination.

POLYETHYLENE GLYCOL ELECTROLYTE PREPARATIONS (Cont.)
DOSAGE: The preparation is not recommended for children. It is given orally. The dosage for adults is as follows: Eight oz. (240ml) every 10 min. until 4 liters are consumed. (The preparation may be given via nasogastric tube at a rate of 20 to 30ml/min.). The first bowel movement usually commences about one hour after administration of the initial dose. Bowel exam is usually scheduled 4 hours after initiation of oral ingestion (3 hours for drinking and 1 hour for complete bowel evacuation).
CONTRAINDICATIONS AND PRECAUTIONS: GI obstruction, gastric retention, bowel perforation, megacolon, or toxic colitis.
ADVERSE EFFECTS: Nausea, vomiting, abdominal bloating or fullness, and cramps occur occasionally but are transient.

POTASSIUM IODIDE (KI)

(Iosat, Lugol's Solution, Pima, Thyro-Block)

USES: Uses of potassium iodide(KI) are given in the next Table:

Uses of Potassium Iodide
Preoperative to Thyroidectomy
Thyrotoxic Crisis
Expectorant: Chronic bronchitis, bronchiectasis, asthma

Preoperative to Thyroidectomy: Potassium iodide(KI) is used preoperatively to reduce vascularity of the thyroid gland prior to thyroidectomy and in the management of thyrotoxic crisis, usually in conjunction with other antithyroid agents, eg, propylthiouracil and/or propranolol.

When used preoperatively, KI is administered after hyperthyroidism is controlled with other agents and for 10-14 days before surgery. KI and propranolol may be preferred for preparation of patients with Grave's disease for surgery.

Thyrotoxicosis: KI is very useful in the treatment of thyrotoxicosis because of its rapid onset of action; KI is administered after the first dose of an antithyroid agent, such as propylthiouracil, to prevent intrathyroidal iodine accumulation.

KI may also be useful for the treatment of persistent or recurrent hyperthyroidism that occurs in patients with Grave's disease after surgery or treatment with radioactive iodine.

Expectorant: KI has been replaced by more effective and safer expectorants, although some expectorant preparations still exist.
DOSAGE FORMS: Tabs: 130mg; Sol'n: 325mg/5ml, 1g/ml; Strong Iodine Sol'n or Lugol's Solution: Iodine 50mg/ml and Potassium Iodide 100mg/ml.
DOSAGE: The dosage of KI is given in the next Table:

Dosage of KI

Condition	Dosage
Reduce Vascularity of Thyroid Gland Preoperatively	Children and Adults: 50-250mg (approx. 1-5 drops of a sol'n containing 1g/ml) 3 times daily for 10-14 days before surgery.
	or Strong iodine sol'n in a dosage of 0.1-0.3ml (approx. 3-5 drops) 3 times daily
Thyrotoxic Crisis	Children: 200-300mg/day divided in 2 or 3 doses.
	Adults: 300-900mg/day divided in 3 doses.
	or 500mg every 4 hours (approx. 10 drops of KI sol'n containing 1g/ml.
	or Strong iodine sol'n in a dosage of 1ml 3 times daily.

ADVERSE EFFECTS: Hypersensitivity. Manifestations of iodism include metallic taste, burning in mouth and throat, soreness of teeth and gums, etc. Gastric irritation is common and diarrhea, sometimes bloody. Prolonged use may result in thyroid dysfunction. In pregnant women, may cause abnormal thyroid function in the neonate.

POTASSIUM SUPPLEMENTS

USES: Potassium supplements are used to treat hypokalemia. There are three mechanisms to consider in hypokalemia (1) gastrointestinal loss, (2) urinary loss and (3) possible movement of potassium from the extracellular to the intracellular fluid. These mechanisms are listed in the next Table: (Bakerman, S. in ABC's of Interpretative Laboratory Data, Published by Interpretive Laboratory Data, Inc., Greenville, N.C., 2nd ed., 1984, pg. 335-336)

Causes of Hypokalemia

G.I. Loss	Urine Loss	Movement into the Intracellular Space
Vomiting	Diuretics (Thiazides)	Diabetic ketoacidosis (treated)
Nasogastric suction	(Chlormetric Sulfonamides):	Familial periodic hypokalemic paralysis
Pyloric obstruction	Furosemide (Lasix);	
Diarrhea	Ethacrynic acid (Edecrin)	
Malabsorption	Magnesium depletion	
Villous adenoma	Antibiotics	
Enema and laxative abuse	Carbenicillin	
	Amphotericin B	**Other**
	Increased mineralocorticoid	Decreased K^+ intake
	Licorice abuse	Acute myeloid leukemia
	Renal tubular acidosis, Type 1 (distal) and type 2 (proximal)	
	Bartter's syndrome	

Diuretic therapy & gastrointestinal loss are major causes of hypokalemia.

Drug-induced hypokalemia is usually due to diuretics or adrenal corticosteroids.

Small potassium supplements do not reliably prevent hypokalemia in patients taking thiazides or loop diuretics. Elderly individuals and patients taking both thiazides or loop diuretics plus digoxin should receive potassium supplements sufficient to maintain a normal plasma potassium concentration. The blood potassium concentration should be checked at least once every 3 months. Generally, serum K^+ reflects K^+ stores; two important exceptions are alkalosis and insulin hypersecretion which promote entry of K^+ into cells resulting in hypokalemia despite adequate or increased intracellular K^+. Excessive cell breakdown, eg, hemolysis, results in a relative excess of extracellular K^+ despite normal stores.

More than 90 percent of potassium is excreted in the urine; it is filtered and totally reabsorbed proximally and is excreted by the distal tubules. The factors that determine the degree of distal tubular secretion are dietary K^+ intake, mineralocorticoid secretion, distal tubular flow and the anion accompanying Na^+ to the distal tubular site.

Both increased dietary K^+ intake and aldosterone promote movement of K^+ into cells and favor secretion into the tubular lumen and subsequent excretion.

Normally, less than 10 percent of potassium that is excreted appears in the stool; however, gastrointestinal abnormalities can cause loss of K^+.

Potassium salts may be used cautiously to abolish arrhythmias of digoxin or digoxin-like compounds precipitated by loss of potassium. Elevation of plasma potassium by 0.5-1.5mEq/liter or to the upper limits of normal may be useful in the managment of tachyarrhythmias following cardiac surgery.

DOSAGE FORMS: Multiple oral and IV preparations contain Potassium Chloride, Potassium Acetate, Potassium Bicarbonate, Potassium Gluconate, Potassium Phosphates, and Potassium Citrate.

Selected Oral Preparations of Potassium Supplements

Produce Name	Composition
Slow-K (Ciba)	Potassium (as chloride) 8mEq; sustained release tabs.
Micro-K (Robbins)	Potassium (as chloride) 8mEq; sustained release caps.
Micro-K-10 (Robbins)	Potassium (as chloride)10mEq; sustained release caps.
K-Tab (Abbott)	Potassium (as chloride)10mEq; sustained release tabs.
Klotrix (Mead Johnson)	Potassium (as chloride)10mEq; sustained release tabs.

POTASSIUM SUPPLEMENTS (Cont.)

Reference Range of Potassium: Adult: 3.5-5.3mmol/liter; premature (48 hours): 3.0-6.0mmol/liter; newborn: 3.7-5.0mmol/liter; infant: 4.1-5.3mmol/liter; child: 3.4-4.7mmol/liter. The following are life-threatening values and, after confirmation, preferably by repeat determination on a different specimen, should be telephoned to the responsible nursing staff or, if unavailable, to the responsible physician so that corrective therapy may be immediately undertaken: serum potassium: <2.5mmol/liters.

The concentration of intracellular K^+ is 130mmol/liter; the serum concentration of K^+ is 3.5 to 5.0 mmol/liter. Thus, only two to three percent of the K^+ is extracellular. Generally, serum K^+ reflects K^+ stores.

DOSAGE: Potassium chloride is usually the salt of choice in the treatment of potassium depletion, since the chloride ion is required to correct hypochloremia which frequently accompanies potassium deficiency. Furthermore, hypochloremia may develop if the acetate, citrate, bicarbonate, gluconate, or other alkalinizing salt of potassium is administered.

If metabolic acidosis exists concurrently with potassium depletion, such as renal tubular acidosis, alkalinizing salts of potassium are preferred.

Oral potassium salts are as follows: chloride, acetate, bicarbonate, citrate and gluconate.

IV potassium salts are as follows: chloride, acetate, and phosphate; administer by IV infusion over a prolonged period. Rapid infusion may result in fatal arrhythmias.

Oral: Whenever possible, potassium supplements should be given orally; slow absorption from the GI tract prevents sudden large increases in plasma potassium concentrations. Give potassium supplements as liquid with or after meals with a full glass of water or fruit juice to minimize the possibility of GI irritation.

IV: Administer slowly as dilute solutions; do not give concentrated solutions. In dehydrated patients, 1 liter of potassium-free fluid should be administered prior to initiating potassium therapy. Generally, potassium concentrations in IV fluids should not exceed 40mEq/liter and the rate of administration should not exceed 20 mEq/hour. In children, max. replacement is 0.5mEq/kg over 1 hr. Oral administration should replace IV potassium therapy as soon as possible.

Daily dietary requirements, for adults are 40-80mEq, for infants, 2-3mEq/kg. The average daily oral dosage of potassium supplements for the prevention of hypokalemia is about 20mEq; the usual oral dosage of potassium for the treatment of potassium depletion is 40-100mEq or more daily.

Forty mEq of potassium is provided by the potassium salts listed in the next Table:

Forty mEq of Potassium Provided by Potassium Salts

Potassium Salt	Amount (grams)
Potassium Chloride	3.0
Potassium Acetate	3.9
Potassium Bicarbonate	4.0
Potassium Citrate	4.3
Potassium Gluconate	9.4
Monobasic Potassium Phosphate	5.4
Dibasic Potassium Phosphate	3.5

Oral potassium supplements are usually administered in 2-4 doses daily. Replacement of potassium deficits is undertaken gradually over a 3-to7-day period.

Daily potassium dosage for adults should not exceed 150 mEq; for children, 3mEq/kg.

MONITOR: Plasma potassium levels and ECG.

ADVERSE EFFECTS: Hyperkalemia may present with cardiac arrhythmias or cardiac arrest. Oral potassium may cause GI disturbances and small bowel ulceration.

PRAZEPAM

(Centrax)

USES: Prazepam is a **benzodiazepine** that is used in the treatment of **situational anxiety** and **generalized anxiety disorder.**

DOSAGE FORMS: Caps: 5, 10, 20mg; Tabs: 10mg.

DOSAGE: Prazepam is administered orally. Dosage is given in the next Table:

Dosage of Prazepam

Condition	Dosage
Anxiety, Adults	Initially: 20mg daily as a single dose at bedtime; if necessary, the dose may be increased to 40 to 60mg daily in divided amounts or as a single dose, usually at bedtime.
Elderly or Debilitated	10 to 15mg daily in divided doses.

PHARMACOKINETICS: Metabolism: Metabolized in the liver to active metabolite, desmethyldiazepam. Peak: 6 hours. Half-Life: 60 hours (50 to 100 hours).

ADVERSE EFFECTS: Abuse potential, drowsiness, dizziness, CNS depression, ataxia, memory impairment, dry mouth, diaphoresis, slurred speech, palpitations, liver disorders, headache, confusion, tremors, vivid dreams.

PRECAUTIONS: Drug or alcohol abuse, suicidal tendencies, depression, renal or liver disease, epilepsy. Withdrawal may occur with abrupt discontinuation after prolonged use.

MONITOR: Liver function tests and blood counts should be performed regularly during long-term therapy.

PRAZIQUANTEL

(Biltricide)

USES: Praziquantel is **an antihelminthic agent.** Uses of praziquantel is given in the following Table (King, C.H. and Mahmond, A.A.F., Annals of Intern. Med. 110, 290-296, 1989; Medical Letter 32, 23-30, March 23, 1990):

Uses of Praziquantel
Shistosomiasis (Blood flukes)
Tissue Flukes
Intestinal Flukes
Tissue Cestodes (Cysticercosis)
Intestinal Cestodes (Tapeworm infection)

DOSAGE FORMS: Tabs: 600mg.

DOSAGE: Praziquantel is administered orally; the dosage of praziquantel in the treatment of various helminthics is given in the next Table (King, C.H. and Mahmond, A.A.F., Annals of Intern. Med. 110, 290-296, 1989; Medical Letter 32, 23-30, March 23, 1990):

Dosage of Praziquantel

Parasite	Dosage
Shistosomiasis	
S. haematobium S. mansoni	20mg/kg 2 times daily for 1 day.
S. japonicum S. mekongi	20mg/kg 3 times daily for 1 day.
S. intercalatum	40mg/kg once.
Tissue Flukes	
Clonorchis Sisensis Paragonimus Westermani	25mg/kg 3 times daily for 2 days.
Opisthorchis viverrini Opisthorchis felineus	25mg/kg 3 times daily for 1 day.
Nanophyetus salmincola	20mg/kg 3 times daily for 1 day.
Intestinal Flukes	
Fasciolopsis buski Heterophyes heterophyes Metagonimus yokogawai	25mg/kg 3 times daily for 1 day.
Tissue Cestatodes	
Cysticercus cellulosae (cysticercosis)	50mg/kg daily in 3 divided doses for 14-30 days.
Intestinal Cestodes (Tapeworms)	
Hymenolepis nana (dwarf)	25mg/kg once.
Diphyllobothrium latum (fish) Taenia sqginata (beef) Taenia solium (pork) Dipylidium caninum (dog)	10-20mg/kg once.

Intestinal cestodes (tapeworms) may be treated with praziquantel or niclosamide.

ADVERSE EFFECTS: Gastrointestinal: pain, anorexia, nausea, vomiting, diarrhea; Neurologic: headache, dizziness, dysphoria; Systemic: fever, urticaria (King, C.H. and Mahmond, A.A.F., Ann. of Intern. Med. 110, 290-296, 1989).

PRAZOSIN

(Minipress)

USES: **Prazosin** is a selective **alpha-1 adrenergic blocking agent,** blocking the effects of norepinephrine on peripheral vasculature. The uses of prazosin are given in the next Table:

Uses of Prazosin
Hypertension
Severe Congestive Heart Failure (CHF)
Raynaud's Disease and Raynaud's Phenomenon associated with Systemic Sclerosis or Ergotamine-Induced Peripheral Ischemia
Urinary Retention

Hypertension: Prazosin is the preferred drug for treating patients with coexisting hypertension and congestive heart failure. Prazosin and hydralazine are equally effective but side effects (dizziness, nightmares, sexual dysfunction) are more common with prazosin (VA Cooperative Study Groups on Antihypertensive Agents, Circulation 64, 772-779, 1981). Treatment of hypertension with prazosin is given in the next Table (The 1988 Report of the Joint National Committee on Detection, Evaluation, and Treatment of High Blood Pressure, Arch. Intern. Med. 148, 1023-1038, 1988):

Treatment of Hypertension with Prazosin

Step 1: Nonpharmacologic Approaches (see **HYPERTENSION**)

↓

Step 2: **Diuretic** or **Beta Blocker** or **Calcium Antagonist** or **ACE Inhibitor**
Observe up to 6 months;if treatment is ineffective,

↓

Step 3: Add a second drug of a different class, eg, prazosin
or Increase the dosage of the first drug
or Substitute another drug

↓

Step 4: Add a third drug of a different class; this may be prazosin depending on the choice in step 3
or Substitute a second drug

↓

Step 5: Consider further evaluation and/or referral
or Add a third or fourth drug

Mechanism of Action: Prazosin reduces arteriolar and venous tone causing a fall in peripheral resistance and hypotension. Prazosin reverses the pressor effects of norepinephrine because beta-2 mediated vasodilator effects are unopposed by alpha-mediated vasoconstriction and the peripheral resistance falls.

Severe Congestive Heart Failure: Prazosin has selective alpha-adrenergic blocking activity with arterial and venous dilator effects. Tolerance to these effects on resting hemodynamics may develop during long-term therapy.

Raynaud's Disease: Prazosin has been used to relieve neurogenic vasoconstriction in patients with Raynaud's disease (Nielsen, S.L. et al., Eur. J. Clin. Pharmacol. 24, 421-423, 1983).

Urinary Retention: Prazosin has been used to treat urinary retention in patients with lower motor neuron lesions and autonomous bladdar (Wein, A.J., in Raz, S. (ed.) Female Urology, New York, W.B. Saunders, 1983, 161-168). Prazosin has fewer side effects as compared to phenoxybenzamine.

DOSAGE FORMS: Caps: 1, 2, 5mg

PRAZOSIN (Cont.)

DOSAGE: Prazosin is administered orally; dosage is given in the next Table:

Dosage of Prazosin

Condition	Age	Dosage
Hypertension	Adults	Give the first dose, 1mg, at bedtime to minimize the danger associated with a syncopal reaction The patient should be instructed to remain in bed for several hours. Thereafter, 1mg may be given two times daily, increased to three times later if required. Maintenance: Dose may be increased gradually to 20mg daily. Concomitant diuretic therapy enhances the therapeutic response. When admisistered with a diuretic and beta blocker, relatively small doses may be sufficient for maintenance.
	Children	Initial: 5 microgram/kg test dose; Maintenance: 25-150 microgram/kg daily in 4 divided doses.
Congestive Heart Failure (CHF)	Adults	2-7mg, four times daily. Initial doses should not exceed 1mg.
Raynaud's	Adults	1mg two or three times daily
Urinary Retention	Adults	Initially, 1mg at bedtime, then 1mg three times daily. Increase at weekly intervals by 1mg/dose until an adequate response in produced or side effects are unacceptable; max. 20mg daily.

PHARMACOKINETICS: Bioavailability: 40-70%; absorption may be delayed by food; Protein Binding: 95%; Volume of Distribution: 0.5 liter/kg. Half-Life: 2.5 hours; prolonged in patients with congestive heart failure and in elderly patients.

ADVERSE EFFECTS: Marked orthostatic hypotension and syncope leading to collapse or loss of consciousness may occur when occasionally started or when dosage is increased. Therefore, first dose should be given at bedtime. Weakness and palpitations may occur.

Prazosin may cause fluid retention and edema if a diuretic is not given concomitantly. Other adverse effects include dryness of the mouth, nasal congestion, headache, nightmares, sexual dysfunction and lethargy.

Adverse effects that occur rarely are as follows: urinary frequency, urinary incontinence, priapism, febrile polyarthritis, hypothermia, urticaria and angioedema.

Prazosin does not adversely affect blood lipid or blood glucose levels.

PRECAUTIONS: Use cautiously in elderly patients because of orthstatic hypotension.

PREDNISOLONE

(Prelone, Cortalone, Delta-Cortef, Others)

USES: Prednisolone is a **glucocorticoid;** uses are given in the next Table:

Uses of Prednisolone
Anti-Inflammatory
Immunosuppressant

Prednisolone has minimal mineralocorticoid properties. If prednisolone is used in the treatment of adrenocortical insufficiency, concomitant therapy with a mineralocorticoid is required. Prednisolone is approximately equivalent to prednisone in its glucocorticoid activity.

DOSAGE FORMS: Tabs: 5mg; Oral Sol'n: 5, 15mg/5ml; Parenteral: 20, 25, 50mg/ml

DOSAGE: The route of administration and dosage of prednisolone and its derivatives are given in the next Table:

Route of Administration and Dosage of Prednisolone and Its Derivatives

Compound	Route	Dosage
Prednisolone	Oral	Adult: 5-60mg daily, in 2-4 divided doses Children:0.14-2mg/kg daily, in 2-4 divided doses
Prednisolone Acetate	IM	Adult: 4-60mg daily, IM at 12-hour intervals Children: 0.04-0.25mg/kg, IM, 1-2 times daily; Doses of 2mg/kg/day may be required.
Prednisolone Sodium Phosphate	Oral, IM, IV Intraarticular Intralesional Soft Tissue, IV Infusion with Dextrose or NaCl	Adult: Oral, IM or IV, initially, 4-60mg; 10-400mg daily Children: Oral, IM or IV, 0.04-0.25mg/kg, 1-2 times daily; Doses of 2mg/kg/day may be required. Intra-Articular, Intralesional or Soft Tissue: 2-30mg repeated at 3 day to 3 week intervals. Larger Joints (eg, Knee): 10-20mg Smaller Joints: 4-5mg Bursae: 10-15mg Ganglia: 5-10mg Soft Tissue; Tendon Sheath: 2-5mg Soft Tissue Infiltration: 10-30mg
Prednisolone Tebutate	Intra-Articular, Intralesional or Soft Tissue	4-40mg repeated at 2-to 3-week intervals. Larger Joints (eg, Knee): 20-40mg Smaller Joints: 8-10mg Bursae: 20-30mg Ganglia: 10-20mg Soft Tissue; Tendon Sheath: 4-10mg Nasal Polyps: 10-20mg; Soft Tissue Infiltration: 20-60mg

ADVERSE EFFECTS: Adrenocortical insufficiency; Musculoskeletal: muscle wasting, delayed wound healing, osteoporosis, etc., increased susceptibility to infection; GI: nausea, vomiting, anorexia, etc., Nervous System: headache, vertigo, insomnia, etc; Dermatologic: skin atrophy and thinning, acne, etc.

See **PREDNISONE** section.

PREDNISONE
(Cortan, Deltasone, Orasone, Others)

USES: Prednisone is a **glucocorticoid**; uses are given in the next Table:

Uses of Prednisone

Rheumatic Disorders and Collagen Disease: Rheumatoid Arthritis, and Rheumatic Carditis and Collagen Diseases, e.g., Dermatomyositis and Polymyositis, Polyarteritis Nodosa, Relapsing Polychondritis Polymyalgia Rheumatica, Giant-Cell (Temporal) Arteritis, Mixed Connective Tissue Diseases.
Dermatologic Diseases: Acute Exacerbations Unresponsive to Conservative Therapy: Pemphigus and Pemphigoid, Exfoliative Dermatitis, Bullous Dermatitis Herpetiformis, Severe Erythema Multiforme (Stevens-Johnson Syndrome), Uncontrollable Eczema, Cutaneous Sarcoidosis, Mycosis Fungoides, Lichen Planus.
Allergic Conditions: Acute Manifestions of: Angioedema, Serum Sickness, Contact Dermatitis, Drug Hypersensitivity, Allergic Symptoms of Trichinosis, Acute Exacerbations of Chronic Allergic Conditions.
Organ Transplants: Used with Other Immunosuppressive Drugs.
Nephrotic Syndrome
Combination with Cytotoxic Drugs for Treatment of Acute Lymphocytic Leukemia, Hodgkin's Disease and Non-Hodgkin's Lymphoma.
Asthma

Prednisone is usually considered the oral glucocorticoid of choice for anti-inflammatory or immunosuppressant effects.

Prednisone has minimal mineralocorticoid properties. If prednisone is used in the treatment of adrenocortical insufficiency, concomitant therapy with mineralocorticoid is required.

Prednisone is converted in the body to the active compound, prednisolone. Patients with liver disease have unpredictable metabolism of prednisone with a variable clinical response.

Mechanism of Action: Like other corticosteroids, prednisone exerts its cellular effects by forming a complex with a specific receptor protein in the cytoplasm; the complex then binds to nuclear chromatin. This is followed by transcription of specific genes of the DNA into corresponding messenger RNA and RNA translation into proteins, including enzymes.

DOSAGE FORMS: Tabs: 1, 2.5, 5, 10, 20, 25, 50mg; Sol'n: 5mg/5ml, 5mg/ml.

DOSAGE: Prednisone is administered orally. The dosage of prednisone in different conditions is given in the next Table:

Dosage of Prednisone in Different Conditions

Condition	Dosage
Physiologic Replacement	Children and Adults: 0.1-0.15mg/kg/day in 2 divided doses or 4-5mg/M^2/day in 2 divided doses.
Anti-Inflammatory or Immunosuppressive	0.5-2mg/kg/day divided in up to 3 divided doses.
Rheumatoid Arthritis	Adults: 7.5mg daily; 5mg in postmenopause women. Adjust amount at 3-7 day intervals depending upon response, to the maintenance level. Discontinuation of therapy should be the gradual with dosage reductions of 1mg/month.
Juvenile Polyarticular Arthritis	Children: Small doses, eg, 2-3mg daily may improve condition.If possible, use 1mg tablets in divided doses during the day. Alternate day therapy is preferred
Polymyositis or Dermatomyositis	1-2mg/kg daily for 2-3 months; the dosage may be reduced gradually after initial response.
Ulcerative Colitis	40-60mg daily initially.
Nephrotic Syndrome	Children: Initial: 2mg/kg/day (max. of 80mg/day) in 3 or 4 divided doses until urine is protein-free for 5 days. (max.of 28 days). If urine is not protein-free within 28 days, dose may be changed to 4mg/kg/day (max. of 120mg/day) given with breakfast on alternate days for up to 28 additional days. Taper over 4-6 weeks. Adults: 60mg daily

PREDNISONE (Cont.)

Dosage of Prednisone in Different Conditions	
Condition	Dosage
Asthma Acute Exacerbation	Children: 1-4 mg/kg/day for 3-5 days. Longer course may be necessary in some cases. Adults: 20-60mg daily as a single morning dose or in divided doses for 3-5 days or until symptoms are controlled.
Severe Refractory Asthma-Chronic Therapy	5-10mg/dose every day. or 10-30mg/dose every other day. An attempt to transfer the patient to inhaled aerosol corticosteroid (beclomethasone)therapy should be done as soon as possible. During transfer to inhaled aerosol, the dose of prednisone is decreased by 2.5mg/dose if on every day schedule or 5mg/dose if on every other day schedule, at intervals of 1 week.

ADVERSE EFFECTS: Dermatologic: acne, thin fragile skin, poor wound healing, petechiae, ecchymoses, facial erythema, diaphoresis. Endocrine: Cushing's syndrome, growth suppression, pituitary-adrenal axis suppression, menstrual changes, glucose intolerance, negative nitrogen balance, decreased protein anabolism. Fluid and Electrolyte Disturbances: salt and water retention, hypertension, congestive heart failure, potassium depletion, hypokalemic alkalosis. Gastrointestinal: peptic ulcers, pancreatitis, esophageal ulceration. Immunologic Suppression: exacerbation of deep fungal or mycobacterial infection or herpes keratitis; chronic use may predispose to infections caused by unusual organisms. Musculoskeletal: weakness, myopathy, decreased muscle mass, osteoporosis, pathologic fractures. Neurologic: increased intracranial pressure (pseudotumor cerebri), vertigo, headache, euphoria, psychosis, convulsions. Ophthalmic: posterior subcapsular cataracts, increased intraocular pressure, glaucoma.

PHARMACOKINETICS: Absorption: Complete; Peak: 1-2 hours; Duration: 1.25-1.5 days; Protein-Binding: 70-95%; Half-Life Prednisone, 3.3-3.8 hours; Prednisolone, 2-4 hours; Metabolism: Prednisone is metabolized in the liver to its active form prednisolone; liver disease does not impair conversion to active metabolites. Patients with liver disease and hypoalbuminemia may develop major side effects as a result of decreased protein binding and delayed clearance of prednisolone.

CONTRAINDICATIONS: Systemic fungal infections.

PRECAUTIONS: Osteoporosis, peptic ulcer, tuberculosis, acute and chronic bacterial, viral and fungal infections, immunizations, liver disease hypoalbuminemia, psychosis, suppression of TB and other skin test reactions.

PREGNANCY CATEGORY

The definitions of the risk factor categories (A,B,C,D,X) are given in the next Table (Federal Register 40, 37434-67, 1980):

Category	Definition
A	Drugs for which adequate and well-controlled human studies have failed to demonstrate a risk to the fetus.
B	Drugs for which human fetal risk is relatively unlikely based upon either negative animal studies and no adequate and well-controlled human studies, or positive animal studies and negative, adequate and well-controlled human studies.
C	Drugs for which human fetal risk is unknown based upon positive animal studies (or no animal studies), and no adequate and well-controlled human studies. Drugs should be given only if the potential benefit justifies the potential risk to the fetus.
D	Drugs for which there is positive human evidence of fetal risk available, but the benefits from use in pregnant women may be acceptable despite the risk.
X	Drugs for which positive animal studies or positive human evidence of fetal risk is available, and whose use in a pregnant woman is contraindicated.

PRIMIDONE

(Mysoline)

USES: Primidone is a **barbiturate,** structurally related to phenobarbital; primidone is used as an **anticonvulsant** in the prophylactic management of the conditions listed in the next Table:

Uses of Primidone as Anticonvulsant
Partial Seizures with Complex Symptomatology (Psychomotor Seizures)
Tonic-Clonic(Grand Mal) Seizures - Refractory to other Anticonvulsant Therapy
Seizures with Autonomic Systems
Akinetic Seizures

Primidone is effective for the same types of seizures as phenobarbital. The anticonvulsant effect is due both to the drug itself and its metabolites, which include phenobarbital. **Some clinicians consider primidone the drug of choice for the prophylactic management of partial seizures with complex symptomatology (psychomotor seizures).**

DOSAGE FORMS: Susp. 250mg/5ml; Tabs: 50mg, 250mg

DOSAGE: Primidone is administered orally; dosage of primidone is given in the next Table:

Age	Dosage
Neonate	Load: 15-25mg/kg Maintenance: 12-20mg/kg/day in 2-4 divided doses
Children <8 years	Initially: 125mg daily as a single dose, usually at bedtime. Increase by 125mg/day at weekly intervals. Maintenance: 10-25mg/kg daily in 3-4 divided doses.
Adults Children >8 years	Initially: 250mg daily as a single dose, usually at bedtime. Increase by 250mg/day at weekly intervals. Maintenance: 750-1500mg/day in 3-4 divided doses.

Table: Dosage of Primidone

ADVERSE EFFECTS: Severe reactions are rare. Mild adverse effects are drowsiness, ataxia, vertigo, anorexia, nausea and vomiting; ataxia and vertigo tend to disappear with continued therapy. Primidone can also cause disturbances in behavior, difficulty in concentration, and loss of libido.

Acute Toxicity: Symptoms similar to those of acute barbiturate intoxication. Treatment is the same as treatment of barbiturate acute toxicity.

MONITOR: Complete blood count (CBC) and SMA-12 every 6 months (manufacturer's recommendation). When monitoring is necessary, both primidone and phenobarbital concentrations should be measured. Therapeutic level: primidone: 8-12mg/L; phenobarbital: 15-40mg/L.

PROBENECID

(Benemid, Probalan)

USES: Probenecid is used to lower serum urate concentrations and is used as an **adjunct to therapy** with **penicillins** to **elevate** and **prolong** the plasma concentrations of these **antibiotics.** Uses are listed in the next Table:

Uses of Probenecid
Hyperuricemia Associated with Gout
Hyperuricemia Secondary to Drugs:
Thiazides, Furosemide, Ethacrynic Acid, Pyrazinamide or Ethambutol
Adjunct to Therapy with Penicillin to Elevate and Prolong the Plasma Concentrations of the Antibiotics

Probenecid should not be used to treat hyperuricemia secondary to cancer chemotherapy, radiation, or myeloproliferative neoplastic diseases because it may increase the risk of uric acid nephropathy.

Mechanism of Action: Probenecid is a renal tubular blocking agent that competitively inhibits active reabsorption of uric acid at the proximal convoluted tubule, thus promoting urinary excretion of uric acid and reducing serum urate concentrations.

Probenecid is used as an adjunct to therapy with penicillin and cephalosporins. Probenecid acts on the proximal and distal renal tubules, competitively inhibiting the secretion of many weak acids including penicillins and cephalosporins. Plasma concentrations of penicillins are more than doubled; the concentration of penicillin in the CSF is also increased. Probenecid also increases the plasma concentrations of most cephalosporins. Half-lives of the penicillins and cephalosporins are prolonged and the volumes of distribution may be reduced.

DOSAGE FORMS: Tabs: 500mg

DOSAGE: Probenecid is administered orally. Adverse GI effects may be minimized by taking the drug with food or antacids, or may require dosage reduction. Daily urine output should be maintained at a minimum of 2-3 liters in all patients; alkalinization of the urine is desirable. Dosage is given in the next Table:

Dosage of Probenecid

Condition	Dosage
Hyperuricemia with Gout	Adult: 250mg, twice daily, for the first week then 500mg twice daily. Serum urate concentrations usually decrease to a minimum within a few days. If symptoms are not controlled or uric acid excretion is not above 700mg/24 hrs, increase daily dosage by 500mg monthly to a max. of 2-3g daily.
Adjunct to Penicillin Therapy	Children (2-14 yrs): Initially, 25mg/kg orally then 40mg/kg daily in 4 divided doses. Adults: 2g daily in 4 divided doses or 1g as a single dose with a penicillin or cephalosporin when treating uncomplicated diseases caused by susceptible strains of N. gonorrhoeae.

ADVERSE EFFECTS: Use with caution in patients with a history of peptic ulcer. Headache, GI symptoms, hypersensitivity, anemia.

CONTRAINDICATIONS: Children less than 2 years of age and patients with renal insufficiency.

PROCAINAMIDE
(Pronestyl, Procan)

USES: **Procainamide** is used in the treatment of **cardiac arrhythmias;** it is most often used to treat life-threatening ventricular arrhythmias resistant to lidocaine and as prophylaxis against ventricular arrhythmias following acute myocardial infarction. Uses are listed in the next Table:

Uses of Procainamide

Use	Comments
Ventricular Premature Contractions	IV or IM lidocaine is the drug of choice. Oral procainamide is frequently used to prevent recurrence of ventricular premature contractions when lidocaine infusion is discontinued. Procainamide is generally not used to treat digitalis-induced ventricular arrhythmias.
Atrial Premature Contractions	Although procainamide can be used for the treatment of atrial contractions, these arrhythmias are usually treated with digitalis
Ventricular Tachycardia Not Torsades de Pointes	Procainamide may be used to treat ventricular tachycardia, but treatment is usually with cardioversion or lidocaine. Procainamide and lidocaine have approximately equivalent activity in the treatment of ventricular arrhythmias and procainamide may be used to prevent recurrence of ventricular tachycardia.
Atrial Fibrillation or Flutter	Treatments of choice are digitalis (alone or with propranolol) or direct current countershock; or digitalis with procainamide or quinidine
Paroxysmal Atrial Tachycardia or AV Junctional Rhythm	Treatments of choice include increase vagal tone (such as carotid sinus massage, Valsalva maneuver, and/or gagging), verapamil, adenosine, digoxin, and beta-blockers as well as cardioversion are usually used for supraventricular tachycardias.

Mechanism of Action: The mechanism of action of procainamide is like that of quinidine and disopyramide except procainamide has weaker anticholinergic effects as compared to quinidine.

Procainamide has a direct action on the cell membrane; it depresses automaticity, especially in ectopic sites. It slows conduction and increases refractoriness of the atria, His-Purkinje system, accessory pathways and ventricles.

DOSAGE FORMS: Caps: 250, 375, 500mg; Tabs: 250, 375, 500mg; Tabs; Extended Release: 250, 500, 750, 1000mg(1g); Parenteral: 100mg/ml, 500mg/ml.

DOSAGE: Procainamide is usually administered orally; oral dosage of procainamide in different conditions is given in the next Table:

Oral Dosage of Procainamide in Different Conditions

Condition	Dosage
Ventricular Tachycardia **Ventricular Premature Contractions**	Adult: 6.25 mg/kg orally every 3 hours. For oral maintenance therapy using extended-release tablets, one-fourth of the required daily dose may be given every 6 hours (50mg/kg daily in equally divided doses at 6-hour intervals).
Atrial Fibrillation and Paroxysmal Atrial Tachycardia	Adult: 1.25g orally; if no change in ECG, 750mg, 1 hr later. Additional doses, 500mg to 1g, may be administered, every 2 hours until normal rhythm or toxic effects. After conversion, maintenance dose, 500mg to 1g every 4-6 hours. When extended-release preparations are used for maintenance therapy, give 1g every 6 hours.
Ventricular Arrhythmias	Children: 15-50mg/kg daily in divided doses every 3-6 hours. Max.: 4g daily.

PROCAINAMIDE (Cont.)

Parenteral dosage is given in the next Table (Textbook of Advanced Cardiac Life Support, American Heart Assoc., 103-104, 1987):

Parenteral Dosage of Procainamide		
Ventricular Tachycardia **Premature Ventricular Complexes**	IV	Adult: 100mg every 5 minutes at a rate of 20mg/min until one of the following: (1) arrhythmia is suppressed; (2) Hypotension; (3) QRS widened by 50%; (4) total of 1g of drug is given. Maintenance infusion: 1-4mg/min.
	or	Loading Dose: 17mg/kg over 1 hr, Maintenance infusion: 2.8mg/kg/hr; Children: Load: 2-6mg/kg over 5 min; Maintenance: 20-80micrograms/kg/min.
	IM	Adult: Load: 500mg to 1g; Maintenance: 250mg to 1gm every 4-6 hours. Children: 20-30mg/kg/day in divided doses every 4-6 hours.

Dosage in Renal Impairment: In patients with renal impairment, the dose of procainamide must be adjusted downward. Dose as follows in patients with renal failure:

Dosage of Procainamide in Renal Failure

Intravenous:
- Loading Dose (Normal): 17mg/kg
  - Moderate Renal Failure (BUN 25 to 40mg/dl): 17mg/kg
  - Severe Renal Failure (BUN >40mg/dl) or pulmonary edema or cardiogenic shock: 12mg/kg
- Maintenance Dose: Normal: 2.8mg/kg/hour
  - Moderate Renal Failure (BUN 25 to 40mg/dl): 2.0mg/kg/hour
  - Severe Renal Failure (BUN >40mg/dl) or pulmonary edema or cardiogenic shock: 1mg/kg/hour

Oral: Normal: 6.25mg/kg every 3 hours to 11.2mg/kg every 4 hours.
- Moderate Renal Failure: Dosing interval, 4 to 6 hours.
- Severe Renal Failure: Dosing interval, 6 to 12 hours.

PHARMACOKINETICS: Bioavailability: 75%-95%; Metabolism: The major metabolite of procainamide is N-acetylprocainamide (NAPA) which also possesses anti-arrhythmic activity. The serum concentration of NAPA is genetically determined by the activity of the hepatic enzyme, N-acetyltransferase; different individuals acetylate procainamide at different rates. Therapeutic: 4-8mcg/ml for procainamide; 10-30mcg/ml for procainamide plus N-acetyl procainamide (NAPA). Toxic: >30mcg/ml for both procainamide plus N-acetyl procainamide (NAPA); up to 30mcg/ml may be tolerated by some individuals. Half-Life: Procainamide: 3 hours in normal subjects; 9 hours with renal impairment. NAPA: 7 hours in normal subjects; 10 hours to 40 hours with renal impairment. Determine creatinine and BUN before starting therapy. Steady State(Time to obtain serum specimens): Oral: 48 hours; Intravenous: 24 hours after loading dose. Excretion: About half of the available dose of procainamide appears in the urine.

ADVERSE EFFECTS: Adverse effects of procainamide are listed in the next Table:

Adverse Effects of Procainamide

Gastrointestinal Disturbances:
- Anorexia, Nausea and Vomiting

Cardiovascular:
- Slow Intraventricular Conduction, A-V Block, Bradycardia, Hypotension, Syncope
- Ventricular Arrhythmias, Increased Ventricular Response to Atrial Flutter or Fibrillation
- QT Prolongation and Widening of the QRS Complex; QRS widening >0.02 seconds suggests toxicity
- Contraindicated in Torsades de Pointes

Adverse Effects of Prolonged Procainamide Therapy:
- Reversible Lupus Erythematosus-Like Syndrome (30% of patients) with Polyarthalgia, Arthritis, Pleuritic Pain, Fever, Rash, Pericarditis, Myocarditis, Thrombocytopenia and Hemolytic Anemia Antinuclear Antibodies: 50% to 80%.

Hypersensitivity with Fever, Rash, Urticaria, Neutropenia

Mental Disturbances

PROCAINAMIDE (Cont.)

Severe neutropenia (granulocytopenia) is associated with procainamide; granulocytopenia generally occurs in the first 3 months and it usually develops rapidly. Therefore, leukocyte determinations should be done at 2-week intervals. Discontinuation of therapy has generally resulted in a prompt return to normal leukocyte counts (Ellrodt, A.G. et al., Ann. Intern. Med. 100, 197-201, 1984; Gabrielson, R.M., ibid 100, 766, 1984).

DRUG INTERACTIONS: Drug interactions of procainamide are shown in the next Table:

Drug Interactions of Procainamide

Drug(s)	Effect
Neuromuscular Blocking Agents, eg, Skeletal Muscle Relaxants	Procainamide may potentiate the effects of skeletal muscle relaxants, e.g.,tubocurarine, succinylcholine, pancuronium.
Anticholinesterase and Anticholinergic Agents	Use with caution, if at all, in patients with myasthenia gravis. The dose of anticholinesterase drugs such as neostigmine and pyridostigmine may have to be increased.
Cardiovascular Drugs	Procainamide may reduce blood pressure; hypotensive effects of other drugs may be additive

MONITOR: The marked variations in absorption, metabolism and elimination are reasons to monitor patients receiving procainamide.

Therapy and Blood Specimens

Intravenous Therapy	Blood Specimens
Loading Dose: 17mg/kg in 100ml D5W given over one hour	First blood specimen obtained at end of Loading Dose
Second Infusion: (Maintenance Dose) 2.8mg/kg/hour (Add total daily dose to 500ml D5W and infuse at 20ml/hour for 24 hours.	Second: Two hours after maintenance infusion begins. Note: Loading infusion level should be higher than maintenance infusion level; neither sample should exceed 15ug/ml. Third: Six to 12 hours after maintenance infusion starts. Fourth: At 24 hours. (This is the time that steady-state is achieved)
Oral Therapy	**Blood Specimens**
Dosing interval should not exceed 4 hours; a sustained release preparation is given every 6 hours. Oral Dose = maintenance infusion rate (see above) x dosing interval in hours. Example: 2.8mg/kg/hr x 4 hrs = 11.2mg/kg/dose	Blood specimens should be obtained as follows: First Blood Specimen: 48 hours after starting oral therapy and when dose is administered. Second Blood Specimen: Middle of same dosing interval. Third Blood Specimen: End of same dosing interval. Obtain second and third blood specimens at equally spaced time intervals.

CONTRAINDICATIONS: Torsades de Pointes.

PROCHLORPERAZINE
(Compazine)

USES: Prochlorperazine is a **phenothiazine;** uses are given in the next Table:

Uses of Prochlorperazine
Control of Severe **Nausea** and **Vomiting**, eg, Postoperative, Toxins, Cytotoxic Drugs, and Radiation
Symptomatic Management of **Psychotic Disorders**
Excessive Anxiety

Mechanism of Action: Prochlorperazine acts as an antiemetic by directly affecting the medullary chemoreceptor trigger zone(CTZ), apparently by blocking dopamine receptors in the CTZ. Antipsychotic effects are most likely due to antidopaminergic effects at the subcortical level (reticular formation, limbic system, and hypothalamus); effects on gamma-aminobutyric acid (GABA), substance P, and endorphins may also play a role.

DOSAGE FORMS: Tabs: 5, 10, 25mg; Sol'n: 5mg/5ml; Caps, Extended Release: 10, 15, 30mg; Supp: 2.5, 5, 25mg; Inject: 5mg/ml.

DOSAGE: The dosage of prochlorperazine is given in the next Table:

Dosage of Prochlorperazine

Condition	Age	Route	Dosage
Nausea and Vomiting	Adult	Oral	5 or 10mg, 3 or 4 times daily or 15mg, extended release once daily upon arising or 10mg, extended release, every 12 hours.
	Adult	Rectal	25mg, twice daily
	Adult	IM	5-10mg; repeat every 3 or 4 hours, but total should not exceed 40mg daily
	Children >2 yrs; >9kg	Oral or Rectal	0.4mg/kg daily, 3 or 4 divided doses.
	Children >2 yrs; >9kg	IM	0.1-0.15mg/kg/dose, 3 or 4 times daily.
Nausea and Vomiting During Surgery	Adult	IM, IV	5-10mg, 1-2 hours (IM) or 15-30 min (IV) before induction of anesthesia. If necessary repeat once, 30 min. later.
			During or after surgery: 5-10mg, repeated once in 30 min. as necessary.
		IV Infusion	20mg/liter, 15-30min. before induction of anesthesia.
Psychotic Disorders	Adult	Oral	Office and outpatients with mild symptoms: 5 or 10mg, 3 or 4 times daily. Hospitalized patients, mod. to severe symptoms: 10mg, 3 or 4 times daily; increase dosage until symptoms controlled or adverse effects occur; up to 150mg daily may be necessary.
	Children 2-12 yrs.	Oral or Rectal	2.5mg, 2 or 3 times daily; do not exceed 10mg on first day. Daily dosage should not exceed 20mg for children 2-5 years and 25mg for children 6-12 years.
	Adult	IM	Severe symptoms: 10-20mg; repeat as necessary every 1-4 hours up to 3 or 4 doses. After control, replace IM by oral dose at same dosage level or higher.
	Children (<12 yrs)	IM	0.1-0.15mg/kg; after control, replace parenteral by oral dose at same dosage level or higher.
Excessive Anxiety	Adult	Oral Rectal, IM	Same dose as for nausea and vomiting.

ADVERSE EFFECTS: Toxicity as for other phenothiazines. The relative freqency of side effects is as follows: sedation, moderate; anticholinergic effects (dryness of the mouth, orthostatic hypotension, blurred vision, urinary retention and constipation), weak; extrapyramidal effects (dystonia, akathisia, parkinsonian signs and symptoms), high. Neuroleptic malignant syndrome (hyperthermia, extrapyramidal dysfunction, and altered mental status) may occur.

PROMETHAZINE
(Anergan, Phenergan, Others)

USES: Promethazine is a **phenothiazine derivative;** uses are given in the next Table:

Uses of Promethazine
Sedative and Antiemetic Effects in Surgery and Obstetrics (during labor)
Reduces Preoperative Tension and Anxiety
Antihistamine
Motion Sickness

DOSAGE FORMS: Oral Sol'n: 6.25, 25mg/5ml; Tabs: 12.5, 25, 50mg; IV Injection: 25mg/ml; IM Injection: 50mg/ml; Rectal Supp.: 12.5, 25, 50mg.

DOSAGE: Promethazine is administered orally, rectally, IV or deep IM injection; dosage by these various routes of administration is identical. Dosage is given in the next Table:

Dosage of Promethazine

Condition	Age	Dosage
Preoperative or Post-operative Sedation, Adjunct to Analgesics	Adult	25-50mg/dose every 4-6 hrs.
	Children	0.5-1mg/kg/dose, every 6 hrs. When used with opiate analgesics, dosage of analgesic should usually be reduced.
Obstetrics		50mg to provide sedation during early labor. 25-75mg when labor is established with reduced dose of opiate agent. 25-50mg doses may be repeated once or twice at 4 hour intervals as necessary. Max. total dose during labor, 100mg
Nausea and Vomiting	Adult	12.5-25mg; doses of 12.5-25mg, every 4 hrs., as necessary.
	Children	0.25-0.5mg/kg, 4-6 times daily.
Antihistamine	Adult	12.5mg before meals and 25mg at bedtime
	Children	0.1mg/kg/dose every 6 hrs and 0.5mg/kg at bedtime.
Motion Sickness		First dose, 30-60 min. prior to departure; second dose 8-12 hrs. later. Additional doses on arising and before evening meal for duration of journey.
	Adult	25mg twice daily.
	Children	0.5mg/kg twice daily.

ADVERSE EFFECTS: Toxicity as for other phenothiazines, side effects include sedation, anticholinergic effects (dryness of the mouth, hypotension, blurred vision, urinary retention and constipation), and extrapyramidal effects (dystonia, akathisia, parkinsonian signs and symptoms. Other effects include arrhythmias, agranulocytosis, lowered seizure threshold, and obstructive jaundice. May potentiate effects of narcotics, sedatives. Neuroleptic malignant syndrome (hyperthermia, extrapyramidal dysfunction, and altered mental status) may occur.

PROPANTHELINE BROMIDE
(Pro-Banthine)

USES: Propantheline bromide is an antimuscarinic agent. Uses of propantheline are given in the next Table:

Uses of Propantheline
Peptic Ulcer Disease
Irritable Bowel Syndrome

DOSAGE FORMS: Tabs: 7.5, 15mg

DOSAGE: Propantheline is given orally; the drug is given 30 minutes before meals and at bedtime. Dosage is given in the next Table:

Dosage of Propantheline

Patient	Dosage
Adults with Mild Symptoms or Geriatric Patients	7.5mg, 3 times daily
Adults	15mg, 3 times daily before meals and 30mg at bedtime (total dosage, 75mg daily)

Safety and efficacy in children has not been established.

ADVERSE EFFECTS: Contraindicated in glaucoma, obstruction of urinary or GI tract and inflammatory bowel disease. May cause sedation, dizziness, mydriasis and cycloplegia.

PROPHYLACTIC USE OF ANTIMICROBIAL AGENTS

Generally accepted prophylactic uses of antimicrobial agents are given in the next Table (Van Scoy, R.E. and Wilkowske, C.J., Mayo Clin. Proc. 62, 1137-1141, 1987):

Generally Accepted Prophylactic Uses of Antimicrobial Agents

Condition	Antimicrobial agent
Tuberculosis	Isoniazid, 300mg/day for 6-12 months (monthly follow-up for toxicity)
Rheumatic fever Prophylaxis	Benzathine penicillin, 1.2 million U/mo intramuscularly; in high risk situations, IM administration should be every 3 weeks or penicillin V 250mg orally twice daily or sulfadiazine 0.5g once daily for patients <27kg, 1.0g once daily for patients >27kg or erythromycin 250mg twice daily (Dajani, A.S. et al., Pediatr. Infect. Dis. J. 8, 263-266, 1989).
Recurrent Cellulitis in Lymphedema	Benzathine penicillin, 1.2 million U/mo intramuscularly, or penicillin V, 250-500mg 4 times/day, for 1 week of each month.
Meningococcal Infections	Adult: Rifampin, 600mg 2 times/day for 2 days. Children: Rifampin 10mg/kg 2 times/day for 2 days. Neonate (0-1 mo.): Rifampin 5mg/kg 2 times/day for 2 days.
Haemophilus Influenza Infections	Adult: Rifampin, 600mg once daily for 4 days. Children: Rifampin, 20mg/kg daily for 4 days. Neonate (0-1 mo.): Rifampin, 10mg/kg daily for 4 days
Plague	Tetracycline, 30mg/kg/day in 4 divided doses for 10 days, or streptomycin, 1g/day for 1 week.
Bite Wounds	Penicillin V, 500mg 4 times/day for 3-5 days, or amoxicillin with clavulanate 500mg 3 times/day for 3-5 days. Children: Pen V, 25-50mg/kg daily in 4 divided doses or amoxicillin with clavulanate 20-40mg/kg daily in 3 divided doses or erythromycin 30-50mg/kg daily in 4 divided doses (Wiley, J.F., Clinical Pediatrics 29, 283-287, May, 1990).
Influenza	Amantadine, 100mg 2 times/day for duration of risk (decrease to 100mg/day if patient is elderly or has renal insufficiency).
Recurrent Cystitis	Trimethoprim-sulfamethoxazole, 40mg + 200mg or trimethoprim, 100mg at bedtime.
Ophthalmia Neonatorum	Topical erythromycin ointment(0.5%), or tetracycline ointment (1%) (Amer. Acad. Ped., Pediatrics 65, 1047-1048, 1980; Laga, M. et al., N. Engl. J. Med. 318, 653-657, 1988).
Herpes Simplex Infections	Acyclovir-400mg orally, 2 times daily(Mertz, G.J. et al., JAMA 260, 201-206, July 8, 1988).See ACYCLOVIR
Otitis Media	Amoxicillin 20mg/kg once daily at bedtime or sulfisoxazole 50mg/kg once daily (Bluestone, C.D., Ped. Infect. Dis. J. 7, S129-S136, 1988).
Endocarditis Prophylaxis	See ENDOCARDITIS PROPHYLAXIS.
Surgical Prophylaxis	See SURGICAL PROPHYLAXIS.

Possible or controversial prophylactic uses of antimicrobial agents are given in the next Table(Van Scoy, R.E. and Wilkowske, C.J., Mayo Clin. Proc. 62, 1137-1141, 1987):

Possible or Controversial Prophylactic Uses of Antimicrobial Agents

Condition	Antimicrobial agent
Traveler's Diarrhea	Trimethoprim-sulfamethoxazole, Bismuth subsalicylate, norfloxacin, others. See TRAVELERS' DIARRHEA, PATHOGENS, PREVENTION, TREATMENT.

PROPOXYPHENE, ACETAMINOPHEN
(Darvocet-N, Others)

USES: Propoxyphene is an analgesic which is used for the relief of mild to moderate pain. Propoxyphene in combination with acetaminophen may result in greater analgesia than propoxyphene alone, but may or may not be more effective than acetaminophen alone.

Propoxyphene is structurally related to the opiate analgesic methadone.

DOSAGE FORMS: Darvocet is available only as tablets. Dosage forms are given in the next Table:

Dosage Forms of Darvocet-N

Form	Propoxyphene (mg)	Acetaminophen (mg)
Darvocet-N 50	50	325
Darvocet-N 100	100	650

Darvocet-N 100 is prescribed more often than Darvocet-N 50.

DOSAGE: Dosage is given in the next Table:

Form	Dosage
Darvocet-N	Two Darvocet-N 50 or one Darvocet-N 100 evert 4 hours as needed. Max. 12 Darvocet-N 50 or 6 Darvocet-N 100 daily.

PHARMACOKINETICS (of Propoxyphene): Onset and Duration: Onset about one hour; Metabolism: Liver; Half-Life: 12 hours.

ADVERSE EFFECTS (of Propoxyphene): Dizziness, sedation, nausea and vomiting are the most frequent adverse effects. Occasionally constipation, euphoria, dysphoria, minor visual disturbances and skin rashes are observed. Chronic ingestion of doses exceeding 800mg/day has caused toxic psychosis and convulsions.

CONTRAINDICATIONS: Suicidal or addiction-prone patients.

PRECAUTIONS: Impaired renal or hepatic function. Elderly or debilitated. Pregnancy, lactation.

DRUG INTERACTIONS: Potentiation with alcohol and CNS depressants. Propoxyphene is metabolized in the liver by cytochrome P-450; multiple potential drug interactions with similarly metabolized agents.

PROPOXYPHENE, ASPIRIN
(Darvon-N with ASA)

USES: Propoxyphene is an **analgesic** which is used for the relief of **mild to moderate pain**. Propoxyphene, in combination with aspirin, may result in greater analgesia than propoxyphene alone, but may or may not be more effective than aspirin alone.

Propoxyphene is structural related to the opiate analgesic methadone.

DOSAGE FORMS and DOSAGE: Darvon-N with ASA is available as tablets and capsules. Dosage forms are given in the next Table:

Dosage Forms of Darvon-N with ASA

Forms	Propoxyphene Napsylate(mg)	Aspirin(mg)	Caffeine(mg)	Dosage
Darvon-N with ASA Tablets	100	325	--	One every 4 hours
Darvon with ASA Caps	65	325	--	One every 4 hours
Darvon Compound 65	65	389	32.4	One every 4 hours
Darvon Compound	32	389	32.4	One every 4 hours

Darvon-N with ASA is not recommended for children:

PHARMACOKINETICS (of Propoxyphene): Onset and Duration: Onset about one hour; Metabolism: Liver; Half-Life: 12 hours.

ADVERSE EFFECTS (of Propoxyphene): Dizziness, sedation, nausea and vomiting are the most frequent adverse effects. Occasionally constipation, euphoria, dysphoria, minor visual disturbances and skin rashes are observed. Chronic ingestion of doses exceeding 800mg/day has caused toxic psychosis and convulsions.

CONTRAINDICATIONS: Suicidal or addiction-prone patients.

PRECAUTIONS: Impaired renal or hepatic function. Elderly or debilitated. Pregnancy, lactation.

DRUG INTERACTION: Potentiated with alcohol and CNS depressants. Propoxyphene is metabolized in the liver by cytochrome P-450; multiple potential drug interactions with similarly metabolized agents.

PROPRANOLOL
(Betachron, Inderal)

USES: Propranolol, a **beta-adrenergic blocking agent,** has been used for the conditions listed in the next Table:

Uses of Propranolol
Hypertension
Angina Pectoris
Cardiac Arrhythmias: Supraventricular Arrhythmias, Ventricular Tachycardias, Tachyarrhythmias assoc. with Digitalis Intox., Resistant Tachyarrhythmias Assoc. with Catecholamine Excess During Anesthesia
Thyrotoxicosis
Hypertrophic Subaortic Stenosis
Pheochromocytoma
Migraine
Myocardial Infarction
Uses not currently approved by U.S. Food and Drug Admin.: Cyanotic Spells Tetralogy of Fallot; Anxiety States; Recurrent GI Bleeding in Patients with Cirrhosis

Hypertension: Propranolol may be used as initial drug therapy or may be given in a subsequent step in the treatment of hypertension. Treatment of hypertension with propranolol is given in the next Table (The 1988 Report of the Joint National Committee on Detection, Evaluation, and Treatment of High Blood Pressure, Arch. Intern. Med. 148, 1023-1038, 1988):

Treatment of Hypertension with Propranolol

Step 1: Nonpharmacologic Approaches (see **HYPERTENSION**)

↓

Step 2: Propranolol (Usual Minimum, 40 mg/day; Usual Maximum, 320 mg/day)
Observe up to 6 months; if ineffective then,

↓

Step 3: Add a second drug of a different class
or Increase the dosage of propranolol
or Substitute another drug

↓

Step 4: Add a third drug of a different class
or Substitute a second drug

↓

Step 5: Consider further evaluation and/or referral
or Add a third or fourth drug

"Step-Down": For patients with mild hypertension, after 1 year of control, consider decreasing or withdrawing propranolol and other hypotensive drugs.

Angina: Propranolol, like other beta-1 blocking agents, reduces heart rate, myocardial contractility, and cardiac output; myocardial oxygen demand is reduced and ischemic pain is relieved.

The reduction in heart rate may increase coronary blood flow and oxygen supply by prolonging the diastolic interval during which coronary flow occurs.

Acute Myocardial Infarction: Propranolol may reduce estimated myocardial infarct size when given IV in the early stages of acute myocardial infarction and may decrease mortality when used for long term therapy.

Mechanism of Action: Propranolol is a beta-blocking agent; it inhibits response to adrenergic stimuli by competitively blocking beta-adrenergic receptors within the myocardium (decreases both heart rate and force of contractions) and within bronchial smooth muscle (constriction of bronchioles) and within vascular smooth muscle (vasoconstriction). Beta-1 receptors are found in the heart and are stimulated by norepinephrine. Propranolol, like other beta-1 blockers, produces a fall in blood pressure by decreasing the cardiac output. With continued treatment, the cardiac output returns to normal but the blood pressure remains low because the peripheral resistance is "reset" at a lower level.

DOSAGE FORMS: Tabs: 10, 20, 40, 60, 80, 90mg; Caps (extended release): 60, 80, 120, 160mg; Solution: 20, 40mg/5ml; Injection: 1mg/ml

PROPRANOLOL (Cont.)

DOSAGE: Conditions and dosages of propranolol are given in the next Table:

Dosage of Propranalol

Condition	Dosages
Hypertension:	Children: Starting dose 0.5-1.0mg/kg/day orally divided every 6-12h (max. dose: 2mg/kg/day) Adults: Initial: 10mg/dose orally, four times daily; Increment: 10-20mg/dose at intervals of 3-7 days, Max. dose: 320-480mg/day, orally
Arrhythmias	Children: 0.01-0.10mg/kg/dose, slow IV push; may repeat every 6-8h as needed(max. single dose:1mg); 0.5-4.0mg/kg/day orally divided every 6-8h (max. daily dose: 60mg) Adults: 1mg/dose IV repeated every 5 min. up to total 5mg; 40-320mg/day orally in divided doses every 6-8 h. Max. rate of infusion: 1mg/min.
Tetralogy Spells	0.15-0.25mg/kg/dose IV slowly - may repeat in 15 min. x 1 (max. single dose: 10mg) then maintenance: 1-2mg/kg/dose every 6h, orally.
Thyrotoxicosis	Neonatal: 2mg/kg/day orally in divided doses every 6h Adolescents and Adults: IV: 1-3mg/dose x 1 over 10min. Orally: 10-40mg every 6h
Migraine Prophylaxis	< 35kg: 10-20mg, orally, three times daily > 35kg: 20-40mg, orally, three times daily Adults: Initially, 80mg/day, orally, in 3-4 divided doses. Usual effective dose range: 160-240mg/day; max.: 320mg/day.

ADVERSE EFFECTS: The most serious adverse effects are secondary to its beta-1 and beta-2 adrenergic blocking activity; these effects are more frequent and may be more severe after IV administration. These effects are summarized in the next Table:

Adverse Effects of Propranolol

System	Effect
Cardiovascular	Bradycardia (atropine may control excessive bradycardia) Hypotension, congestive heart failure, Raynaud's
Respiratory System	Inc. airway resist. and may provoke asthmatic attacks
G.I. Effects	Nausea, vomiting, diarrhea, flatulence
Metabolic Effects	Hypoglycemia; decreased HDL cholesterol, increased serum triglyceride, increased uric acid
Neurologic, Psychiatric Effects	Fatigue and lethargy (most common CNS effects), depression, insomnia,vivid dreams or hallucinations, organic brain syndrome
Allergic Reactions	Severe, epinephrine resistant anaphylactic reactions
Other	Impotence, loss of libido, psoriasis, transient hearing loss, blood dyscrasias

Sudden withdrawal is dangerous.

PHARMACOKINETICS: Absorption: Almost complete; a large hepatic first-pass effect occurs, limiting systemic availability; Bioavailability: 30%; Protein-Binding: 93%; Metabolism: Liver; an active metabolite, 4-hydroxypropranolol is formed after oral but not IV administration; Half-Life: 4-6 hours for propranolol(oral) and 2 hrs. for 4-hydroxypropranolol; Duration: 6 to at least 12 hours.

CONTRAINDICATIONS: Abrupt withdrawal, asthma, sinus node dysfunction, second or third degree heart failure, cardiogenic shock or severe heart failure, concomitant MAO inhibitor therapy.

DRUG INTERACTIONS: Drug interactions are given in the next Table:

Drug Interactions of Propranolol

Drug	Effect
Phenothiazines, eg, **Chlorpromazine, Perphenazine, Prochlorperazine, Promethazone, Thioridazine**	May have additive hypotensive effects.
Sympathomimetics, eg, **Dopamine Isoproterenol**	Antagonized by propranolol.
Antimuscarinics, eg, **Atropine**	May counteract bradycardia caused by propranolol
Other Antiarrhythmic Drugs, eg, **Lidocaine, Phenytoin, Procainamide, Quinidine**	Cardiac effects may be additive or antagonistic

PROPYLTHIOURACIL
(PTU)

USES: Uses of propylthiouracil are given in the next Table:

Uses of Propylthiouracil
Palliative treatment of hyperthyroidism
Ameliorate hyperthyroidism in preparation for surgical treatment or radioactive iodine therapy

Propylthiouracil is used to control the symptoms of hyperthyroidism associated with Grave's disease and maintain the patient in a euthyroid state for about 1 to 2 years until a spontaneous remission occurs; however, spontaneous remission may not occur and the patient may require ablative therapy, such as surgery or radioactive iodine.

Mechanism of Action: Propylthiouracil inhibits the synthesis of thyroid hormones by blocking the incorporation of iodine into tyrosyl residues of thyroglobulin and by inhibiting the coupling of these iodotyrosyl residues to form iodothyronine.

DOSAGE FORMS: Tabs: 50mg

DOSAGE: Propylthiouracil is given orally, daily in 3 equally divided doses at about 8-hour intervals. Dosage in different hyperthyroid conditions in adults is given in the next Table:

Adult Dosage of Propylthiouracil

Condition	Dosage
Mild Hyperthyroidism	Adult, initial: 300-450mg daily
Moderate Hyperthyroidism and Very Large Goiters	Adult, initial: 600-1200mg daily
Thyrotoxic Crisis	Adult, initial: 200mg every 4-6 hours on the first day

In general, once full control of symptoms have been achieved, therapy is continued at initial dosage levels for about 2 months. Subsequent dosage should be adjusted according to the patient's tolerance and therapeutic response.

Adult maintenance dose ranges from 100-150mg daily in divided doses every 8 hours.

For the treatment of hyperthyroidism in children, dosage of propylthiouracil is given in the next Table:

Pediatric Dosage of Propylthiouracil

Age	Dosage
Neonate	5-10mg/kg daily
6-10 yrs.	50-150mg daily
>10 yrs.	150-300mg or 150mg/m^2 daily

Maintenance dosage is determined by the patient's response, usually one-third or two-thirds of the initial dose.

Note that 100mg PTU is equal to 10mg methimazole.

REFERENCE VALUES: Peak: 1-1.5 hour; half-life: 1-2 hours; excreted in urine.

ADVERSE EFFECTS: Adverse effects occur in less than 1% of patients and are listed in the next Table:

Adverse Effects of Propylthiouracil
Agranulocytosis
Pancytopenia
Exfoliative Dermatitis
Hepatitis

Dermatologic effects are most common with rash, uriticaria, pruritis, abnormal hair loss, skin pigmentation.

Inhibition of myelopoiesis with resultant agranulocytosis, granulocytopenia and thrombocytopenia may occur; most cases appear in the first two months of therapy and rarely after 4 months. The risk is increased in patients older than 40 years of age and in patients receiving dosages greater than 40mg daily.

MONITOR: Patients should be instructed to contact their physician immediately if the following signs or symptoms develop: sore throat, skin eruptions, fever, chills, headache or general malaise.

Leukocyte and differential counts must be done in patients with fever or sore throat.

Monitor T3, T4 and TSH levels, maintain in the normal range.

PROSTAGLANDIN E1

(Alprostadil, PGE_1, Prostin VR)

USES: Palliative, not definitive, therapy to temporarily maintain patency of ductus arteriosus until corrective or palliative surgery can be performed in neonates who have congenital heart disease and depend upon the patent ductus for survival (pulmonary atresia, pulmonary stenosis, tricuspid atresia, tetrology of Fallot, interruption aortic arch, coarctation of aorta or transposition of great vessels with or without other defects).

DOSAGE FORMS: Amps: 500mcg/ml

DOSAGE: Neonates: Initial: 0.05-0.1mcg/kg/min. Advance to 0.2mcg/kg/min as necessary.

Maintenance: When increase in pO_2 is noted, decrease to lowest effective dose (eg, 0.01mcg/kg/min). Administer in large vein or umbilical artery catheter at ductal opening. Must be infused continuously because rapidly metabolized.

Comments: Continuous vital sign monitoring is essential. Should not be used in respiratory distress syndrome(RDS). Cyanosis (pO_2<40mmHg) and restricted pulmonary blood flow by x-ray are appropriate indicators of cong. heart defects. Monitor: Arterial blood pressure by umbilical artery catheter, auscultation or Doppler Transducer. Restricted Pulmonary Blood Flow: Monitor pO_2. Restricted Systemic Blood Flow: Monitor pO_2 and blood pressure. Respiratory status must be monitored; ventilatory assistance must be immediately available due to the risk of apnea.

ADVERSE EFFECTS: Apnea(12%); fever(14%); seizures(4%); cerebral bleeding (1%); flushing(10%), bradycardia(7%); hypertension(4%); tachycardia (3%); cardiac arrest(1%); diarrhea(2%); DIC(1%).

PROSTATE GLAND, PATHOGENS, TREATMENT

Pathogens: The pathogens that cause prostatitis are given in the next Table (Meares, E.M.,Jr., Infect. Dis. Clin. No. Amer. 1, No. 4, 855-873, Dec.1987):

Pathogens that Cause Prostatitis
Coliform Bacteria:
E. coli (56%)
Klebsiella (20%)
P. mirabilis (8%)
E. aerogenes
P. morganii
Pseudomonas aeruginosa (8%)
Enterococcus (26%)
S. aureus
Chlamydiae

The pathogens that cause acute and chronic prostatitis are similar to those that cause urinary tract infection. In nonhospitalized patients, the most common pathogens are pansensitive E. coli or other coliforms. In hospitalized patients, the most common pathogens are more resistant coliforms, Pseudomonas, enterococcus or Staphylococcus aureus.

Treatment: If the infecting pathogen is identified and antimicrobial susceptibility tests are performed, pathogen specific therapy should be administered. Pending results, treatment of acute bacterial prostatitis is based on the presence of the most likely bacteria being present, that is, coliform bacteria. Outpatient treatment of acute bacterial prostatitis is given in the next Table (Meares, E.M.,Jr., Infect. Dis. Clin. No. Amer. 1, No. 4, 855-873, Dec., 1987; Fuselier, H.A., Jr. et al., Patient Care, pgs. 43-53, April 30, 1985):

Outpatient Treatment of Acute Bacterial Prostatitis

Medication	Dosage
Trimethoprim (TMP)/Sulfamethoxazole (SMX)	Oral: One double-strength tablet (160mg TMP and 800mg SMX) every 12 hours for at least 30 days.
Doxycycline hyclate (Vibramycin, Vibra-Tabs)	Oral: 100mg twice daily for 14 days.
Amoxicillin	Oral: 500mg, four times daily for 14 days
Ciprofloxacin (Malinverni, R. and Glauser, M.P., Rev. Infect. Dis. 10, S153-S163, 1988).	Oral: 1000mg daily (500mg twice daily) for at least 28 days.
Norfloxacin (Malinverni, R. and Glauser, M.P., Rev. Infect. Dis. 10, S153-S163, 1988).	Oral: 800mg daily (400mg twice daily) for at least 28 days.

PROSTATE GLAND, PATHOGENS, TREATMENT (Cont.)

During therapy, give analgesics, antipyretics and stool softeners. Use a punch suprapubic catheter under local anaesthetic to relieve acute urinary retention.

Rarely, hospitalization may be required for acute prostatitis; this may be necessary in patients who don't respond to therapy, and in older males who have difficulty urinating. Inpatient treatment of acute prostatitis is given in the next Table (Meares, E.M., Jr., Infect. Dis. Clin. North Am. 1, 855-873, Dec. 1987):

Inpatient Treatment of Acute Bacterial Prostatitis

Medication	Dosage
Trimethoprim (TMP)/Sulfamethoxazole (SMX)	IV: 8 to 10mg per kg daily (based on the TMP component) in 2-4 divided doses every 6, 8, or 12 hours. Within 48 hours after fever subsides, convert to oral preparation.
Gentamicin plus Ampicillin	IV: Gentamicin, 3 to 5mg/kg daily divided into 3 IV doses; Ampicillin: 2gm daily in 4 divided doses. If appropriate, after one week, start oral antibiotic. Continue therapy for at least 30 days.
Doxycycline hyclate	IV: 100mg every 12 hours.

The treatment of chronic bacterial prostatitis is given in the next Table (Meares, E.M.,Jr., Infect. Dis. Clin. North Am. 1, No. 4, 855-873, Dec. 1987):

Treatment of Chronic Bacterial Prostatitis

Medication	Dosage
Trimethoprim (TMP)/Sulfamethoxazole (SMX)	Oral: One double strength tablet (160mg TMP and 800mg SMX) every 12 hours for 4-16 weeks.
Kanamycin (Pfau, A., Urol. Clin. North Am. 13, 695, 1986)	1000mg IM twice daily for 3 days followed by 500mg twice daily for 11 days.

Other drugs that have been used in the treatment of chronic bacterial prostatitis are carbenicillin, erythromycin, minocycline, doxycycline, and cephalexin; these drugs have not been successful.

The antimicrobial spectrum of activity of drugs used for therapy of prostatitis is given in the next Table:

Antimicrobial Therapy of Prostatitis

	Gram-positive cocci			Gram-negative bacilli						Anaerobes	
Classification	S. aureus	Strep	Enterococci	H. influenzae	E. coli	Klebsiella	P. mirabilis	Other enterics	Pseudomonas a.	B. fragilis	Others
Trimethoprim (TMP)/ Sulfamethoxazole(SMX)	4	3		4	3	3	4	3			
Doxycycline		3		2	3	3		2		2	2
Amoxicillin		4	4	4*	2		4			2	3
Ciprofloxacin	4	±	4	4	4	4	4	4	3		
Gentamicin plus	2			3	4	4	4	4	3		
Ampicillin		4	4	4*	2		4			2	3

4 = best activity; 3 = good activity; 2 = some activity
* = Beta-lactamase negative

PROTAMINE SULFATE

USES: Protamine sulfate is used in the treatment of severe **heparin calcium** or **heparin sodium overdose** or for **reversal of heparinization** following cardiac surgery.

Mechanism of Action: Protamine sulfate is a strongly basic protein which complexes with strongly acidic heparin sodium or heparin calcium; the protamine-heparin complex has no anticoagulant activity. Neutralization of heparin occurs within 30-60 seconds.

DOSAGE FORMS: Injection: 10mg/ml

DOSAGE: Protamine sulfate is given by very slow IV injection over 1-3 minutes; the drug has also been given by continuous IV infusion. Dosage of protamine sulfate is determined by the dose of heparin, the time elapsed since it was given and the route of administration. One mg of protamine sulfate will neutralize approximately 90 units of heparin sodium derived from bovine lung tissue, 100 units of heparin calcium derived from porcine intestinal mucosa or 115 units of heparin sodium derived from porcine intestinal mucosa. Dosage is given in the next Table:

Dosage of Protamine Sulfate

Time Post-IV Heparin Calcium or Heparin Sodium	Mg of Protamine Sulfate Required to Neutralize Every 100 units of Heparin
Few Minutes	1-1.5mg
30-60 Minutes	0.5-0.75mg
2 Hours or More	0.25-0.375

If heparin was given by IV infusion, a dose of 25-50mg of protamine sulfate is given after stopping the infusion.

If heparin was given by deep subcutaneous injection, give 1-1.5mg protamine sulfate for each 100 units of heparin.

Do not give more than 50mg of protamine in any 10 minute period.

ADVERSE EFFECTS: Hypotension, bradycardia, dyspnea, transient flushing may occur with rapid IV infusion. Be prepared to treat shock. Fatal hypersensitivity reactions have been reported. Protamine is derived from salmon sperm; patients with allergy to fish and vasectomized or infertile males may have a higher rate of allergic reaction to protamine.

MONITOR: Activated partial thromboplastin time(APTT) or the activated coagulation time(ACT) should be used to monitor the effect of protamine sulfate in neutralizing heparin. Coagulation tests are usually performed 5-15 minutes after giving the drug. Because heparin may rebound, another test in 2-8 hours is done.

PSEUDOEPHEDRINE, AZATADINE

(Trinalin)

USES: Trinalin is commonly used for **rhinitis** or the **common cold.** Trinalin has two components, **pseudoephedrine,** a **decongestant** and **azatadine,** an **antihistamine.**

DOSAGE FORMS: Each tablet (timed release) contains pseudoephedrine, 120mg and azatadine, 1mg.

DOSAGE: One tablet every 12 hours; not recommended for children.

ADVERSE EFFECTS: Drowsiness, sedation, anticholinergic effects, (eg, dry mouth, blurred vision, urinary retention), dizziness, anxiety, weakness, lightheadedness, insomnia, thickening of bronchial secretions, hypotension, arrhythmias, respiratory depression or difficulty, palpitations, blood dyscrasias.

CONTRAINDICATIONS: Severe hypertension, coronary artery disease, bronchospasm, glaucoma, GI or urinary obstruction, lactation.

PRECAUTIONS: Hypertension, angina, urinary retention, thyroid disease, diabetes, history of bronchospasm, pregnancy.

PYRANTEL PAMOATE
(Antiminth)
USES: Pyrantel pamoate, a pyrimidine derivative, is an **anthelmintic agent**; uses are given in the next Table (The Medical Letter 32, 23-30, March 23, 1990):

Uses of Pyrantel Pamoate
Enterobius Vermicularis (Pinworm)
Ascaris lumbricoides (Roundworm)
Ancyclostoma Duodenale (Hookworm)
Necator Americanus (Hookworm)
Trichostrongylus Orientalis (Hairworm)

Pyrantel pamoate, like mebendazole, is considered one of the drugs of choice in pinworm, roundworm and hookworm infections. However, pyrantel has been reported to produce more adverse effects than mebendazole. Pyrantel is also the drug of choice for the treatment of trichostrongyliasis.
DOSAGE FORMS: Susp: 250mg/5ml
DOSAGE: Pyrantel pamoate is given orally; it may be mixed with milk or fruit juice. Dosage of the drug in mg/kg is the same for adults and children; dosage is given in the next Table:

Dosage of Pyrantel Pamoate

Condition	Dosage
Pinworm, Roundworm, Hairworm Infection	11mg/kg (max. dose 1g) given as a single dose; dose repeated after 2 weeks in patients with pinworm.
Hookworm	11mg/kg (max. dose 1g) given daily for 3 consecutive days; treatment repeated in one month as necessary.

ADVERSE EFFECTS: Usually mild, infrequent, and transient, disappearing when drug is discontinued. Most common adverse effects are GI disturbances, including nausea, vomiting, tenesmus, anorexia, diarrhea, abdominal cramps.
SGOT elevations; use with caution in patients with preexisting hepatic dysfunction.

PYRETHRINS WITH PIPERONYL BUTOXIDE
(A-200, Pronto, Pyrinal, Pyrinyl, RID)
USES: Pyrethrins are used for topical treatment of **arthropods**; uses are given in the next Table:

Uses of Pyrethrins
Pediculus Capitis (Head Lice)
Pediculus Corporis (Body Lice)
Phthirus Pubis (Crab Lice)

DOSAGE FORMS: Topical: Gel, Shampoo, Sol'n.
DOSAGE: Do not administer orally; do not allow inhalation. Avoid contact with eyes.
For treatment of pediculosis, cover affected area (avoid face and urethral meatus). After 10 minutes, the hair is washed thoroughly with soap or plain shampoo and water, dried with a clean towel, and combed with a fine tooth comb to remove remaining nit shells.
Repeat after 7-10 days to kill any newly hatched lice.
All contaminated clothing and bed linen should be machine-washed in hot water and hot-dried for at least 20 minutes.
ADVERSE EFFECTS: Local irritation.

PYRIDOXINE HYDROCHLORIDE

(Vitamin B-6, Hexa-Betalin, Rodex, Beesix)

USES: Pyridoxine (vitamin B-6) is a water soluble vitamin; uses are given in the next Table:

Uses of Pyridoxine

Pyridoxine deficiency - often associated with uremia, alcoholism, cirrhosis, congestive heart failure, malabsorption, hyperthyroidism or drugs (isoniazid, cycloserine, ethionamide, hydralazine, penicillamine or pyrazinamide).

Pyridoxine-dependent infants - Infants exposed to large doses of pyridoxine may develop pyridoxine dependency. Presentation is seizures unresponsive to usual therapy.

Metabolic disorders - Homocystinuria, xanthuric aciduria, cystathioninuria, hyperoxaluria.

Drug toxicity - Isoniazid, cycloserine or hydralazine overdosage.

Sideroblastic anemia

Isoniazid overdose causes seizures and coma. Isoniazid induces pyridoxine deficiency; pyridoxine reverses isoniazid-induced seizures and coma (Brent, J. et al., Arch. Intern. Med. 150, 1751-1753, August, 1990).

DOSAGE FORMS: Caps: 500mg; Caps (extended-release): 100, 150mg; Tabs: 10, 25, 50, 100, 200, 250, 500mg; Tabs (extended release): 500mg; Injection: 100mg/ml.

DOSAGE: Pyridoxine is usually administered orally but may be given IM, IV or subcutaneously. The dosage of pyridoxine is given in the next Table:

Dosage of Pyridoxine

Condition	Age	Route	Dosage
Pyridoxine Recommended Daily Allowance	Children	Oral	0.3-2mg daily.
	Adult	Oral	1.6-2mg daily; 2.1-2.2mg in pregnant or lactating women.
Pyridoxine Deficiency	Children Adult	Oral	2.5-10mg daily for several weeks.
Drug-Induced Anemia or Neuritis	Children	Oral	Prophylaxis: 1-2mg/kg/day; Treatment: 10-50mg/day
	Adult	Oral	Prophylaxis: 25-100mg/day; Treatment: 100-200mg/day
Pyridoxine-Dependent Infants	Infant	IV or IM	10-100mg; seizures should stop. Long-term therapy: 2-100mg daily orally.
Metabolic Disorders	Children Adult	Oral	100-500mg daily; type I primary hyperoxaluria may require lower doses.
Drug Toxicity Prophylaxis	Adult	Oral	Isoniazid or penicillamine: 10-50mg/day; cycloserine: 100-300mg/day.
Drug Toxicity Treatment	Adult	IV then IM	Isoniazid toxicity, given pyridoxine dose equal to amount of isoniazid ingested; Pyridoxine 1-4g IV then 1g IM every 30 min until entire dose is given.
Sideroblastic Anemia	Children Adult	Oral	200-600mg daily for 1-2 months, then 30-50mg/day for life.

ADVERSE EFFECTS: Generally nontoxic. Chronic, large doses may cause neuropathy. Seizures have occurred following large IV doses.

QUINACRINE
(Atabrine)

USES: **Quinacine** is an acridine dye derivative, structurally related to primaquine, and is used as an **anthelmintic.** Uses of quinacrine, compared to other drugs, are given in the next Table:

Uses of Quinacrine and Other Drugs

Infection	Drugs of Choice	Other Drugs
Giardia Lamblia	**Quinicrine**	Metronidazole may be better tolerated, especially in children
Cestodes (Tapeworms)	**Niclosamide** **Praziquantel** **Paromomycin**	Quinacrine
Malaria	**Chloroquine**	Quinacrine

Quinicrine is the drug of choice for the treatment of giardiasis.

DOSAGE FORMS: Tabs: 100mg

DOSAGE: Quinacine is administered orally or through a duodenal tube. Only the treatment of giardiasis will be given. Quinacrine should be taken after meals with a full glass of water, tea, or fruit juice. Dosage of quinacrine for the treatment of giardiasis is given in the next Table:

Dosage of Quinacrine for Treatment of Giardiasis

Age	Dosage
Adults	100mg, 3 times daily, 5-7 days
Children	2mg/kg, 3 times daily, (max. 300mg/day for 5 days)

The stool should be examined 2 weeks later and a repeat course given if indicated.

ADVERSE EFFECTS: GI disturbances, toxic psychosis, yellow color (not jaundice) of skin, bone marrow depression. Corneal and retinal changes may occur.

Use with caution in patients with severe renal or cardiac disease or hepatic disease or alcohol dependence or a history of psychosis and in patients older than 60 or younger than 1 year of age. Use with caution in G6PD deficiency. May exacerbate psoriasis or porphyria. May cause disulfiram-like reaction with alcohol ingestion.

CONTRAINDICATIONS: Concomitant primaquine use.

QUINIDINE

Quinidine Sulfate (Cin-Quin, Quinidex);
Quinidine Gluconate (Duraquin, Quinaglute, Quinalan, Quinatime);
Quinidine Polygalacturonate (Cardioquin)

USES: Quinidine depresses the excitability of cardiac muscle and slows the heart rate; uses are given in the next Table:

Uses of Quinidine

Prophylactic Therapy to Maintain Normal Sinus Rhythm after Conversion of Atrial Fibrillation and/or Flutter by other methods
Prevent Recurrence:
- **Paroxysmal Atrial Fibrillation**
- **Paroxysmal Atrial Tachycardia**
- **Paroxysmal AV Junctional Rhythm**
- **Paroxysmal Ventricular Tachycardia**

Treatment of Severe Malaria, eg, Cerebral Malaria, caused by Plasmodium Falciparum - use is investigational.

When quinidine is given to a patient with atrial fibrillation, the ventricular rate may occasionally increase as the atrial rate slows. For this reason, digitalis, verapamil, or propranolol, each of which increases atrioventricular block, is usually given first.

Mechanism of Action: The mechanism of action of quinidine is like that of procainamide and disopyramide. Quinidine has a direct action on the cell membrane; it depresses automaticity, especially in ectopic sites. It slows conduction and increases refractoriness of the atria, His-Purkinje system, accessory pathways and ventricles.

Quinidine has anticholinergic effects and combined with the reduction in atrial impulses, it may facilitate A-V conduction in patients with atrial fibrillation or flutter.

The mechanism of action of quinidine's antimalarial activity is unknown, but it may interfere with plasmodial DNA function.

DOSAGE FORMS: Quinidine Sulfate (83% Quinidine); Caps: 300mg; Tabs: 100, 200, 300mg; Tabs (timed-release): 300mg. Quinidine Gluconate (62% Quinidine); Tabs (timed-release): 324, 330mg; Injection: 80mg/ml; Quinidine Polygalacturonate (73% Qunindine); Tabs: 275mg.

DOSAGE: Idiosyncratic and Hypersensitivity Reactions: Idiosyncratic hypersensitivity reactions to quinidine may occur; a test for these reactions in adults is done as follows: Give test dose several hours prior to full dosage; give 200mg of quinidine sulfate, orally, or 200mg of quinidine gluconate, IM. For children, give 2mg/kg of either quinidine sulfate orally or quinidine gluconate, IM.

Quinidine gluconate, quinidine polygalacturonate, and quinidine sulfate are administered orally; quinidine gluconate is also administered by IM injection or IV infusion. Dosage is given in the next Table:

Dosage of Quinidine

Drug	Condition	Age	Route	Dosage
Quinidine Sulfate	Maintain Normal Sinus Rhythm after Conversion	Adult	Oral	Loading Dose: 200mg every 2-3 h titrate to desired effect(often, 5-8 doses). Maintenance Dose:200-600mg every 6-8 h. Slow-release products may be given every 12 h.
		Child.	Oral	Maintenance Dose: 15-60mg/kg daily in 4-5 divided doses.
Quinidine Polygalacturonate	Maintenance	Adult	Oral	275mg, 2 or 3 times daily
Quinidine Gluconate	Maintain Normal Sinus Rhythm	Adult	IV	200-400mg/dose
			Oral	100-600mg/dose every 4-6 h. Initial dose: 200mg
		Child.	Oral	15-60mg/kg daily in 4-5 divided doses.
			IV	Not recommended, but 2-10mg/kg/dose every 3-6 h. has been given.

Active metabolites accumulate in patients with renal failure and adjustment of dosage may be necessary.

ADVERSE EFFECTS: Toxicity may occur if serum levels exceed 5mcg/ml. The common toxic effects of quinidine are listed in the next Table:

QUINIDINE (Cont.)

Common Toxic Effects of Quinidine
Gastrointestinal Disturbances:
Nausea, Vomiting, Anorexia, Diarrhea
Cardiovascular:
Slow Intraventricular Conduction
Bradycardia, Hypotension, Syncope
Cinchonism:
Headache "Tinnitus, Light-Headedness, Giddiness", etc.
Eighth Cranial Nerve Damage

Adverse cardiovascular effects, eg, vasodilatation and hypotension, are more common with IV and less common with oral administration. Serious ventricular tacharrhythmias associated with excessive QT prolongation (eg, Torsade de Pointes) are the likely cause of "quinidine syncope," potentiated by hypokalemia.

Digoxin concentration increases 2-3 fold when quinidine therapy is initiated. Therefore, digoxin dose must be reduced (eg, by half) and digoxin levels must be monitored carefully.

Reversible hepatitis and a lupus-like syndrome have been reported (Knobler, H. et al., Arch. Intern. Med. 146, 526, 1986; Lavie, C.J. et al., Arch. Intern. Med. 145, 446, 1985).

The major route of elimination is hepatic; renal failure does not generally lead to toxicity on the usual doses; however, active metabolites may accumulate and dosage adjustment may be required.

Quinidine can cause cinchonism, headache, visual and auditory disturbances.

Hypoglycemia and thrombocytopenia may occur.

Quinidine has numerous adverse effects and drug interactions, not all of which are listed here. Physicians should be familiar with these effects and interactions prior to administering this drug.

PHARMACOKINETICS: Absorption: Rapid; Peak: 90 min. (sulfate); 4 hour (gluconate); Quinidine is metabolized in the liver and excreted by the kidneys. Therapeutic: 2.0-5.0mcg/ml; Toxic: >5.0mcg/ml; Half-Life: 6 hours; Steady State: 24 to 42 hours (4 to 7 half-lives).

Conditions which alter the half-life of quinidine are listed in the next Table:

Conditions Which Alter Half-Life of Quinidine
Decrease: Phenobarbital, Phenytoin, Nifedipine, Primidone, Rifampin
Increase: End Stage Liver Disease, Severe Heart Failure

The drugs, phenobarbital, phenytoin, nifedipine, primidone, rifampin, stimulate hepatic metabolism of quinidine, decreasing plasma concentrations and antiarrhythmic effect; discontinuing these drugs that stimulate hepatic metabolism may lead to quinidine toxicity.

Potentiation of Effects of Other Drugs: Quinidine can increase the effects and possible toxicity of drugs listed in the next Table:

Potentiation of Effects of Other Drugs by Quinidine
Oral Anticoagulants
Neuromuscular Blockers
Digoxin

The effects of quinidine can be increased by concurrent use of antacids, amiodarone, carbonic anhydrase inhibitors, and cimetidine. Hypotension can occur with IV verapamil.

MONITOR: Monitor serum levels of quinidine as follows:

The first serum specimen should be obtained when first initiating quinidine therapy after 24 to 42 hours (4 to 7 half-lives) following initial dose and just prior to the next dose (trough). Trough concentration should be above the minimum effective concentration to maintain the desired therapeutic effect (2.0mcg/ml).

Different preparations peak at different times; quinidine sulfate peaks in 1.5 hours; quinidine gluconate peaks in 4-5 hours.

If it is necessary to determine the half-life of quinidine, collect at least 3 timed specimens 30-60 min apart, and plot log concentration vs. time.

CONTRAINDICATIONS: A-V block, incomplete or complete; when used in patients with incomplete heart block, complete heart block may occur. Use with extreme caution if at all in patients with digitalis toxicity. Use cautiously, if at all, in patients with congestive heart failure, preexisting hypotension, or G6PD deficiency. Contraindicated in myasthenia gravis.

QUININE

(Legatrin, Quinamm, Strema, Others)

USES: Quinine is used to relieve nocturnal leg cramps. Nocturnal leg cramps most often involve the calf and foot area. Etiology is usually unknown; arterial insufficiency or electrolyte abnormalities are rarely found. The treatment of choice has been quinine but quinine may be poorly tolerated and is often ineffective; verapamil may be an alternative treatment (Baltodano, N. et al., Arch. Intern. Med. 148, 1969-1970, 1988).

Quinine sulfate, in combination with pyrimethamine-sulfadoxine or tetracycline or clindamycin, is the drug of choice for treatment of chloroquine-resistant Plasmodium falciparum. Quinine dihydrochloride (available from the CDC at 404-488-4046 or 404-639-2888) or quinidine gluconate are parenteral drugs of choice for all Plasmodium, including chloroquine-resistant P. falciparum (Medical Letter 32, 23-32, March 23, 1990).

Mechanism of Action: Unknown. Antimalarial activity may be due to interference with plasmodial DNA function.

DOSAGE FORMS: Powder: 130, 200, 300, 325mg; Tabs: 260, 325mg.

DOSAGE: Nocturnal leg cramps: 200-300mg at bedtime. Increase dosage if necessary.

Dosage of quinine for treatment of malaria is given in the following Table:

Dosage of Quinine for Malaria

Drug	Route	Age	Dosage
Quinine Sulfate	Oral	Children	25mg/kg daily in 3 divided doses for 3 days (max: 650mg/dose).
		Adult	650mg three times a day for 3 days.
Quinine Dihydrochloride	IV	Children	25mg/kg daily in 3 divided doses. Infuse doses over 2-4 hrs. Max: 1800mg/day.
		Adult	600mg in 300ml normal saline over 2-4 hrs. Repeat doses three times a day. Max: 1800mg/day.

ADVERSE EFFECTS: Adverse effects are as follows: CNS disturbances; headache; tinnitus; impaired vision rash; GI disturbances; nausea; angina-like symptoms; blood dyscrasias, particularly thrombocytopenia. Hypoglycemia may occur.

The Public Citizen Health Research Group petitioned the Food and Drug Administration to ban the over-the-counter sales of quinine products such as, Q-vel and Legatrin, citing an FDA list of eight deaths linked to the use of quinine. In addition, there have been numerous cases of adverse reactions including vomiting, deafness, serious blood disorders and severe allergic reactions associated with its use. Several countries, Denmark, Hungary, Israel and Columbia have banned over-the-counter sale of quinine for leg cramps (Ingersoll, B., Wall Street Journal, pg. B4, Dec. 2, 1988).

CONTRAINDICATIONS: Pregnancy, blood dyscrasias; G6PD deficiency; tinnitus; optic neuritis.

PRECAUTIONS: Atrial fibrillation.

DRUG INTERACTIONS: Quinine potentiates the effects of the following: digitalis, anticoagulants and neuromuscular blocking agents.

RABIES IMMUNE GLOBULIN
(RIG, Hyperab, Imogam Rabies)

USES: Rabies immune globulin(RIG) is prepared from plasma or serum of healthy adults hyperimmunized with rabies vaccine.

RIG, which contains **rabies antibody,** is used to provide passive immunity to rabies in individuals exposed to the disease or virus. The rabies antibody neutralizes rabies virus so that spread of the virus is slowed and its infective or pathogenic properties are inhibited.

Both RIG and rabies vaccine are given following exposure to disease or virus.

DOSAGE FORMS: Injection (IM): 150 IU/ml

DOSAGE: RIG is given by IM injection and local wound infiltration. RIG must not be given by IV.

In adults and older children, injection of RIG preferably is made into the deltoid muscle or the anterolateral aspect of the thigh. In infants and small children, IM injections with RIG preferably should be made into the anterolateral aspect of the thigh.

Up to 50% of the dose of RIG should be infiltrated locally at the wound and the remainder administered IM. For wounds involving mucous membranes, give entire dose IM. Do not give more than 5ml at one IM injection site.

To reduce possibility of neutralization, inject IM portion of RIG in gluteal region and vaccine in deltoid region.

Give both RIG and rabies vaccine regardless of the interval between exposure and treatment.

Prophylaxis should be initiated as soon as possible; results of direct fluorescent antibody test of the animal's brain tissue may be available within 24 hours.

RIG should not be given to individuals who have been immunized with rabies vaccine.

If vaccine therapy is given without RIG, RIG may be given up to 8 days after the first dose of vaccine; after the eighth day, sufficient antibody will probably have developed.

For postexposure prophylaxis, the usual dose of RIG in adults and children is 20 IU/kg administered at the same time as the first dose of rabies vaccine (Immunization Practices Advisory Committee, **MMWR** 40 (RR-3), 1-19, March 22, 1991).

ADVERSE EFECTS: Local pain at injection site; urticaria, anaphylaxis.

Serious systemic reactions could occur following inadvertent IV injection.

RABIES VACCINE, HUMAN DIPLOID CELL (HDCV)
(Imovax Rabies)

USES: Rabies postexposure prophylaxis guide is given in the next Table; (Centers for Disease Control, Immunization Practices Advisory Committee, MMWR 40 (RR-3), 4, March 22, 1991):

Rabies Postexposure Prophylaxis Guide

Animal Species	Condition of Animal at time of attack	Treatment of Exposed Person
Domestic Dog and Cat	Healthy and available for 10 days of observation	None, unless animal develops rabies. Begin treatment with rabies immune globulin(RIG) and HDCV at first sign of rabies in a dog or cat during the usual 10-day observation period. If the animal shows signs of rabies, it should be killed immediately & tested
	Rabid or suspected rabid	Give RIG and HDCV. When RIG is not available, antirabies serum (equine) can be used. However, antirabies serum (equine) is associated with a high incidence of adverse reactions (eg, serum sickness). Do not use more than the recommended dosage.
	Unknown (escaped)	Consult public health officials. If treatment is indicated, give RIG and HDCV.
Wild: Skunk, bat, fox, coyote, raccoon, bobcat, and other carnivores	Regard as rabid unless proven otherwise by laboratory tests.	Give RIG and HDCV.
Other: Livestock, rodents and lagomorphs (rabbits and hares)	Consider individually. Local or state public health officials should be consulted regarding the need for rabies prophylaxis. Provoked bites of squirrels, hamsters, guinea pigs, gerbils, chipmunks, rats, mice, other rodents, rabbits, or hares almost never require rabies prophylaxis.	

DOSAGE FORMS: IM or intradermal Injection: 2.5 IU

DOSAGE: The vaccine is administered by IM injection or intradermal injection.

Postexposure prophylaxis: For postexposure prophylaxis, a total of 5 doses of HDCV are given. HDCV is given in conjunction with RIG; the remaining doses of HDCV are given at 3, 7, 14 and 28 days after the first dose.

HDCV is given IM to adults and children in 1ml doses.

Preexposure prophylaxis: For preexposure prophylaxis, 3 doses of HDCV are given: day 0 and 7 and 21 or 28 days after the first dose.

ADVERSE EFFECTS: Infrequent local or mild systemic reactions. Local reactions to vaccines are common and do not contraindicate continuing treatment. Discontinue vaccine if direct fluorescent antibody testing of the animal does not show rabies.

DRUG INTERACTIONS: Concomittant administration of chloroquine for malaria suppression or prophylaxis may interfere with the development of antibodies to rabies vaccine - particularly when given by the intradermal route. The IM route is recommended in this setting.

MONITOR: Collect serum for rabies titers on day 28 (indicated only if patient is immunosuppressed).

RADIOGRAPHIC CONTRAST AGENTS

Types, examples and osmolality of radiologic contrast media are given in the next Table (Bettmann, M.A. and Morris, T.W., Radiol. Clin. N.Am. 24, 347-357, 1986):

Types, Examples and Osmolality of Radiologic Contrast Media

Type and Examples	Osmolality (mOsm/liter)
Conventional Ionic Monomer	
Diatrizoate (Renografin, Hypaque)	1570
Meglumine Iothalamate (Conray)	750-1500
Ionic Dimer	
Ioxaglate (Hexabrix)	560
Nonionic Formulations	
Iopamidol (Isovue, Niopam)	616
Iohexol (Omnipaque)	690
Metrizamide (Amipaque)	480

Osmolality: The conventional ionic monomers have significantly higher osmolality as compared to the ionic dimer, ioxaglate, or the nonionic formulations. Normal serum osmolality is 285-295 mOsm/liter. The higher osmolality of the conventional ionic monomers may be partially responsible for some of the adverse effects associated with these contrast media.

Deaths Associated with Contrast Media: There are about 5.2 million contrast studies per year with 300-600 deaths and 1,800 major life-threatening reactions per year (Wolf, G.L., Radiology 159, 557-558, 1986). The incidence of death related to contrast material in studies with conventional agents is 1 per 15,000 to 40,000 examinations (Hartman, B.W. et al. A.J.R. 139, 919-929, 1982; Shehadi, W.H., Radiology 143, 11-17, 1982). The most serious reaction to contrast media is anaphylaxis or an anaphylactoid-like reaction with sudden death. Ioxaglate ionic dimer, iopamidol and iohexol nonionic formulations have been used in more than 1 million examinations, and the death rate appears to be much lower than 1 in 40,000 (Bettmann, M.A. and Morris, T.W., Radiolog. Clin. N.Am 24, 347-357, 1986).

Other Adverse Reactions with Contrast Media: Transient symptoms of nausea, vomiting, and heat sensation or pain are statistically more common with the high osmolality contrast media (conventional ionic monomers) as compared to the low osmolality contrast media (ionic dimer, nonionic formulations).

Results of studies with the newer contrast media indicate significant decreases in dermal reactions, in cardiovascular reactions (transient bradycardia, lowering of blood pressure, left ventricular contractility) during coronary and left ventricular angiography and CNS symptoms eg, less pain.

For renal studies the advantages for using low osmolality contrast media over high osmolality contrast media are not as apparent (Bettmann, M.A. and Higgins, C.B., Invest. Radiol. 20, 565-569, 1985).

Expenses for Contrast Media: The newer contrast media (low osmolality) costs are about twenty times that of conventional high-osmolality contrast media.

RANITIDINE
(Zantac)

USES: Uses of ranitidine are given in the next Table:

Uses of Ranitidine
Active Duodenal Ulcers
Prophylaxis of Recurrent Duodenal Ulcers
Treatment of Active Gastric Ulcers
Pathologic Hypersecretory Conditions, eg, Zollinger-Ellison Syndrome, Systemic Mastocytosis and Multiple Endocrine Adenomas

Ranitidine and antacids may be administered concomitantly but not simultaneously since antacids interfere with absorption of ranitidine (Hansten, P.D., Drug Interact. Newslett 5, 11-14, 1985).

Antacids used for the relief of pain may be taken if at least an interval of 1 hr. has elapsed between the administration of antacid and ranitidine.

Ranitidine is used in pathologic hypersecretory conditions, eg, Zollinger-Ellison syndrome, systemic mastocytosis and multiple endocrine adenomas. Ranitidine reduces diarrhea, anorexia and pain and promotes healing of intractable ulcers in patients with these conditions.

Ranitidine is preferred to cimetidine in the conditions listed in the next Table:

Conditions in Which Ranitidine is Preferred to Cimetidine
Peptic Ulcers Refractory to Cimetidine
Patients taking Multiple Drugs
Patients requiring very Large Doses of Cimetidine
Patients who cannot Tolerate Cimetidine's Adverse Effects, eg, Geriatric Patients
Patients with Severe Liver or Kidney Impairment

The major differences between ranitidine and cimetidine are as follows: ranitidine has a 12 hour duration of action and may be taken twice-a-day rather than four times a day for cimetidine. Ranitidine does not inhibit hepatic microsomal enzymes and causes fewer drug interactions.

Mechanism of Action: Ranitidine competitively **inhibits** the action of **histamine** on **H_2 receptors** of parietal cells, thus reduces acid secretion by parietal cells of the stomach; it acts like the other H_2 receptor antagonist, i.e., cimetidine (Tagamet), famotidine (Pepcid) and nizatidine (Axid).

DOSAGE FORMS: Tabs: 150, 300mg; Sol'n: 75mg/5ml; Inject: 25mg/ml.

DOSAGE: Ranitidine is usually administered orally. The drug may also be given by IM or slow IV injection or by slow IV infusion in hospitalized patients with pathologic hypersecretory conditions or intractable duodenal ulcer, or when oral therapy is not feasible. Dosage is given in the next Table:

Dosage of Ranitidine

Condition	Age	Route	Dosage
Duodenal or Gastric Ulcer and Reflux Esophagitis	Adult	Oral	150mg, twice daily. For duodenal ulcer, 300mg once daily at bedtime is as effective as twice daily administration. Duodenal ulcers usually heals in 4-6 weeks; gastric ulcers usually heal in 8-12 wks. Maintenance: 150mg at bedtime.
	Children	Oral	2-4mg/kg/day divided every 12 hours.
Hypersecretion Syndromes, eg, Zollinger-Ellison Syndrome	Adult	Oral	150mg twice daily or more frequently; max. 6g/day
		IV	1mg/kg/hr; increase by 0.5mg/kg/hr every 4 hours if acid secretion >10 mEq/hr. Max: 2.5mg/kg/hr or 220mg/hr.
Hypersecretory Syndromes or Peptic Ulcer Refractory to Oral medication or Patients unable to Tolerate Oral Medication	Adult	IV IM	50mg every 6-8 h., increase as necessary. Max: 400mg/day, or IV infusion at 6.25-12.5mg/hr*.
	Children	IV	1-2mg/kg/day divided every 6-8 hours.

*Continuous IV infusion of ranitidine is more effective in maintaining a higher gastric pH than intermittent bolus method (Ballesteros, M.A. et al., Ann. Intern. Med. 112, 334-339, 1990).

RANITIDINE (Cont.)

Duodenal ulcers usually heals in four to six weeks with daily treatment; gastric ulcer usually requires 8 to 12 weeks. Endoscopy or x-rays are used to verify healing of a gastric ulcer. In patients with duodenal ulcer, relief of symptoms after four to six weeks may be considered the endpoint of initial therapy.

Renal Impairment: Ranitidine is excreted primarily by the kidneys; 150mg once orally every 24 h. and an IM or IV dosage of 50mg every 18-24 h. in patients with creatinine clearance <50ml/min.

PHARMACOKINETICS: Oral Absorption:50%; Metabolized: Liver; Excretion: Principally in urine; Half-Life: 1.7 to 3 h.; prolonged in geriatric patients and those with liver or kidney disease; Plasma Protein Binding: 15%; Apparent Volume Distribution: 1.2 to 1.9 liter/kg.

ADVERSE EFFECTS: Minor adverse effects occur infrequently(<3%). Headache(3%) usually subsides with continued therapy. Malaise, dizziness, constipation, nausea, abdominal pain, and rash occur in <1% of patients.

Reversible leukopenia, granulocytopenia, thrombocytopenia and pancytopenia are rare; hepatitis, rare.

See **H_2 ANTAGONISTS** section for additional information.

RESERPINE

(Serpasil, Serpalan)

USES: **Reserpine** is a **rauwolfia alkaloid;** it is a peripheral-acting adrenergic antagonist. Uses are given in the next Table:

Uses of Reserpine
Hypertension
Psychotic Disorders

Hypertension: Reserpine is used in the management of mild to moderate hypertension. Treatment of hypertension with reserpine is given in the next Table (The 1988 Report of the Joint National Committee on Detection, Evaluation, and Treatment of High Blood Pressure, Arch. Intern. Med. 148, 1023-1038, 1988):

Treatment of Hypertension with Reserpine

Step 1: Nonpharmacologic Approaches (see **HYPERTENSION**)

↓

Step 2: **Diuretic** or **Beta Blocker** or **Calcium Antagonists** or **ACE Inhibitor**

Observe up to 6 months; if treatment ineffective

↓

Step 3: Add a second drug of a different class; this may be reserpine

or Increase the dosage of the first drug

or Substitute another drug

↓

Step 4: Add a third drug of a different class

or Substitute a second drug

↓

Step 5: Consider further evaluation and/or referral

or Add a third or fourth drug

"Step-Down": For patients with mild hypertension, after 1 year of control, consider decreasing or withdrawing reserpine and other hypotensive drugs.

Psychotic Disorders: Reserpine has been used in the symptomatic treatment of agitated psychotic states such as schizophrenic disorders.

DOSAGE FORMS: Tabs: 0.1, 0.25mg.

DOSAGE: Reserpine is given orally in a single daily dose or divided into 2 doses daily. The initial daily dose for adults is 0.1-0.5mg; the maintenance dose is 0.1-0.25mg.

ADVERSE EFFECTS: Lethargy, nasal congestion, depression

CONTRAINDICATIONS: Contraindicated in patients with history of mental depression; use with caution in patients with history of peptic ulcer.

RIBAVIRIN

(Virazole)

USES: Ribavirin is used in the treatment of lower respiratory infections due to respiratory syncytial virus (RSV) in hospitalized infants and young children. Ribavirin therapy is most effective when therapy is initiated within the first 3 days following onset of infection, and may reduce the morbidity from RSV in young children, especially those with bronchopulmonary dysplasia (BPD) and congenital heart disease (CHD)(Groothuis, J.R. et al., J. Pediatr. 117, 792-798, Nov. 1990). Ribavirin has been shown to decrease the duration of intubation, oxygen requirement, and hospital stay in young infants with respiratory failure due to RSV (Smith, D.W., et al., N. Engl. J. Med., 325, 24-29, July 4, 1991).

Current recommendations of the American Academy of Pediatrics for treatment of RSV infection with ribaviron include the patients at high risk for morbidity and mortality as listed in the following Table(American Acedemy of Pediatrics Infections Disease Committee, Pediatrics 79, 475-478, 1987):

Clinical Use of Ribavirin in Patients with RSV Infection
Congenital Heart Disease
Bronchopulmonary Dysplasia
Other Chronic Lung Diseases (eg, Cystic Fibrosis)
Prematurity
Immunodeficiency (AIDS, Severe combined immunodeficiency syndrome, Transplant, Malignancy)
Hypoxia (PaO_2 < 65mmHg)
Increasing $PaCO_2$
Age <6 weeks
Multiple Congenital Anomalies, Neurologic, Metabolic Diseases

Ribavirin is effective by oral or I.V. routes as treatment and post-exposure prophylaxis in Lassa fever. Ribavirin has shown promise in the treatment of herpes and influenza A and B infections; use in HIV infections is currently under investigation.

Mechanism of Action: The exact mechanism of action of ribavirin is unknown but ribavirin appears to mediate its antiviral activity by interfering with RNA and DNA synthesis; it is thought to inhibit either reverse transcriptase or viral mRNA synthesis. The chemical structure of ribavirin is shown in the next Figure:

Chemical Structure of Ribavirin

Guanosine **Ribavirin**

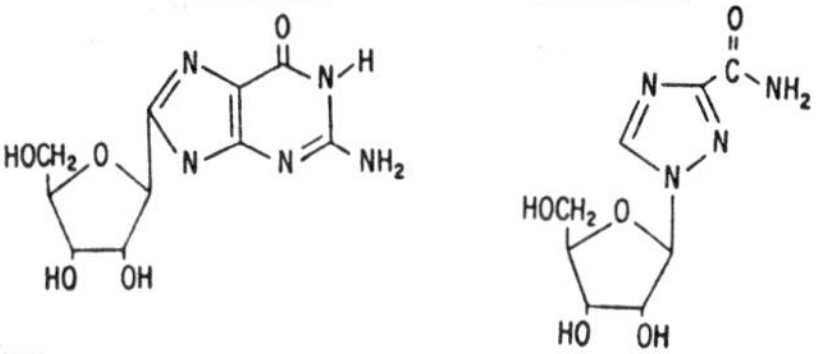

Ribavirin resembles guanosine chemically.

DOSAGE FORMS: Ribavirin 6g; powder for reconstitution and aerosol inhalation.

DOSAGE: Children: Use only recommended SPAG-2 nebulizer for administration.

When a 20mg/ml ribavirin solution is used as the starting solution in the SPAG-2 reservoir, the SPAG-2 aerosol generator delivers a mist containing about 190 microgram of ribavirin per liter; dose is estimated using the following equation:

$$\text{Dose delivered to Respiratory Tract} = \text{Minute Volume (liters)} \times \text{Duration of Inhalation (minutes)} \times \text{0.19mg/liter (nebulized ribavirin concentration)} \times \text{0.7(fraction of inhaled dose deposited in respiratory tract)}$$

Patients should have 12.5 liter of mist per minute delivered for 12-18 hrs. daily for 3-7 days.

The manufacturer does not recommend the use of ribavirin in intubated, mechanically ventilated patients due to the risk of drug precipitation in the ventilator circuit or endotracheal tube. Ribavirin has been administered safely to mechanically ventilated patients when appropriate protocols are in place and ventilator modifications are made (Adderley, R.J., Pediatr. Infect. Dis. J. 9, S112-S114, Sept., 1990).

RIBAVIRIN (Cont.)
ADVERSE EFFECTS: The most common adverse effects associated with inhalation of ribavirin are respiratory and cardiovascular effects; these occur infrequently.
Respiratory Effects: Pulmonary function deterioration, pneumonia, pneumothorax, apnea, ventilator malfunction.
Cardiovascular Effects: Cardiac arrest and hypotension.
Other Adverse Effects: Reticulocytosis, rash, conjunctivitis.
PRECAUTIONS: Monitor respiratory and fluid status. Discontinue if pulmonary function deteriorates.

Environmental exposure of health care personnel and visitors to ribavirin is an area of concern due to potential risks. Because of animal evidence of teratogenic potential, hospitals should develop policies regarding exposure. Environmental exposure should be minimized, particularly in pregnant caregivers.
INTERACTIONS: Ribavirin antagonizes the antiviral activity of zidovudine in-vitro.

RIFAMPIN
(Rimactane, Rifadin)
USES: Rifampin is an antibiotic; uses are given in the next Table:

Antibiotic Uses of Rifampin
Treatment of clinical tuberculosis, given in combination with at least one other antituberculosis drug.
Treatment of asymptomatic meningococcus carriers.
Prophylaxis of Haemophilus influenza type b.
Treatment of leprosy

Tuberculosis: Rifampin is used in the prevention and treatment of tuberculosis. It is used for the prophylaxis of subclinical infection to prevent active disease in patients with a positive tuberculin skin test but no evidence of active disease on chest x-ray; however, isoniazid is the drug of choice. It is also used with isoniazid in the treatment of active tuberculosis.
Contacts of Patients with Meningococcal Meningitis: Rifampin is the preferred drug for chemoprophylaxis of close contacts of patients with meningococcal meningitis; it eliminates nasopharyngeal carriage of Neisseria meningitidis.
Prophylaxis of Haemophilus Influenzae Type B: Rifampin is the preferred drug for the elimination of oropharyngeal carriage of Haemophilus influenzae, type B.
Mechanism of Action: Rifampin binds to the beta subunit of bacterial DNA-dependent RNA poly-merase and blocks initiation of RNA synthesis in susceptible bacteria.

RIFAMPIN (Cont.)

DOSAGE FORMS: Caps: 150, 300mg; Parenteral: 600mg.

DOSAGE: Rifampin is usually administered orally, one hour before or two hours after ingestion of food. Contents of capsules may be mixed with applesauce or jelly. IV infusion may be given when oral therapy is not possible. IV and oral doses are identical. Dosage is given in the next Table:

Dosage of Rifampin

Condition	Age	Dosage
Tuberculosis (Prophylaxis, positive tuberculin skin test, no evidence of active disease on chest x-ray)	Adults	10 to 20mg/kg daily or 600mg daily. Continue therapy for 12 months.
	Children	10 to 20mg/kg daily or 600mg daily. Continue therapy for 12 months.
Tuberculosis, Active	Adult	600mg, once daily and 300mg of isoniazid, daily plus pyrazinamide 30mg/kg daily for 8 weeks followed by isoniazid and rifampin for an additional 16 weeks. Ethambutal 15mg/kg is added if patient has had previous isoniazid therapy or had immigrated from a country where drug resistance is common (Combs, D.L. et al., Ann. Intern. Med. 112, 397-406, 1990).
	Children	Rifampin: 10-20mg/kg (up to 600mg) and Isoniazid 10-20mg/kg (up to 300mg) both for 1-2 months followed by twice-weekly rifampin, 10-20mg/kg, up to 600mg and isoniazid, 20-40mg/kg (up to 900mg) for the next 7-8 months (9 month course).
Asymptomatic Meningococcus Carriers	Adult	10mg/kg (up to 600mg) twice daily for 2 days.
	Children	
	Up to 1 mo.	5mg/kg, twice daily for 2 days.
Prophylaxis of Haemophilus Influenzae, type b	Adult Children	20mg/kg (up to 600mg) daily as a single dose for 4 consecutive days.
	Up to 1 month	10mg/kg daily as a single dose for 4 consecutive days.
Leprosy	Adult	100mg of dapsone daily for a minimum of 6 months in conjunction with rifampin (600mg once daily for 6 months).

PHARMACOKINETICS: Absorption: 90-95%; Peak: 1-3 hours; Half-Life: 2-4 hours; Protein-Binding: 80%; Metabolism: Liver; Elimination: Deacetylation in the liver to partially active metabolite which is extensively enterohepatically recirculated. Half-Life: 1.5-5 hours; increased by liver disease or biliary obstruction; Excretion: Fecus, 50-60% and partially in urine.

ADVERSE EFFECTS: Patients taking rifampin should be advised that rifampin reduces the effectiveness of oral contraceptives; other methods of birth control should be used. Urine, saliva, tears, and other body secretions develop red discoloration. Contact lenses may be permanently stained red. Rifampin has other drug interactions which may be important in certain individuals. Rifampin has teratogenic potential and should not be used for Haemophilus Influenzae Type B prophylaxis in pregnant women. In other conditions, risks must be weighed against benefits. Use with caution in patients with preexisting liver disease; rifampin is hepatotoxic and may add to the risk of isoniazid-induced hepatitis. Rifampin has been associated with adrenocortical insufficiency. GI Effects: Heartburn, epigastric distress, nausea, vomiting, anorexia, abdominal cramps, flatulence, and diarrhea. Nervous System Effects: Headache, drowsiness, fatigue, ataxia, etc. Hypersensitivity Reactions: Flu-like syndrome with fever, chills, headache, rashes. Urine: Red discoloration of the urine is common. Hematologic: Thrombocytopenic purpura.

DRUG INTERACTIONS: Rifampin interferes with the effectiveness of digoxin, theophylline, phenytoin, oral contraceptives, corticosteroids, sulfonylureas, quinidine, oral hypoglycemics, ketoconazole, dapsone, disopyramide, warfarin and methadone. These effects are probably secondary to the induction of hepatic cytochrome P-450 enzymes and alterations in absorption and hepatic uptake. Increased doses of digoxin, theophylline, phenytoin, and other drugs may be necessary. Rifampin interferes with the absorption of ketoconazole and increases its metabolism, resulting in low serum levels. The manufacturer of ketoconazole recommends against concomitant administration of these drugs.

SCOPOLAMINE HYDROBROMIDE
(Hyoscine Hydrobromide, Transderm Scop)

USES: **Scopolamine** is a belladonna **alkaloid;** its uses are given in the next Table:

Uses of Scopolamine
Prevention of Nausea and Vomiting induced by Motion
Adjunct to Anesthesia
Applied to Eye to produce **Mydriasis** (Pupillary Dilation) and Cycloplegia for Refraction and for the Treatment of Acute Inflammatory Conditions of the Iris and Uveal Tract

Scopolamine is considered the single most effective drug in preventing nausea and vomiting induced by motion. However, adverse effects are associated with oral scopolamine therapy, and antihistamines, e.g., dimenhydrinate, or other drugs are preferred for prevention of motion sickness in patients with prolonged exposure to mild to moderate motion.

DOSAGE FORMS: Injection: 0.3, 0.4, 0.86, 1mg/ml; Ophthalmic: 0.25%; Transdermal: 0.5mg/72hrs.

DOSAGE: Scopolamine hydrobromide is administered orally or by IM, direct IV or subcutaneous injection; it is administered percutaneously by topical application of a transdermal system (Transderm Scop). Many combination preparations contain scopolamine hydrobromide (Donnagel-PG; Donnatal Capsules, elixir, extentabs and tablets, Donnazymne tablets, Ru-Tuss tablets). Dosage is given in the next Table:

Dosage of Scopolamine

Condition	Age	Route	Dosage
Self-Medication in Prevention of Motion Sickness	Adult	Oral	0.4-0.8mg, repeated as necessary 3 or 4 times daily
	Adult	IM,IV or Subcut.	0.3-0.65mg, repeat as necessary 3 or 4 times daily
	Children	IM,IV or Subcut.	0.006mg/kg/dose
Antiemetic	Adult	IM,IV or Subcut.	0.2-1mg
Inhibition of Salivation	Adult	IM,IV or Subcut.	0.2-0.6mg
Amnestic Effect	Adult	IM,IV or Subcut.	0.32-0.65mg
Sedation or Tranquilization	Adult	IM,IV or Subcut.	0.6mg
Prevention of Motion Sickness	Adult	Transdermal Patch	0.5mg per 72 hours; apply at least 4 hrs prior to exposure.
Mydriasis and Cycloplegia for Refraction	Adult	Topical	1 or 2 drops of a 0.25% sol'n. into the eyes before the procedure; to avoid excessive systemic absorption, apply finger pressure on lacrimal sac for 1-2 minutes.
	Children	Topical	1 drop of a 0.25% sol'n onto the eye(s) twice daily for 2 days before the procedure.
Pupillary Dilation in Treat. of Acute Inflam. Conditions of Iris & Uveal Tract	Adult	Topical	1 or 2 drops of a 0.25% sol'n. onto the eyes up to 3 times daily
	Children	Topical	1 drop of a 0.25% sol'n. up to 3 times daily.

ADVERSE EFFECTS: SEE ATROPINE; contraindicated in urinary or GI obstruction and glaucoma.

SECOBARBITAL
(Seconal)

USES: **Secobarbital** is a **barbiturate;** uses are given in the next Table:

Uses of Secobarbital
Hypnotic in Short Term Treatment of Insomnia
Preoperatively to Relieve Anxiety and Provide Sedation
Status Epilepticus or Acute Seizure Episodes

DOSAGE FORMS: Caps: 50, 100mg; Injection: 50mg/ml; Rectal Supp.: No longer available. Injectable preparation has been given rectally.

DOSAGE: Secobarbital sodium may be administered orally, rectally, deep IM or slow-IV injection. Dosages are given in the next Table:

Dosage of Secobarbital

Condition	Age	Route	Dosage
Hypnotic for Insomnia	Adult	Oral or IM	100-200mg
	Children	IM	3-5mg/kg/dose to max. of 100mg Do not exceed two weeks of therapy; Withdraw slowly
Sedation	Adult	Oral	100-300mg,1-2 hrs. prior to surgery
	Children	Oral, IM or Rectal	4-6mg/kg daily in 3 divided doses.
Acute Seizure Episodes		IM or IV	5.5mg/kg; repeat every 3-4 hrs. as necessary
Status Epilepticus		IM or IV	250-350mg

ADVERSE EFFECTS: Similar to other barbiturates - see **PHENOBARBITAL.** Acute toxicity includes CNS depression and respiratory depression.

SEIZURES, TREATMENT

Epilepsy affects more than 2 million Americans.

The initial drug selection depends on the accurate diagnosis of the seizure disorder which is based on clinical presentation and electroencephalographic(EEG) studies. For a review of the evaluation and treatment of seizures, see Scheuer, M.L. and Pedley, T.A., N. Engl. J. Med. 323, 1468-1474, 1990.

Classification of Seizures: A classification of seizures, adapted from the Commission on Classification and Terminology of the International League Against Epilepsy, is given in the next Table; (Epilepsia 22, 489-501, 1981):

Classification of Seizures

I. **Partial (Focal, Local) Seizures**
   A. **Simple Partial** (Consciousness is not Impaired)
      1. With Motor Signs (Includes Jacksonian Seizures)
      2. With Somatosensory or Special Sensory Symptoms
      3. With Autonomic Symptoms or Signs
      4. With Disturbance of Higher Cortical Function
   B. **Complex Partial** (Psychomotor or Temporal Lobe) (Consciousness is Impaired)
      1. Simple Partial Onset Followed by Impairment of Consciousness
      2. With Impairment of Consciousness at Onset
   C. **Partial Seizures Evolving to Secondarily Generalized Seizures**
      1. Simple Partial (A) Evolving to Generalized Seizures
      2. Complex Partial (B) Evolving into Generalized Seizures
      3. Simple Partial Seizures (A), Evolving to Complex Partial Seizures (B), Evolving to Generalized Seizures

II. **Generalized Seizures**
   A. Absence (Petit Mal) Seizures
   B. Myoclonic (Petit Mal Variant, Lennox-Gastaut) Seizures
   C. Clonic Seizures (Clonic=Muscle Activity Intermittent)
   D. Tonic Seizures (Tonic=Muscle Activity Sustained)
   E. Tonic-Clonic (Grand Mal) Seizures
   F. Atonic Seizures

III. **Unclassified Epileptic Seizures**

The types of seizures, most often recognized in infants and children, are given in the next Table:

Seizures in Infants and Children

I. Partial (Focal, Local) Seizures:
   Complex Partial (Psychomotor or Temporal Lobe)

II. Generalized Seizures:
   Absence (Petit Mal)
   Myoclonic (Petit Mal Variant, Lennox-Gastaut)
   Tonic-Clonic (Grand Mal)

Partial or generalized seizures are terms that describe the extent of involvement of the brain in the seizure activity.

Partial (Focal, Local) Seizures: Partial seizures are the most common form of seizure disorder, occurring in about 40% of all children with epilepsy. Complex partial seizures usually last longer than 10 seconds. The psychomotor symptoms last an average of three minutes. Almost 50% of patients have an aura and full consciousness develops slowly.

Treatment of Epilepsies: Almost all forms of seizure disorders should be treated with an antiepileptic drug.

SEIZURES, TREATMENT (Cont.)

The characteristics and treatment of the common types of seizures are given in the next Table (Barkin, R.M. and Rosen, P. eds, Emergency Pediatrics, The C.V. Mosby Company, St. Louis, pg. 606, 1990; Medical Letter 31, 1-4, Jan. 13, 1989):

Characteristics of Common Types of Seizures

Types of Seizure; Etiology	Diagnostic Findings	Treatment
Complex Partial (Temporal Lobe Psychomotor) Etiology: Idiopathic, Hypoxia, Birth Trauma, Infection (Herpes), Temporal Lobe Mass	Aura: Fear, Abdominal Pain, Smell; Automatisms: Rubbing, Chewing, Staring, Salivation; Seizure Occurs Singly (Min.); Psychic: (Fearful, Anger, Hallucination), Sensory (Numbness, Tingling), Motor (Purposeless Movement). Comments: Distinguish from Petit Mal and Behavior Disorder.	Drugs of Choice: Carbamazepine or Phenytoin Alternatives: Phenobarbital Primidone
Absence (Petit Mal) Etiology: Idiopathic Genetic	No Aura: Transient (5-20 sec) Lapses of Consciousness, Appearing to be Daydreaming, Disinterested, Staring, Immobile; Rhythmic Blinking Movement; Not Postictal; EEG 3-sec Wave and Spike; Evoked by Hyperventilation. Comments: Common in 4-10 yr-olds;	Drugs of Choice: Ethosuximide or Valproate(2) Alternative: Clonazepam
Myoclonic (Petit Mal Variant, Lennox-Gastaut) Etiology: Degenerative CNS Infection, Lead, Subacute Sclerosing Parencephalitis, Retarded Children	Sudden Spasmodic Contraction of Extremities (Few Sec) - Single or Repetitive; May Also Have Akinetic Spells (Drop Fits) with Sudden Loss of Muscle Tone. Comments: Very Rare, Usually Accompanied by Grand Mal	Drugs of Choice: Valproate(1) Alternative: Clonazepam
Tonic-Clonic (Grand Mal) Etiology: Idiopathic, Genetic, Trauma, Infection, Intoxication, Endocrine/Metabolic, Metabolic Degenerative, Tumor	Aura(50%): Motor, Sensory (Smell, Taste), Visceral (Abdominal Pain); Crying; Loss of Consciousness; Tonic (Stiffening)-Clonic (Rhythmic Jerking, Twitching); Involuntary Urination & Defecation; Postictal Rare Transient Paresis (Todd's Paralysis).	Drugs of Choice: Carbamazepine or Phenytoin or Valproate(1) Alternatives: Phenobarbital Primidone

(1) Not FDA approved unless absence involved.
(2) First choice if primary generalized tonic-clonic also present.

STATUS EPILEPTICUS: The drugs that are used to treat status epilepticus are given in the next Table (Medical Letter 31, 1-4, Jan. 13, 1989):

Treatment of Status Epilepticus

Drugs of Choice		Usual Initial Dose	Usual Rate	Repeat Doses PRN	Maximum /24hrs
Diazepam, IV	Adults	5-10mg	1-2mg/min*	5-10mg q20-30min	100mg
	Children	0.1-0.2mg/kg**	(See footnote*)	0.1-0.2mg/kg** q20-30min	40mg
Phenytoin, IV	Adults	15-20mg/kg	30-50mg/min	100-150mg q30min	1.5grams
	Children	15-20mg/kg	0.5-1.5mg/kg/min	1.5mg/kg q30min	20mg/kg
Phenobarbital, IV	Adults	10-20mg/kg	25-50mg/min	120-240mg q20min	1-2grams
	Children	20mg/kg	1mg/kg/min	5-10mg/kg q20min	40mg/kg

*Slower rates of administration should be used for children;
**To a maximum of 5-10mg.

Diazepam is the drug of choice for termination of status epilepticus. The usefulness of phenytoin is limited by the need for slow administration and its slow onset of action. Concurrent IV phenytoin and diazepam is the treatment of choice for status epilepticus by some clinicians.

SELENIUM SULFIDE
(Selsun Blue, Exsel)

USES: Selenium sulfide is an **anti-infective agent** having antibacterial and antifungal activity when used **topically;** uses are given in the next Table:

Uses of Selenium Sulfide
Dandruff with Itching and Flaking of Scalp
Seborrheic Dermatitis
Tinea Versicolor

DOSAGE FORMS: Topical Lotion: 1%, 2.5%

DOSAGE: Dandruff or Seborrheic Dermatitis: Selenium sulfide lotion, (5-10ml of the 2.5% lotion) is massaged into the wet scalp as a shampoo. The lotion is allowed to remain on the scalp for 2-3 minutes; rinse thoroughly and repeat. Initially, the lotion is applied as a shampoo twice weekly for 2 weeks. Subsequently, the frequency of application is determined by response; for maintenance therapy, the lotion is applied once every 1 to 4 weeks.

Tinea Versicolor: Selenium sulfide lotion (2.5%) is applied to the skin and allowed to remain for 10 minutes, then rinsed. Repeat daily for 7 days.

Dandruff: A 1% lotion is available over the counter for control of dandruff.

ADVERSE EFFECTS: Irritation when contact with mucous membranes of the eye. Skin irritation, discoloration of the hair, hair loss.

SEPTICEMIA, PATHOGENS, TREATMENT

Pathogens: The pathogens that are most likely to cause septicemia are given in the next Table (Handbook of Antimicrobial Therapy, The Medical Letter, 1990):

Pathogens Causing Septicemia		
Newborn Infants	**Children**	**Adults**
1. Escherichia coli (or other gram-negative bacilli)	1. Strep. pneumoniae	1. Escherichia coli (or other gram-negative bacilli)
2. Strep. Group B	2. Neisseria meningitidis	2. Staph. aureus
3. Listeria monocytogenes	3. Haemophilus influenzae	3. Strep. pneumoniae
4. Staph. aureus	4. Staph. aureus	4. Bacteroides
5. Strep. pyogenes Group A)	5. Strep. pyogenes (Group A)	5. Strep. pyogenes (Group A)
6. Enterococci	6. Escherichia coli (or other gram-negative bacilli)	6. Staph. epidermidis
7. Strep. pneumoniae		7. Neisseria meningitidis
8. Salmonella		8. Candida albicans
		9. Neisseria gonorrhoeae
		10. Other Candida species

The organisms causing septicemia in a large tertiary care hospital are given in the next Table (Geddes, A.M., Lancet 1, 286-289, Feb. 6, 1988):

Organisms Causing Septicemia			
Gram-Negative		**Gram-Positive**	
Organism	**%**	**Organism**	**%**
Escherichia coli	16%	Staphylococcus aureus	12%
Proteus mirabilis	6%	Staph epidermidis	9%
Pseudomonas aeruginosa	5%	Streptococcus pneumoniae	9%
Klebsiella aerogenes	4%	Strep pyogenes	4%
Neisseria meningitis	4%	Strep faecalis	4%
Haemophilus influenzae	3%	Strep milleri	2%
Bacteroides fragilis	3%	Strep sanguis	2%
Enterobacter cloacae	2%	Other streptococci	4%
Salmonella spp	2%	Clostridia	1%
Enterbacter aerogenes	1%		45%
Salmonella typhi	1%		
Salmonella paratyphi A	1%		
Campylobacter spp	1%		
Other organisms	6%		
	55%		

Gram-Negative Bacteria: About half the gram-negative bacteria are common enterobacteria such as Escherichia coli.

Gram-Positive Bacteria: Ninety-eight percent of the gram-positive bacteria are either staphylococci or streptococci, most being Staphylococcus aureus, Streptococcus pneumoniae, or haemolytic streptococci.

SEPTICEMIA (Cont.)

In septicemia, the results of culture and antimicrobial susceptibility tests are usually obtained 36 to 48 hours after the institution of empirical antimicrobial therapy. Choice of drugs should be based on the probable anatomic focus of infection, such as the lungs or kidneys, on gram-stained smears of appropriate clinical specimens and on the immune status of the patient. All hospitals should monitor the organisms causing bacteremia so as to alert clinicians to changing patterns of infection and to indicate a suitable strategy for blind therapy of suspected septicemia. Most febrile patients with neutropenia have infections from which no organisms are isolated, gram-positive infections, or fevers of unknown origin (Anaissie, E. et al., N. Engl. J. Med. 318, 1694-1695, June 23, 1988).

Treatment: Empirical antimicrobial therapy is given in the next Table (Handbook of Antimicrobial Therapy, The Medical Letter, 1990):

Empirical Antimicrobial Therapy of Septicemia

Probable Cause	Drug Treatment
Gram-Negative Bacilli	"Third-generation" cephalosporins (cefotaxime, or ceftizoxime, or ceftriaxone or ceftazidime); or Imipenem or Aztreonam
Sepsis in Infants <1 mon.	Ampicillin plus aminoglycoside or Ampicillin plus cefotaxime
Pseudomonas Aeruginosa	Extended-spectrum penicillin (carbenicillin, ticarcillin, mezlocillin, azlocillin or piperacillin) plus aminoglycoside. or "Third-generation" cephalosporins (ceftazidime, cefoperzone) or Imipenem or Aztreonam
Life-Threatening Bacteremia	"Third-generation" cephalosporins (cefotaxime, ceftizoxime, or ceftriaxone) or Ticarcillin-clavulanic acid or Imipenem Together With Aminoglycosides (gentamicin, tobramycin, or amikacin)
Bacterial Endocarditis	Penicillin G (or ampicillin) plus gentamicin plus vancomycin
Methicillin-Resistant Staphylococci	Vancomycin plus gentamicin
Intra-abdominal or Pelvic Infections likely to involve Anaerobes	Clindamycin or metronidazole plus Aminoglycoside or Ticarcillin-clavulanic acid or Imipenem or Cefoxitin (2nd generation cephalosporin)
Biliary Tract	Ampicillin or Cephalosporin plus Aminoglycoside (gentamicin, tobramycin or amikacin) possibly also with Anti-anaerobe, eg., metronidazole
Antibiotic-Resistant (Gentamicin, Tobramycin Netilmicin) Gram-Negative Bacilli	Amikacin or cefotaxime, or ceftizoxime or ceftriaxone or ceftazidime or imipenem or aztreonam
Neutropenic Patients (Pseudomonas occur commonly)	Aminoglycoside plus Ticarcillin, or azlocillin, or mezlocillin or piperacillin or ceftazidime or Imipenem with Aminoglycoside Add Vancomycin when methicillin-resistant staphylococci are a consideration.

SEXUALLY TRANSMITTED DISEASES, PATHOGENS, TREATMENT

Sexually transmitted diseases and their treatment are listed in the next Table (Handbook of Antimicrobial Therapy, The Medical Letter, 1990; Centers for Disease Control," 1989 Sexually Transmitted Diseases Treatment Guidelines," MMWR 38(S-8), 1-40, Sept. 1, 1989):

Treatment of Sexually Transmitted Diseases

Type or Stage	Drug of Choice (Dosage)	Alternatives
GONORRHEA (TREAT FOR CHLAMYDIA)		
Urethritis or Cervicitis or Rectal	Ceftriaxone 250mg IM once.	Spectinomycin 2 grams IM once. Ciprofloxacin 500mg orally once.
Pharyngeal	Ceftriaxone 250mg IM once.	Ciprofloxacin 500mg orally once.
Ophthalmia adults	Ceftriaxone (1 gram IM once) plus saline irrigation.	Ceftriaxone (1 gram IV or IM daily x5 days) plus saline irrigation.
Bacteremia and arthritis (Disseminated Gonococcal Infection	Ceftriaxone (1 gram IV or IM daily x7-10 days)	Ceftizoxime or cefotaxime (1 gram IV every 8 hours for 2-3 days) followed by cefuroxime axetil 500mg orally twice daily for total of 7-10 day course.
Meningitis	Ceftriaxone (2 grams IV daily for at least 10 days)(Medical Letter); (1-2 grams IV every 12 hours for 10-14 days) (CDC).	Penicillin G at least 10 million Units IV daily in divided doses for at least 10 days (susceptible strains). Chloramphenicol 4-6 grams/day in divided doses for at least 10 days (susceptible strains).
Endocarditis	Ceftriaxone (2 grams IV daily for at least 4 weeks).	Penicillin G at least 10 million Units IV daily in divided doses for at least 4 weeks.
Neonatal Infant born to mother with Gonococcal Infection	Ceftriaxone 50mg/kg IV or IM once. (Max: 125mg). (Not in hyperbilirubinemic infants).	
Neonatal Ophthalmia	Cefotaxime (25mg/kg IV q8-12 hours x7 days) plus saline irrigation. OR Ceftriaxone (25-50mg/kg, max. 125mg IM or IV once daily for 7 days) plus saline irrigation.	Penicillin G 100,000 U/kg/day IV in 4 doses x 7 days susceptible strains plus saline irrigation. Ceftriaxone 50mg/kg, max. 125mg as a single injection.
Neonatal Arthritis and septicemia	Cefotaxime (25-50mg/kg IV q8-12h x 10-14 days).	Penicillin G 75,000 to 100,000 U/kg/day IV in 4 doses x 7 days (susceptible strains).
Neonatal Meningitis	Cefotaxime (50mg/kg q8-12h x 10-14 days).	Penicillin G 100,000-150,000 U/kg/day IV in 3 or 4 doses for at least 10 days(susceptible strains)
Children (under 45kg) Urogenital, rectal and pharyngeal	Ceftriaxone (125mg IM once).	Spectinomycin 40mg/kg IM once (Not for pharyngeal infection). Amoxicillin 50mg/kg oral once plus probenecid 25mg/kg (max. 1 gram) oral once (susceptible strains). Penicillin G procaine 100,000 U/kg IM once plus probenecid 25mg/kg (max. 1 gram) once (susceptible strains).

SEXUALLY TRANSMITTED DISEASES, PATHOGENS, TREATMENT (Cont.)

Table cont.

Type or Stage	Drug of Choice (Dosage)	Alternatives
Bacteremia or Arthritis	Ceftriaxone [50mg/kg/day (max. 2 grams) IV x 7 days].	Penicillin G 150,000 U/kg/day in 6 divided doses IV x 7 days (susceptible strains).
Meningitis	Ceftriaxone [100mg/kg/day (max. 2 grams) IV x 7-14 days].	Penicillin G 250,000 U/kg/day IV in 6 divided doses for at least 10-14 days (susceptible strains)
	OR Cefotaxime (200mg/kg/day IV in divided doses every 6 h for 10-14 days.	Chloramphenicol 100 mg/kg/day in 4 divided doses IV for at least 10-14 days (susceptible strains)
CHLAMYDIA TRACHOMATIS		
Urethritis or cervicitis OR **Oculogenital syndrome** OR **Proctitis**	Doxycycline 100mg bid x 7 days or Tetracycline, 500mg, qid x 7 days. Erythromycin base (500mg oral qid x 7 days).	Sulfisoxazole 500mg oral qid x 10 days.
Neonatal		
Ophthalmia	Erythromycin (12.5mg/kg oral or IV qid x 14 days).	
Pneumonia	Erythromycin (12.5mg/kg oral or IV qid x 14 days).	Sulfisoxazole 100mg/kg/day oral or IV in divided doses (after 4 weeks of age) x 14 days.
Lymphogranuloma venereum	Doxycycline 100mg bid x 21 days.	Erythromycin (500mg oral qid x 21 days).
VAGINAL INFECTIONS		
Trichomoniasis	Metronidazole (2 grams oral once).	Metronidazole 500mg twice daily for 7 days.
in pregnancy	Consider metronidazole 2 grams orally once (Contraind. in the first trimester).	
Bacterial vaginosis	Metronidazole(500mg oral bid x 7 days)	Clindamycin 300mg orally bid x 7 days.
Vulvovaginal candidiasis	Miconazole (Monistat) [100mg intravaginally at bedtime x 7 days, or 200 x 3 days).	Butoconazole (5 grams of 2% cream intravaginally at bedtime for 3-6 days.
	OR Clotrimazole (100mg intravaginally at bedtime x 7 days, or 200mg x 3 days).	OR Terconazole (80mg supp. intravaginally at bedtime for 3 days or 5 grams of 0.4% cream for 7 days).
SYPHILIS		
Early (Primary, secondary, or latent less than one yr.)	Penicillin G benzathine (2.4 million U IM once)	Doxycycline 100mg oral bid or Tetracycline 500mg oral qid x 14 days. Erythromycin 500mg oral qid x 14 days. Ceftriaxone 250mg IM once daily for 10 days.

SEXUALLY TRANSMITTED DISEASES, PATHOGENS, TREATMENT (Cont.)

table cont.

Type or Stage	Drug of Choice (Dosage)	Alternatives
Late (more than one year's duration, cardiovascular)	Penicillin G benzathine (2.4 million U IM weekly x 3 weeks).	Doxycycline 100mg oral bid or Tetracycline 500mg oral qid x 30 days.
Neurosyphilis	Penicillin G (2 to 4 million U IV q4h x 10-14 days)	No proven alternative; penicillin allergic patients should be desensitized.
OR	Penicillin G procaine (2.4 million U IM daily) plus probenicid (500mg qid orally) both x 10-14 days	
	either one followed by penicillin G benzathine (2.4 million U IM weekly x 3 weeks.)	
Congenital	Penicillin G (50,000 U/kg IM or IV every 8-12 hours for 10-14 days).	
OR	Penicillin G procaine (50,000 U/kg IM daily for 10-14 days).	
CHANCROID (Schmid, G.P., JAMA 255, 1757-1762, 1986) (Haemophilus ducreyi)	Ceftriaxone (250mg IM once) OR Erythromycin (500mg oral qid x 7 days).	Trimethoprim-sulfamethoxazole 2 tablets (80mg TMP/400mg SMX) bid x 7 days. Ciprofloxacin 0.5g orally bid x 3 days.
HERPES SIMPLEX VIRUS (genital)	Acyclovir (See **ACYCLOVIR** for drug dosage).	
(encephalitis	Acyclovir (See **ACYCLOVIR** for drug dosage).	Vidarabine
(neonatal)	Acyclovir (See **ACYCLOVIR** for drug dosage).	Vidarabine
(disseminated, adult)	Acyclovir (See **ACYCLOVIR** for drug dosage).	Vidarabine
(keratitis)	Trifluridine (topical)	Vidarabine (topical) idoxuridine (topical)
UREAPLASMA UREALYTICUM	Doxycycline 100mg orally bid or Tetracycline 500mg orally qid for 7 days.	Erythromycin base 500mg or Erythromycin ethylsuccinate 800mg orally qid for 7 days.
PEDICULOSIS PUBIS	Lindane (Kwell, Scarbene)	Apply for 4 minutes then wash.
OR	Permethrin (Nix)	Apply for 10 minutes then wash.
OR	Pyrethrins with piperonyl butoxide (Rid and others)	Apply for 10 minutes then wash.
	Treat sexual partners. Wash bedding and clothing. Retreat in 1 week if necessary.	
VENEREAL WARTS	Podophyllin Alpha interferon (Eron, L.J. et al., N. Engl. J. Med. 315, 1059, 1986) Fluorouracil, topical (Krebs, H-B, Obstet. Gynecol 70, 68, 1987)	
GRANULOMA INGUINALE (Calymmatobacterium, (Donovan bodies) granulomatis)	A Tetracycline	Streptomycin

SEXUALLY TRANSMITTED DISEASES, PATHOGENS, TREATMENT (Cont.)

Other sexually transmitted conditions include scabies, pubic lice, human immunodeficiency virus (HIV), hepatitis B, cytomegalovirus infection

SYPHILIS: The recommended treatment of primary and secondary syphilis is 2.4 million units of penicillin G benzathine. There is no simple test to determine cure of syphilis. To assess treatment, serological testing is done at 3-,6-,and 12-month visits. When serological results revert to negative, the patient is considered cured.

Criteria for determining treatment failures are given in the next Table (Guinan, M.E., JAMA 257, 359-360, 1987):

Criteria for Determining Treatment Failures for Syphilis

1. The patient has clinical signs or symptoms suggestive of syphilis.
2. Fourfold rise in serum titer of the nontreponemal test for syphilis (VDRL or RPR) and
3. A positive VDRL or RPR test result persists after one year in patients treated for primary syphilis or after two years in patients treated for secondary syphilis.

FEMALE GENITAL TRACT, VAGINA; PATHOGENS, TREATMENT

Pathogens: The pathogens that cause infection of the vagina are given in the next Table (Handbook of Antimicrobial Therapy, The Medical Letter, 1990):

Pathogens that Cause Infection of the Vagina

- Trichomonas vaginalis (a protozoan)
- Candida albicans (a yeast)
- Bacterial vaginosis:
  - Gardnerella vaginalis (a bacterium)
  - Mycoplasma hominis
  - Various anaerobes
- Neisseria gonorrhoeae
- Streptococcus pyogenes (Group A)
- Treponema pallidum

The three most common organisms causing vaginitis are Trichomonas vaginalis (a protozoan), Candida albicans (a yeast) and Gardnerella vaginalis (previously called Haemophilus vaginalis, a bacterium).

Diagnosis of suspected vaginal infections is done usually by microscopic examination of discharge. The methods for diagnosing these three pathogens are given in the next Table (Kaufman, R.H., Hospital Medicine, pgs. 23-44, Nov. 1986):

Methods for Diagnosing Vaginal Pathogens

Pathogen	Saline Wet-Mount	20% KOH Wet Mount	Vaginal pH (Normal 3.8-4.2)
Trichomonas vaginalis	Motile ovoid to pear-shaped trichomonads with flagellae		>5.0
Candida albicans	Spores and filaments	Spores and filaments	
Gardnerella vaginalis	"Clue cells"		>5.0

Bacterial Vaginosis: Bacterial vaginosis (formerly called nonspecific vaginitis) is associated with characteristics as given in the next Table:

Characteristics of Bacterial Vaginosis

- Vaginal discharge and odor
- Elevated vaginal fluid pH > 4.5
- Wet mount of vaginal fluid showing "Clue cells" (epithelial cells heavily coated with bacteria)
- "Fishy" odor when 10% KOH is added to vaginal secretions (Spiegel, C.A. et al., J. Infect. Dis. 148, 817, 1983).

SEXUALLY TRANSMITTED DISEASES, PATHOGENS, TREATMENT (Cont.)

Gardnerella vaginalis occurs in about one-third of women with vaginitis; it is present in about 10% of truly asymptomatic women (West, R.R. et al., Brit. Med. J. 296, 1163-1164, 1988).

Treatment: Treatment of infection of the vagina is given in the next Table:

Treatment of Infection of the Vagina

Pathogen	Treatment	Dosage
Trichomonas vaginalis (a protozoan)	Metronidazole (Flagyl and others).	2gms oral once or 500mg orally every 12 hours for 5-7 days.
in pregnancy	Consider metronidazole (contraind. in first trimester).	2 gms oral once.
Candida albicans (a yeast)	Clotrimazole (Gyne-Lotrimin; Mycelex G).	100mg intravaginally at bedtime for 7 days or 200mg for 3 days.
	or Miconazole (Monistat)	100mg intravaginally at bedtime for 7 days or 200mg for 3 days.
Bacterial vaginosis: Gardnerella vaginalis Mycoplasma hominis Various anaerobes	Metronidazole (Flagyl and others)	500mg oral twice daily for 7 days.
Neisseria gonorrhoeae	Ceftriaxone	250mg IM once
Treponema pallidum, early	Penicillin G benzathine	2.4 million Units, IM, once.

Trichomoniasis: The most effective therapy is the 5 day regimen as compared to the single-dose regimen. In the compliant patient who does not respond to standard therapy, the dose should be increased to 500mg three times daily for 10 to 14 days.

Bacterial Vaginosis: The seven day course of 500mg given twice daily is more effective therapy for Gardnerella vaginalis as compared to a single 2g dose (Swedberg, J. et al., JAMA 254, 1046-1049, 1985).

VULVOVAGINAL CANDIDIASIS

Topical drugs for the treatment of vaginal candidiasis are given in the next Table (The Medical Letter, 28, 68, July 4, 1986):

Treatment of Vaginal Candidiasis

Drug	Formulation	Dosage
Butoconazole		
Femstat-Syntex	2% Cream	5 grams at bedtime x 3 days (nonpregnant) x 6 days (pregnant)
Clotrimazole		
Gyne-Lotrimin-Schering	100-mg vaginal tablet	1 tablet at bedtime x 7 days. 2 tablets at bedtime x 3 days (nonpregnant)
Mycelex-G-Miles	100-mg vaginal tablet	1 tablet at bedtime x 7 days. 2 tablets at bedtime x 3 days (nonpregnant)
Gyne-Lotrimin-Schering	500-mg vaginal tablet	1 tablet once
Mycelex-G-Miles	500-mg vaginal tablet	1 tablet once
Gyne-Lotrimin-Schering	1% cream	5 grams at bedtime x 7-14 days.
Mycelex-G-Miles	1% cream	5 grams at bedtime x 7-14 days.

SEXUALLY TRANSMITTED DISEASES, PATHOGENS, TREATMENT (Cont.)

Table cont.

Drug	Formulation	Dosage
Miconazole		
Monistat 7-Ortho	2% cream	5 grams at bedtime x 7 days.
Monistat 7-Ortho	100-mg vaginal suppository	1 suppository at bedtime x 7 days.
Monistat 3-Ortho	200-mg vaginal suppository	1 suppository at bedtime x 3 days.
Nystatin		
Mycostatin-Squibb	100,000-U vaginal tablet.	1 tablet at bedtime x 14 days.
Nilstat-Lederle	100,000-U vaginal tablet.	1 tablet at bedtime x 14 days.
generic	100,000-U vaginal tablet.	1 tablet at bedtime x 14 days.

Butoconazole, clotrimazole or miconazole are more effective and convenient than nystatin. Prophylactic oral ketoconazole (Nizoral) may be effective in women with frequent, persistent recurrences (Sobel, J.D., N. Engl. J. Med. 315, 1455, 1986).

FEMALE GENITAL TRACT, UTERUS, PATHOGENS, TREATMENT

Pathogens: The pathogens that cause infection of the uterus are given in the next Table (Handbook of Antimicrobial Therapy, The Medical Letter, 1990):

Pathogens that Cause Infection of the Uterus
Anaerobic streptococci
Bacteroides
Neisseria gonorrhoeae (cervix)
Clostridia
Escherichia coli (or other gram-negative bacilli)
Herpes virus, type II (cervix)
Streptococcus, Group A
Streptococcus, Groups B and C
Treponema pallidum
Staphylococcus aureus
Enterococci
Chlamydia trachomatis
Mycoplasma hominis

FEMALE GENITAL TRACT, FALLOPIAN TUBES, PATHOGENS, TREATMENT

Pathogens: The pathogens that cause infection of fallopian tubes are given in the next Table (Stanton, S.L., Brit. Med. J. 295, 621-622, Sept. 12, 1987; Handbook of Antimicrobial Therapy, The Medical Letter, 1990):

Pathogens that Cause Infection of Fallopian Tubes
Chlamydia trachomatis
Neisseria gonorrhoeae
Escherichia coli (or other gram-negative bacilli)
Anaerobic streptococci
Bacteroides
Mycoplasma

Chlamydia is the most common infecting bacteria, implicated in almost two-thirds of cases; the gonococcus is isolated in over half the cases. Other organisms implicated include enterobacteria, mycoplasma and anaerobic bacteria, that is, anaerobic streptococci and bacteroides.

Treatment: See Treatment of Pelvic Inflammatory Disease, below. Doxycycline should be avoided during pregnancy.

**SEXUALLY TRANSMITTED DISEASES,
PATHOGENS, TREATMENT** (Cont.)

PELVIC INFLAMMATORY DISEASE (PID), PATHOGENS, TREATMENT

Pathogens: The pathogens that cause pelvic inflammatory disease (PID) are given in the next Table (Thompson, S.E. et al., Am. J. Obstet. Gynecol. 136, 179, 1980):

Pathogens that Cause Pelvic Inflammatory Disease (PID)

Pathogen	Cervix (%)	Peritoneal Cavity (%)
Neisseria gonorrhoeae	80 (27-80%)*	33
Ureaplasma urealyticum	60	17
Mycoplasma hominis	33	20
Streptococci	27	23
Candida species	23	0
Trichomonas vaginalis	23	0
Enterobacteriaceae	20	17
Chlamydia trachomatis	10 (5-39%)*	10
Corynebacterium vaginalis	10	7
Anaerobic species	Not done	63

*Pelvic Inflammatory Disease: Guidelines for Prevention and Management. MMWR 40, RR-5, 1991.

There is a polymicrobial nature of pelvic inflammatory disease (PID).

The incidence of gonorrhea cases has reached a plateau while the incidence of cases caused by C. trachomatis are increasing.

Treatment: Treatment of acute and subacute pelvic inflammatory disease (PID) is given in the next Table (Handbook of Antimicrobial Therapy, The Medical Letter, 1990; CDC "1989 Sexually Transmitted Diseases Treatment Guidelines", MMWR 38(S-8), 1-40, Sept. 1, 1989; Pelvic Inflammatory Disease: Guidelines for Prevention and Management, MMWR 40, RR-5, 1991):

Treatment of Acute and Subacute Pelvic Inflammatory Disease (PID)

Condition	Drug of Choice	Dosage	Alternative
Outpatients	Cefoxitin	2 grams IM once	
	plus probenecid	1 gram oral once	
	or Ceftriaxone	250mg IM once	
	either one followed by doxycycline.	100mg oral bid x 10-14 days.	Tetracycline 500mg oral qid x 10-14 days. Erythromycin 500mg oral qid x 10-14 days.
Hospitalized Patients	Cefoxitin	2 grams IV every 6 hours.	Clindamycin 900mg IV every 8 hours plus gentamicin 2mg/kg IV once, then 1.5mg/kg IV q 8 h.
	or Cefotetan	2 grams IV every 12 hours.	
	plus doxycycline followed by doxycycline.	100mg IV bid until improvement 100mg oral bid to complete 10-14 days.	followed by clindamycin 450mg oral qid to complete 10-14 days.

In the treatment of pelvic inflammatory disease (PID), use a combination of a cephalosporin (cefoxitin or cefotetan or ceftriaxone) plus doxycycline. The cephalosporins have a broad spectrum of antibacterial activity but are ineffective against Chlamydia trachomatis infections; Clindamycin may be effective against chlamydia, but doxycycline is the drug of choice (Wolner-Hanssen, P. et al, JAMA 256, 3262-3263, Dec. 19, 1986; Grimes, D.A. et al., JAMA 256, 3223-3226, 1986; Chlamydia trachomatis infections: Policy guidelines for prevention and control. MMWR 34, 53S-74S, 1985; Burnakis, T.G. and Hildebrandt. N.B., Rev. Infect. Dis. 8, 86, 1986; Bell T.A. and Grayston, J.T., Ann. Intern. Med. 104, 524-526, 1986; Sanders, L.L. et al., JAMA 255, 1750-1756, 1986; MMWR 40, RR-5, 1991).

Doxycycline should be avoided during pregnancy and childhood. Erythromycin is the drug of choice for treating chlamydial infections during pregnancy. Erythromycin ethylsuccinate (400mg four times a day for seven days) is effective for eradicating chlamydial infection in pregnant women and for preventing perinatal transmission to their infants (Schachter, J. et al., N. Engl. J. Med. 314, 276-279, 1986). Erythromycin estolate has been associated with hepatotoxicity and is not recommended for use during pregnancy (Chow, A.W. and Jewesson, P.J., Rev. Infect. Dis. 7, 287-313, 1985).

For treating chronic pelvic inflammatory disease, the same antibiotics are used through 2-3 menses.

SEXUALLY TRANSMITTED DISEASES, PATHOGENS, TREATMENT (Cont.)

MALE GENITAL TRACT, EPIDIDYMITIS, SEMINAL VESICLES, PATHOGENS, TREATMENT

The pathogens that cause infection of seminal vesicles are given in the next Table (Handbook of Antimicrobial Therapy, The Medical Letter, 1990):

Pathogens that Cause Infection of Seminal Vesicles
Gram-negative bacilli
Neisseria gonorrhoeae

EPIDIDYMITIS

Pathogens: The pathogens that cause infection of the epididymis are given in the next Table (Handbook of Antimicrobial Therapy, The Medical Letter, 1990):

Pathogens that Cause Infection of the Epididymis
Chlamydia
Gram-negative bacilli
Neisseria gonorrhoeae
Mycobacterium tuberculosis

Treatment: The treatment of epididymitis is given in the next Table:

Treatment of Epididymitis

Drug of Choice	Dosage
Ceftriaxone followed by	250mg IM once.
doxycycline	100mg oral bid x 10 days.

URETHRITIS, PATHOGENS, TREATMENT

Pathogens: The pathogens that cause infection of the urethra in men are given in the next Table (Krieger, J.N. et al., Arch. Intern. Med. 148, 703-707, 1988):

Pathogens that Cause Infection of the Urethra in Men
Neisseria gonorrhoeae
Chlamydia Trachomatis
Ureaplasma urealyticum
Trichomonas vaginalis
Herpes simplex virus
Human papilloma virus

Treatment: See **Sexually Transmitted Diseases, Pathogens, Treatment.** Refer to individual pathogens. The treatment of nongonococcal urethritis (NGU) is given in the following Table (CDC, "1989 Sexually Transmitted Diseases Treatment Guidelines," MMWR 38(S-8), 1-40, Sept. 1, 1989):

Treatment of Nongonococcal Urethritis

Drug of Choice	Dosage	Alternative
Doxycycline	100mg oral bid x 7 days	Erythromycin base 500mg oral qid for 7 days or
or Tetracycline	500mg oral qid x 7 days	Erythromycin ethylsuccinate 800mg oral qid for 7 days.
		Use half dose for twice as long for patients who do not tolerate higher doses of erythromycin.

SINUSITIS

Pathogens: The pathogens that cause acute sinusitis are given in the next Table(Handbook of Antimicrobial Therapy, The Medical Letter, 1990; Wald, E.R., Pediatr. Infect. Dis. J. 7, S150-S153, Nov. 1988):

Pathogens Causing Acute Sinusitis

Organism	Percent
Streptococcus pneumoniae	25-30
Moraxella (Branhamella) catarrhalis	15-20
Haemophilus influenzae	15-20
Streptococcus pyogenes (Group A)	2-5
Anaerobes	2-5
Sterile	20-35
Other: Klebsiella (or other gram-negative bacilli)	
Alpha-hemolytic streptococcus	
Staphyloccus aureus (acute and chronic sinusitis)	
Mucor, Aspergillus (especially in diabetics)	
Virus: Rhinovirus, Influenza A, Parainfluenza virus, Adenovirus	

Acute Sinusitis: In adults, Haemophilus influenzae and Streptococcus pneumoniae are the most common pathogens, accounting for about 65% of all significant bacterial strains. In children, these bacteria are also most commonly isolated (Wald, E.R. et al., Pediatrics 77, 795-800, 1986).

Sites; The anatomy of the paranasal sinuses are given in the next Figure:

Anatomy and Development of the Paranasal Sinuses

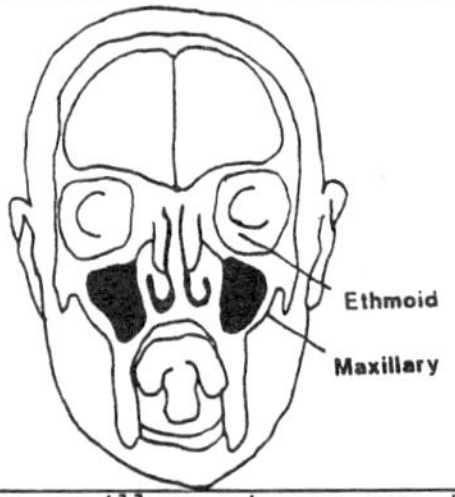

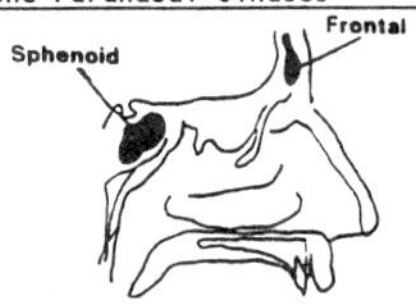

Development

Sinus	Age
Maxillary	Present at birth
Ethmoid	Present at birth
Sphenoid	3-7 years
Frontal	3 years

The maxillary sinuses are the most common sites of infection; the ethmoid and frontal sinuses are also prone to infection. The incidence of sphenoid sinusitis is 7 percent of all sinus infections (Lew, D. et al., N. Engl. J. Med. 309, 1149-1154, 1983).

Complications of Acute Bacterial Sinusitis: Bacteria sinusitis can lead to serious complications including osteomyelitis, orbital cellulitis, meningitis, venous sinus thrombosis, epidural or cerebral abscess or subdural empyema.

Treatment: The recommended antibiotic regimens are similar in type and duration to those used to treat **acute otitis media.**

Current recommendations are for 10-14 days of oral therapy: however, treatment may be continued for another week if symptoms are only partially resolved. Oral agents for the treatment of acute bacterial sinusitis are given in the next Table (Gleckman, R.A. Hosp. Pract., Jan. 30, 1986, Wald, E.R. Pediatr. Infect. Dis. J. 7, S150-S153, Nov. 1988):

Oral Agents for Acute Bacterial Sinusitis

	Dosage	
Drug	Children	Adults
Amoxicillin	40mg/kg/day in 3 divided doses.	500mg every 8 hrs.
Amoxicilin/potassium clavulanate	40/10mg/kg/day in 3 divided doses.	500mg Amoxicillin and 125mg Clavulanic Acid every 8 hrs.
Erythromycin/sulfis-oxazole	50/150mg/kg/day in 4 divided doses.	
Trimethoprim/sulfame-thoxazole	8/40mg/kg/day in 2 divided doses.	160mg of Trimethoprim, 800mg of Sulfameth-oxazole every 12 hrs.
Cefaclor	40mg/kg/day in 3 divided doses.	500mg every 6 hrs.

SINUITIS (Cont.)

No single antibiotic is effective against all possible pathogens and no single antibiotic has emerged as the preferred drug. Antibiotics other than those listed in the previous Table that are potentially effective in the treatment of acute bacterial sinusitis are doxycycline, and cephalexin(Keflex) (Sotomayor, J.L. et al., Hosp. Pract. pgs. 129-136, April 15, 1986; Frazier, L.M. and Corey, G.R., North Carolina Med. J. 47, 115-117, March, 1986; Minor, M.W. and Lockey, R.F. Southern Med. J. 80, 1141-1147, 1987).

Efficacy of selected antibiotics for the common pathogens in acute sinusitis is given in the next Table (Minor, M.W. and Lockey, R.F., Southern Med. J. 80, 1141-1147, 1987; Bluestone, C.D., Pediatr. Infect. Dis. J. 7, No. 11, S129-S136, Nov. 1988):

Efficacy of Selected Antibiotics for Common Pathogens in Acute Sinusitis

Antimicrobial Agents	Strep. pneumoniae	Haemophilus influenzae	Moraxella catarrhalis	Strep. pyogenes	Staph. aureus
Ampicillin or amoxicillin	(+)	(+,-)	(+,-)	(+)	(+,-)
Amoxicillin-clavulanate	(+)	(+)	(+)	(+)	(+)
Erythromycin-sulfamethoxazole	(+)	(+)	(+)	(+)	(+)
Trimethoprim-sulfamethoxazole	(+)	(+)	(+)	(-)	(+)
Cefaclor	(+)	(+)	(+,-)	(+)	(+)
Cefuroxime axetil	(+)	(+)	(+)	(+)	(+)

(+),Effective; (+,-), Effective for strains not producing beta-lactamase; (-), not effective.

The most commonly used antibiotic for initial empirical treatment of sinusitis is amoxicillin. The combination, amoxicillin-clavulanic acid (Augmentin) is FDA-approved for the treatment of sinusitis; Augmentin provides broader anti-bacterial activity against the major bacterial pathogens bound in acute sinusitis. However, the comparative cure rate of amoxicillin and amoxicillin-clavulanate in acute paranasal sinus infections in children is about equal (Wald, E.R. et al., Pediatrics 77, 795-800, 1986).

In patients who have beta-lactamase positive H. influenzae and M. catarrhalis or who are allergic to penicillin or have failed to respond to it, then the combination drug sulfamethoxazole-trimethoprim (co-trimoxazole) (Septra, Bactrim, generic) may be effective.

Amoxicillin and cefaclor have similar cure rates of approximately 80% in children with acute maxillary sinusitis (Wald, E.R. et al., J. Peds. 104, 297-302, 1984).

Clinical improvement with appropriate antibiotics usually occurs within 2-5 days. If the patient does not improve, then change in antibiotic should be considered.

Cost is a major consideration when treating acute sinusitis. Cefaclor, a second generation cephalosporin, costs approximately eight times that of amoxicillin or trimethoprim-sulfamethoxazole and twice as costly as amoxicillin-clavulanic acid (Augmentin).

Oral or topical decongestants, antihistamines, and corticosteroids have controversial, essentially unstudied use in sinusitis. However, nasal decongestants have been found by some clinicians to be an important component of therapy; Neosynephrine nose drops, 1/4% or 1/2%, or Afrin spray, applied several times per day during the first five days of therapy, decreases mucosal edema and promotes sinus drainage (Frazier, L.M. and Corey, G.R. North Carolina Med. J. 47, 115-117, 1986). Antihistamines should not be used because they thicken purulent sinus fluid and impair drainage.

A glucocorticosteroid aerosol, such as Decadron Phosphate Turbinaire (dexamethasone sodium phosphate) decreases inflammation; it is particularly useful when sinusitis is associated with allergic rhinitis. (Minor, M.W. and Lockey, R.F., Southern Med. J. 80, 1141-1147, 1987).

Rhinocerebral mucormycosis, caused by mycelial elements of pathogenic fungi of the order Mucorales causes progressive infection of the sinus and orbit in diabetics with ketoacidosis; it is treated with amphotericin B.

SKIN AND SUBCUTANEOUS TISSUES, PATHOGENS, TREATMENT

Pathogens: The pathogens that are most likely to cause infection of skin and subcutaneous tissues are given in the next Table (Handbook of Antimicrobial Therapy, The Medical Letter, 1990):

Pathogens Causing Infection of Skin and Subcutaneous Tissues

Burns	Skin Infections	Decubitus Wound Infections	Traumatic and Surgical Wounds
1. Staphylococcus aureus	1. Staphylococcus aureus	1. Staphylococcus aureus	1. Staphylococcus aureus
2. Streptococcus pyogenes (Group A)	2. Streptococcus pyogenes (Group A)	2. Escherichia coli (or other gram-negative bacilli)	2. Anaerobic streptococci
3. Pseudomonas aeruginosa (or other gram-negative bacilli)	3. Dermatophytes	3. Streptococcus pyogenes (Group A)	3. Gram-negative bacilli
	4. Candida albicans	4. Anaerobic streptococci	4. Clostridia
	5. Herpes simplex or zoster	5. Clostridia	5. Streptococus pyogenes (Group A)
	6. Gram-negative bacilli	6. Enterococci	6. Enterococci
	7. Treponema pallidum	7. Bacteroides	

Treatment: The treatment of different conditions involving the skin and subcutaneous tissues is given in the next Table:

Treatment of Different Skin Infections

Condition	Organism(s)	Treatment
Impetigo	Streptococcus pyogenes	Penicillin V or Erythromycin
	Staphylococcus aureus	Dicloxacillin or Cephalexin
Cellulitis	same as above	
	Haemophilus influenzae (facial cellulitis)	Cefuroxime or A third generation cephalosporin
Bite Wound Infections Animal Bites	Anaerobes Streptococci Staphylococci Pasteurella multocida Gram-negative bacilli	Oral Amoxicillin plus Clavulanic Acid (Augmentin) or Parenteral Ampicillin plus Sulbactam (Unasyn) or In the penicillin-allergic patient, use an oral cephalosporin or tetracycline
Burns	Staphylococcus aureus Streptococcus pyogenes (Group A) Pseudomonas aeruginosa (or other gram-negative bacilli)	Ticarcillin plus Clavulanic Acid (Timentin) with or without an Aminoglycoside antibiotic
Diabetic Foot frequently with osteomyelitis	Streptococci Anaerobes such as Bacteroides fragilis Aerobic gram-negative bacilli Staphylococci (uncommon)	Ticarcillin plus Clavulanic Acid (Timentin) Aminoglycoside Metronidazole Clindamycin
Acne	Propionobacterium acne	Oral antibiotics: Tetracycline, Clindamycin, Erythromycin

SODIUM POLYSTYRENE SULFONATE
(Kayexalate, SPS)

USES: Sodium **polystyrene sulfonate** is a sulfonated **cation-exchange resin** which is used to **remove excess potassium from the blood.**

DOSAGE FORMS: Suspension: 1.25g/5ml; contains sorbital. Powder, for suspension.

DOSAGE: Sodium polystyrene sulfonate is administered orally or rectally; the drug should be given with a laxative, such as sorbitol. One gram of resin binds approximately 1 mEq of potassium. Dosage is given in the next Table:

Dosage of Sodium Polystyrene Sulfonate

Age	Route	Dosage
Adult	Oral	15-60g, 1-4 times daily (approx. 4 level teaspoonfuls of powder or 60ml of commercial suspension).
	Rectal	30-60g as needed (eg, at 1-to 2-hour intervals initially and then every 6 hours or as necessary.
Children	Oral	1gm/kg/dose, every 6 hours
	Rectal	1gm/kg/dose, every 2-6 hours

Rectal use should be by retention enema - the suspension should be retained for at least 30-60 minutes, and longer if possible.

ADVERSE EFFECTS: GI: anorexia, nausea, vomiting, and constipation; large oral doses of the drug may cause fecal impaction, especially in geriatric patients.

Use cautiously in presence of renal failure. Do not administer with antacids or laxatives containing Mg^{++} or Al^{+++}. Systemic alkalosis may result.

MONITOR: Serum potassium, calcium, magnesium and sodium at least daily.

Electrocardiogram(ECG) monitoring for hypokalemia: lengthened QT intervals; widened, flat or inverted T waves and prominent U waves.

SOMATREM
(Protropin)

USES: Somatrem is identical to human growth hormone(GH) except for the addition of methionine on the N-terminus of the molecule; it is prepared by recombinant DNA technology (192 amino acids, mol. wt. 22,000 daltons). The biological effects are identical to those of naturally occurring growth hormone derived from the pituitary glands.

Somatrem is used for the treatment of proven **growth hormone deficiency.** (see Bakerman, S., "ABC's of Interpretive Laboratory Data" 2nd Ed., 1984, pg. 223 for evaluation of growth hormone deficiency).

DOSAGE FORMS: 5mg (approx. 13 IU) or 10mg (approx. 26 IU)/container.

DOSAGE: Somatrem is administered intramuscularly or subcutaneously; the subcutaneous route is safe, effective, less painful and may be preferable to the intramuscular route. (Russo, L. and Moore, W.V., J. Clin. Endocrinol. Metab. 55, 1003-1006, 1982; Wilson, D.M. et al., Pediatrics 76, 361-364, 1985). Dosage is given in the next Table:

Dosage of Somatrem

Condition	Route	Dosage
Growth Hormone Deficiency	IM	Max. dosage: 0.1mg/kg (0.26 IU/kg) three times per week.

The recombinant DNA synthesized growth hormone is produced by Genentech, Inc. 460 Point San Bruno Blvd., South San Francisco, CA 94080, Tel. No. 415-266-1015. Somatrem costs $10,000-$20,000 per year to treat a child with growth hormone deficiency.

PHARMACOKINETICS: Half-Life: 20 minutes; Duration(Target Tissues): Prolonged.

ADVERSE EFFECTS: Antibodies to somatrem; hyperglycemia and ketosis; hypothyroidism. Slipped capital femoral epiphysis may occur more frequently.

MONITOR: Thyroid function tests for hypothyroidism; tests for glycosuria and hyperglycemia.

SPECTINOMYCIN
(Trobicin)

USES: Spectinomycin is an antibiotic used in the treatment of uncomplicated **gonorrhea** caused by susceptible Neisseria gonorrhoeae. The uses of spectinomycin in the treatment of gonorrhea are given in the next Table:

Uses of Spectinomycin in Treatment of Gonorrhea
Patients Allergic to Penicillins, Cephalosporins or Probenecid
and Allergic to Tetracycline or who are Unlikely to complete a Multiple-Dose Tetracycline Regimen
or Penicillin or Cephalosporin Therapy has been Ineffective, e.g., Penicillinase-Producing Strains of N. Gonorrhoeae(PPNG)

Spectinomycin is effective in the treatment of urethral and anorectal gonococcal infections; it is ineffective in treatment of pharyngeal gonococcal infections. It is not effective in the treatment of syphilis. Spectinomycin may be used in the treatment of disseminated gonococcal infections caused by PPNG.

Spectinomycin, like penicillins and cephalosporins, is ineffective in the treatment of chlamydial and mycoplasmal infections; these infections are treated with oral doxycyline therapy or, alternately, oral tetracycline hydrochloride therapy whenever the latter drug is used in the treatment of gonorrhea (except in homosexual men and pregnant women).

In neonates, PPNG is treated with cefotaxime or gentamicin.

DOSAGE FORMS: Injection: 2, 4 grams.

DOSAGE: Spectinomycin is administered by deep IM injection into the upper outer quadrant of the gluteal muscle using a 20-gauge needle. Dosage is given in the next Table:

Dosage of Spectinomycin in Treatment of Gonorrhea

Condition	Age	Dosage
Uncomplicated Gonorrhea	Adult	2g as single dose
	Children	40mg/kg as a single dose
Acute, Sexually Transmitted Epididymo-Orchitis	Adult	2g of Spectinomycin followed by Oral Tetracycline or Erythromycin
Disseminated Gonococcal Infections	Adult	2g of Spectinomycin twice daily for 7-10 days

ADVERSE EFFECTS: Low order of toxicity. The most frequent adverse effect is pain at the injection site. Occasional adverse effects following single dose as follows: urticaria, transient rash, pruritus, dizziness, headache, nausea, vomiting, chills, fever, nervousness and insomnia. Rarely, increased BUN and ALT (SGPT).

MONITOR: Cultures from all sites of gonococcal infections 3-7 days after completion of spectinomycin treatment to verify infection has been eradicated.

All patients being treated for gonorrhea with spectinomycin should receive a serologic test for syphilis at the time of diagnosis and 3 months later.

SPIRONOLACTONE
(Aldactone)

USES: **Spironolactone** is a synthetic steroid **aldosterone antagonist.** Spironolactone competitively inhibits the physiologic effects of the adrenocortical hormone aldosterone on the distal renal tubules, thereby producing increased excretion of sodium chloride and water and decreased excretion of potassium, ammonium, titratable acid and phosphate. Since most sodium is reabsorbed in the proximal renal tubules, spironolactone is relatively ineffective when administered alone, and concomitant administration of a diuretic (such as thiazide diuretic, ethacrynic acid, or furosemide) which blocks reabsorption of sodium proximal to the distal portion of the nephron, is required for maximum diuretic effects. The uses of spironolactone are given in the next Table:

Uses of Spironolactone
Edema: Cirrhosis of the Liver, Nephrotic Syndrome, Congestive Heart Failure
Hypertension
Diagnosis of Primary Aldosteronism
Hypokalemia, Diuretic-Induced

DOSAGE FORMS: Tabs: 25, 50, 100mg

DOSAGE: Spironolactone is administered orally. For children, spironolactone tablets are pulverized and administered as an oral suspension. Dosage is given in the next Table:

Dosage of Spironolactone

Condition	Age	Dosage
Edema	Adult	100mg (25-200mg) daily, single dose or in divided doses. When used alone, administer spironolactone for at least five days; if response is satisfactory, dosage may be adjusted to optimal therapeutic or maintenance dosage. If results are not satisfactory after 5 days, add thiazide diuretic or loop diuretic (furosemide or ethacrynic acid).
	Children	1.0-3.3mg/kg daily in 2-4 divided doses.
Hypertension	Adult	25-100mg daily, single dose or in divided doses alone or with a thiazide diuretic for a minimum of 2 weeks.
	Children	1.0-3.3mg/kg daily in 2-4 divided doses.
Diagnosis of Primary Aldosteronism	Adult	Administer 80-160mEq supplemental potassium daily for 5 days; if serum potassium does not rise to normal, place patient on a normal diet with normal sodium intake (150 mEq) and normal potassium intake (75-100mEq) daily. Spironolactone is then administered in a dosage of 400mg daily for 3-4 weeks. A rise in serum potassium to within normal limits and correction of hypertension indicates diagnosis of primary aldosteronism
	Children	125-375mg/m^2 in divided doses over 24 hours
Test for Response to Adrenalectomy in Primary Aldosteronism	Adult	100mg, 4 times daily for 3-5 weeks. Potassium, sodium, chloride and bicarbonate concentrations return to normal, but only those who patients who subsequently had a successful response to adrenalectomy had a return of blood pressure to within normal limits.
Hypokalemia, Diuretic-Induced	Adult	25-100mg daily
	Children	1.0-3.3mg/kg daily in 2-4 divided doses.

ADVERSE EFFECTS: The most serious adverse effect is hyperkalemia which occurs most frequently in patients receiving potassium supplements and those with renal insufficiency. Gynecomastia and amenorrhea may occur.

STEROID WITHDRAWAL

Suppression of Hypothalamus-Pituitary-Adrenal (HPA) Axis: The hypothalamus-pituitary-adrenal axis and the effect of exogenous steroids are shown in the next Figures:

Hypothalamus-Pituitary-Adrenal (HPA) Axis and Effect of Exogenous Steroids

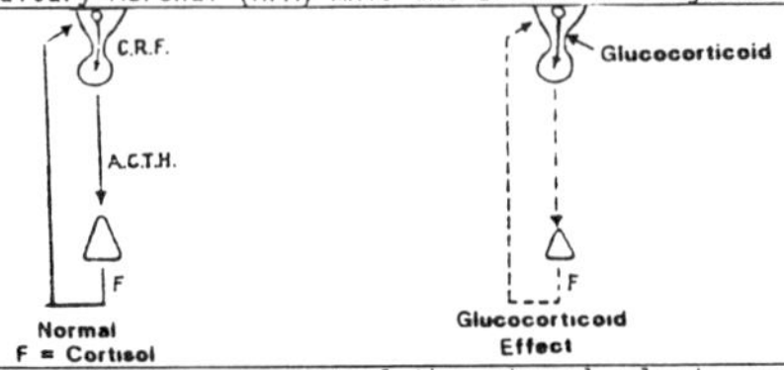

If suppression continues, atrophy of the adrenal glands and decreased responsiveness of the pituitary gland occur.

Tests to Measure Steroid Suppression: Tests to measure steroid suppression are given in the next Table:

ACTH Suppression Test

(a) Withhold glucocorticoids for 12-24 hours.
(b) Obtain a blood specimen (green top vacutainer) for plasma cortisol assay (time 0).
(c) Give 0.25mg of alpha 1-24 corticotropin (Cortrosyn) I.V. or I.M. (in patients less than 2 years old, give 0.125mg). An occasional allergic reaction has been reported to synthetic corticotropin.
(d) Collect blood at 30, 60 and 120 minutes.

The results for normal subjects and for patients receiving glucocorticoids in HPA suppressive quantities are given in the next Figures:

Effect of ACTH on Plasma Cortisol in Normal Subjects and Patients whose Hypothalamic-Pituitary-Adrenal (HPA) Axis is Suppressed

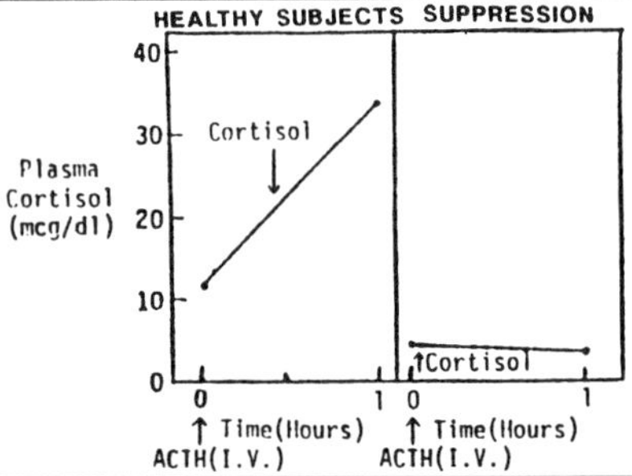

Healthy Subjects: Following I.V. ACTH, a normal response is an increment of plasma cortisol greater than 10mcg/dl.

Suppression: Following suppression, there is no increase in plasma cortisol.

Modes of Reduction of Glucocorticoid Dosage: Following control of the disease state with steroid therapy, it is important to taper the glucocorticoids. The methods of tapering glucocorticoid dosage are given in the next Table (Nelson, A.M. and Conn, D.L., Mayo Clin. Proc. 55, 758-769, 1980):

Tapering Glucocorticoid Dosage
Switch to Alternate-Day Dosage
Keep Dosage Divided and Reduce by Decrements

To taper glucocorticoid dosage, switch to an alternate-day dosage or keep the dosage divided and reduce by decrements.

Switch to Alternate Day Therapy: Alternate day therapy is less suppressive than daily therapy. The steroids that have an intermediate duration of action (24-36 hours), eg, prednisone, prednisolone, methylprednisolone or triamcino-

STEROID WITHDRAWAL (Cont.)
lone, can be given in alternate day doses. Hydrocortisone and cortisone have short duration of action and cannot be given in alternate day doses. Longer-acting steroids, such as dexamethasone and betamethasone have a duration of action of 24 to 48 hours and alternate-day therapy is not done for these latter steroids.

Keep Dosage Divided and Reduce by Decrements: Tapering regimens of glucocorticoid therapy are given in the next Table:

Tapering Regimens of Glucocorticoid Therapy

Glucocorticoid Therapy	Tapering Regimens
Short Term (8 days) combined IV and oral (high dose)	Short Term Tapering: Reduce initial 45mg prednisone dose by 5mg daily for seven days. Long-Term Tapering: Reduce initial 45mg prednisone dose by 5mg weekly for seven weeks.
Long-Term Steroid Therapy; Daily Dose > 40mg Prednisone	Decrease prednisone by 5-10mg per week. When prednisone dose has been reduced to less than 20mg/day, decrease the dose by 1 to 2.5mg every 2 to 3 weeks.
Long-Term Steroid Therapy; Daily Dose < 40mg Prednisone	Decrease prednisone by 2.5-5mg per week. When prednisone dose has been reduced to less than 20mg/day, decrease the dose by 1 to 2.5mg every 2 to 3 weeks.

Short-Term, High Dosage Steroid Therapy: The relapse rate is high regardless of the corticosteroid tapering regimen used; a long taper does not appear to provide enough benefit to justify its routine use (Lederle, F.A. et al., Arch. Intern. Med. 147, 2201-2203, 1987).

A protocol for glucocorticoid withdrawal is given in the next Table (Byyny, R.L., N. Engl. J. Med. 295, 30-32, 1976):

Protocol for Glucocorticoid Withdrawal

Step	Interval	Observation	Result	Glucocorticoid & Dose
I	Variable	Underlying disease	Worsening of underlying disease Symptoms & signs of steroid withdrawal	Variable; gradual decrements in dose to biologic equivalent of hydrocortisone,20mg/day Raise dosage for flare-up of disease; continue if disease quiescent; supplement for stress
II	4 wk	8 a.m. plasma cortisol	Plasma cortisol; When < 10mcg/dl	Begin hydrocortisone, 20mg/day & then taper by 2.5mg/day once/week to 10mg each morning & continue this dosage; supplement for stress.
			When > 10mcg/dl	Stop maintenance hydrocortisone; supplement for stress
III	4 wk - indefinite	8 a.m. 250mcg IM cosyntropin test	When plasma cortisol increment <6 mcg/dl or maximum <20 mcg/dl (or both)	Supplement for stress
IV	4 wk - indefinite	8 a.m. 250mcg IM cosyntropin test	When plasma cortisol increment >6 mcg/dl & maximum ≥20 mcg/dl	Stop; Supplement for stress
V	Indefinite	Routine		As indicated

Withdrawal Syndrome: Typical symptoms associated with too rapid withdrawal of steroids are given in the next Table:

Withdrawal Syndrome
Fatique
Weakness
Arthralgias
Anorexia and Nausea
Orthostatic Hypotension
Hypoglycemia

STREPTOKINASE
(Kabikinase, Streptase)

USES: **Streptokinase** is a bacterial protein derived from group C beta-hemolytic streptococci; uses as a **thrombolytic agent** are given in the next Table:

Uses of Streptokinase

Acute Coronary Artery Thrombosis and Myocardial Infarction
Acute Massive Pulmonary Embolism
Acute Deep-Vein Thrombosis
Acute Arterial Thrombosis and Embolism
Occluded Arteriovenous Cannulae

Acute Coronary Artery Thrombosis and Myocardial Infarction: Intracoronary route: Therapy with streptokinase should be started within 4 hours after onset of symptoms; this route has largely been abandoned for the IV route due to the delay in therapy involved, limited availability, expense, and conflicting results - probably as a result of delay in therapy (Marder, V.J. and Sherry, S., "Thrombolytic Therapy: Current Status" NEJM 318, 1585-1595, 1988). Intravenous route: Use of this method avoids the complications associated with intracoronary catheterization.
Acute Massive Pulmonary Embolism: Embolism should first be confirmed by pulmonary angiography. Heparin may be given while the diagnosis is being confirmed but is discontinued prior to infusion of streptokinase; streptokinase may be useful up to 7 days after embolism has occurred.
Acute Deep-Vein Thrombosis: Streptokinase should be used within 72 hours after thrombosis has occurred; two-thirds of thrombi can be dissolved.
Peripheral Artery Thrombosis: Thrombolytic therapy may be effective in the first 72 hrs.
Mechanism of Action: Thrombolytic agents, eg, streptokinase or urokinase, dissolve existing thrombi through a proteolytic action in the supporting fibrin network; the fibrinolytic system is illustrated in the next Figure:

Fibrinolytic System

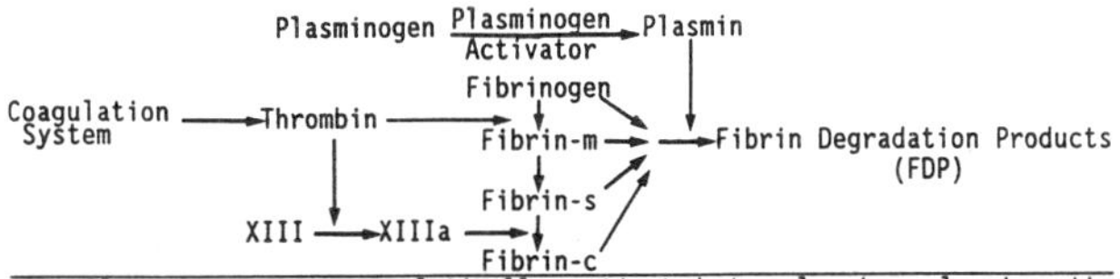

Plasminogen is proteolytically activated to plasmin; plasmin attacks fibrinogen and fibrin to produce fibrin degradation products(FDP). Streptokinase acts indirectly initially combining with plasminogen to form a streptokinase-plasminogen complex. This complex then activates plasminogen to form plasmin. Plasmin is a protease which digests fibrin and fibrinogen to produce fibrin degradation products(FDP). FDP inhibit thrombin's conversion of fibrinogen to fibrin and thereby become circulating anticoagulants themselves. Plasmin also hydrolyzes prothrombin, factors V, VIII, and XII, the first component of complement and prekallikrein.

Both streptokinase and t-PA are equally effective in reperfusing occluded coronary arteries in patients with acute myocardial infarction; however, streptokinase cost much less than t-PA - see **TISSUE PLASMINOGEN ACTIVATOR** section for discussion and references.
DOSAGE FORMS: Injection: 250,000; 600,000; 750,000 and 1,500,000 IU.
DOSAGE: Streptokinase is administered IV, intracoronary and intra-arterial; dosage is given in the next Table:

Dosage of Streptokinase

Condition	Route	Dosage
Acute Myocardial Infarction	IV	1.5 million IU over 1 hour. Other dosage regimens have been used.
	Intra-coronary	Prior to angiography, 5,000 to 10,000 units of heparin is administered intra-arterially. The obstructed vessel is identified by angiography. Then, 15,000-20,000 IU of streptokinase is administered over 15-120 sec,

STREPTOKINASE (Cont.)

Dosage of Streptokinase		
Condition	Route	Dosage
		usually by ostial infusion through the angiographic catheter; some angiographic equipment permits a catheter to be passed down the coronary artery to the site of the clot. Then 2,000-4,000 units/min are infused with interruption of infusion every 15 min to monitor the progress of clot lysis. Infusion is continued until reperfusion occurs usually to a total dose of 150,000 to 500,000 units and for 30 to 60 min. thereafter, total infusion time is usually 60-90 min. Following streptokinase treatment, heparin is administered IV; maintain clotting time 2-3 times normal. Other dosage regimens have been used.
Acute Massive Pulmonary Embolism; Acute Deep-Vein Thrombosis; Arterial Thrombosis or Embolism	IV	Initially, a loading dose of 250,000 IU is infused over 30 minutes, followed by 100,000 IU/hr. Duration: Pulmonary Embolism: 24hrs.; Arterial Thrombosis or embolism: 24 to 72 hrs.; Deep Vein Thrombosis: 72 hrs. After treatment is discontinued and thrombin time(TT) has decreased to less than twice the normal control value (usually after 2-4 hrs.), heparin is given by continuous infusion in a dose that prolongs the APTT by 20 to 30 seconds.
Occluded Arteriovenous Cannulae	Intra-Arterial	250,000 IU diluted to 2ml into each occluded limb of the cannula over 30 min.; then clamp cannula for two hrs. Cannula contents are aspirated and the cannula is flushed with normal saline and reconnected.

An increase in dosage is sometimes necessary in patients with high titer antistreptokinase antibodies, eg, recent streptococcal infection or recent treatment with streptokinase.

PHARMACOKINETICS: Half-Life: Biphasic; "fast" half-life 11 to 13 minutes due to action of antibodies and a "slow" half-life of 83 minutes in absence of antibodies. Duration: Activity ceases shortly after therapy is discontinued.

ADVERSE EFFECTS: Bleeding is the most common adverse effect. Severe internal bleeding occurs occasionally; rarely cerebral hemorrhage occurs. Anaphylactoid reactions are rare. Streptokinase is antigenic; this means that patients have antibody-mediated resistance to streptokinase because of prior exposure to infection with streptococci. Fever, chills, rash, or urticaria occur in abcut 5% of patients; anaphylactoid reactions develop in only 0.1% of patients receiving streptokinase (Marder, V.J. and Sherry, S., N. Engl. J. Med. 318, 1512, 1988).

CONTRAINDICATIONS: Active internal bleeding, history of cerebrovascular accident, recent intracranial or intraspinal surgery of trauma, intracranial neoplasm, arteriovenous malformation, intracranial aneurysm, known bleeding diathesis, severe uncontrolled hypertension.

MONITOR: The tests that are done to monitor thrombolytic therapy (streptokinase or urokinase) are given in the next Table; (Sharma, G.V.R.K. et al., N. Engl. J. Med. 306, 1268-1276, 1982):

Tests to Monitor Thrombolytic Activity	
Tests	Comment
Euglobulin Lysis Time	Most sensitive test but is not available in most laboratories
Thrombin Time	Next most sensitive test
Partial Thromboplastin Time(PTT)	Less Sensitive
Prothrombin Time(PT)	Less sensitive
Fibrin Degradation Products(FDP)	Less sensitive

The timing of the tests is given in the next Table; (Sharma, G.V.R.K. et al., already cited):

STREPTOKINASE (Cont.)

Timing of Testing and Objective
Before Therapy
Detect and correct coagulation defects (determine thrombin, partial thromboplastin, and prothrombin times)
Determine base line or control for fibrinolysis (any of the above tests; euglobulin lysis time or fibrin(ogen) degradation products if patient has been receiving heparin)
Drug Therapy (3-4 hr after start)
Use same test(s) used for establishing base line or control
After Therapy
Use partial thromboplastin time if heparin therapy is to begin
Objective
Ensure establishment of fibrinolytic state:
Determine whether values have marked prolongation over control value
Administer streptokinase:
If values not changed from control at 3-4 hr, give another loading dose (250,000 units) and continue infusion (standard, 100,000 units per hr).
Recheck in another 3-4 hr. If still no change, discontinue streptokinase and switch to urokinase, or begin heparin therapy.

STREPTOMYCIN

USES: Streptomycin is an **aminoglycoside** antibiotic; it is not used today for those bacterial infections that are most commonly treated with aminoglycosides because of the widespread emergence of resistant strains to this drug. It is used for the treatment of the conditions listed in the next Table:

Uses of Streptomycin
Tularemia
Plague
Severe Brucellosis (In Combination with a Tetracycline or Chloramphenicol)
Glanders (In Combination with a Tetracycline or Chloramphenicol)
Alternative Drug in Rat Bite Fever (Preferred Therapy, Penicillin G)
Endocarditis caused by Viridans Streptococci (with Penicillin G)
Tuberculosis (Organisms Resistant to Isoniazid, Rifampin or Ethambutol

Streptomycin is the preferred drug for the treatment of tularemia and plague; it is the preferred drug, in combination with a tetracycline or chloramphenicol, for the treatment of severe brucellosis and glanders.

Streptomycin is used with penicillin G or ampicillin for treatment of endocarditis caused by susceptible strains of enterococci.

Mechanism of Action: The mechanism of action of Streptomycin is like other aminoglycosides in that it binds to the bacterial 30S ribosomal subunit to produce a non-functional 70S initiation complex that results in the inhibition of bacterial cell protein synthesis and misreading of the genetic code.

DOSAGE FORMS: One gram and 5 gram solutions.

DOSAGE: Streptomycin is administered only by deep IM injection into a large muscle mass; injection sites should be alternated. Dosage should be based on ideal body weight. Dosage of streptomycin is given in the next Table:

Dosage of Streptomycin

Condition	Age	Dosage
Usual	Adults	15mg/kg daily in divided doses every 6-12 hours for 7-10 days. Max: 2g daily.
	Children	20-30mg/kg daily in divided doses every 6-12 hrs
	Premature and Newborns	10-20mg/kg daily in divided doses every 6-12 hours.
Tularemia	Adults	1-2g daily in divided doses every 12 hours for 7-10 days or until patient is afebrile 5-7days
Plague	Adults	2-4 g daily in divided doses until the patient is afebrile for at least 3 days.
Tuberculosis (See note below)	Adults	1g or 15mg/kg daily.
	Children	20-50mg/kg daily.
	Adults	Intermittent Therapy: 25mg/kg 2-3 times weekly.
Endocarditis; Pen. Susc. Streptococcae (Viridans Gr.)	Adults	Give with a penicillin; 1g twice daily for 7 d followed by 500mg twice daily for 7 d.
	Adults (>60yrs)	500mg twice daily
Endocarditis, Enterococcae	Adults	1g twice daily for 2 weeks followed by 500mg twice daily for 4 weeks.

Note on Treatment of Tuberculosis: When streptomycin is used daily in an anti-tuberculosis regimen, the drug is discontinued after the first few months or when bacteriologic smears or cultures become negative; the other drugs are continued for the full length of therapy.

Dose must be decreased in patients with impaired renal function. Estimate creatinine clearance based on formula in **AMINOGLYCOSIDES** section. Load with 1g, subsequent doses of 7.5mg/kg every 24h (CrCl 50-80ml/min), every 24-72h (CrCl 10-50ml/min), every 72-96h (CrCl < 10ml/min).

PHARMACOKINETICS: Peak: 2 hours; Half-Life: 5 hours; Protein-Binding: 30% Excretion: Kidney.

ADVERSE EFFECTS: Toxicity and untoward effects are listed in the next Table:

Toxicity of Streptomycin

Major:	Renal Toxicity
	Vestibular Toxicity (Equilibrium)
	Auditory Toxicity (Cochlear)
	Neuromuscular Blockage
Minor:	Skin Rash, Drug-Induced Fever

Hematopoietic reactions, eg, neutropenia, and, rarely, agranulocytosis, aplastic anemia, or thrombocytopenic purpura, have ocurred.

MONITOR: Renal function (BUN, creatinine) and peak (5-25mcg/ml) and trough (<5mcg/ml) every few days.

SUCCINYLCHOLINE

(Anectine, Quelicin, Sucostrin)

USES: **Succinylcholine** is a **depolarizing neuromuscular blocking agent** used principally to produce **skeletal muscle relaxation** during procedures of short duration; uses are given in the next Table:

Uses of Succinylcholine
Endotracheal Intubation
Endoscopic Examination
Electric or Pharmacologically Induced Convulsive Therapy
Skeletal Muscle Relaxation During Orthopedic Manipulations

Succinylcholine has a rapid onset and a short duration of action. Following IV administration, complete muscle relaxation occurs within 1 minute, persists for about 2-3 minutes, and gradually dissipates within 10 minutes.

Following IM administration, the onset of action occurs in 2-3 minutes; the duration of action ranges from 10-30 minutes.

Succinylcholine is metabolized rapidly, mainly by plasma pseudocholinesterase, to succinylmonocholine and choline.

DOSAGE FORMS: Injection: 20, 50, 100mg/ml; IV Infusion: 500mg, 1g.

DOSAGE: Succinylcholine is usually administered IV; the drug may be administered by deep IM injection, preferably high into the deltoid muscle in patients in whom a suitable vein is not accessible. Dosage is given in the next Table:

Dosage of Succinylcholine

Condition	Age	Dosage
After Anesthesia has been Induced, to assess ability to metabolize succinylcholine		Test Dose: 0.1mg/kg (up to 10mg) Normal: Little or no respiratory depression within five minutes. Abnormal: Respiratory paralysis sufficient to permit endotracheal intubation; recovery generally occurs in 30-60 min.
Short Surgical Procedures	Adult	Give test dose IV. Usual dose: 0.6mg/kg (0.3-1.1mg/kg) given IV over 10-30 seconds. If test dose produces moderate muscle relaxation, 20mg is usually adequate. If test dose produces minimum relaxation, 30mg will be needed.
Electroconvulsive Therapy		Give succinylcholine; administer shock about about 1 minute later.
Pediatric	Children	1-2mg/kg
Prolonged Procedures	Adult	0.5-10mg/minute by continuous IV infusion; or 0.3-1.1mg/kg by intermittent IV injection followed by 0.04-0.07mg/kg as necessary to maintain adequate relaxation.
	Neonates and Children	Continuous IV infusions are considered unsafe in neonates and children because of the risk of malignant hyperthermia
IM Dose	Adult Children	2.5-4mg/kg. Do not exceed 150mg

CONTRAINDICATIONS: Any condition in which hyperkalemia may be exaggerated (preexisting hyperkalemia, paraplegia, extensive burns, extensive trauma). Any condition in which increasing intracranial or intraocular pressure is contraindicated (head trauma, ocular surgery, glaucoma, open globe injury). History of malignant hyperthermia.

ADVERSE EFFECTS: Bradycardia, hypotension, arrhythmia. Prolonged respiratory depresssion may occur in patients with liver disease, malnutrition, pseudocholinesterase deficiency and hyperkalemia. Malignant hyperthermia in susceptible individuals.

SUCRALFATE
(Carafate)

USES: Uses are given in the next Table:

Duodenal Ulcer
Gastric Ulcer

Sucralfate is an inhibitor of pepsin and is an antiulcer agent. The therapeutic effects of sucralfate result from local, ie, at the ulcer site, rather than systemic activity.

Sucralfate is as effective as cimetidine or antacids in healing duodenal and gastric ulcers.

Mechanism of Action: Sucralfate is a complex of sulfated sucrose and aluminum hydroxide which is not absorbed from the GI tract. It forms a complex with albumin and fibrinogen that adheres to the ulcer to form a barrier against acid, pepsin and bile acid penetration.

DOSAGE FORMS: Tabs: 1g

DOSAGE: Sucralfate is administered orally. The drug is taken on an empty stomach, 1 hour before each meal and at bedtime. Antacids may be used as needed for relief of pain but should not be taken within 30 minutes before of after sucralfate. Dosage is given in the next Table:

Dosage of Sucralfate

Condition	Age	Dosage
Duodenal Ulcer	Adult	1g, 4 times daily for 4-8 weeks unless healing is verified by radiographic or endoscopic exam
Gastric Ulcer	Adult	1g, 4 times daily

Although sucralfate is not approved for children <12 years old, some clinicians use a dose of approximately 250mg 4 times daily for each 10kg of weight up to 1 gram 4 times daily for patients weighing 40kg or more.

ADVERSE EFFECTS: The incidence of adverse reactions is 5%; the most common side effect is constipation. G.I. distress occurs rarely.

DRUG INTERACTIONS: Sucralfate may interfere with the absorption of tetracycline, warfarin, phenytoin, cimetidine, digoxin, and fluoroquinolones. Sucralfate and these drugs should be given two hours apart.

SULFACETAMIDE SODIUM
(Sulamyd, Sulfair, AK-Sulf, others)

USES: Sulfacetamide is used as a topical ophthalmic antibiotic; uses are given in the next Table:

Uses of Sulfacetamide, A Topical Ophthalmic Antibiotic
Conjunctivitis
Corneal Ulcers
Prevent Infections after Removal of Foreign Bodies or Injuries to the Eye

DOSAGE FORMS: Ophthalmic Ointment: 10%; Ophthalmic Sol'n: 10%, 15%, 30%

DOSAGE: Sulfacetamide is applied topically to the eye. Ointment should be applied 4 times daily; solution should be used every 1-3 hours while awake. Usual infections are treated with 10% ointment or 10-15% solution. More serious infections are treated with 30% solution.

ADVERSE EFFECTS: Topical application of sulfonamides may produce sensitization and preclude later systemic use of these drugs. Patients who are sensitized may develop hypersensitivity reactions. 30% solution may cause transient stinging or burning.

SULFADIAZINE

(Microsulfon)

USES: Uses of sulfadiazine are given in the next Table:

Uses of Sulfadiazine
Prophylaxis of Recurrent Rheumatic Fever
Nocardiosis
Asymptomatic Meningococcal Carriers
Malaria
Toxoplasmosis

Sulfadiazine is an intermediate-acting antibacterial sulfonamide.

DOSAGE FORMS: Tabs: 500mg. Many combination preparations.

DOSAGE: Sulfadiazine is administered orally; dosage is given in the next Table:

Dosage of Sulfadiazine

Condition	Age	Dosage
Usual Dose	Adult	2-4g initially, followed by 2-4g daily, administered in 3-6 equally divided doses
	Children >2 months	75mg/kg initially, followed by 150mg/kg daily administered in 4 equally divided doses. Total daily pediatric dosage should not exceed 6g.
Prophylaxis of Recurrent Rheumatic Fever	<30kg	500mg, once daily
	>30kg	1g, once daily
Nocardiosis	Adult	4-8g, daily, for minimum of 6 weeks
Asymptomatic Meningococcal Carriers	Adult	1g, twice daily, for 2 days
	2-12 mos.	500mg, once daily, for 2 days
	1-12 yrs.	500mg, twice daily, for 2 days
Malaria		For Chloroquine-resistant Plasmodium falciparum when sulfadoxine and pyrimethamine cannot be used. Use in conjunction with quinine sulfate and pyrimethamine.
	Adult	500mg, 4 times daily for 5 days
	Children	25-50mg/kg, 4 times daily (up to 2g daily) for 5 days
Toxoplasmosis		Pyrimethamine, in conjunction with trisulfapyrimidines or with sulfadiazine, is treatment of choice for toxoplasmosis.
	Adult	2-8g daily in 4 divided doses for 3-4 wks. in immunocompetent patients and up to 6 months in immunocompromised patients.
	Children	100-200mg/kg daily in 4 divided doses for 3-4 weeks in immunocompetent patients and up to 6 months in immunocompromised patients.
	Infant	100mg/kg daily in 4 divided doses.

ADVERSE EFFECTS: Maintain adequate fluid intake to reduce the risk of crystalluria. Fever, rash, hepatitis, vasculitis, bone marrow suppression. Hemolysis in patients with G-6PD deficiency. Turns alkaline urine orange-yellow. Hypersensitivity reactions may occur.

CONTRAINDICATIONS: Infants <2 months due to potential for displacement of bilirubin from binding sites.

SULFASALAZINE

(Azulfidine, Salicylazosulfapyridine)

USES: Sulfasalazine is a combination of sulfapyridine and 5-aminosalicylic acid. Uses of sulfasalazine are given in the next Table (Klotz, V. et al., N. Engl. J. Med 303, 1499-1502, 1980):

Uses of Sulfasalazine
Ulcerative Colitis
Crohn's Disease

Sulfasalazine is the most commonly used drug for ulcerative colitis; it is effective both to induce remission of mildly to moderately active disease (Dissanayake, A.S. and Truelove, S.C., Gut 14, 923-926, 1973), and for long-term maintenance therapy (Azad Khan, A.K. et al., Gut 21, 232-240, 1980).

Addition of steroids to sulfasalazine results in faster improvement in symptoms in all patients, but at 4 months, disease activity is significantly better only in patients with severe disease (Rijk, M.C.M. et al., Ann. Intern. Med. 114, 445-450, 1991).

SULFASALAZINE (Cont.)
Metabolism: Oral sulfasalazine undergoes minimal metabolism or absorption in the upper gastrointestinal tract; colonic bacteria degrade the diazo bond to release free 5-aminosalicylic Acid (5-ASA) and sulfapyridine(Klotz, U. et al., N. Engl. J. Med 303, 1499-1502, 1980). Some sulfapyridine is absorbed and appears responsible for most adverse reactions (Taffet, S.L. and Das, K.M. Dig. Dis. Sci., 28, 833-842, 1983), whereas 5-ASA is the therapeutically active component (Biddle. W.L. et al., Gastroenterology 94, 1075-1079, 1988).
DOSAGE FORMS: Tabs: 500mg, Tabs, Enteric Coated: 500mg; Sol'n: 250mg/5ml
DOSAGE: The drug is given orally; the interval between doses should not exceed 8 hours; the drug should be administered after food. Dosage of sulfasalazine is given in the next Table:

Dosage of Sulfasalazine

Condition	Age	Dosage
Ulcerative Colitis	Adult	Initial: 3-6g daily in equally divided doses
		Maintenance: 2g daily in 4 divided doses
	Children	Initial: 40-60mg/kg daily in 3-6 divided doses
	(>2 yrs)	Maintenance: 30mg/kg daily in 4 divided doses

ADVERSE EFFECTS: The sulfapyridine component of sulfasalazine is primarily responsible for the drug's adverse effects. GI: Nausea, vomiting, diarrhea, anorexia. Orange-yellow color to alkaline urine and skin. Hypersensitivity reactions. Hematologic: anemia, thrombocytopenia and leukopenia.

SULFISOXAZOLE
(Gantrisin)
USES: Sulfisoxanzole is a short-acting sulfonamide; uses are that of sulfonamides.
DOSAGE FORMS: Tabs: 500mg; Susp or Solution: 500mg/5ml; Syrup: 500mg/5ml; Ophth. Sol'n: 40mg/ml; Ophth. Ointments: 40mg/gm.
DOSAGE: Sulfisoxazole and sulfisoxazole acetyl are administered orally. Dosage of sulfisoxazole is given in the next Table:

Dosage of Sulfisoxazole

Route	Age	Dosage
Oral	Adult	2-4g initially, followed by 4-8g daily in 4-6 equally divided doses.
	>2 months	75mg/kg initially followed by 150mg/kg daily administered in 4-6 equally divided doses. Total daily pediatric dose should not exceed 6g/day.
Intravaginal		One applicatorful of cream or one suppository intravaginally once or twice daily, through one complete menstrual cycle.

The oral dosage of sulfisoxazole in different conditions is given in the next Table:

Oral Dosage of Sulfisoxazole in Different Conditions

Condition	Age	Dosage
Lymphogranuloma Venereum or Chancroid	Adults	500mg-1g, 4 times daily for 3 weeks
Acute Pelvic Inflammatory Disease(PID)	Pre-pubertal	100mg/kg daily in 4 equally divided doses in combination with IV ceftriaxone or cefuroxime for at least 4 days and for at least 2 days after patient shows marked improvement; thereafter, oral sulfisoxazole is given to complete at least 14 days of therapy.
Otitis Media Prophylaxis	Children	50-75mg/kg daily in 2 divided doses.
Rheumatic Fever Prophylaxis	Children	<30kg: 500mg daily as a single dose.
		>30kg: 1 gram daily as a single dose.

ADVERSE EFFECTS: Contraindicated in infants <2 mos., near-term pregnant or nursing mothers. Use cautiously in presence of renal or liver disease, or G6PD deficiency. Maintain adequate fluid intake.

SULINDAC
(Clinoril)

USES: Sulindac is a nonsteroidal anti-inflammatory drug (NSAID) which like other NSAIDs, exhibits analgesic, antipyretic, anti-inflammatory activity, and inhibits platelet aggregation; uses are given in the next Table:

Uses of Sulindac

Anti-Inflammatory: Rheumatoid Arthritis, Osteoarthritis, Ankylosing Spondylitis, Psoriatic Arthritis, Reiter's Syndrome, Acute Gouty Arthritis and Acute Painful Shoulder (Bursitis or Tendinitis)

Sulindac, like other non-steroidal anti-inflammatory drugs (NSAIDs), is used for the treatment of arthritic conditions; it may be useful as an alternative drug in these conditions.

Sulindac, is as effective as aspirin in rheumatoid arthritis and osteoarthritis; it may be comparable to phenylbutazone in alkylosing spondylitis.

Mechanism of Action: The mechanism of action of sulindac is similar to that of aspirin in that it inhibits the activity of cyclo-oxygenase in the pathway for the synthesis of prostaglandins. See ASPIRIN.

DOSAGE FORMS: Tabs: 150mg and 200mg.

DOSAGE: Dosage for children has not been established. Sulindac should be taken with food to reduce G.I. effects. Dosage is given in the next Table:

Dosage of Sulindac

Condition	Dosage
Rheumatoid Arthritis, Osteoarthritis, Ankylosing Spondylitis	Initial: 150mg twice daily. max. 400mg daily. Symptomatic improvement may occur in 1 week or longer. Maintenance: Patients with rheumatoid arthritis usually require 200mg twice daily.
Acute Painful Shoulder (Bursitis and/or Tendinitis) or **Acute Gouty Arthritis**	200mg twice daily. In acute painful shoulder, 7-14 days of therapy is usually adequate. In acute gouty arthritis, 7 days is usually adequate.

ADVERSE EFFECTS: Adverse effects of sulindac are like that of aspirin and other non-steroidal anti-inflammatory drugs (NSAIDs). see ASPIRIN, INDOMETHACIN, IBUPROFEN; adverse reactions of sulindac are given in the next Table:

Adverse Effects of Sulindac

System	Effects
Gastrointestinal	Nausea, dyspepsia, abdominal pain, constipation and diarrhea; sulindac causes less G.I. bleeding than aspirin but peptic ulceration may occur.
Central Nervous System	Headache, drowsiness and dizziness.
Platelets	Inhibits platelet aggregation and prolongs bleeding time.
Liver	Hepatitis
Kidney	Acute renal failure has been reported;use cautiously in patients with renal impairment.
Other	Hypersensitivity, toxic epidermal necrolysis, Stevens-Johnson syndrome, pancreatitis.

The most common reactions are abdominal pain, dyspepsia, nausea, constipation, and diarrhea. The incidence of gastrointesinal disturbances generally is lower than with aspirin. Peptic ulcer and G.I. bleeding may occur.

Central nervous system effects include dizziness, drowsiness, and headache and tinnitus.

Other common adverse reactions are rash, pruritis and edema.

Platelet aggregation and prolonged bleeding time may occur. Therefore, sulindac should be used cautiously in patients with bleeding disorders.

Other serious adverse effects include acute renal failure, hepatotoxicity, toxic epidermal necrolysis, Stevens-Johnson syndrome, pancreatitis and hypersensitivity reactions.

CONTRAINDICATIONS: Pregnant and nursing women.

PHARMACOKINETICS: Absorption: Rapid and almost complete; Metabolism: The parent drug is inactive but is reduced reversibly to the active metabolite, the sulfide, and oxidized irreversibly to the inactive metabolite, the sulfone; Half-Life: 16 hours; Protein Bound: 98%. Excretion: Urine.

DRUG INTERACTIONS: Drug interactions of sulindac are given in the next Table:

Drug Interactions of Sulindac

Drug	Effect
Warfarin	Enhances hypoprothrombinemic effect.
Oral Hypoglycemics	No clinically significant interaction.

Therapeutic effects of these drugs as well as other drugs that are highly protein bound should be monitored during concomittant administration of sulindac.

SURGICAL PROPHYLAXIS

Surgical antimicrobial prophylaxis is intended to prevent or reduce the incidence of wound infection and sepsis. Likely pathogens and recommended adult doses for antimicrobial prophylaxis for some of the more commonly performed surgical procedures are listed in the following Table (The Medical Letter, Handbook of Antimicrobial Therapy, 76-83, 1990):

Antimicrobial Prophylaxis for Surgical Patients

Surgery	Likely Pathogens	Drug and Dosage
General Surgery		
Appendectomy	Enteric G - bacilli Anaerobes	Cefoxitin 1 gram IV.
Cholecystectomy	Enteric G - bacilli Enterococci Clostridia	Cefazolin 1 gram IV in high risk patients only(>70 years, acute cholecystitis, obstructive jaundice or common duct stones)
Colorectal	Enteric G - bacilli Anaerobes	Cefoxitin 1 gram IV plus Neomycin 1 gram and erythromycin base 1 gram orally at 1 P.M., 2 P.M., 11 P.M. on day preceeding surgery.
Gastroduodenal	Enteric G - bacilli G + cocci	Cefazolin 1 gram IV for percutaneous endoscopic endoscopy & gastric bypass for obesity. Prophylaxis indicated in other surgeries in high risk patients (obstruction, hemorrhage, gastric ulcer, malignancy).
Ruptured Viscus	Enteric G - bacilli Anaerobes Enterococci	Cefoxitin 1 gram IV every 6 hours with or without gentamicin 1.5mg/kg IV every 8 hrs. or Clindamycin 600mg IV every 6 hours plus gentamicin.
Traumatic Wound	S. Aureus, Group A Strep., Clostridia	Cefazolin 1 gram IV every 8 hours.
Gynecologic Surgery		
Cesarean Section	Enteric G - bacilli Anaerobes Group B Strep., Enterococci	Cefazolin 1 gram IV, high risk patients only (active labor, premature rupture of membranes)
Abortion First Trimester	Same as above	Patients with previous pelvic inflammatory disease: Penicillin G 1 million units IV or doxycycline 300mg orally.
Abortion Second Trimester	Same as above	Cefazolin 1 gram IV.
Hysterectomy Vaginal or Abdominal	Same as above	Cefazolin 1 gram IV.
Head and Neck Surgery-Entering Oral Cavity	S. aureus Streptococci Anaerobes	Cefazolin 2 grams IV.
Cardiac Surgery		
Open Heart Surgery, Coronary Artery Bypass	S. Epidermidis, S. Aureus, Corynebact., Enteric G. - bacilli	Cefazolin 1 gram IV or Vancomycin 1 gram IV.
Vascular Surgery		
Abdominal Aorta	S. Aureus, S. Epidermidis, Enteric G-bacilli	Cefazolin 1 gram IV or Vancomycin 1 gram IV.
Lower Extremity Amputation for Ischemia	S. Aureus, S. Epidermidis, Enteric G - bacilli, Clostridia	Cefazolin 1 gram IV.
Orthopedic Surgery		
Total Joint Replacement or Internal Fixation of Fractures	S. Aureus S. Epidermidis	Cefazolin 1 gram IV or Vancomycin 1 gram IV.
Neurosurgery		
Craniotomy		Controversial; possibly antistaphylococcal antibiotics
Spinal Surgery		Not indicated
Thoracic, Non-Cardiac		Controversial

SURGICAL PROPHYLAXIS (Cont.)

Parenteral prophylactic antibiotics should generally be given just prior to surgery. Cefoxitin is used for certain surgeries to provide better gram negative and anaerobic coverage, whereas cefazolin has better gram positive coverage. Many alternative regimens are used and are probably effective for surgical prophylaxis. As a general rule, antibiotic prophylaxis should be initiated shortly before or at the start of surgery. Duration of prophylaxis is controversial; antibiotics are often used only in the perioperative period or for 24 hours. In operations in which a foreign body is inserted, antibiotics are often continued for 48 hours or longer.

SYMPATHOMIMETICS

The sympathomimetics are used to treat shock; shock is characterized by inadequate tissue perfusion. Sympathomimetics are used only when volume replacement and treatment of etiologic factors fail to maintain the circulation. The purpose of employing these drugs is to improve tissue perfusion. The effects of the sympathomimetics on alpha, beta-1 (heart) and beta-2 receptors, dosage, and "problems" are given in the next Table:

Effects of Sympathomimetics on Alpha, Beta-1 (Heart) and Beta-2 Receptors

Drug (Use)	Alpha: Constrict. of Pulmonary & Renal Arterioles	Beta-1: Heart - Inc. Rate	Beta-1: Heart - Inc. Contractility	Beta-1: Inc. A-V Conduction	Beta-1: Inc. Automaticity	Beta-2: Bronchial Ms. Relaxation	Beta-2: Arteriolar (Renal & ? Pulmonary) Dilatation	Dopamine: Increase in Renal Blood Flow	Problems
Epinephrine (Shock - 2nd Drug) 0.1-1.0mcg/kg/min	3+*	3+	3+	3+	3+	3+	3+*	0	Renal Vasoconstriction
Norepinephrine (Refractory Hypotension;"Warm Shock") 0.1-1.0mcg/kg/min	4+	3+	3+	3+	3+	0	0	0	Reflex Dec. H.R.; Renal Vasoconstrict.
Isoproterenol (Refractory Bradycardia; Status Asthmaticus) 0.1-1.0mcg/kg/min	0	4+	4+	4+	4+	4+	4+	0	Tachycardia, Arrhythmias
Dopamine (Shock - 1st Drug) 1-20mcg/kg/min	1+** 2+	2+	2+	2+	2+	0	0	4+	
Dobutamine (Myocarditis; Post-Cardiac Surgery) 1-20mcg/kg/min	0	1+	2+	1+	1+	0	0	0	

*Vasoconstriction, high dose; vasodilation, low dose.
**Children have very little alpha effect.

The effects of the sympathomimetics on body function are given in the next Table:

Effects of Sympathomimetics on Body Function

Drug	Heart	Vascular Bed	Lungs	Kidneys
Epinephrine	Inc. cardiac output(C.O.); Arrhythmias.	B.P. effects variable.	Relieves bronchospasm.	Variable effects: Urinary output may increase sec. to improved C.O.
Norepinephrine	C.O. effects variable; Arrhythmias.	Systolic and diastolic B.P. increased.	-	Variable; renal vasoconstriction and decreased urine output is common.
Isoproterenol	Inc. C.O.; Arrhythmias frequent.	B.P. variable	Relieves bronchospasm; May inc. shunt.	Variable
Dopamine	Inc. C.O.; Arrhythmias.	Inc. B.P.	-	Urinary output usually increased
Dobutamine	Inc. C.O.; Arrhythmias rarely.	B.P. variable	-	Urinary output often increased.

SYMPATHOMIMETICS (Cont.)

Physiologic response to sympathomimetic agents is variable and dosage must be individualized. The overall goal is to improve oxygen delivery to tissues and thus improve the shock state. Significant toxicity may occur within the therapeutic range. All of these drugs increase myocardial oxygen requirements which may lead to myocardial ischemia, particularly in patients with coronary artery disease. Arrhythmias may also occur. Alpha adrenergic stimulation may lead to renal vasoconstriction and acute renal failure. Dosage must be titrated to obtain the desired therapeutic effects while minimizing adverse effects.

TAMOXIFEN

(Nolvadex)

USES: Tamoxifen is a **nonsteroidal antiestrogenic drug** which is the drug of choice for the palliative treatment of **advanced breast cancer** in pre- and postmenopausal women with estrogen-receptor(ER)-positive breast cancer.

Overall response rates in postmenopausal women with advanced ER-positive breast cancer were 60% (range, 4 to 40 months, median 8 months).

Mechanism of Action: Tamoxifen forms a stable complex with the estrogen receptor; this complex is transported to the nucleus; this tamoxifen-estrogen receptor complex does not stimulate RNA, which is required for protein synthesis to occur.

DOSAGE FORMS: Tabs: 10mg (protect from heat and light)

DOSAGE: 10mg two or three times daily.

ADVERSE EFFECTS: Life-threatening adverse effects have not been reported. Adverse effects are given in the next Table:

Adverse Effects of Tamoxifen

System	Effect
Gastrointestinal	Nausea, vomiting.
Metabolic	Hot flashes
Hematologic	Transient decrease in platelet count not associated with bleeding; transient decrease in leukocyte count
Other less frequent effects	Vaginal bleeding or discharge, menstrual irregularities, skin rashes, hypercalcemia (osseous lesions), peripheral edema, anorexia, pruritus vulvae, depression, dizziness, lightheadedness, headache.
Liver	Hepatitis; this occurs rarely.

PHARMACOKINETICS: Peak: 4-7 hours; Half-Life: 7-14 hours. Excretion: Mostly in feces. Metabolism: Undergoes enterohepatic circulation.

PRECAUTIONS: Leukopenia, thrombocytopenia, bone metastases.

MONITOR: Complete blood count periodically.

TEMAZEPAM

(Restoril)

USES: Temazepam is a short acting **benzodiazepine** which is used in the treatment of **insomnia**; it has hypnotic and antianxiety activity.

Temazepam does not affect the onset of sleep probably because temazepam is absorbed slowly. It decreases the total number of awakenings, increases total sleep time, and improves the subjective quality of sleep.

Other drugs such as flurazepam and triazolam are generally preferred in patients have trouble falling asleep.

DOSAGE FORMS: Caps: 15, 30mg

DOSAGE: Adults: 15 or 30mg at bedtime; in elderly or debilitated, 15mg.

PHARMACOKINETICS: Oral Bioavailability: 100%; Absorption: Slow; Half-Life: 15 hours; Major Active Metabolites: none.
Volume of Distribution: 1.5 liter/kg

ADVERSE EFFECTS: Morning drowsiness (17%), dizziness (7%), lethargy (5%), confusion (3%), anorexia, diarrhea (1-2%). Adverse effects that occur infrequently include vertigo, dryness of the mouth, paresthesias, tachycardia, panic reaction, nystagmus, paradoxical excitement, hallucinations. Withdrawal may occur with prolonged use.

TERBUTALINE

(Brethaire, Brethine, Bricanyl)

USES: Terbutaline, a selective beta-2 agonist, is used as a **bronchodilator** in the symptomatic treatment of **bronchial asthma** and **reversible bronchospasm** which may occur in association with chronic obstructive pulmonary diseases such as chronic bronchitis, pulmonary emphysema and bronchiectasis.

Terbutaline is a synthetic sympathomimetic drug which is similar to albuterol and metaproterenol in chemical structure and in pharmacologic action.

Mechanism of Action: Terbutaline, like albuterol, isoproterenol, and metaproterenol, is a beta-2 stimulant (beta-2 agonist). It stimulates the beta-2 receptors on smooth muscle of the airway; terbutaline activates the enzyme adenyl cyclase which catalyzes the reaction ATP to cyclic AMP. Increased cellular concentration of cyclic AMP occurs; cyclic AMP acts as a "second messenger". The concentration of calcium in bronchial smooth muscle is affected causing relaxation and bronchodilation.

Beta-2 receptors are found on bronchial, vascular and uterine smooth muscle.

DOSAGE FORMS: Tabs: 2.5, 5mg; Injection: 1mg/ml; Oral Inhalation: 200 micrograms/spray.

DOSAGE: Terbutaline is administered by oral inhalation, orally, and subcutaneously. Dosage by different is given in the next Table:

Dosage of Terbutaline

Route	Age	Dosage
Oral Inhalation	Adults, Children >12 yrs.	400 micrograms (2 inhalations) every 4-6 hours; one minute elapse between inhalations.
Nebulization	Children	0.1mg/kg/dose (max. 2.5mg)
	<2 yrs	0.5mg in 2cc NS
	2-9 yrs	1.0mg in 2cc NS
	>9 yrs	1.5mg in 2cc NS
Oral	Adult Children >12 years	2.5-5mg, 3 times daily, max. 15mg daily.
	Children <12 years	Initial: 0.05mg/kg/dose three times daily; increase dose as needed to 0.15mg/kg/dose; usual maximum, 5mg daily.
Subcutaneous	Adult	0.25mg. Wait 15-30 minutes; if the patient fails to respond, repeat. Max. 0.5mg within 4 hours.
	Children	5-10 micrograms/kg (0.005-0.010mg/kg). Max: 0.5mg/dose.

PHARMACOKINETICS: Absorption: 35% to 50% of an oral dose is absorbed; well absorbed following subcutaneous administration. A comparison of the action of terbutaline by different routes of administration is given in the next Table:

Actions of Terbutaline by Routes of Administration

Route	Onset	Peak	Duration
Subcutaneous	15 min.	30-60 min.	1.5-4 hours
Oral	30 min.	2-3 hours	4-8 hours
Oral Inhalation	5-30 min.	1-2 hours	3-6 hours

Metabolism: Partially metabolized in the liver, mainly to inactive sulfate conjugate. Elimination: Following subcutaneous administration, 60% excreted in urine.

ADVERSE EFFECTS: Adverse effects include fine tremor, nervousness, dizziness, tachycardia, and palpitations; these effects are not usually troublesome when terbutaline is given by inhalation. The increase in heart rate may persist for a relatively long time.

Other adverse effects that may occur include headache, nauea, vomiting, lethargy, drowsiness, sweating, nausea, and muscle cramps.

The incidence and severity of adverse effects with subcutaneous terbutaline are similar to those associated with subcutaneous epinephrine; terbutaline is less beta-2 selective when given by this route.

TERFENADINE
(Seldane)

USES: Terfenadine is a specific, selective, **histamine antagonist** at the **H-1 histamine receptor**. Terfenadine is the antihistamine now most commonly prescribed in the United States; sedation does not occur as often with terfenadine as with other antihistamines. Uses are given in the next Table:

Uses of Terfenadine
Seasonal Allergic Rhinitis, eg, Hay Fever
Perennial (Nonseasonal) Allergic Rhinitis

DOSAGE FORMS: Tabs: 60mg

DOSAGE: Terfenadine is administered orally. Dosage is given in the next Table:

Dosage of Terfenadine

Age	Dosage
Adults and Children >12 years	60mg every 12 hrs (Range: 10-300mg/dose)
Children 7-12 years	30mg every 12 hrs
Children 3-6 years	15mg every 12 hrs

PHARMACOKINETICS: Rapidly absorbed; Peak: 1-2 hrs; Therapeutic Effects: 1-2 hrs.; Metabolism: Liver; Half-Life: Distribution phase, 3.5 hrs.; Terminal phase, 16-23 hrs.; Excretion: Feces and urine.

ADVERSE EFFECTS: Adverse effects are given in the next Table:

Adverse Effects of Terfenadine

System	Effects
Nervous System	Sedation, eg, drowsiness, tiredness, sleepiness, fatigue; headache; dizziness, nervousness, and weakness. Occasionally, mental depression and insomnia have ocurred.
G.I. Effects	Abdominal distress, nausea and vomiting.
Oronasopharyngeal Effects	Dry mouth, nose, throat, lips; cough; sore throat.
Cardiovascular	Rarely causes arrhythmias (ventricular tachycardia, Torsade de pointes, ventricular fibrillation).
Other	Skin eruptions or dryness and itching; rarely hepatitis.

The most frequent adverse effects are related to the CNS: sedation (5-15%), eg, drowsiness, tiredness, sleepiness, fatigue, and headache. Other less frequent CNS adverse effects include dizziness, nervousness and weakness. Rare CNS adverse effects include mental depression, insomnia, paresthesia, tremor, decreased concentrating ability, nightmares, irritability incoordination and vertigo.

Adverse GI effects (5-8%) include abdominal distress, nausea, vomiting, constipation or diarrhea, increased appetite and weight gain.

Oronasopharyngeal effects (<5%) include dry mouth, nose throat and/or lips; cough, sore throat and epistaxis.

Cardiovascular effects occur rarely, but may include life-threatening arrhythmias including ventricular tachycardia, both typical and atypical (torsades de pointes) and ventricular fibrillation. These effects usually occur at very high daily dosages (eg, 900mg daily).

DRUG INTERACTIONS: Terfenadine is metabolized in the liver, presumably by the P-450 metabolic pathway. There is a single case report of torsades de pointes in a patient receiving terfenadine 60mg twice daily as well as ketoconazole, an inhibitor of P-450 (Monahan, B.P. et al., JAMA 264, 2788-2790, 1990). Other P-450 inhibitors (eg, erythromycin, cimetidine, etc) may predispose to terfenadine toxicity.

TETRACYCLINE

(Achromycin, Sumycin, Tetralan, Others)

USES: Tetracycline(s) in different conditions, either as drug of choice or as an alternative drug, is given in the next Table.

Tetracycline, in Different Conditions, as Drug of Choice or (Alternative)

Condition	Drug of Choice or (Alternative)
Brucellosis	Yes, combine with streptomycin
Cholera	Yes
Relapsing Fever	Yes
Melioidosis	Yes; combine with chloramphenicol in seriously ill pts.
Glanders (Pseudomonas mallei)	Yes; combine with streptomycin
Leptospirosis	(Yes)
Lyme Disease (Borrelia burgdorferi)	Early stages
Mycoplasma Pneumoniae	Yes; but erythromycin preferred by some
Rickettsial Infections: Rocky Mountain Spotted Fever, Typhus Fever, Q Fever, Rickettsialpox	Yes; but chloramphenicol preferred by some
Chlamydial Infections	Yes
Granuloma Inguinal	Yes
Urethritis due to Ureaplasma	Yes, but erythromycin preferred by some
Chancroid	(Yes)
Neisseria Gonorrhoeae	(Yes)
Syphilis	(Yes)
Acne	Yes
Other Conditions: Actinomycosis, Tularemia, Anthrax, Yaws, Plague, Pasteurella multocida, Yersinia Enterolitica gastroenteritis, Campylobacter jejuni, E. coli, Clostridium perfringens tetani, Moraxella (Branhamella) catarrhalis, Klebsiella pneumoniae, proteus, Aeromonas, Eikenella corrondens, Rat bite fever.	(Yes)

Tetracycline should not be used in children less than 8 years of age unless other appropriate drugs are ineffective or are contraindicated.

Tetracycline has also been used for intrapleural instillation in patients with chronic or recurrent pleural effusions (Oszko, M.A., Drug. Intell. Clin. Pharm. 22, 15-20, 1988) and to prevent recurrent pneumothorax (Light, R.W. et al., JAMA 264, 2224-2230, 1990). Tetracycline is irritating to the pleural surfaces and leads to the formation of adhesions between the visceral and parietal pleural surfaces.

Mechanism of Action: Tetracycline is bacteriostatic. Tetracycline interferes with protein synthesis by binding to the bacterial 30S ribosomal subunit preventing the attachment of aminoacyl transfer RNA to the acceptor site on the messenger RNA-ribosome complex.

DOSAGE FORMS: Tabs: 250, 500mg; Caps: 100, 250, 500mg; Suspension: 125mg/5ml; Parenteral (IM): 250 (with procaine HCl 40mg); Parenteral (IV): 500mg; Ophth. Oint: 1%; Ophth. Susp: 1%

DOSAGE: Tetracycline is administered orally. When oral therapy is not feasible, tetracycline hydrochloride may be administered by IM injection or, preferably, by slow IV injection or infusion.

TETRACYCLINE (Cont.)

Food and/or milk reduce GI absorption of tetracycline and tetracycline hydrochloride; therefore, oral preparations of the drugs should be given 1 hour before or 2 hours after meals and/or milk. Administer with adequate amounts of fluid. Do not give at bedtime or to patients with esophageal obstruction or compression. Dosage is given in the next Table:

Dosage of Tetracycline Hydrochloride

Condition	Route	Dosage
Severe Systemic Illness	IV	Adult: 250-500mg/dose every 6-12 hrs. Children: 20-30mg/kg/day in 2-3 divided doses.
	IM	Adult: 250-300mg/day in 2-3 divided doses. Children: 15-25mg/kg/day in 2-3 divided doses.
Chlamydial Infections, eg, Psittacosis	Oral	2-3g daily, in 4 divided doses, continue for 1-2 weeks after fever has subsided
Chlamydial Infections, Trachomatis, Genital, Inguinal or Anorectal	Oral	500mg, 4 times daily for at least 2 weeks
Trachoma	Oral	1-2g, daily in 2-4 divided doses for 3 weeks or 25-50mg/kg daily in 2-4 divided doses
Rickettsial Infections [Rocky Mountain Spotted Fever; Louse-Borne (Epidemic) Typhus; Q Fever; & Rickettsialpox]	Oral	1-2g daily in 2-4 divided doses for 12-14 days. or 25-50mg/kg daily in 2-4 divided doses. Note: A single dose of doxycycline is usually effective for the treatment of epidemic typhus, Brill-Zinsser disease & scrub typhus.
Mycoplasma Pneumoniae	Oral	1-2g daily in 2-4 divided doses for 1-4 wks. or 25-50mg/kg daily in 2-4 doses for 1-4 wks.
Gonorrhea Infections, Uncomplicated		Tetracycline or doxycycline alone is not considered adequate therapy for gonococcal infections. These drugs are added for treatment of coexisting chlamydial infections.
Gonorrhea plus Coexisting Chlamydial and Mycoplasmal Infections		Penicillins, cephalosporins and spectinomycin are ineffective for treatment of chlamydial and mycoplasmal infections. The CDC currently recommends that most adults with uncomplicated or disseminated gonococcal infections receive oral tetracycline,500mg 4 times daily or doxycycline 100mg twice daily for 7 days as follow-up cephalosporin or spectinomycin.
Epididymo-Orchitis caused by N. Gonorrhoeae and/or C. Trachoma		Adults: 500mg, 4 times daily or doxycycline 100mg twice daily for 10 days as follow-up to single-dose cephalosporin or spectinomycin therapy.
Acute Pelvic Inflammatory Disease(PID) in Adults		Ambulatory Adults: Single dose cephalosporin followed preferably by oral doxycycline in a dosage of 100mg twice daily for 10-14 days or alternatively, oral tetracycline in a dosage of 500mg, 4 times daily for 10-14 days. Hospitalized Patients: Doxycycline plus cefoxitin or cefotetan. See SEXUALLY TRANSMITTED DISEASES.
Brucellosis		1-2g orally, daily in 2-4 divided doses for at least 2-4 weeks. If streptomycin is given in conjunction, 1g of streptomycin should be given IM twice daily during first week and once daily during second week.

TETRACYCLINE (Cont.)

ADVERSE EFFECTS: Tetracycline should not be used in children less than 8 years of age because it may cause tooth staining and decreased bone growth.

Adverse effects are given in the next Table:

Adverse Effects of Tetracycline

System	Effect
Bones and Teeth	Tetracycline chelates calcium in bone and teeth. In the fetus, infancy and children, bone growth may be depressed and tooth development may be inhibited; in addition, permanent discoloration of teeth may occur. Because of these effects, tetracycline should not be used in the last half of pregnancy or in children less than 8 years.
Gastrointestinal	G.I. effects occur more often following oral administration. The most common effects (10% of patients) are anorexia, nausea, vomiting, flatulence and diarrhea. G.I. effects are usually dose related.
Renal	Tetracyclines except doxycycline may exacerbate renal impairment.
Liver	Drug induced hepatitis, especially in pregnancy.
Skin	Photosensitivity reaction; rash.

CONTRAINDICATIONS: Tetracyclines are generally not recommended for pregnant women, infants or children eight years old or younger, or patients with liver damage or biliary obstruction.

DRUG INTERACTIONS: Drug interactions are given in the next Table:

Drug Interactions of Tetracycline

Drug	Effect
Penicillin	Tetracycline interferes with the actions of penicillin. If it is necessary to give both drugs, give penicillin several hours before giving tetracycline.
Coumarin	Action potentiated.
Antacids, Vitamins Minerals, Milk, Milk Products	Tetracycline chelates divalent Ca^{++}, Mg^{++}, Zn^{++}, Fe^{++} and trivalent (Al^{+++}) ions forming an insoluble complex.

PHARMACOKINETICS: Oral Dose Absorption: 75%; Half-Life: 8 hours; the half-life is prolonged in patients with renal insufficiency but not in those with hepatic failure; Protein-Binding: 65%; Distribution: Affinity for rapidly growing or metabolizing tissue, eg, liver, teeth and new bone; tetracycline crosses the placenta and appears in the milk of lactating women; Metabolism: Liver (40%); enterohepatic circulation with 90% fecal excretion; Excretion: 60% excreted in urine and 40% by hepatic metabolism.

THEOPHYLLINE

(Aminophylline, Theo-Dur, Slo-bid, others)

USES: Theophylline, like caffeine and theobromine, is structurally classified as a xanthine derivative; uses are given in the next Table:

Uses of Theophylline

Asthma:
- **Treatment of Acute Asthma**
- **"Prophylactic" Drug for Controlling Symptoms and Signs of Chronic Asthma**
- **Alleviation of Signs and Symptoms During Periods of Remission**

Patients with Chronic Bronchitis who have Bronchospasm

Some Patients with Emphysema

Control of Apnea of Prematurity

The use of theophylline in the acute (and possibly the chronic) management of asthma is controversial. In acute bronchospasm, IV aminophylline may not provide additional bronchodilatation compared to treatment with beta-adrenergic agents alone, and side effects may be increased with combined therapy (Siegel, D. et al., Am. Rev. Respir. Dis. 132, 283-286, 1985).

Theophylline is the most widely prescribed bronchodilator in the United States for maintenance therapy in patients with chronic asthma.

Theophylline stimulates the central nervous system at the medullary level and is used to treat apnea of prematurity.

In addition to its bronchodilator effect, theophylline has positive cardiac, inotropic effect (increase in strength of contraction of the heart), vasodilatory and diuretic actions. It also stimulates diaphragmatic contraction in normal subjects (Aubier, M., et al., N. Engl. J. Med. 305, 249-252, 1981) and in patients with chronic obstructive pulmonary disease, theophylline improves the contractile properties of the diaphragm and prevents the occurrence of diaphragmatic fatigue.

Effects of theophylline on different systems are given in the next Table:

Effects of Theophylline on Different Systems

Respiratory System:

Relaxation of Smooth Muscle with Bronchodilation: Relief of bronchospasm and increased flow rates and vital capacity; dilates pulmonary arterioles, reduces pulmonary hypertension, and reduces alveolar carbon dioxide tension and increases pulmonary blood flow.

Nervous System:

Stimulates all Levels of the CNS but to a lesser extent than does caffeine. In the medulla, lowers the threshold of the respiratory center to carbon dioxide but significant increases in rate & depth of respiration occur only if respiration is depressed. Alleviation of neonatal apnea and apnea of Cheyne-Stokes Respiration may be caused by direct stimulation of the medullary respiratory center.

Cardiovascular System:

Produces inotropic effect (increase in strength of contraction of the heart) and a positive chronotropic effect at the sinoatrial node (increase in heart rate), particularly at higher doses.

Renal Effects: Diuretic effect is usually mild

Mechanism of Action: The mechanism of action is not clear. It has been thought that theophylline inhibits the enzyme phosphodiesterase which metabolizes cyclic AMP. This compound acts as a "second messenger" in the cell, and its action upon smooth muscle is to decrease tension or motility, causing relaxation of smooth muscle and bronchodilation. More recent data suggests that this effect does not account for the bronchodilator properties of theophylline. Other theories relate to the effects on intracellular calcium and prostaglandin antagonism.

THEOPHYLLINE (Cont.)

DOSAGE FORMS: Oral: Numerous oral theophylline preparations are available; preparations are classified as immediate release (q6h dosing) or sustained release (q8, 12 or 24 h dosing). Immediate release preparations are listed in the following Table (Harriet Lane Handbook, 246-247, 1991):

Oral Theophylline Preparations - Immediate Release (Q6h Dosing)

Generic Name	Brand Name	Preparations
Aminophylline	Generic	Tabs: 100, 200mg (79% Theoph)
	Somophyllin	Liq.: 105mg/5ml (86% Theoph)
Oxtriphylline (64% Theoph)	Choledyl	Elixir: 100mg/5ml Syrup: 50mg/5ml Tabs: 100, 200mg
Theophylline	Accurbron	Elixir: 50mg/5ml
	Aerolate	Liq.: 150mg/15ml
	Bronkodyl	Caps: 100, 200mg
	Elixophyllin	Caps: 100, 200mg Elixir: 80mg/15ml
	Slo-Phyllin	Tabs: 100, 200mg
	Slo-Phyllin-80	Syrup: 80mg/15ml
	Somophyllin-T	Caps: 100, 200, 250mg
	Theoclear-80	Syrup: 80mg/15ml
	Theolair	Liq: 80mg/15ml Tabs: 125, 250mg
	Generic	Tabs: 100, 200, 300mg Elixir: 80mg/15ml Sol'n: 80mg/15ml

Sustained release preparations are listed in the following Table:

Oral Theophylline Preparations - Sustained Release

Generic Name	Brand Name	Preparations
Oxtriphylline (64% Theoph)(Q8-12h Dosing)	Choledyl SA	Tabs: 400, 600mg
Theophylline (Q8-12h Dosing)	Elixophyllin SR	Caps: 125, 250mg
	Slo-Bid Gyrocaps	Caps: 50, 75, 100, 125, 200,300mg
	Slo-Phyllin Gyrocaps	Caps: 60, 125, 250mg
	Theobid Duracaps	Caps: 260mg
	Theo-Dur	Tabs: 100, 200, 300, 450mg
	Theo-Dur Sprinkle	Caps: 50, 75, 125, 200mg
	Theolair-SR	Tabs: 200, 250, 300, 500mg
	Theophylline SR	Tabs: 100, 200, 300mg
Theophylline	Theo-24(Q24h Dosing)	Caps: 100, 200, 300mg
	Uniphyl(Q12-24h Dosing)	Tabs: 400mg

Intravenous (aminophylline): 25mg/ml (19.7mg Theophylline = 79%)

DOSAGE: Theophyllines can be given only orally.

Aminophylline is theophylline ethylene diamine; aminophylline and other theophylline salts can be given orally or parenterally. Aminophylline formulations vary in their equivalence to anhydrous theophylline from 79% to 86%.

For faster absorption of theophyllines, take conventional dosage forms with a full glass of water on an empty stomach 30-60 minutes before meals or 2 hours after meals.

To minimize local GI irritation, oral theophyllines may be taken with meals or immediately after meals with a full glass of liquid or with antacids.

Extended-release theophylline preparations are indicated in patients with relatively continuous or frequently recurring asthma symptoms.

Aminophylline may be administered undiluted by slow IV injection or preferably, in large volume parenteral fluids by slow IV infusion.

IM injection of aminophylline causes intense local pain and is not recommended.

Dosage of Aminophylline for Acute Therapy: For acute therapy, an intravenous loading dose of about 6mg/kg aminophylline, if ideal body weight, will usually yield a serum concentration in the range 10 to 15mcg/ml in patients who have previously taken no theophylline. The intravenous loading dose should be infused over a period of at least 30 minutes to minimize the probability of serious arrhythmias.

THEOPHYLLINE (Cont.)

A protocol for aminophylline therapy for acute asthmatic attack is given in the next Figure (Hendeles, L. and Weinberger, M. in Individualizing Drug Therapy, Vol. I, Taylor, W.J. and Finn, A.L., eds., Gross, Townsend and Frank, Inc., N.Y., N.Y., 1981, pgs. 32-65):

Aminophylline Therapy for Asthma

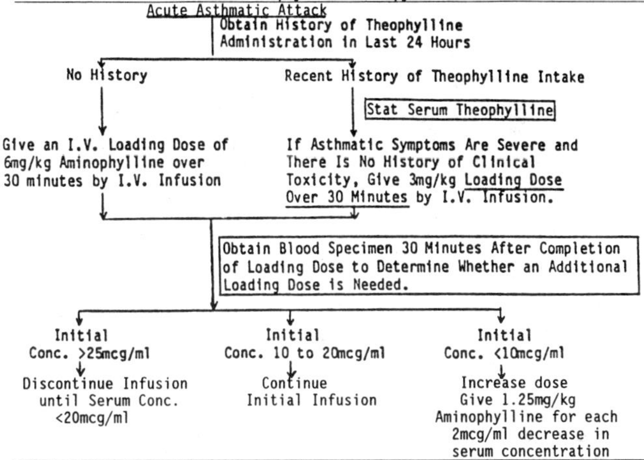

Acute Asthmatic Attack
Obtain History of Theophylline Administration in Last 24 Hours
No History
Recent History of Theophylline Intake
Stat Serum Theophylline
Give an I.V. Loading Dose of 6mg/kg Aminophylline over 30 minutes by I.V. Infusion
If Asthmatic Symptoms Are Severe and There Is No History of Clinical Toxicity, Give 3mg/kg Loading Dose Over 30 Minutes by I.V. Infusion.
Obtain Blood Specimen 30 Minutes After Completion of Loading Dose to Determine Whether an Additional Loading Dose is Needed.
Initial Conc. >25mcg/ml
Initial Conc. 10 to 20mcg/ml
Initial Conc. <10mcg/ml
Discontinue Infusion until Serum Conc. <20mcg/ml
Continue Initial Infusion
Increase dose Give 1.25mg/kg Aminophylline for each 2mcg/ml decrease in serum concentration

Blood Specimen: (Loading Dose in Hospital) A blood sample for aminophylline assay should be drawn prior to loading dose if the patient has a history of theophylline therapy; then obtain a blood specimen 30 minutes after completion of loading dose.

Maintenance Dose: The aminophylline infusion rate necessary to attain a serum level of 10mcg/ml for different conditions is as follows (Powell, R., School of Pharmacy, Univ. N.C.):

Aminophylline Infusion Rate

Adults:

Characteristic	0.5mg/kg/hr x Factor	Aminophylline Infusion Rate
Nonsmoker	0.5mg/kg/hr x 1 =	0.5 (mg/kg/hr)
Smoker (within last 3 mos > 1 pack/day) Plus ages 10-16	0.5mg/kg/hr x 1.6 =	0.8 (mg/kg/hr)
CHF (edema, x-ray)	0.5mg/kg/hr x 0.4 =	0.2 (mg/kg/hr)
Pneumonia, Viral Respiratory Infection	0.5mg/kg/hr x 0.4 =	0.2 (mg/kg/hr)
Cirrhosis	0.5mg/kg/hr x 0.4 =	0.2 (mg/kg/hr)
Severe hepatic obstruction (PEER < 100L/min or PCO_2 > 45mmHg)	0.5mg/kg/hr x 0.8 =	0.4 (mg/kg/hr)

Example. The aminophylline infusion rate in a 60kg male who smokes 2 packs of cigarettes per day and currently has signs and symptoms of CHF: Aminophylline infusion rate = 0.5mg/kg/hr · 60kg · 1.6 · 0.4 = 19.2mg/hr

Premature Infants and Neonates: Aminophylline Infusion Rate = 0.19mg/kg/hr

Infants 4 to 52 Weeks: Aminophylline Infusion Rate=0.37 + (0.012 x Age in Wks)

Children (1 to 9 Years of Age): Aminophylline Infusion Rate = 1.0mg/kg/hr. Interindividual and intraindividual differences or changes in theophylline clearance in children necessitates frequent therapeutic drug monitoring (Kubo, M., et al., J. Pediatr. 108, 1011-1015, 1986).

Blood Specimen (Inpatient Maintenance Dose): Obtain a blood specimen 4 to 8 hours after start of maintenance I.V. infusion and 18 to 30 hours after starting the infusion and at 12 to 24 hour intervals thereafter for possible adjustment of the infusion rate until the infusion is discontinued. As a function of results, the dose may be altered appropriately.

THEOPHYLLINE (Cont.)

Outpatient Maintenance Dose: Maintenance dose to achieve a peak level of 10 to 20mg/L is given in the next Table (Powell, R.):

Maintenance Dose of Theophylline or Aminophylline (mg/kg/day) Ideal Body Wt.

	Theophylline (mg/kg/day)	Aminophylline (mg/kg/day)
Adult - Nonsmoker	10	12
Smoker	15	19
Cirrhotic	4	5
Children (1-8)	12-24	15-30
Children (9-12)	10-20	12.5-25
Children (12-16)	8-18	10-22.5

MONITOR: Blood Specimens (Outpatient Maintenance Dose): Blood specimens should be obtained at about 3 day intervals and at the time of peak concentration or about 2 to 4 hours after a scheduled dose depending on the product formulation.

Concentrations of 5 to 10 mcg/ml may be effective for some patients, particularly children.

ADVERSE EFFECTS: Adverse effects usually are seen when serum levels rise above 20mg/liter. Early signs of toxicity are nausea, vomiting and headache. Toxic reactions are listed in the next Table:

Toxic Reactions of Theophylline

Gastrointestinal: Abdominal Pain, Nausea, Vomiting
Cardiovascular: Tachycardia, Arrhythmias
Blood Pressure: Elevated
Central Nervous System: Agitation, Irritability, Insomnia, Tremor, Seizures, Convulsions, Coma.
Occasionally: Hyperthermia, Diuresis, Ketosis, Hyperglycemia

An acute oral overdose should be treated by induced emesis, followed by oral administration of activated charcoal (repeat every two hours). Obtain blood for assay of electrolytes, glucose, urea, arterial gases and theophylline; repeat every six hours. Correct dehydration and hypokalemia. Treat seizures with intravenous benzodiazepines; monitor with ECG. Correct hypokalemia, acidosis and hypoxia. Consider hemodialysis or hemoperfusion.

PHARMACOKINETICS: Oral Absorption: Rapid and complete; Therapeutic Range: 10 to 20mcg/ml (10 to 20mg/liter). Toxicity: >20mcg/ml (20mg/liter). Half-Life: The serum half-life for different age groups is given in the next Table:

Change of Plasma Half-Life with Age

Age Group	Half-Life (Hours)
Adult (Healthy Non-Smoker)	8.7 (4 to 16)
Adult (Cigarette or Marijuana Smoker)	4.4 (3.0 to 9.5)
Children (1 to 9)	3.7 (2 to 10)
Premature Infants	30
Term Infants (under 3 months)	24
Infants beyond Neonatal Period	Gradually decreases from newborn value to childhood levels by year one.
Children (10-16)	Increases with age beyond nine years to adult values.

Note that cigarette smoking shortens the half-life of theophylline. Conditions that lengthen the half-life of theophylline are given in the next Table:

Conditions that Lengthen Half-Life of Theophylline

Chronic Liver Diseease
Congestive Heart Failure (CHF)
Severe Obstructive Pulmonary Disease

The plasma half-life is prolonged (20-30 hours) by the following conditions: Chronic liver disease, congestive heart failure and severe obstructive pulmonary disease. Metabolism: Liver (90%) to 1,3 dimethyl uric acid; Excretion: 10% excreted unchanged.

DRUG INTERACTIONS: Theophylline decreases lithium levels. Drugs that alter the metabolism of theophylline are given in the next Table:

Drugs and Metabolism of Theophylline

Decreased Clearance (Prolonged Half-Life)	Increased Clearance (Decreased Half-Life)
Cimetidine (Tagamet)	**Phenytoin**
Propranolol (Inderal)	**Barbituates**
Allopurinol (Zyloprim, others)	
Erythromycin	
Calcium Channel Blockers (Verapamil, others)	
Fluoroquinolones	

Serum concentrations of theophylline should be monitored in patients taking these drugs concurrently with theophylline, especially when these drugs are introduced or discontinued (The Medical Letter 26, 1-3, Jan. 6, 1984).

THIOPENTAL SODIUM
(Pentothal)

USES: **Thiopental sodium** is an **ultrashort-acting barbiturate;** uses are given in the next Table:

Uses of Thiopental Sodium
Induction of Anesthesia
Anesthesia for Short Procedures with Minimal Pain
Sedation for Intubation - especially when elevated intracranial pressure is expected
Treatment of Increased Intracranial Pressure

Thiopental produces rapid induction of anesthesia, unconsciousness occurs in 10-20 seconds. Thiopental is a good amnestic and sedative, but does not provide analgesia. Therefore, thiopental must be supplemented with other anesthetic agents except for short procedures with minimal pain. Thiopental, like other barbiturates, reduces cerebral blood flow, cerebral metabolic rate, and intracranial pressure. Thiopental is used to facilitate intubation in patients with suspected elevation of intracranial pressure.

DOSAGE FORMS: Injection: 250, 400, 500mg syringes; 0.5, 1.0gm vials; 1, 2.5, 5gm kits. Usual dilution: 2.5% solution (25mg/ml).

DOSAGE: Thiopental is administered IV; dosage is given in the next Table:

Condition	Age	Dosage
Intubation Anesthesia Induction	Adults	150-250mg or 3-5mg/kg.
	Children	2mg/kg.
Anesthesia Maintenance	Adults	50-100mg as needed.
	Children	1mg/kg as needed.
Intracranial Pressure	Adults Children	1.5-5.0mg/kg/dose as needed.

PHARMACOKINETICS: Onset of Action: 10-20 second; Duration of Effect: 20-30 minutes; more prolonged when large doses are used; Plasma Half-Life: 3 minutes; Elimination Half-Life: 9 hours; Metabolism: Liver; Excretion: Renal. Rapid onset of action is due to initial distribution of thiopental into the brain. Recovery of consciousness is due to redistribution into other tissues. If large doses are given, tissues will be saturated and duration of sedation will be prolonged.

ADVERSE EFFECTS: Profound respiratory depression. Laryngospasm may occur. Cardiovascular: Normal adults may have mild, transient hypotension. Severe hypotension and cardiac arrest may occur in patients with hypovolemia, sepsis, or shock.

CONTRAINDICATIONS: Variagate porphyria or acute intermittent porphyria (AIP). In this disease, barbiturates may lead to demyelinization of peripheral and cranial nerves resulting in pain, weakness and paralysis.

THIORIDAZINE
(Mellaril)

USES: **Thioridazine** is a piperazine derivative of **phenothiazine** with pharmacologic effects similar to those of chlorpromazine; it is used for the symptomatic management of **psychotic disorders.** Uses of thioridazine are given in the next Table:

Uses of Thioridazine in Management of Psychotic Disorders
Psychotic Disorders
Short-Term Treatment of anxiety associated with Major Depression in Adults
Severe Behavioral Problems in Children
Short-Term Treatment of Hyperactive Children

DOSAGE FORMS: Tabs: 10, 15, 25, 50, 100, 150, 200mg; Susp: 5, 20, 30, 100mg/ml.

DOSAGE: Thioridazine is administered orally; dosage is given in the next Table:

Dosage of Thioridazine

Condition	Age	Dosage
Psychotic Disorders	Adult	50-100mg, 3 times daily; dosages up to 800mg daily in 2-4 divided doses may be required in severely psychotic adults. Max. 800mg. Maintain dosage at lowest effective level.
Short-Term Treatment of Adults with Major Depression	Adult	25mg, 3 times daily (range, 20-200mg daily)
Psychotic Disorders	Children (2-12 yrs)	0.5-3mg/kg daily in 2-4 divided doses.
Moderate Behavioral Problems in Child.	Children (2-12 yrs)	Usual dose: 10mg, 2 or 3 times daily

ADVERSE EFFECTS: Drowsiness, extrapyramidal reactions, autonomic symptoms, paradoxical reactions, endocrine disturbances. More serious reactions include cardiac effects (Q-T abnormalities, hypotension, cardiac arrest) and neuroleptic malignant syndrome. Seizure threshold may be lowered. See also CHLORPROMAZINE section.

DRUG INTERACTIONS: Thioridazine may enhance the action of other central nervous system depressants such as antianxiety agents, hypnotics, analgesics or alcohol. Combined with lithium, may cause encephalopathic syndrome rarely. Increased seizure risk with metrizamide. Decreased metabolism of phenytoin.

THIOTHIXENE
(Navane)

USES: Thiothix is indicated in the management of the **psychotic disorders** including those listed in the next Table:

Uses of Thiothixene
Schizophenia
Psychoses
Severe Psychomotor Excitement
Mental Retardation with Behavior Complications (?)

Mechanism of Action: Thiothixene, like other antipsychotic drugs, blocks dopamine receptors.

DOSAGE FORMS: Caps: 1,2,5,10 and 20mg; thiothixene (as HCl) 5mg/ml; Navane injection, thiothixene (as HCl) 2mg/ml.

DOSAGE: Thiothixene is administered orally; thiothixene HCl is administered orally or IM. Dosage of thiothixene is given in the next Table:

Dosage of Thiothixene

Condition	Age	Route	Dosage
Mild to Moderate Psychotic Conditions	Adults	Oral	2mg, 3 times daily. If necessary, gradually increase to 15mg daily.
Severe Psychoses	Adults	Oral	5mg, twice daily. If necessary, gradually increase dosage; usual optimal dose, 20-30mg daily. Max: 60mg daily.
Acute Agitated Patients	Adults	IM	4mg, 2-4 times daily; optimal dosage, 16-20mg daily. As control is obtained, start oral therapy.

PHARMACOKINETICS: Absorption: Well absorbed from GI tract and from parenteral sites; Response: IM, 1-6 hours; orally, few days to weeks. Metabolism: Liver. Excretion: Mainly in bile.

ADVERSE EFFECTS: The most common adverse effects are given in the next Table:

Adverse Effects of Thiothixene
Extrapyramidal Side Effects
Sedation
Autonomic Activity (Alpha Antiadrenergic and Anticholinergic Actions)

Thiothixene is associated with a high incidence of extrapyramidal side effects but has little sedative and autonomic activity (alpha antiadrenergic and anticholinergic actions).

Extrapyramidal side effects include dystonia, akathisia, Parkinsonism, tardive dyskinesia, and neuroleptic malignant syndrome. Three of these reactions, dystonia, akathisia and Parkinsonism, occur within hours to weeks after initiation of therapy. Tardive dyskinesia usually is not observed for months to years after initiation of therapy.

Sedation is common but decreases during lòng-term treatment and tolerance may develop. Seizure threshold is decreased.

Autonomic activities are alpha antiadrenergic and anticholinergic actions. These effects are more common after parenteral administration. The antiadrenergic effect that causes the most difficulty is orthstatic hypotension and acute hypotensive crisis that tends to occur in elderly or debilitated patients after large parenteral doses.

Anticholinergic effects include dryness of the mouth, tachycardia, blurred vision, urinary retention and constipation.

Other adverse effects include cutaneous allergic reactions, photosensitivity and sexual dysfunction.

DRUG INTERACTIONS: Potentiates CNS depression with alcohol and other CNS depressants. Decreased guanethidine effects.

PRECAUTIONS: Cardiovascular disease, epilepsy, elderly pregnancy, lactation.

THROMBOSIS, PREVENTION AND TREATMENT

Thrombosis, Prevention and Treatment
Antiplatelet Drugs
Aspirin
Dipyridamole
Sulfinpyrazone
Anticoagulants:
Heparin
Warfarin
Thrombolytic Therapy
Streptokinase
Urokinase
Tissue Plasminogen Activator (t-PA)
Alteplase (Activase)

Comparison of Efficacy Streptokinase and Tissue Plasminogen Activator (t-PA): In a 12,490 patient comparison of streptokinase with t-PA, each given with or without heparin, there was no difference between the two agents with regard to the end-point (severe left ventricular damage or death). Heparin therapy did not show additional benefit; all patients received atenolol and aspirin (GISSI-2, Lancet 336, 65-71, 1990). For review of streptokinase vs t-PA literature, see Sherry, S. and Marder, V.J., Ann. Intern. Med. 114, 417-423, 1991.

t-PA costs 10 times as much as streptokinase; the price of a 100mg dose to the pharmacist is $2,300. A DRG allotment is around $4,000. Therefore, t-PA can consume more than one-half of the DRG allotment.

t-PA may be more useful than streptokinase in patients who present relatively late after the onset of myocardial infarction (Sheehan, F.H. et al., Circulation 75, 817-829, 1987).

Streptokinase is antigenic; this means that patients have antibody-mediated resistance to streptokinase because of prior exposure to infection with streptococci. Fever, chills, rash, or urtica occur in about 5% of patients; anaphylactoid reactions develop in only 0.1% of patients receiving streptokinase (Marder, V.J. and Sherry, S., N. Engl. J. Med. 318, 1512, 1988). It may be that these patients should receive t-PA if thrombolytic therapy is required for a second time.

See also **ANTICOAGULANTS.**

TICARCILLIN

(Ticar)

USES: Ticarcillin is an alpha-carboxypenicillin that is closely related to carbenicillin; it is not absorbed orally and must be given either IV or IM. The indications for ticarcillin are similar to those for carbenicillin with the **primary use** being suspected or proven infections caused by **P. aeruginosa**; it is 2 to 4 times more active against P. aeruginosa than is carbenicillin; activities of ticarcillin are given in the next Table (Wilkowske, C.J. and Hermans, P.E., Mayo Clin. Proc. 62, 789-798, 1987; Parry, M.F., Med. Clin. No. Am. 71, 1093-1112, Nov. 1987; Adams, H.G., Personal Comm.):

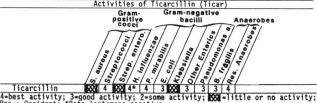

Activities of Ticarcillin (Ticar)

	Gram-positive cocci			Gram-negative bacilli						Anaerobes	
	S. aureus	Streptococci	Strep. entero.	H. influenzae	P. mirabilis	E. coli	Klebsiella	Other Enterics	Pseudomonas a.	B. fragilis	Res. Anaerobes
Ticarcillin	▩	4	▩	4*	4	3	▩	3	3	3	4

4=best activity; 3=good activity; 2=some activity; ▩=little or no activity; Res.= Resident; *Beta-lactamase negative.

TICARCILLIN (Cont.)

Ticarcillin is frequently preferred over carbenicillin in the treatment of serious gram-negative infections because of its greater activity and lower incidence of adverse effects.

Some consultants to the Medical Letter recommend concurrent use of ticarcillin together with an aminoglycoside (gentamicin, tobramycin or amikacin) for treatment of Pseudomonas meningitis and for treatment of Pseudomonas in neutropenic patients (The Medical Letter 30, 33-40, Mar 25, 1988).

The Medical Letter published a list of antimicrobial drugs of choice. Ticarcillin was not a drug of first choice but it was one of several alternative drugs of choice for treatment of bacterial infections as given in the next Table (Medical Letter 30, 33-40, Mar. 25, 1988):

Spectrum of Gram-Negative Antimicrobial Activity of Ticarcillin

Enteric Bacilli: Bacteroides(Gastrointestinal strains); Enterobacter; Escherichia Coli; Proteus Mirabilis; Proteus, Indole-positive(Providencia Rettgeri, Morganella Morganii, Proteus Vulgaris); Providencia Stuartii; Serratia

Other Bacilli: Acinetobacter (Mima, Herellea)

Resistant strains of Pseudomonas aeruginosa are common.

DOSAGE FORMS: Powder: 1, 3 and 6g (equivalent to base)(sodium, 5.2mEq/gram).

DOSAGE: Ticarcillin is administered IM or IV; dosage is given in the next Table:

Dosage of Ticarcillin

Condition	Age	Route	Dosage
Uncomplicated Urinary Tract Infection	Adults	IM or IV	4g daily in divided doses every 6 hours.
	Children <40kg	IM or IV	50 to 100mg/kg daily in divided doses every 6 to 8 hours.
Urinary Tract Infect. with Complications	Adults & Children	IV	150 to 200mg/kg daily in divided doses every 4 to 6 hours.
Severe Systemic Infections (eg, Septicemia, Respiratory Tract, Skin and Soft Tissue, Intra-Abdominal and Female Pelvic and Genital Tract Infections	Adults Children	IV	200 to 300mg/kg daily in divided doses every 4 or 6 hours (Max. 24-30gm daily).
	Infants >2kg & 0-7 days	IV	225mg/kg daily in divided doses every 8 hours.
	Infants >2kg & >7 days	IV	300mg/kg daily in divided doses every 6 hours.
	Infants <2kg & 0-7 days	IV	150mg/kg daily in divided doses every 12 hours.
	Infants <2kg & >7 days	IV	225mg/kg daily in divided doses every 8 hours.

Dosage must be adjusted downward in patients with renal impairment, as given in the following Table:

Dosage of Ticarcillin in Renal Failure

Loading Dose	Creatinine Clearance (ml/min) 60-30	30-10	<10
3gm	2gm IV every 4 hrs	2gm IV every 8 hrs	2gm IV every 12 hrs or 1gm IM every 6 hrs

PHARMACOKINETICS: Peak: IM, one hour; Protein-Binding: 50-60%; Excretion: Renal tubular secretion; probenecid delays excretion; between 75% and 85% of a dose is recovered as unchanged in the urine: Half-Life: 1.2 hours, prolonged in renal impairment.

ADVERSE EFFECTS: The adverse effects of ticarcillin, like those shared by all penicillin, and those associated specifically with ticarcillin, are given in the next Table (Wright, A.J. and Wilkowske, C.J., Mayo Clin. Proc. 62, 806-820, 1987):

Adverse Effects of Ticarcillin

Shared by All Penicillins:

- Allergic reactions (rarely anaphylactic)
- Skin rashes
- Diarrhea
- Neuromuscular irritability, including seizures associated with large doses or renal failure.
- Hematologic changes such as neutropenia and anemia (at times hemolytic)
- Drug-induced fever
- Nephropathy (as component of serum sickness-type reaction) or interstitial nephritis.

Adverse Effects Associated Specifically with Ticarcillin:

- Hypokalemic alkalosis
- Sodium overload
- Platelet dysfunction

TICARCILLIN/CLAVULANATE
(Timentin)

USES: Ticarcillin/clavulanate is a fixed combination of **ticarcillin** with the **beta-lactamase inhibitor**, potassium **clavulanate** which extends the antibacterial spectrum of ticarcillin to include beta-lactamase producing strain of *S. aureus*, *H. influenzae*, *Citrobacter*, *Enterobacter*, *E. coli*, *Klebsiella*, *Pseudomonas*, *Serratia* and *B. fragilis*; activities of ticarcillin/clavulanate (Timentin) are given in the next Table (Allan, J.D., Med. Clin. No. Am. 71, 1079-1091, Nov. 1987; Parry, M.F., Med. Clin. No. Am. 71, 1093-1112, Nov. 1987; Adams, H.G., Personal Comm.):

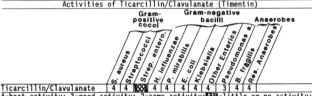

Activities of Ticarcillin/Clavulanate (Timentin)

	Gram-positive cocci			Gram-negative bacilli						Anaerobes	
	S. aureus	Streptococci	Strep. entero.	H. influenzae	P. mirabilis	E. coli	Klebsiella	Other Enterics	Pseudomonas a.	B. fragilis	Res. Anaerobes
Ticarcillin/Clavulanate	4	4	▩	4	4	4	4	4	3	4	4

4=best activity; 3=good activity; 2=some activity; ▩=little or no activity; Res.= Resident

The drug may be particularly useful for the empiric treatment of nosocomial (pertaining to or originating in a hospital or infirmary) urinary or respiratory tract infections or peritonitis.

DOSAGE FORMS: Vials: 3.1gm.(30:1 fixed ratio: 3.0gm. ticarcillin and 0.1gm. clavulanate); 3.2gm(15:1 fixed ratio: 3.0gm ticarcillin & 0.2gm(clavulanate). The 15:1 fixed ratio preparation is not available in the United States.

DOSAGE: Ticarcillin/potassium clavulanate should be administered by intermittent infusion over 30 minutes. See manufacturer's literature for appropriate dilution of the drug, compatible diluents and intravenous solutions. Dosage is given in the next Table:

Dosage of Ticarcillin/Clavulanate

Condition	Age	Dosage
Systemic Infections and Urinary Tract Infections	Adults (>60kg)	3.1gm of the 30:1 fixed-ratio combination (3.0gm ticarcillin and 0.1gm clavulanate) every 4-6 hours.
	Adults and Children	200-300mg/kg of the 30:1 fixed ratio combination(3.0gm. ticarcillon and 0.1gm. (3.0gm ticarcillin and 0.1gm clavulanate) daily given in divided doses every 4-6 hours.

For infants and children under 12, safety and efficacy has not been established.

Dosage in renal failure is given in the next Table:

Dosage of Ticarcillin/Clavulanate in Renal Failure

	Creatinine Clearance (ml/min)		
Loading Dose	60-30	30-10	<10
3.1gm	2gm every 4 hours	2gm every 8 hours	2gm every 12 hours

PHARMACOKINETICS: After intravenous infusion, peak serium concentrations of ticarcillin/clavulanate are attained immediately after completion of the infusion.

Protein-Binding: Ticarcillin, 45%; clavulanic acid, 10%. Excretion: Kidney. Elimination Half-Life: 1.1 hours.

ADVERSE EFFECTS: Patients allergic to any penicillin should be considered allergic to ticarcillin/clavulanate. Adverse reactions are similar to those seen with ticarcillin alone (see TICARCILLIN). These may include hypersensitivity reactions (eg, skin rash), central nervous system disturbances (eg, headache), gastrointestinal disturbances (eg, nausea, diarrhea), hematologic abnormalities (eg, platelet dysfunction with potential for bleeding) and hypokalemia.

TIMOLOL

(Blocadren, Timoptic)

USES: Timolol is a nonselective beta-adrenergic blocking agent. Timolol lowers **intraocular pressure** and is the **drug of choice** in **open-angle glaucoma.** Ophthalmic uses of timolol are given in the next Table:

Ophthalmic Uses of Timolol
Primary Open Angle Glaucoma
Some Secondary Glaucomas
Chronic Glaucoma in Aphakia (Developmental Absence of the Lens)
Prevent of Treat Glaucoma Induced by Alpha Chymotrypsin, Sodium Hyaluronate or Laser Procedures
Emergency Treatment of Acute Angle-Closure Glaucoma when given with Systemic Ocular Hypotensive Drugs and Pilocarpine

Uses of orally administered Timolol are given in the following Table:

Oral Uses of Timolol
Hypertension
Angina Pectoris
Myocardial Infarction

Hypertension: Timolol may be used as initial drug therapy or may be given in a subsequent step in the treatment of hypertension. Treatment of hypertension with Timolol is given in the next Table (The 1988 Report of the Joint National Committee on Detection, Evaluation, and Treatment of High Blood Pressure, Arch. Intern. Med. 148, 1023-1038, 1988):

Treatment of Hypertension with Propranolol

Step 1: Nonpharmacologic Approaches (see **HYPERTENSION**)

↓

Step 2: Timolol (Usual Minimum, 20mg/day; Usual Maximum, 80mg/day)
Observe up to 6 months; if ineffective then,

↓

Step 3: Add a second drug of a different class
or Increase the dosage of Timolol
or Substitute another drug

↓

Step 4: Add a third drug of a different class
or Substitute a second drug

↓

Step 5: Consider further evaluation and/or referral
or Add a third or fourth drug

"Step-Down": For patients with mild hypertension, after 1 year of control, consider decreasing or withdrawing timolol and other hypotensive drugs.

Angina: Timolol, like other beta-1 blocking agents, reduces heart rate, myocardial contractility, and cardiac output; myocardial oxygen demand is reduced and ischemic pain is relieved.

The reduction in heart rate may increase coronary blood flow and oxygen supply by prolonging the diastolic interval during which coronary flow occurs.

Acute Myocardial Infarction: Timolol may reduce estimated myocardial infarct size when given IV in the early stages of acute myocardial infarction and may decrease mortality when used for long term therapy.

Mechanism of Action: Timolol is a beta-blocking agent; it inhibits response to adrenergic stimuli by competitively blocking beta-adrenergic receptors within the myocardium (decreases both heart rate and force of contractions) and within bronchial smooth muscle (constriction of bronchioles) and within vascular smooth muscle (vasoconstriction). Beta-1 receptors are found in the heart and are stimulated by norepinephrine. Timolol, like other beta-1 blockers, produces a fall in blood pressure by decreasing the cardiac output. With continued treatment, the cardiac output returns to normal but the blood pressure remains low because the peripheral resistance is "reset" at a lower level.

TIMOLOL (Cont.)
Ophthalmic Effects: Timolol blocks beta-2 receptors on the ciliary processes and thus reduces aqueous secretion. In addition, timolol may block beta-receptors causing vasoconstriction in the afferent blood vessels supplying the ciliary processes. The vasoconstriction results in reduced ultrafiltration and aqueous formation.
DOSAGE FORMS: Ophthalmic: Timoptic solution 0.25% and 0.5% preservative free or with benzalkonium chloride 0.1%. Oral: 5, 10, 20mg.
DOSAGE: Ophthalmic: Initially 1 drop of 0.25% twice daily; if necessary, adjust dosage based on response to maximum of 1 drop of 0.5% twice daily. Occasionally, once-daily application of the 0.5% solution may be sufficient for maintenance. If there is a change in treatment from some other antiglaucoma drug, the previously used drug should not be discontinued for three weeks or longer and the pressure should be checked to confirm that an abrupt rise has not occurred.
Oral: The oral dosage of Timolol in various conditions is given in the following Table:

Oral Dosage of Timolol

Condition	Dosage
Hypertension	Initial: 10mg twice daily; Increment: increase dosage at weekly intervals to a maximum of 60mg daily.
Myocardial Infarction	Usual: 10mg twice daily.
Angina	15-45mg daily in 3-4 divided doses.

ADVERSE EFFECTS: Ophthalmic Use: Blurred vision is the most common reason for discontinuation of timolol therapy. Other reactions include mild ocular irritation, conjunctival hyperemia, ocular pain, headache, corneal anesthesia, transitory dry-eye syndrome, local hypersensitivity reactions, superficial punctate keratitis, blepharoptosis. Timolol is absorbed into the systemic circulation resulting in blockage of cardiac and non-cardiac beta receptors.
Systemic Effects: Systemic effects may occur with ophthalmic use, but are more common with the oral preparations. Systemic effects are similar to other beta-adrenergic blocking agents (see PROPRANOLOL). Most common side effects are cardiovascular (bradycardia, hypotension, congestive heart failure), respiratory (bronchospasm), GI (nausea, vomiting), and neurologic (lethargy, fatigue, dizziness, headache).

TISSUE PLASMINOGEN ACTIVATOR (t-PA, Alteplase)
(Activase)

USES: Tissue plasminogen activator (t-PA, alteplase) is a thrombolytic drug; uses are given in the next Table (Loscalzo, J. and Braunwald, E., N. Engl. J. Med. 319, 925-931, Oct. 6, 1988; Wilcox, R.G. et al., Lancet ii, 525-530, Sept. 3, 1988):

Uses of Tissue Plasminogen Activator (t-PA, Alteplase)
Acute Coronary Artery Thrombosis and Myocardial Infarction
Acute Pulmonary Embolism
Unstable Angina
Deep Venous Thrombosis
Peripheral Arterial Thromboembolic Disease
Nonhemorrhagic Cerebrovascular Thrombotic Occlusion

Alteplase has been approved by the FDA for use in improving ventricular function and reducing the incidence of congestive heart failure in patients with acute myocardial infarction.

Acute Coronary Artery Thrombosis and Myocardial Infarction: Therapy with t-PA given within five hours of onset of pain in patients with suspected myocardial infarction reduces the one-month mortality by 26% and the 6-month mortality by 21% (ASSET Study Group, Lancet ii, 525-530, 1988; ASSET Study Group, Lancet 335, 1175-1178, May 19, 1990). Other studies using t-PA also show a decrease in mortality following acute myocardial infarction (O'Rourke, M. and Norris, R., J. Am. Coll. Cardiol. 11, 105A, 1988; Guerci, A.D. et al., N. Engl. J. Med. 317, 1613-1618, 1987). t-PA increases artery patency (Topol, E.J. et al., J. Am. Coll. Cardiol. 10, 1205-1213, 1987; Mueller, H. et al., J. Am. Coll. Cardiol. 10, 479-490, 1987).

In other studies, comparing alteplase to placebo, each infused within 4 hours of onset of symptoms, examination of ejection fraction on the 10th day after infarction showed significantly better left ventricular function in the alteplase group; in addition, there was a lower incidence of clinical congestive heart failure in the treated group. (GISSI Study, Lancet ii, 871-874, Oct. 1987).

Comparing t-PA to streptokinase in patients with acute myocardial infarction treated within 6 hours of onset of symptoms, no significant difference in mortality rate, late congestive heart failure, and extensive left ventricular damage could be demonstrated. There was a significantly higher incidence of major bleeds in streptokinase treated patients compared to tPA (1.0% vs. 0.5%) but the incidence of stroke was similar. Streptokinase allergic reactions and hypotensive episodes resulted in no serious clinical consequences (GISSI-2, Lancet 336, 65-71, July 14, 1990; GISSI-2, Lancet 336, 71-75, May 14, 1990). There is no difference in angiographic patency in t-PA treated vs. streptokinase treated patients (Hogg, K.J. et al., Lancet 335, 254-258, Feb. 3, 1990). For review of streptokinase vs t-PA literature, see Sherry, S. and Marder, V.J., Ann. Intern. Med. 114, 417-423, 1991.

Acute Pulmonary Embolism: t-PA can lyse pulmonary emboli; lysis of pulmonary emboli occurred in 95% of patients (Goldhaber, S.Z. et al., Lancet 2, 886-889, 1986) and 82% of patients (Goldhaber, S.Z. et al., Lancet 2, 293-298, Aug. 6, 1988).

Unstable Angina: Coronary thrombi may be responsible for unstable angina (Sherman, C.T. et al., N. Engl. J. Med. 315, 913-919, 1986). Unstable angina was treated successfully in some patients using t-PA; however, prolonged therapy with t-PA may be associated with bleeding (Gold, H.K. et al., Circulation 75, 1192-1199, 1987).

TISSUE PLASMINOGEN ACTIVATOR (Cont.)

Mechanism of Action: The fibrinolytic system is illustrated in the next Figure:

Fibrinolytic System

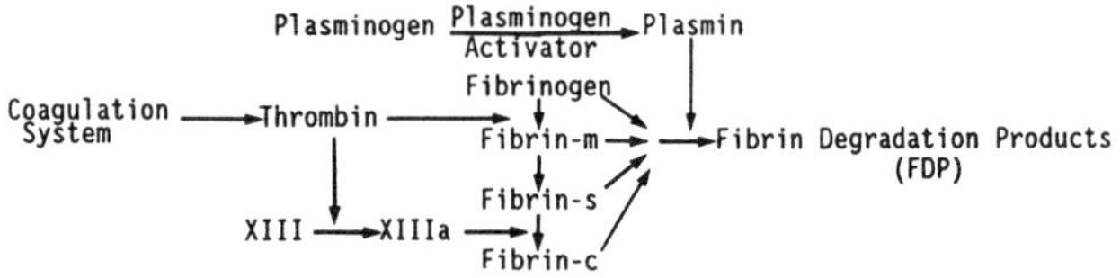

Tissue plasminogen activator (t-PA) is an enzyme that catalyzes the conversion of the inactive proenzyme plasminogen into the active protease plasmin; plasmin attacks fibrinogen and fibrin to produce fibrin degradation products (FDP).

Alteplase is an enzyme with the property of fibrin-enhanced conversion of plasminogen to plasmin. In the absence of fibrin, there is limited conversion of plasminogen. When introduced into the systemic circulation, it binds to fibrin in a thrombus and converts the entrapped plasminogen to plasmin. This initiates local fibrinolysis.

DOSAGE FORMS: Activase is supplied as a sterile, lyophilized powder in 20mg and 50mg vials containing vacuum. Each 20mg Activase vial (11.6 million IU) is packaged with diluent for reconstitution. (20mL sterile water for injection, USP). Each 50mg Activase vial (29.0 million IU) is packaged with diluent for reconstitution. (50 mL sterile water for injection, USP).

DOSAGE: Tissue plasminogen activator (t-PA) is given intravenously as soon as possible after onset of symptoms. Dosage is given in the next Table (Vogel, J.H.K., Emergency Med. Reports 9, 77-84, Nov. 7, 1988):

Dosage of Tissue Plasminogen Activator (t-PA)

Bolus injection: 10mg IV; then,
1st hour: 50mg IV given by continuous infusion over the 1-hour period; then,
Subsequent 2-4 hours: 40mg IV given by continuous infusion at a rate of 10-20mg/hour (total dose: 100mg over 3 hours).

OR

1st hour: 1mg/kg (up to 90mg) given over the first hour, with 10% administered as a bolus injection.
Subsequent 3 hours: 0.5mg/kg (up to a total combined dose of 135mg) given by continuous infusion over the 3-hour period.

The use of a transfer filter or intravenous tubing with an in-line filter decreases the amount of t-PA delivered to the patient. These should not be used when mixing or administering t-PA.

CAUTION: Intramuscular, intravenous and intraarterial punctures should be performed only when required. Pressure should be applied to arterial puncture sites for at least 30 minutes.

TISSUE PLASMINOGEN ACTIVATOR (Cont.)

Contraindications: Contraindications to thrombolytic therapy are given in the next Table (Vogel, J.H., Emerg. Med. Reports 9, 77-84, Nov. 7, 1988):

Contraindications to Thrombolytic Therapy

Absolute
- Active internal hemorrhage (i.e., peptic ulcer)
- History of a cerebrovascular event (<2 months)
- Intracranial or intraspinal surgery (< 2 months)
- Intracranial neoplasm, arteriovenous malformation, or aneurysm
- Known clotting disorder
- Severe, uncontrolled hypertension (systolic BP > 200mm Hg or diastolic BP > 120mm Hg)
- Recent CPR with possible chest trauma (not CPR alone)
- Terminal illness

Relative
- Major surgery within the last 20 days
  - Coronary artery bypass graft
  - Obstetrical delivery
  - Organ biopsy
  - Puncture of a noncompressible vessel
- Cerebrovascular disease
- Hypertension (systolic BP > 180mm Hg or diastolic BP > 110mm Hg)
- Gastrointestinal bleeding within the last 10 days
- Genitourinary bleeding within the last 10 days
- Traumatic bleeding within the last 10 days
- High likelihood of a left ventricular thrombus
  - Mitral stenosis with atrial fibrillation
  - Chronic atrial fibrillation
- Acute pericarditis
- Subacute bacterial endocarditis
- Possible clotting defects secondary to renal or hepatic disease
- Pregnancy
- Hemorrhagic ophthalmic conditions (eg, diabetic retinopathy)
- Septic thrombophlebitis
- Advanced age: >75 years old
- Patients currently on anticoagulant therapy
- Severe renal disease
- Severe hepatic disease
- Any other condition in which bleeding is a serious risk or would be difficult to manage

ADVERSE EFFECTS: Bleeding is the most common complication of alteplase therapy. Bleeding is divided into two broad categories as given in the next Table

Bleeding with Alteplase

Internal Bleeding: Gastrointestinal tract, genitourinary tract, retroperitoneal sites or intracranial sites.

Superficial Bleeding: Invaded or disturbed sites, e.g., catheter insertion sites, arterial and venous puncture sites, cutdown and needle puncture sites.

In cases of serious internal bleeding, concomitant infusion of heparin should be stopped immediately.

PHARMACOKINETICS: Initial Half-Life: 3.6-4.6 min; Terminal Half-Life: 39-53 min. However, the half-life in-vivo is longer because t-PA binds to thrombi and because of the effects and longer half-life of its product, plasmin; Volume of Distribution: 27 to 40 liters; Metabolism: Liver.

Molecular Properties: The gene coding for human t-PA is on chromosome 8. Mol. wt.: 65,000 daltons. Alteplase is synthesized by vascular endothelial cells.

Alteplase is produced by Genentech Inc., San Francisco, CA, as follows: The complementary DNA coding for t-PA is isolated from a human melanoma cell line; it is inserted into the genome of Chinese hamster ovary cells. Alteplase is collected in suspension cultures of these cells. The product is predominantly (60 to 80%) a single-chain species and is called alteplase.

FDA Approval of TPA: The Cardiovascular and Renal Drugs Advisory Committee on May 29, 1987, considered the application submitted to the FDA for the approval of IV recombinant tissue plasminogen activator (rt-PA) for treatment of patients with acute myocardial infarction. The committee recommended postponement of approval pending further data analysis; rt-PA was approved six months later after further data were submitted. The committee thought it necessary to justify their original decision (Kowey, P.R. et al., JAMA 260, 2250-2252, Oct. 21, 1988).

TOBRAMYCIN

(Nebcin)

USES: **Tobramycin** is an **aminoglycoside** antibiotic (gentamicin, streptomycin, amikacin, tobramycin, kanamycin, netilmicin, sisomicin) and is used frequently in hospitals for parenteral treatment of patients who have serious infections caused by **aerobic gram-negative bacilli** (eg, a number of the Enterobacteriaceae, P. aeruginosa). Activities of tobramycin are given in the next Table (Pancoast, S.J., Med. Clin. No. Am. 72, 581-612, May, 1988; Adams, H.G., Personal Comm.):

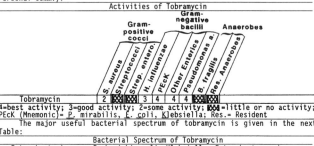

Activities of Tobramycin

	Gram-positive cocci			Gram-negative bacilli				Anaerobes	
	S. aureus	Streptococci	Strep. entero.	H. influenzae	PEcK	Other Enterics	Pseudomonas a.	B. fragilis	Res. Anaerobes
Tobramycin	2	▩	▩	3	4	4	4	▩	▩

4=best activity; 3=good activity; 2=some activity; ▩=little or no activity; PEcK (Mnemonic)= P. mirabilis, E. coli, Klebsiella; Res.= Resident

The major useful bacterial spectrum of tobramycin is given in the next Table:

Bacterial Spectrum of Tobramycin

Enterobacteriaceae: Escherichia coli, Klebsiella, Enterobacter and Serratia species, Proteus mirabilis, indole-positive Proteus (Providencia rettgeri, Morganella morganii, Proteus vulgaris), Providencia stuartii and Citrobacter species. Salmonella and Shigella species are usually susceptible but other effective and less toxic antibiotics are used.

Pseudomonas aeruginosa: (Note: Tobramycin is most effective). Aminoglycosides are usually combined with a penicillin, eg, carbenicillin, or cephalosporin, eg, ceftazidime.

Enterococci, eg, Streptococcus faecalis: Gentamicin plus penicillin G or ampicillin is frequently treatment of choice for enterococcal endocarditis (synergistic effect).

Prophylaxis of Endocarditis: Gentamicin plus ampicillin is the standard parenteral regimen for high risk patients.

Staphylococci, eg, S. aureus and S. epidermidis

Tobramycin frequently is the aminoglycoside of choice for infections caused by P. aeruginosa because of its greater in-vitro activity; however, superior in-vivo efficacy is not proven. For the treatment of infections caused by P. aeruginosa, tobramycin usually is given in **combination** with a cephalosporin or penicillin, eg, carbenicillin.

There is controversy regarding the use of gentamicin versus tobramycin for treatment of infections caused by susceptible organisms; the considerations for use of gentamicin versus tobramycin are given in the next Table:

Gentamicin versus Tobramycin

Consideration	Comments
Cost of Ten Day Therapy	Gentamicin: $28.50/day; Tobramycin: $52.50/day
Nephrotoxicity	Tobramicin is probably less nephrotoxic than gentamicin. However, nephrotoxicity usually is mild and reversible and seldom requires additional hospitalization or dialysis. Tobramycin may be preferable in patients at increased risk for nephrotoxicity, eg, elderly or those requiring prolonged therapy.
Tobramycin is more Potent against P. aeruginosa	In-vitro studies indicate that this is true; however, it is not proven that the in-vitro activity translates into in-vivo activity

TOBRAMYCIN (Cont.)

DOSAGE FORMS: Inj: 10mg/ml (pediatric) and 40mg/ml; powder 1.2g.

DOSAGE: Tobramycin sulfate is administered by IM injection or IV infusion; dosage is identical for either route of administration. Dosage is given in the next Table:

Dosage of Tobramycin Sulfate			
Condition	Age	Route	Dosage
Usual	Adults,	IM or IV	3-5mg/kg daily in equally divided doses at 8-hr. intervals.
	Children	IM or IV	6-7.5mg/kg daily in equally divided doses at 8-hr. intervals.
	Neonate	IM or IV	2.5mg/kg/dose <7 days, <28 weeks: Q 24h <7 days, 28-34 weeks: Q 18h <7 days, term: Q 12h >7 days, <28 weeks: Q 18h >7 days, 28-34 weeks: Q 12h >7 days, term: Q 8h

Dosage Adjustment in Renal Failure: When serum tobramycin concentrations cannot be measured, dosage guidelines based on predictive nomograms are used (Sarubbi, F.A., Jr. and Hull, J.H., Ann. Intern. Med. 89, 612-618, 1978).

(1) Loading Dose: The usual loading dose for tobramycin is 1.5 to 2.0mg/kg (IDEAL WEIGHT) for expected peak serum level of 4 to 10mcg/ml.

(2) Calculate creatinine clearance using the formula:

$$\text{Creatinine Clearance*} = \frac{\text{Wt}(140\text{-age})}{72(\text{Serum Creatinine})}\text{; *85\% for females}$$

(3) Select maintenance dose (as percentage of chosen loading dose) to continue peak serum concentrations indicated above according to desired dosing interval and the patients corrected creatinine clearance as given in the next Table:

Percentage of Loading Dose Required for Dosage Interval Selected				
CrCl(ml/min)	Estimated Half-life* (hrs.)	8hrs.	12hrs.	24hrs.
90	3.1	84%	-	-
80	3.4	80	91%	-
70	3.9	76	88	-
60	4.5	71	84	-
50	5.3	65	79	0
40	6.5	57	72	92%
30	8.4	48	63	86
25	9.9	43	57	81
20	11.9	37	50	75
17	13.6	33	46	70
15	15.1	31	42	67
12	17.9	27	37	61
10**	20.4	24	34	56
7	25.9	19	28	47
5	31.5	16	23	41
2	46.8	11	16	30
0	69.3	8	11	21

*Alternatively, one-half of the chosen loading dose may be given at an interval approximately equal to the estimated half-life.

**Dosing for patients with creatinine clearance 10ml/min should be assisted by measured serum levels.

Example:

58 y/o male, 5 ft.11 inches, Actual Body Weight = 200lbs.(91kg), Serum Creatinine = 1.6

Lean Body Weight (LBW) = 50kg + 2.3 (11 inches) = 75kg

$$\text{CrCl} = \frac{75(140-58)}{72\ (1.6)} = 53\ \text{ml/min.}$$

Loading Dose (LD) of Tobramycin = 2mg/kg X 75kg = 150mg

Maintenance Dose = 65% of LD (150mg) q 8hrs.; i.e. 100mg q 8hrs. or
79% of LD (150mg) q 12hrs.; i.e. 120mg q 12hrs.

Then: At steady state, draw trough just prior to dose; draw peak 30 minutes after tobramycin infusion is completed. Recheck serum creatinine every 3-5 days.

TOBRAMYCIN (Cont.)
ADVERSE EFFECTS: Toxicity and untoward effects are listed in the next Table (Edson, R.S. and Keys, T.F., Mayo Clin. Proc. 58, 99-102, 1983):

Toxicity of Aminoglycosides
Major:
Renal Toxicity
Vestibular Toxicity
Auditory Toxicity
Neuromuscular Blockade
Minor: Skin Rash, Drug-Induced Fever

The three main toxic side effects of tobramycin are ototoxicity, nephrotoxicity, and neuromuscular blockage (Smith, C.R. et al., N. Engl. J. Med. 302, 1106, May 15, 1980); it is important to control the dose given by monitoring peak and trough levels of the drug, particularly in patients with any degree of renal failure. As renal function declines, drug half-life increases to 70 hours.

Nephrotoxicity is usually mild. Irreversible ototoxicity may occur; both the hearing(cochlear) and equilibrium(vestibular) functions may be affected.

Electrolyte disturbances are given in the next Table:

Electrolyte Disturbances
Hypomagnesemia
Hypocalcemia
Hypokalemia

Hypomagnesemia (<1.6mg/dl) is observed in almost 40% of patients; hypocalcemia and hypokalemia may also occur. It may be advisable to monitor serum magnesium and use replacement therapy (Zaloga, G.P. et al., Surg. Gynecol. Obstet. 158, 561-565, 1984).

PHARMACOKINETICS: Therapeutic Range: 4-10mcg/ml; Toxic Level Peak: >12mcg/ml; Trough: <2mcg/ml; Toxic Level, Trough: >2mcg/ml; Half-Life: 2-3 hrs (adults); 5-70 hrs. (adults with renal impairment); 4.6 hrs. (full-term infants); 8.7 hrs in low birth-weight infants; Excretion: renal, unchanged.

MONITOR: Monitor parameters given in the next Table:

Monitor Parameters, Tobramycin Treatment

Parameter	Comment
Serum Tobramycin Levels	Initially and every 2-3 days during therapy
Serum Creatinine or BUN	Before and every 2-3 days during therapy
Audiograms	Baseline and weekly in patients with preexisting renal, auditory or vestibular impairment or in patients who receive prolonged, high-dose therapy
Tinnitus or Vertigo	Daily

Serum Tobramycin Levels: Red top tube, separate serum and freeze. Obtain serum specimens as follows:
(1) 24-48 hours after starting therapy if loading dose is not given.
(2) 5 to 30 minutes before I.V. tobramycin (trough)
(3) 30 minutes following completion of a 30 minute I.V. infusion of tobramycin (peak)

The first serum level of tobramycin is obtained when tobramycin has reached steady-state serum concentrations; steady-state is reached in 24 to 48 hours after starting therapy if the patient has not received a loading dose (steady state = 5-7 drug half-lives; half-life of tobramycin is 2 to 3 hours). The following times should be recorded on the laboratory requisition form and on the patient's chart:

Trough Speciment Drawn ________(Time) (5 to 30 minutes before Tobramycin)
Tobramycin Started ________(Time) (30 minutes I.V. infusion)
Tobramycin Completed ________(Time)
Peak Specimen Drawn ________(Time) (30 minutes after I.V. Tobramycin)

DRUG INTERACTIONS: High concentrations of beta-lactam antibiotics inactivate aminoglycosides (gentamicin, streptomycin, amikacin, tobramycin & kanamycin); to reduce this interaction, specimens containing both classes of antibiotics should either be assayed immediately using a rapid method or stored frozen.

TOLAZAMIDE
(Tolinase)

USES: Tolazamide is a "first" generation **sulfonylurea compound** which is used to **lower glucose levels** in patients with **non-insulin dependent diabetes mellitus** (NIDDM; Type II diabetes mellitus). Tolazamide is only used following dietary management; dietary management is continued during therapy.
Mechanism of Action: Sulfonylureas act by stimulating the release of insulin from pancreatic islets by increasing the sensitivity of the beta cells to glucose, which stimulates insulin secretion. Sulfonylureas may suppress the secretion of glucagon and the production of hepatic glucose and potentiate insulin-stimulated glucose transport in adipose tissue and across skeletal muscle membrane.
DOSAGE FORMS: Tabs: 100, 250, 500mg.
DOSAGE: Initially, 100-250mg daily with breakfast; the amount is adjusted every 4-6 days as needed. If fasting glucose is <200mg/dl, begin with 100mg/day; if fasting glucose is >200mg/dl, begin with 250mg/day. Adjust by increments of 100-250mg/day (50-125mg in geriatric patients). A single dose is effective in most patients;if 500mg or more is required daily, the drug is given in two doses. Max. 1g daily.
PHARMACOKINETICS: Absorption: Slow but well absorbed; Peak: 4-8 hrs.; Metabolism: By liver to partially active metabolites; Half-Life: 7 hrs.; Duration: 12-24 hrs.; Excretion: Urine.
ADVERSE EFFECTS: Similar to other sulfonylureas: hypoglycemia; GI disturbances; allergic skin reactions; photosensitivity, cholestasis; blood dyscrasias. Disulfiram-like reactions may occur with alcohol.
MONITOR: Blood glucose is monitored every one to two weeks until the dosage of tolazamide is established and monthly thereafter; therapy is continued if the response is satisfactory.

TOLAZOLINE
(Priscoline)

USES: Uses are given in the next Table:

Uses of Tolazoline
Treatment of Persistent Pulmonary Hypertension of the Newborn (Persistent Fetal Circulation)
Other Uses: Adjunctive Therapy in the Treatment of Peripheral Vasospastic Disease associated with Acrocyanosis, Acroparesthesia, Arteriosclerosis Obliterans, Thromboangitis Obliterans (Buerger's Disease), Causalgia, Diabetic Arteriosclerosis, Gangrene, Endarteritis, Frostbite Sequelae, Post-Thrombotic Conditions (Thrombophlebitis), Raynaud's Disease and Scleroderma)

Treatment of Persistent Pulmonary Vasoconstriction and Hypertension of the Newborn (Persistent Fetal Circulation): Tolazoline may improve oxygenation when systemic arterial oxygenation cannot be adequately maintained by supplemental oxygen and/or mechanical ventilation. Monitor vital signs, arterial blood gases including acid-base status, fluid and electrolyte balance.
Mechanism of Action: Tolazoline causes **perphipheral vasodilation** and decreases peripheral resistance primarily by direct relaxation of vascular smooth muscle.
DOSAGE FORMS: Parenteral: 25mg/ml.
DOSAGE: Tolazoline hydrochloride is usually administered IV; it may be administered subcutaneously, IM or intra-arterially. Dosage is given in the next Table:

Condition	Dosage
Persistent Pulmonary Hypertension of the Neonate	1-2mg/kg is given IV over a 10-minute period followed by IV infusion of 1-2mg/kg per hour. Response should be evident within 30 minutes.
Peripheral Vasospastic Dis.	IV, IM or Subcutaneously: 10-50mg, 4 times daily

Dosage of Tolazoline

CONTRAINDICATIONS: Active bleeding, hypotension, cerebrovascular accident and coronary artery disease.
ADVERSE EFFECTS: Monitor blood pressure, renal status and bone marrow status (agranulocytosis, thrombocytopenia, and pancytopenia have been reported). GI and pulmonary hemorrhage have been observed. Hypotension may be dramatic; volume expanders should be available. Severe hypotension should be treated with ephedrine or dopamine. Concurrent administration of epinephrine or norepinephrine may cause paradoxical hypotension followed by exaggerated rebound hypertension. Arrhythmias may occur. Adjust dosage downward in renal failure or oliguria.

TOLMETIN SODIUM

(Tolectin)

USES: Tolmetin is a **nonsteroidal anti-inflammatory drug(NSAID)**; it exhibits **anti-inflammatory analgesic** and **antipyretic activity**. Uses of tolmetin, as an anti-inflammatory agent, are given in the next Table:

Uses of Tolmetin as an Anti-Inflammatory Agent
Rheumatoid Arthritis
Juvenile Rheumatoid Arthritis
Osteoarthritis
Other Uses: Ankylosing Spondylitis in Adults; Adhesive Capsulitis Shoulder (Frozen Shoulder); Radiohumeral Bursitis (Tennis Elbow), or Local Trauma, eg, Recent Sprains

When used in the treatment of rheumatoid arthritis or juvenile arthritis, tolmetin has relieved pain and stiffness, reduced swelling, tenderness and the number of joints involved, improved mobility, grip strengthand knee joint function; in osteoarthritis, tolmetin and other NSAID are used principally for their analgesic rather than anti-inflammatory effect.

Mechanism of Action: The anti-inflammatory effect of tolmetin, like other NSAIDs, may be due in part to inhibition of prostaglandin synthesis and release during inflammation.

DOSAGE FORMS: Tabs: 200, 600mg; Caps: 400mg.

DOSAGE: Tolmetin is administered orally. Dosage is given in the next Table:

Dosage of Tolmetin

Condition	Age	Dosage
Rheumatoid Arthritis Osteoarthritis	Adults	400mg, 3 times daily, preferably a dose on arising and at bedtime. Subsequent Dosage: 600mg to 1.8g daily in 3 or 4 divided doses.
Juvenile Rheumatoid Arthritis	Children (>2 yrs.)	15mg/kg daily in 3 divided doses Subsequent Dosage: 15-30mg/kg daily

Symptomatic improvement usually begins in a few days to 1 week after initiating therapy with progressive improvement during succeeding weeks of therapy.

ADVERSE EFFECTS: GI Effects: The most frequent adverse effects is nausea which occurs in about 10% of patients. GI bleeding may occur. Nervous System Effects: The most common adverse nervous system effects include headache, dizziness, lightheadedness, tension or nervousness, drowsiness and mental depression. Hematologic Effects: Anemia; Renal Effects: Hematuria, proteinuria, dysuria, elevations in BUN. May cause false-positive test for proteinuria by acid precipitation, but not by dipstick.

TOLNAFTATE

(Aftate, Tinactin)

USES: Tolnaftate is an **antifungal agent**; uses of tolnaftate are given in the next Table:

Uses of Tolnaftate
Tinea Pedis; T. Cruris; T. Corporis and T. Manuum caused by:
Trychophyton Rubrum
T. Mentagrophytes
T. Tonsurans
M. Canis
M. Audoninii
E. Floccosum
Aspergillus associated with otitis externa.

Tolnaftate will control tinea capitis or tinea unguium if the infection is very superficial; however, if hair follicles or nail beds are infected, concomitant treatment with a systemic antifungal agent, such as griseofulvin, will be needed.

Tolnaftate, 4 drops applied 4 times a day for 3 weeks is effective in the treatment of otitis externa caused by Aspergillus (Liston, S.L. and Siegel, L.G., Laryngoscope 96, 699, 1986).

DOSAGE FORMS: Cream: 1%; Sol'n: 1%; Powder: 1%; Liquid Aerosol: 1%; Powder Aerosol: 1%.

DOSAGE: Tolnaftate preparations are applied topically.

ADVERSE EFFECTS: Slight local irritation may occur.

TRAVELERS' DIARRHEA, PATHOGENS, PREVENTION, TREATMENT

Pathogens: The pathogens that usually cause travelers' diarrhea are given in the next Table (Editorial, The Lancet, 2, 144, July 16, 1988):

Pathogens that Usually Cause Travelers' Diarrhea
Enterotoxigenic Escherichia coli(ETEC)
Shigellae
Giardia lamblia
Entamoeba histolytica

The most common cause of travelers' diarrhea is infection with enterotoxigenic E. coli. Infection with Shigellae is also common. Other possible pathogens are Salmonella, Campylobacter, other bacteria, viruses, and parasites. Use of prophylaxis is controversial; traveler's diarrhea is usually self-limiting and easily treated. Side effects of these therapies include Stevens-Johnson syndrome and hematologic reactions (trimethoprim-sulfamethoxazole), photosensitivity (doxycycline), and black tongue and stools (Pepto-Bismol). Quinolones (ciprofloxacin, norfloxacin) are contraindicated in children under 12 years.

Prevention: Drugs used to prevent travelers' diarrhea are given in the next Table (The Medical Letter, Handbook of Antimicrobial Therapy, 1990):

Drugs Used to Prevent Travelers' Diarrhea

Drug	Dosage
Pepto-Bismol Liquid (Bismuth Subsalicylate)	60ml, four times daily (one 240-ml bottle per day) (Dupont, H.L. et al, JAMA 243, 237, 1980).
Bismuth Subsalicylate Tablets	0.5-1.0 gram, twice daily (Stoffen, R. et al., Antimicrob. Agents Chemother. 29, 625, 1986)
Trimethoprim-Sulfamethoxazole (Septra DS, Bactrim DS and generics).	Double strength, one tablet daily, (Dupont, H.L. et al., Gastroenterology 84, 75, 1983).
Trimethoprim (Proloprim and others)	200mg once daily
Doxycycline (Vibramycin and others)	Doxycycline is a long-acting tetracycline. Give 100 mg. once daily.
Ciprofloxacin (Cipro)	A quinolone; not recommended for children under 12. 500mg once daily
Norfloxacin (Noroxin)	A quinolone; not recommended for children under 12. 400mg once daily.

Pepto-Bismol (bismuth subsalicylate) liquid and bismuth subsalicylate tablets are non-prescription drugs. Prophylactic bismuth subsalicylate at a dose of 524mg daily will reduce the attack rate by 65% (Dupont, H.L. et al., JAMA 257, 1347-1350, 1987).

Drugs, other than those listed in the previous Table, that are used to prevent travelers' diarrhea are neomycin and non-absorbable sulphonamides. These antibiotics reduce the attack rate by up to 90% (Dupont, H.L., Am. J. Med. 78, 81, 1987).

Treatment: The antibiotics that are used to prevent travelers' diarrhea will reduce the duration of illness from up to five days to one or two days when taken at the first sign of diarrhea (Gorbach, S.L., Lancet 2, 1378-1382, 1987).

Treatment of travelers' diarrhea is given in the next Table:

Treatment of Travelers' Diarrhea

Drug	Dosage
Trimethoprim-Sulfamethoxazole (Septra DS, Bactrim DS, and generics)	Double strength, 1 tablet every 12 hours for five days.
Trimethoprim (Proloprim and others)	200mg, twice daily for five days.
Ciprofloxacin (Cipro)	500mg, twice daily for five days.

TRAZODONE

(Desyrel)

USES: **Trazodone** is used in the treatment of **major depression** and is especially effective in reducing signs and symptoms of depression and in reducing associated **anxiety.** Trazodone has been used as an adjunct to anti-psychotic therapy in schizophrenia. Trazodone has also been used to reduce tremor, depression, and anxiety associated with treatment for alcohol dependence.

Compared to tricyclic antidepressants, trazodone has much lower anticholinergic activity (lower incidence of diaphoresis, dryness of the mouth, blurred vision, constipation), less cardiotoxic effects (lower incidence of tachycardia) and has a moderate sedative effect.

DOSAGE FORMS: Tabs: 50, 100, 150, 300mg.

DOSAGE: Trazodone is administered orally. The drug is taken shortly after a meal or light snack. If drowsiness occurs, a major portion of the drug is taken at bedtime or dosage may be reduced. Optimal response occurs in 2-4 weeks. In order to avoid recurrence of depressive symptoms, therapy may be required for several months after optimum therapeutic response.

Dosage is as follows: Initially, 150mg daily in divided doses. Then, increase if needed by 50mg daily every 3-4 days. Usual max. 600mg daily in divided doses. Trials using trazodone as an antianxiety drug employ doses of 50-200mg daily.

PHARMACOKINETICS: Rapidly absorbed; Peak: One hour on empty stomach or 2 hours with food. Half-Life: Initial phase, 3-6 hours; terminal phase, 5-9 hours. Steady state, 2-4 days. Crosses blood-brain barrier; metabolized in liver; excreted in urine.

ADVERSE EFFECTS: As opposed to doxepin (Adapin, Sinequan) and amitriptyline (Elavil, Endep), anticholinergic activity is minimal. Adverse effects, arranged in decreasing order of incidence, are as follows: somnolence, headache, nausea/vomiting, dizziness, dry mouth, constipation, myalgia, chest pain and back pain (Debus, J.R. et al., J. Clin. Psychiatry 49, 422-426, 1988). Other adverse effects include CNS overstimulation, cardiac arrhythmias, hypotension, fatigue, headache, impotence, seizures, altered liver function tests, priapism (Medical Letter 26, 35, 1984).

TRETINOIN

(Retin-A)

USES: The uses of Tretinoin, a vitamin A derivative, are given in the next Table:

Uses of Tretinoin
Acne Vulgaris (FDA approved)
Investigational:
Wrinkles
Actinic Keratosis
Other Uses:
Disorders of Keratinization, eg, Flat Warts
Keratosis Follicularis (Darier's Disease)
Lamellar Ichthyosis

Tretinoin is FDA approved for the treatment of acne vulgaris.

Acne Vulgaris: Acne vulgaris is a chronic inflammatory disorder, very common in the mid to late teenage years and characterized clinically by comedones, papules, nodules and cysts.

Tretinoin is used topically to treat **acne vulgaris.** Acne may be aggravated during the first six weeks of therapy; good results are noted after 3 or 4 months in most patients.

Actinic Keratosis: Actinic keratosis is a premalignant skin lesion characterized by focal areas of epidermal atypia; it is common among fair-complexioned persons who have a history of chronic sun exposure.

Preliminary findings in 10 medical centers indicate that tretinoin inhibits the transformation of cells in the actinic keratosis lesions to tumor.

Wrinkles: Tretinoin has anti-wrinkling effects and may lighten so-called liver spots.

DOSAGE FORMS: Cream: 0.025%, 0.05%, 0.1%; Gel: 0.01%, 0.025%; Solution: 0.05%.

DOSAGE: Tretinoin is not used for children. Initially apply to cleansed and completely dry skin once daily at bedtime; then, adjust strength or frequency to minimize irritation while maintaining effective comedolytic action. The liquid preparation is generally more irritating.

TRETINOIN (Cont.)
ADVERSE EFFECTS: Skin irritation with redness and peeling; stinging on application; aggravation of acne during first six weeks of therapy.
PRECAUTIONS: Minimize exposure to sun or U.V. light; avoid eyes, mouth, angles of nose, mucous membranes.
CONTRAINDICATIONS: Eczema, sunburn.

TRIAMTERENE
(Dyrenium; with Hydrochlorothiazide: Dyazide, Maxzide)
USES: **Triamterene** is a **potassium-sparing diuretic;** triamterene is similar to amiloride but differs from spironolactone in that triamterene does not inhibit aldosterone. Triamterene acts directly on the distal renal tabules, thereby producing increased sodium excretion and decreased potassium excretion. Calcium, magnesium, and bicarbonate excretion are also increased. Since most sodium is reabsorbed in the proximal renal tubules, triamterene is relatively ineffective when administered alone, and concomitant administration of a diuretic (such as a thiazide diuretic, ethacrynic acid, or furosemide) which blocks reabsorption of sodium proximal to the distal portion of the nephron, is required for maximal diuretic effects. The uses of triamterene are given in the next Table:

Uses of Triamterene
Edema: Congestive Heart Failure, Nephrotic Syndrome, Cirrhosis of the Liver
Hypertension: Usually combined with other diuretics
Hypokalemia, Diuretic-Induced

DOSAGE FORMS: Caps: Dyrenium: 50, 100mg; Combination preparations containing triamterene and hydrochlorothiazide (HCTZ) are given in the following Table:

Triamterene/Hydrochlorothiazide Combinations

Product	Triamterene(mg)	HCTZ(mg)
Dyazide	50	25
Maxzide 25	37.5	25
Maxzide	75	50

DOSAGE: Triamterene is administered orally; dosage is given in the next Table:

Dosage of Triamterene

Condition	Age	Dosage
Usual	Adult	Initially, 100mg twice daily after meals; Usual maintenance: 100mg daily or every other day. Maximum daily dose: 300mg.
	Children	2-4mg/kg daily in 2 divided doses; increase to 6mg/kg daily as needed.

Triamterene is often administered with hydrochlorothiazide. Generally, dosage requirements for each drug should be adjusted independently prior to initiating therapy with a fixed combination. For further discussion of combination preparations, see HYDROCHLOROTHIAZIDE AND TRIAMTERENE section.
PHARMACOKINETICS: Absorption: 50%; Peak Effect: 2-4 hrs.; Duration of Action: 8-24 hrs.; Half-Life: 100-150 min.; Metabolism: Liver.
ADVERSE EFFECTS: Hyperkalemia may occur. Adverse effects are infrequent; most commonly, nausea, vomiting, dizziness and leg cramps. Nephrolithiasis occurs in 1 in 1500 patients.
CONTRAINDICATIONS: Indomethacin-Triamterene combination may lead to nephrotoxicity, even in patients with normal renal function.

TRIAZOLAM
(Halcion)
USES: Triazolam is a benzodiazepine used in the treatment of **insomnia;** it is used for used in transient insomnia and for intermittent administration in short-term insomnia. It may also be used as a preanesthetic medication. It does not have daytime sedation or antianxiety actions. Triazolam is the most frequently prescribed hypnotic agent in the United States.
DOSAGE FORMS: Tabs: 0.125mg, 0.25mg.
DOSAGE: Triazolam is administered orally at bedtime. Adults: Initially, 0.25mg or less (range, 0.125 to 0.5mg); elderly patients should receive, on average, 50 percent of the dose used in young patients, since a given dose will produce a greater degree of sedation and psychomotor impairment (Greenblatt, D.J. et al., N. Engl. J. Med. 324, 1691-1698, 1991). Dosage for children under 18 years is not established.
PHARMACOKINETICS: Absorption: rapid; Time to Peak: 1.25 hours; Protein Binding: 90%; Volume of Distribution: 0.8-1.3 liter/kg.
Clearance: 3.7-10.6ml/min/kg. Half-Life: 2.6 hours. Excretion:Excreted in urine as a hydroxylated or glucuronide conjugate.
ADVERSE EFFECTS: The most common side effects are drowsiness, dizziness and headache. Next day memory impairment/amnesia is a prominent feature of this drug, even with intermittent, short term use; prevalence is 5 out of 6 subjects, with impairment reported on 40% of subject-days in patients given 0.5mg dose at bedtime (Bixler, E.O. et al., Lancet 337, 827-831, 1991). This serious and common adverse effect should be considered prior to prescribing this drug. Other less common side effects include hallucinations (0.1%) and confusion and possibly intrahepatic cholestasis. With overdose, there is respiratory depression, hypotension and coma. Withdrawal may occur with prolonged use.
DRUG INTERACTIONS: Additive sedation with alcohol and other CNS depressant drugs.

TRIMETHAPHAN

(Arfonad)

USES: Trimethaphan is a hypotensive agent used for temporary immediate reduction of blood pressure in patients with hypertensive emergencies; uses are given in the next Table:

Uses of Trimethaphan
Severe Hypertension and Hypertensive Emergencies
Controlled Hypotension During Anesthesia

Trimethaphan blocks transmission of impulses at both sympathetic and parasympathetic ganglia by competing with acetylcholine for cholinergic receptors at the autonomic ganglia and by stabilizing the postsynaptic membranes against the action of acetylcholine released from presynaptic nerve endings.

IV infusion of trimethaphan produces almost immediate reduction in blood pressure. Blood pressure begins to rise when the infusion is slowed or stopped and usually returns to pretreatment levels within 10 minutes after the infusion is discontinued.

DOSAGE FORMS: Injection: 50mg/ml

DOSAGE: Trimethaphan is administered by IV infusion using an infusion pump that will allow precise measurement of the flow rate. A solution of 1mg/ml for IV infusion may be prepared by adding 500mg of trimethaphan to 500ml of 5% dextrose. Dosage is given in the next Table:

Dosage of Trimethaphan

Condition	Dosage
Severe Hypertension	Initial Rate: 0.5-1mg/min. with subsequent gradual increases in the rate of infusion until the desired blood pressure response is achieved (blood pressure achieved not less than 2/3 of the pretreatment level).
Hypertension Associated with Acute Dissecting Aneurysms of the Aorta	1-2mg/minute with adjustments as needed to maintain a systolic blood pressure of 100-120mmHg
Controlled Hypotension During Anesthesia to Reduce Bleeding	Trimethaphan is administered after the patient is anesthetized; the drug is stopped prior to wound closure. Maintain systolic blood pressure above 60mmHg. Initial Rate: 3-4mg/minute; Maintenance Rate: 0.3-6mg/minute

CONTRAINDICATIONS: Glaucoma; use cautiously if at all in pregnancy, arteriosclerosis, cardiac, renal or hepatic disease, elderly patients or children.

ADVERSE EFFECTS: Urinary retention, orthostatic hypotension, tachycardia, precipitation of angina, anorexia, nausea, vomiting, dry mouth, extreme weakness, restlessness, cycloplegia, urticaria and itching.

Excessive hypotension may be reversed by tilting the head to the head-down position or elevating the extremities.

Causes histamine release.

TRIMETHOBENZAMIDE

(Tigan)

USES: **Trimethobenzamide** is used for the control of nausea and vomiting. The drug is less effective as an antiemetic than phenothiazines but may be associated with fewer adverse effects than phenothiazine therapy.

DOSAGE FORMS: Caps: 100, 250mg; Supp: 100, 200mg; Injection: 100mg/ml.

DOSAGE: Trimethobenzamide·HCl is administered orally, rectally, or by IM injection. Dosage is given in the next Table:

Dosage of Trimethobenzamide·HCl

Age	Route	Dosage
Adult	Oral	250mg, 3 or 4 times daily
Child, 15-40kg	Oral	100 or 200mg, 3 or 4 times daily
Child, by wt.	Oral	20mg/kg daily in 3 or 4 divided doses
Adult	Rectal	200mg, 3 or 4 times daily
Child, 15-40kg	Rectal	100-200mg, 3 or 4 times daily
Child, <15kg	Rectal	100mg, 3 or 4 times daily
Child, by wt.	Rectal	15mg/kg daily in 3 or 4 divided doses
Adult	IM	200mg, 3 or 4 times daily
Child	IM	Not recommended

ADVERSE EFFECTS: CNS disturbances are common in children (eg, extrapyramidal reactions, drowsiness, dizziness, confusion, opisthotonus, seizures and coma).

TRIMETHOPRIM

(Proloprim, Trimpex)

USES: Trimethoprim is used to treat acute uncomplicated urinary tract infections; it is also used in the prophylaxis of chronic and recurrent urinary tract infections.

Trimethoprim is active against common gram-negative bacteria associated with urinary tract infection as given in the next Table:

Antimicrobial Activity of Trimethoprim

Gram-Negative Aerobic Bacteria	Gram-Positive Aerobic Bacteria
E. coli	Staphylococci, coagulase negative
Klebsiella pneumoniae	Strep. pneumoniae
Proteus mirabilis	Strep. pyogenes
Other enterics	
H. influenzae	

Trimethoprim is inactive against Pseudomonas aeruginosa, anaerobic bacteria such as B. fragilis, and other anaerobes, and enterococci.

Mechanism of Action: Bacteria require tetrahydrofolic acid as a cofactor in the synthesis of thymidine, purines and ultimately DNA. Trimethoprim inhibits the enzyme dihydrofolate reductase, an enzyme required for the synthesis of tetrahydrofolic acid. See Mechanism of Action under **TRIMETHOPRIM AND SULFAMETHOXAZOLE** (Co-Trimoxazole).

DOSAGE FORMS: Tabs: 100mg, 200mg.

DOSAGE: Trimethoprim is administered orally; dosage for adults is given in the next Table (Johnson, J.R. and Stamm, W.E., Infect. Dis. Clin. North Am. 1, 773-791, Dec. 1987):

Dosage of Trimethoprim

Condition	Dosage
Cystitis	Single Dose Therapy: 400mg Three-Day Regimen: 100mg every 12 hours for three days or 200mg every 24 hours for three days.
Cystitis, complicating factors present	Seven-Day Regimen: Same dosage as three day regimen.
Pyelonephritis, Mild	Fourteen-Day Regimen: Same dosage as three-day regimen.
Prophylaxis against recurrent urinary tract infection	50-100mg every evening.

ADVERSE EFFECTS: The incidence and severity of adverse reactions to trimethoprim are generally dose-related and may be decreased by a reduction in dosage; adverse effects are given in the next Table:

Adverse Effects of Trimethoprim

System	Effect
Skin	Rash and pruritus; 5% appearing in 7-14 days at 200mg or less daily; 25% at 400mg for 14 days.
G.I. System	6%;Epigastric discomfort, nausea, vomiting, glossitis and abnormal taste sensation.
Hematologic	Rare; thrombocytopenia, neutropenia, megaloblastic anemia, and methemoglobinemia. Folic acid administered during trimethoprim therapy will not interfere with the drug's antibacterial effect. Hematologic abnormalities usually resolve following administration of 3-6mg of leucovorin (folinic acid) for 3 days or until normal hematopoiesis is restored.
Other	Fever; elevation of transaminases, bilirubin, creatinine, urea.

PRECAUTIONS: Impaired renal function; impaired hepatic function; suspected folate deficiency; pregnancy.

TRIMETHOPRIM AND SULFAMETHOXAZOLE (Co-Trimoxazole)
(Bactrim, Septra, TMP-SMZ)

USES: Trimethoprim(TMP)/sulfamethoxazole(SMZ) is prepared in a fixed combination containing 5:1 ratio of sulfamethoxazole to trimethoprim. Activities of trimethoprim/sulfamethoxazole are given in the next Table (Foltzer, M.A. and Reese, F.E., Med. Clin. No. Am. 71, 1177-1194, Nov. 1987; Adams, H.G., Personal Comm.):

Activities of Trimethoprim/Sulfamethoxazole (Co-Trimoxazole)

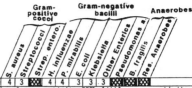

	Gram-positive cocci			Gram-negative bacilli						Anaerobes	
	S. aureus	Streptococci	Strep. entero.	H. influenzae	P. mirabilis	E. coli	Klebsiella	Other Enterics	Pseudomonas a.	B. fragilis	Res. Anaerobes
Trimethoprim/Sulfamethoxazole	4	3	▨	4	4	3	3	3	▨	▨	▨

4=best activity; 3=good activity; 2=some activity; ▨ =little or no activity; Res.= Resident

Uses of trimethoprim/sulfamethoxazole are given in the next Table:

Uses of Trimethoprim(TMP)/Sulfamethoxazole(SMZ)

Chronic or Recurrent Urinary Tract Infections(UTI): Susceptible strains of E. coli, Proteus (indole-positive or -negative). Klebsiella, or Enterobacter (Culture, start therapy, evaluate sensitivity data).

Acute Uncomplicated UTI: Use less expensive and as effective as amoxicillin, or ampicillin, or sulfisoxazole, or trimethoprim.

Acute Complicated UTI (Abnormalities of Urinary Tract or Neurogenic Bladder): Use less expensive and as effective as amoxicillin, or ampicillin or sulfisoxazole, or trimethoprim.

Acute Pyelonephritis: Single anti-infective IV regimen, eg, gentamicin for 4-7 days followed by single anti-infective oral antibiotic therapy.

Pneumocystis Carinii Pneumonia(PCP): TMP/SMZ is at least as effective as pentamidine.

Prophylaxis of Pneumocystis Carinii Infections

Enteritis caused by susceptible strains of Shigella flexneri or S. sonnei. When susceptibility of the isolate is unknown,TMP/SMZ is the drug of choice Oral TMP/SMZ has been used to treat enterotoxigenic E. coli and to prevent traveler's diarrhea.

Otitis Media: TMP/SMZ is used to treat ampicillin-resistant Haemophilus influenzae or in pencillin-allergic patients.

Bronchitis: TMP/SMZ is as effective as amoxicillin, ampicillin, erythromycin or tetracycline in treatment or prophylaxis of acute exacerbations of chronic bronchitis; choice of antibiotic depends on bacterial resistance.

Infection in Granulocytopenic Patients

Nocardia Infections: Sulfonamides are usually drugs of first choice.

Other Uses: TMP/SMX may be effective in the treatment of pertussis. TMP/SMZ is one of several alternatives to erythromycin or ceftriaxone in the treatment of genital ulcers caused by susceptible H. ducreyi (chancroid).

Mechanism of Action: Bacteria require tetrahydrofolic acid, a derivative of folic acid, as a cofactor in the synthesis of thymidine, purines and ultimately, DNA.

The combination of trimethoprim with sulfamethoxazole inhibits enzymes and results in a blockage of two steps in the biosynthetic pathway for the

TRIMETHOPRIM AND SULFAMETHOXAZOLE (Cont.)
synthesis of tetrahydrofolic acid as illustrated in the next Figure (Drug Evaluations, 6th ed., Am. Med. Assoc. Chicago, Illinois, 1986):

Synthesis of Tetrahydrofolic Acid and Sites of Inhibition by Trimethoprim and Sulfamethoxazole

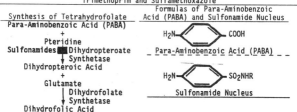

Synthesis of Tetrahydrofolate

Para-Aminobenzoic Acid (PABA)
+
Pteridine
Sulfonamides ■ **Dihydropteroate Synthetase** ↓
Dihydropteroic Acid
+
Glutamate
↓ **Dihydrofolate Synthetase**
Dihydrofolic Acid
+2NADPH
Trimethoprim ■ **Dihydrofolate Reductase** ↓
Tetrahydrofolic Acid
+2NADP

Formulas of Para-Aminobenzoic Acid (PABA) and Sulfonamide Nucleus

Para-Aminobenzoic Acid (PABA)

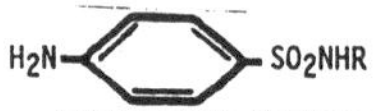

Sulfonamide Nucleus

Sulfonamides: Most bacterial cells are impermeable to folic acid and must synthesize it from para-aminobenzoic acid (PABA). The sulfonamides are structural analogues of PABA and competitively inhibit the synthesis of dihydropteroic acid, the immediate precursor of dihydrofolic acid, from PABA and pteridine.
Trimethoprim: Trimethoprim, a 2,4 - diaminopyrimidine, inhibits dihydrofolate reductases of bacterial and protozoal but not mammalian cells, thus preventing the formation of tetrahydrofolic acid.
DOSAGE FORMS: (Bactrim,Septra,TMP-SMZ) Tabs: Reg. Strength: 80mg Trimethoprim plus 400mg Sulfamethoxazole; Double Strength: 160mg Trimethoprim plus 800mg Sulfamethoxazole; Susp.:40mg Trimethoprim plus 200mg Sulfamethoxazole per 5ml; Injection for IV Infusion:16mg Trimethoprim plus 80mg Sulfamethoxazole per ml.
DOSAGE: TMP/SMZ is administered orally or by IV infusion and not by IM.

For IV infusion, dilute 5ml of IV concentrate with 125ml of 5% dextrose or with 75ml of 5% dextrose. Infuse over a period of 60-90 minutes; avoid rapid or direct IV injection.

Dosage in different conditions is given in the next Table:

Dosage of TMP/SMZ in Different Conditions

Condition	Age	Route	Dosage
Chronic or Recurrent Urinary Tract Infection (UTI)	Adults	Oral	160mg TMP/800mg SMZ, (double strength) every 12 hours, 10-14 days
	Children (2 mos. or older)	Oral	8-10mg TMP/40-50mg SMZ/kg daily in 2 divided doses every 12 hours, 10-14 days
Severe Urinary Tract Infection (UTI)	Adults or Children (2 mos. or older)	IV	8-10mg TMP/40-50mg SMZ/kg administered in 2-4 equally divided doses daily for up to 14 days (Max: 0.96g TMP/4.8g SMZ daily).
Prophylaxis of Chronic or Recurrent UTI's	Adults	Oral	40mg TMP/200mg SMZ or 80mg TMP/400mg SMZ (single strength) daily or 3 times weekly for 3-6 months
Prostatitis	Men	Oral	160mg TMP/800mg SMZ (double strength) every 12 hours, 3-6 months.
Enteritis caused by Shigella flexneri or Shigella sonnei	Adults	Oral	160mg TMP/800mg SMZ (double strength) every 12 hours, 7 days.
	Children (2 mos. or older)	Oral	8-10mg TMP/40-50mg SMZ/kg daily in 2 divided doses every 12 hours, for 5 days
Severe Enteritis Caused by Shigella flexneri or Shigella sonnei	Adults or Children (2 mos. or older)	IV	8-10mg TMP/40-50mg SMZ/kg administered in 2-4 equally divided doses daily for up to 5 days (Max: 0.96g TMP/4.8g SMZ daily).

Dosage of TMP/SMZ in Different Conditions

Condition	Age	Route	Dosage
Bronchitis	Adults	Oral	160mg TMP/800mg SMZ (double strength) 12 hours, 7-10 days
Otitis Media	Children (2 mos. or older)	Oral	8-10mg TMP/40-50mg SMZ/kg daily in 2 divided doses every 12 hours for 10 days.
Prophylaxis of Traveler's Diarrhea	Adults	Oral	160mg TMP/800mg SMZ (double strength) once daily during period of risk (up to 2 weeks), beginning the day of travel and continuing for 2 days after returning home.
Treatment of Traveler's Diarrhea	Adults	Oral	160mg TMP/800mg SMZ (double strength) twice daily for 3-5 days
Pneumocystis carinii pneumonia	Adults or Children (Older than 2 months)	Oral	20mg TMP/100mg SMZ/kg daily 4 equally divided doses every 6 hours.
		IV	15-20mg TMP/75-100mg SMZ/kg daily, in 3 or 4 equally divided doses every 6 or 8 hours for at least 14 days.
Prophylaxis of P. carinii Pneumonia	Adults Children	Oral	150mg TMP/750mg SMZ/m^2 given either as a single dose or in divided doses twice daily, 7 days/week or 3 days/week (M-T-W or M-W-F)(MMWR 40, No. RR-2, 1-13, 1991).
Sepsis in Granulocytopenic Adults	Adults	IV	10mg TMP/50mg SMZ/kg in 4 divided doses daily
Prophylaxis of Gram-Negative Bacteremias in Granulocytopenic Adults	Adults	Oral	160-320mg TMP/800-1600mg SMZ, in 2 divided doses daily
Nocardia	Adults	Oral	640mg TMP/3200mg SMZ daily for months
Chancroid	Adults	Oral	160mg TMP/800mg SMZ twice daily for at least 7 days or 640mg TMP/3200 SMZ, single dose

Dosage in Renal Impairment: The usual adult daily dosage should be reduced 50% in patients with creatine clearances of 15-30ml/minute.

PHARMACOKINETICS: Absorption: Rapid and efficient from the upper intestinal tract; Peak: 1-4 hours; Protein-Binding: Trimethoprim, 45%; sulfamethoxazole, 70%; Half-Life: Trimethoprim, 10 hours; sulfamethoxazole, 10-12 hours; Excretion: Kidneys.

ADVERSE EFFECTS: Hypersensitivity and hematologic reactions are the most serious adverse effects.

Skin rashes (mild, diffuse, maculopapular) are the most common (6%-8%) adverse effects and are usually due to hypersensitivity to the sulfonamide component; these are reversible upon discontinuation of the drug. More serious skin reactions (eg, Stevens-Johnson syndrome) are rare.

Gastrointestinal effects, eg, anorexia, nausea, and vomiting are common; diarrhea is relatively rare. Glossitis and stomatitis may occur.

Hematologic effects, eg, thrombocytopenia, eosinophilia, agranulocytosis, aplastic anemia and neutropenia may occur. Hemolytic anemia due to hypersensitivity reactions and secondary to G6PD deficiency has been reported.

IV administration may cause pain, local irritation and rarely, thrombophlebitis.

TRIMETHOPRIM AND SULFAMETHOXAZOLE (Cont.)

Trimethoprim has caused megaloblastosis which is probably secondary to interference with folate metabolism; megaloblastosis occurs most often in patients who are prone to folate deficiency, eg, alcoholics, patients receiving phenytoin, pregnant women, and patients with malabsorption syndromes. The administration of leucovorin prevents or reverses these effects.

Headache, neuritis and hallucinations have been reported.

Drug Interactions: Drug interactions are given in the next Table:

Drug Interactions of Trimethoprim/Sulfamethoxazole

Drugs	Effect
Warfarin	Potentiates anticoagulant effect; measure PT.
Oral Hypoglycemics, eg, Chlorpropamide, Tolbutamide, Acetohexamide	Oral hypoglycemic effect potentiated.
Methotrexate	Bone marrow depressant effect potentiated.
Phenytoin	Half-life prolonged

CONTRAINDICATIONS: Modify dosage in patients with renal impairment, patients with folate deficiency and G6PD deficiency.

TRIMETREXATE

USES: Trimetrexate is an investigational antifolate drug; similar to methotrexate, that has been used in conditions listed in the next Table:

Uses of Trimetrexate

Pneumocystis Carinii Pneumonia (PCP) in patients with Acquired Immunodeficiency Syndrome (AIDS)
Experimental Treatment of certain carcinomas

Pneumocystis Carinii Pneumonia (PCP) in Patients with AIDS: Trimetrexate with leucovorin rescue has shown initial promise in treating PCP infections in patients with AIDS (Allegra, C.J. N. Engl. J. Med. 317, 978-985, Oct. 15, 1987). This drug is currently available from Warner-Lambert (1-800-426-7527 outside Michigan, 1-800-833-0014 inside Michigan); use is restricted to AIDS patients with Pneumocystis carinii pneumonia who are unable to tolerate or fail to respond to trimethoprim-sulfamethoxazole and pentamidine. Patients must have a neutrophil count greater than 1000, platelet count greater than 50,000/mm^3, and serum creatinine less than 2.5mg/dl (The Medical Letter 31, 5-6, January 27, 1989).

Experimental Treatment of Certain Carcinomas: The activity of trimetrexate, alone and in combination with other drugs, in patients with cancer of the head and neck, nonsmall cell lung cancer and breast cancer, is being evaluated (Yarbro, J.W. ed., Seminars in Oncology 15, No.2, Suppl.2, April, 1988).

Dosage in Patients with PCP: Trimetrexate: 30mg per sq. meter, IV bolus daily; duration: 21 days. Leucovorin Rescue: 20mg per sq. meter; IV bolus or orally every six hours; duration: 23 days.

ADVERSE EFFECTS: (Based on article by Allegra, C.N. Engl. J. Med. 317, 978-985, Oct. 15, 1987; leucovorin rescue was used): Minimal toxicity with transient neutropenia or thrombocytopenia and transaminase elevation.

ULCERATIVE COLITIS

Sulfasalazine is the most commonly used drug for **ulcerative colitis**; it is effective both to induce remission of mildly to moderately active disease (Dissanayake, A.S. and Truelove, S.C., Gut 14, 923-926, 1973), and for long-term maintenance therapy (Azad Khan, A.K. et al., Gut 21, 232-240, 1980).

Metabolism: Oral sulfasalazine undergoes minimal metabolism or absorption in the upper gastrointestinal tract; colonic bacteria degrade the diazo bond to release free 5-aminosalicylic Acid (5-ASA) and sulfapyridine (Klotz,U. et al., N. Engl. J. Med. 303, 1499-1502, 1980). Some sulfapyridine is absorbed and appears responsible for most adverse reactions (Taffet, S.L. and Das, K.M, Dig. Dis. Sci., 28, 833-842, 1983), whereas 5-ASA is therapeutically active component. See also SULFASALAZINE.

UPPER AIRWAY; PATHOGENS, TREATMENT

UPPER AIRWAY OBSTRUCTION: Upper airway obstruction is usually caused by conditions listed in the next Table:

Upper Airway Obstruction

Condition	Pathogen(s)
EPIGLOTTITIS	Haemophilus influenzae
CROUP (Laryngotracheo-bronchitis)	Parainfluenza virus types 1, 2 and 3 Respiratory syncytial virus Influenza virus types A and B
TRACHEITIS	Staphylococcus aureus Haemophilus influenzae Others (Group A Streptococcus, Strep. Pneumoniae, Moraxella [Branhamella] Catarrhalis)

EPIGLOTTITIS; PATHOGENS, TREATMENT

Pathogens: H. influenza causes epiglottitis in infants and young children; acute epiglottitis in adults is unusual but not rare (Mayo-Smith, M.F., et al., N. Engl. J. Med. 314, 1133-1139, 1986; Baker, A.S. and Eavey, R.D., ibid, 1185-1186, 1986). There is sudden onset of fever; hyperemia and edema of the epiglottis may lead to respiratory obstruction.

Bacteremia occurs in 65 to 90% of children with acute epiglottitis. Cultures of the pharynx do not reliably identify the causative organism. However, in 75% of children with epiglottitis, H. influenza grows from direct culture of the epiglottis (Wetmore, R.F. and Handler, S.D., Ann. Otolaryngol. 88, 822-826, 1979; Lewis, J.K., et al., Clin. Pediatr. 17, 494-496, 1978).

In adults, acute epiglottitis with systemic involvement and bacteremia is also almost invariably due to H. influenza, type b (Tveteras, K. and Kristensen, S., Clin. Otolaryngol. 12, 337-343, 1987).

Treatment: In any child with epiglottitis, endotracheal intubation should be performed urgently or emergently. Ideally, intubation is performed in the operating room by an anesthesiologist or other person experienced in the management of pediatric airways. Provisions should be available for emergency tracheostomy. After intubation, subsequent management should be in a pediatric intensive care unit.

Since H. influenza is the predominant organism in acute epiglottitis, I.V. antibiotic therapy is directed against this organism. Initial antibiotic choice should cover H. influenza, including beta-lactamase producing strains. Possibilities include a suitable second-generation cephalosporin (Cefuroxime) or third generation cephalosporin, or ampicillin plus chloramphenicol. Antibiotics are given for several days (as necessary) in the hospital and then taken orally for 10-14 days at home.

Prevention: H. influenzae type b conjugate vaccine is being offered to children; vaccination is performed at 2, 4 and 6 months with a booster at 15 months (HbOC schedule; see IMMUNIZATIONS for details and PRP-OMP schedule). Most epiglottitis usually occurs between the ages of two and six years; thus, epiglottitis may nearly vanish within a few years (Cochi, S.L. and Broome, C.V., Ped. Inf. Dis. 5, 12-19, 1986).

CROUP; PATHOGENS, TREATMENT

Pathogens: Laryngotracheobronchitis or croup is most often caused by parainfluenza virus. This virus accounts for 75% of cases; two-thirds of these or 50% of all cases are caused by parainfluenza type 1. Other important etiologic agents include respiratory syncytial virus (10%), influenza types A and B (7%) and Mycoplasma pneumoniae (4%)(Denny, F.W., et al., Pediatrics 71, 871-876, 1983).

Diagnosis: Croup is a clinical syndrome that is characterized by a barking cough, often accompanied by stridor, respiratory distress and retractions. Wheezing may be present as well. The disease primarily affects children 3 months to 3 years and tends to be seasonal. Patients usually present with mild to moderate fever and respiratory symptoms that wax and wane. In the absence of complications, symptoms usually resolve in 3 days. Differential diagnosis includes foreign body and epiglottitis; drooling, agitation, and absence of cough are more predictive of epiglottitis than croup (Mauro, R.D., et al., AJDC 142, 679-682, 1988).

Treatment: The treatment of viral laryngotracheobronchitis is usually symptomatic relief of the upper airway obstruction: humidification of inspired air; nebulized diluted solution of racemic epinephrine (0.25-0.5ml in 2.5ml normal saline); short-course relatively high doses of steroids may be beneficial (eg, dexamethasone 0.6mg/kg IV or IM once)(Super, D.M. et al., J. Pediatr. 115, 323-329, 1989) although steroid therapy remains controversial (Smith, D.S., J. Pediatr. 115, 256-257, 1989). Patients who do not respond to medical therapy may require intubation.

UPPER AIRWAY: PATHOGENS, TREATMENT (Cont.)
TRACHEITIS; PATHOGENS, TREATMENT
Pathogens: The causes of acute bacterial tracheitis are given in the next Table:

Causes of Acute Bacterial Tracheitis
Staphylococcus aureus
Haemophilus influenzae
Group A Streptococci
Strep. Pneumoniae
Moraxella (Branhamella) catarrhalis

Tracheitis is less common than either croup or epiglottitis and shares many of the same clinical features. Patients generally present with high fever, systemic toxicity, elevated neutrophil count with bandemia, and poor response to racemic epinephrine inhalation or systemic steroids. Compared to epiglottitis, onset is not as acute and stridor is both inspiratory and expiratory.
Treatment: Nasotracheal intubation should be performed and the patient should remain sedated. Since Staphylococcus aureus accounts for about half of the cases, antistaphylococcal coverage should be included in empiric IV antibiotic therapy. Cefuroxime has been suggested (Kasian, G.F., et al., Can. Med. Assoc. J. 140, 46-50, 1989); alternatively, nafcillin plus a third generation cephalosporin may be used initially and replaced with a more specific antibiotic following identification of the pathogen.

URINARY TRACT; PATHOGENS, TREATMENT
Pathogens: The pathogens that cause urinary tract infection are given in the next Table:

Pathogens that Cause Urinary Tract Infection	
Gram-Negative Bacteria	**Gram-Positive Bacteria**
Enteric Bacilli	**Cocci**
E. coli	Staphylococcus aureus
Proteus mirabilis	or epidermidis
Proteus, indole positive	Streptococcus, enterococci
and other Enterobacteriaceae	**Other Pathogens**
Klebsiella pneumoniae	**Mycoplasma**
Bacteriodes (Anaerobic)	Ureaplasma urealyticum
Other Bacilli	**Fungi**
Pseudomonas aeruginosa	Candida albicans

Urethritis: The sexually transmitted diseases that cause urethritis are Chlamydia trachomatis (CT), N. gonorrhoeae, Herpes simplex virus (HSV), Treponema pallidum. Trichomonas vaginalis also causes urethritis.

The etiologic agent most commonly identified in patients with pyelonephritis is Escherichia coli. There are numerous other urinary pathogens, eg., Proteus vulgaris, Pseudomonas aeruginosa, Klebsiella pneumoniae, Salmonella, the enterococci and the hemolytic staphylococci. With anatomical lesions of the urinary tract, there is a higher incidence of infections caused by Klebsiella, Enterobacter, Proteus and Pseudomonas.
Female Adolescents: First urinary tract infections in female adolescents tend to be associated with the occurrence of sexual activity, menstruation or contraceptive use (Nicolle, L.E. et al., J. Infect. Dis. 146, 579-583, 1982).

Organisms isolated in acute urinary tract infection in female non-pregnant adolescents, age range 12 to 18 years, are given in the next Table; (Fine, J.S. and Jacobson, M.S., Pediatrics 75, 916-920, 1985):

Organisms Isolated in Acute Urinary Tract Infection in Female Adolescents

Organism	Percent(%)
Escherichia Coli	74
Proteus Mirabilis	16
Staphylococcus Coagulase Negative	65
Enterobacter Cloacae	3.5

Nosocomial Urinary Tract Infections: Urinary tract infections account for 30% to 40% of all hospital-acquired infections; up to 85% of nosocomial urinary tract infections follow genitourinary instrumentation, most often urethral catherization (Krieger, J.N., et al., J. Infect. Dis. 148, 57-62, 1983).
Treatment: Oral Antibiotic therapy for acute urinary tract infections is given as single dose therapy, 3 day therapy, 7 day therapy and 14 day therapy; these regimens are given in the next Tables (Johnson, J.R. and Stamm, W.E., Infect. Dis. Clin. North Am. 1, 773-791, Dec. 1987; Wilhelm, M.P. and Edson, R.S., Mayo Clin. Proc. 62, 1025-1031, 1987; Koffer, K.F., American Druggist, pgs. 81-87, June 1988).

Single Oral Antibiotic Therapy: Acute cystitis occurs most frequently in women of childbearing age and is often related to sexual activity and use of a diaphragm (Ann. Intern. Med. 107, 816-823, 1987).

Single oral antibiotic therapy for cystitis with no complicating factors present is given in the next Table:

Single Oral Antibiotic Therapy for Acute Uncomplicated Cystitis

Preferred Single Oral Dose Therapies:
- Trimethoprim (TMP); 400mg (4 tabs, 100mg each).
- TMP/Sulfamethoxazole (SMZ); 320mg TMP/ 1600mg SMZ (2 tablets, double-strength).
- Nitrofurantoin (Macrodantin); 200mg (2 tabs, 100mg each)

Other Recommended Single Oral Dose Therapies:
- Amoxicillin; 3g (6 caps, 500mg each)
- Amoxicillin plus Clavulanate (Augmentin); (1 tab., 500mg amoxicillin).
- First Generation Cephalosporin, eg., Cephalexin (Keflex); 2g (2 tabs., 1g. each).
- Sulfisoxazole (Gantrisin); 2g. (2 tabs, 1g each)

Single-dose treatment with amoxicillin is less effective than longer durations of treatment. Single-dose treatment with trimethoprim-sulfamethoxazole is less effective than 10 day treatment with respect to cure rates at 2 weeks after the start of treatment but by 6 weeks the advantage of longer treatment no longer exists. An intermediate duration of treatment, eg., 3 day may be optimal (Fihn, S.D. et al., Ann. Intern. Med. 108, 350-357, 1988).

The effectiveness of single dose of trimethoprim-sulfamethoxazole, as compared to multidose regimens, for treatment of acute urinary tract infection in children is given in the next Table (Madrigal, G. et al., Pediatr. Infect. Dis. J. 7, 316-319, 1988):

Single versus Multi-Dose Regimens of Trimethoprim-Sulfamethoxazole for Treatment of Acute Urinary Tract Infection in Children

Rates	One Dose	Two Doses/Day 3 Days	Two Doses/Day 7 Days
Cure Rates (%)	93%	96%	96%
Recurrence Rate (%)	20.5%	5.6%	8%

There is no significant difference in the cure rates for the single dose regimen (93%) and multidose regimens (96%). However, single dose therapy is not as effective as multidose regimens in preventing recurrent urinary tract infections in children; recurrent infection was defined as culture positive urine at the time of follow-up visits (10th-12th days or 28th-37th days).

Three Day Therapy: Three-day oral antibiotic therapy for acute cystitis with no complicating factors present is given in the next Table:

Three-day Oral Antibiotic Therapy for Acute Uncomplicated Cystitis

Medication	Dose	Interval (hours)
Preferred Three-Day Oral Antibiotic Therapies:		
Trimethoprim (TMP)	100 (200)mg	12 (24)
TMP/Sulfamethoxazole	160/800mg (double strength tab.)	12
Nitrofurantoin	100mg	6
Other Recommended Three-Day Oral Antibiotic Therapies		
Amoxicillin	500mg	8
Amoxicillin plus Clavulanate (Augmentin)	500mg	8
First Gen. Cephalosporin eg., Cephalexin (Keflex)	500mg	6
Norfloxacin	400mg	12
Sulfisoxazole (Gantrisin)	500mg	6
Tetracycline	500mg	6

URINARY TRACT; PATHOGENS, TREATMENT (Cont.)

Cytitis with Complicating Factors: In patients with cystitis with complicating factors, antibiotic therapy is continued for at least 7 days.

Pyelonephritis Mild: The treatment of mild pyelonephritis, using oral antibiotics for 14 days, is given in the next Table:

Treatment of Mild Pyelonephritis

Medication	Dose	Interval (Hours)
Preferred Oral Antibiotic Therapies		
Trimethoprim (TMP)	100(200mg)	12(24)
TMP/Sulfamethoxazole	160/800mg	12
First Gen. Cephalosporin, eg, Cephalexin (Keflex)	500mg	6
Norfloxacin	400mg	12
Ciprofloxacin	250	12
Other Recommended Oral Antibiotic Therapies:		
Amoxicillin	500mg	8
Amoxicillin plus Clavulanate	500mg	8

Candida vaginitis occurs in 20% of patients following conventional dose (10 day) therapy(Fine, J.S. and Jacobson, M.S., Pediatrics 75, 916-920, 1985.)

Drugs used in treatment of urinary tract infections in children are given in the next Table (Sidor, T.A. and Resnick, M.I., Pediatr. Clin. N.Am. 30, No. 2, 323-331, Apr. 1983):

Treatment of Urinary Tract Infections in Children

Drug	Route of Administration	Dosage
Amoxicillin	Oral, Parenteral	30-50mg/kg/day Divided q 8 h
Cephalexin(Keflex)	Oral	25-100mg/kg/day Divided q 6 h
Cefazolin(Ancef)	Parenteral	25-100mg/kg/day Divided q 6-8 h
Nitrofuratoin	Oral	3-8mg/kg/day Divided q 6 h
Tobramycin	Parenteral	5-7.5mg/kg/day Divided q 8 h
Trimethoprim-Sulfamethoxazole	Oral	8-10mg/kg/day Trimethoprim and 40-50mg/kg/day Sulfamethoxazole Divided q 12 h

The antimicrobial spectrum of activity of drugs used for therapy of urinary tract infections is given in the next Table (Adams, H. G., Personal Communication):

Antimicrobial Therapy for Urinary Tract Infections

	Gram-positive cocci			Gram-negative cocci					Anaerobes		
Drug	*S. aureus*	*Strep*	*Enterococci*	*E. coli*	*Klebsiella*	*P. mirabilis*	*Other enterics*	*Pseudomonas a.*	*B. fragilis*	*Others*	*H. influenzae*
Trimethoprim (Trimpex, Proloprim)	3	3		3	3	4	3				3
Trimethoprim-Sulfamethoxazole (Co-Trimoxazole)(Bactrim, Septra)	4	3		3	3	4	3				4
Nitrofurantoin (Macrodantin)	4	3	4	4	2						
Amoxicillin		4	4	2		4			2	3	4*
Norfloxacin	4	±	4	4	4	4	4	3			4
Ciprofloxacin	4	±	4	4	4	4	4	3			4
Sulfisoxazole (Gantrisin)	3	3		3	3	4	3				
Cephalexin (Ist Gen. Ceph.) (Keflex)	4	4		4	4	4				3	
Tetracycline		3		3	3		2		2	2	2
Amoxicillin plus Clavulanate (Augmentin)	4	4	4	3	4	4	3			4	4

4 = best activity; 3 = good activity; 2 = some activity
* = beta-lactamase negative

URINARY TRACT; PATHOGENS, TREATMENT (Cont.)

Treatment of Severe Upper Urinary tract Infections (Pyelonephritis): Patients with severe pyelonephritis require hospitalization. Intravenous antibiotic therapy is usually required. Drug treatment of severe upper urinary tract infections (pyelonephritis) is given in the next Table (Koffer, K.F., American Druggist, pgs. 81-87, June, 1988; Johnson, J.R. and Stamm, W.E., Infect. Dis. North Amer. 1, 773-791, 1987):

Drug Treatment of Severe Upper Urinary Tract Infections (Pyelonephritis)

Medication	Dose	Interval (hours)
Preferred Antibiotic Therapies:		
Third Generation Cephalosporin, eg, Cefotaxime, Ceftazadime or Ceftriaxone.	Varies	Varies
Trimethoprim (TMP)/Sulfamethoxazole	160/800mg	12 hrs., I.V.
Other Recommended Antibiotic Therapies:		
Ampicillin plus	1 gram	6 hrs., I.V.
Gentamicin	1mg/kg	8 hrs., I.V.
First Generation Cephalosporin, eg, Cefazolin (Ancef, Kefzol)	1 gram	8 hrs., I.V.
Mezlocillin (Mezlin)	1 gram	6 hrs., I.V.
Norfloxacin	400mg	12 hrs. (Oral)
Ciprofloxacin	500mg	12 hrs. (Oral)

Therapy is given intravenously until symptoms have improved and the patient is afebrile and able to take oral medication.

The antimicrobial spectrum of activity of drugs used for the therapy of severe upper urinary tract infections (pyelonephritis) is given in the next Table:

Antimicrobial Therapy of Severe Upper Urinary Tract Infections(Pyelonephritis)

	Gram-positive cocci			Gram-negative cocci					Anaerobes		
Classification	*S. aureus*	*Strep*	*Enterococci*	*E. coli*	*Klebsiella*	*P. mirabilis*	*Other enterics*	*Pseudomonas a.*	*B. fragilis*	*Others*	*H. influenzae*
Third Gen. Cephalosporin: eg, Cefotaxime (Claforan)	3	3		4	4	4	4			3	4
Third Gen. Cephalosporin: eg, Ceftazidime (Fortaz)		2		4	4	4	4	4		2	4
Third Gen. Cephalosporin: eg, Ceftriaxone (Rocephin)	2	3		4	4	4	4			3	4
Trimethoprim (TMP)/Sulfamethoxazole (SMX) (Septra, Bactrim)	4	3		3	3	4	3				4
Ampicillin plus		4	4	2		4			2	3	4*
Gentamicin	2			4	4	4	4	3			3
First Gen. Cephalosporin: eg, Cefazolin (Ancef, Kefzol)	4	4		4	4	4				3	
Mezlocillin (Mezlin)		4	3	2	4	4	4	3	4	4	4*
Norfloxacin	4	±	4	4	4	4	4	4			4
Ciprofloxacin	4	±	4	4	4	4	4	4			4

4 = best activity; 3 = good activity; 2 = some activity

* = Beta-lactamase negative

URINARY TRACT; PATHOGENS, TREATMENT (Cont.)

Prophylaxis: Antibiotics for long-term prophylaxis against recurrent urinary tract infection are given in the next Table (Wilhelm, M.P. and Edson, R.S., Mayo Clin. Proc. 62, 1025-1031, 1987; Kopper, K.F., American Druggist, pgs. 81-87, June, 1988):

Prophylaxis Against Recurrent Urinary Tract Infection

Choice	Antibiotic	Dosage	Time	Duration
First-choice agents	Trimethoprim-sulfamethoxazole, single-strength tablet	1/2 or 1 tablet	Every evening	≥ 6 mo.
	Nitrofurantoin (Macrodantin)50mg capsule	1 capsule	Every evening	≥ 6 mo.
	Trimethoprim, 100mg tablet	1/2 tablet	Every evening	≥ 6 mo.
Alternatives	Cephalexin, 250mg capsule	1 capsule	Every evening	≥ 6 mo.
	Methenamine mandelate, 1g tablet	1 tablet	Every 6 h	≥ 6 mo.
	Methenamine hippurate, 1g tablet	1 tablet	Every 12 h	≥ 6 mo.

Each single-strength trimethoprim-sulfamethoxazole tablet consists of 80mg of trimethoprim and 400mg of sulfamethoxazole.

Low-dose trimethoprim-sulfamethoxazole (40/200mg), three times per week at bedtime, proved effective as prophylaxis for urinary tract infection over a period of five years (Nicolle, L.E. et al., J. Infect. Dis. 157, 1239-1242, 1988).

Trimethoprim-Sulfamethoxazole(Septra, Bactrim): This combination is effective in single-dose, 3 day, and conventional treatment regimens for lower urinary tract infections (Gossius, G. and Vorland, L., Scand. J. Infect. Dis. 16, 373-379, 1984): This combination is the "gold standard" single-dose drug (Wilhelm, M.P. and Edson, R.S., Mayo Clin. Proc. 62, 1025-1031, 1987).

The advantages of using this combination is that they act synergistically and emergence of resistant bacteria is decreased. Each double-strength tablet consists of 160mg of trimethoprim and 800mg of sulfamethoxazole. Each single-strength tablet consists of 80mg of trimethoprim and 400mg of sulfamethoxazole.

Trimethoprim(TMP): Trimethoprim, when used alone, is as effective as trimethoprim/sulfamethoxazole in the treatment of cystitis and is associated with fewer side effects, presumable because of the absence of the sulfa component (Harbord, R.B. and Gruneberg, R.N., Br. Med. J. 283, 1301, 1981).

Nitrofurantoin: Nitrofurantoin is available in two forms: microcystalline (Furadantin) and macrocrystalline (Macrodantin); the macrocrystalline form is preferred because it is absorbed and excreted more slowly. Nitrofurantoin is active only in the urinary tract and will not affect vaginal flora.

Amoxicillin: Orally administered amoxicillin is preferred over oral ampicillin because it is more completely absorbed and may be given every 8hrs.

A single 3-g dose (six 500-g capsules) is effective for the treatment of uncomplicated lower urinary tract infection in women (Rubin, R. H. et al., JAMA 244, 561-564, 1980).

Amoxicillin plus Clavulanate: The combination of clavulanate (a beta-lactamase inhibitor) and amoxicillin which is marketed as Augmentin results in a considerable antimicrobial spectrum with activity against penicillin-resistant S. aureus and beta-lactamase producing E. coli, Klebsiella, and Proteus.

Cephalosporin: Ceftriaxone, A Third Generation Cephalosporin: Once daily intramuscular ceftriaxone (initial dose of 75mg/kg/day followed by 50mg/kg/day, max. 1.5g/day) was successfully in treating serious community-acquired pediatric infections, including urinary tract infections; four patients had E. coli and one patient had K. pneumoniae. Clinical improvement occurred within 36 hours. There was very significant saving in hospitalization (Dagan, R. et al., Pediatr. Infect. Dis. J. 6, 1080-1084, 1987).

Fluoroquinolones: The fluoroquinolones, norfloxacin and ciprofloxacin, produce very high concentrations of drug in the urine. It has been shown that these two fluoroquinolones are at least as effective as trimethoprim/sulfamethoxazole (TMP/SMZ) and amoxicillin in the treatment of uncomplicated or complicated urinary tract infection. (Malinverni, R. and Glauser, M.P. Reviews Infect. Dis. 10, Suppl. 1, S153-S163, Jan.-Feb. 1988; Neu, H.C., Med. Clin. No. Amer. 72, No. 3, 623-636, 1988; Walker, R.C. and Wright, A.J., Mayo Clin. Proc. 62, 1007-1012, 1987).

The fluoroquinolones may be highly effective in patients with urinary tract infections due to P. aeruginosa. These drugs are effective in the treatment of pyelonephritis and cystitis.

UROKINASE

(Abbokinase)

USES: Urokinase is an enzyme produced by human renal parenchymal cells and is isolated from human urine or tissue cultures of human kidneys; it is used as a **thrombolytic agent** in the conditions given in the next Table:

Uses of Urokinase
Acute Coronary Artery Thrombosis and Myocardial Infarction
Acute Massive Pulmonary Embolism
Acute Deep-Vein Thrombosis
Acute Arterial Thrombosis and Embolism
Occluded Arteriovenous Cannulae

Acute Coronary Artery Thrombosis and Myocardial Infarction: Intracoronary route: Therapy with urokinase should be started within 4 hours after onset of symptoms; this route has largely been abandoned for the IV route due to the delay in therapy involved; limited availability, expense, and conflicting results - probably as a result of delay in therapy (Marder, V.J. and Sherry, S., "Thrombolytic Therapy: Current Status," NEJM 318, 1585-1595, 1988). Intravenous route: Use of this method avoids the complications associated with intracoronary catheterization.

Urokinase is the least studied thrombolytic agent. It is currently approved only for intracoronary administration, not for intravenous administration. Intravenous use is currently under investigation (Anderson, J.L., J. of Critical Illness 5, 77-84, January, 1990).

Acute Massive Pulmonary Embolism: Embolism should first be confirmed by pulmonary angiography. Heparin may be given while the diagnosis is being confirmed but is discontinued prior to infusion of urokinase; urokinase may be useful up to 7 days after embolism has occurred. tPA acts more rapidly and is safer than urokinase in the treatment of acute pulmonary embolism (Goldhaber, S.Z., et al., Lancet, 293-298, 1988).

Acute Deep-Vein Thrombosis: Urokinase should be used within 72 hours after thrombosis has occurred; two-thirds of thrombi can be dissolved.

Peripheral Artery Thrombosis: Thrombolytic therapy may be effective in the first 72 hrs.

Mechanism of Action: Thrombolytic agents, e.g., streptokinase or urokinase dissolve existing thrombi through a proteolytic action in the supporting fibrin network; the fibrinolytic system is illustrated in the next Figure:

Fibrinolytic System

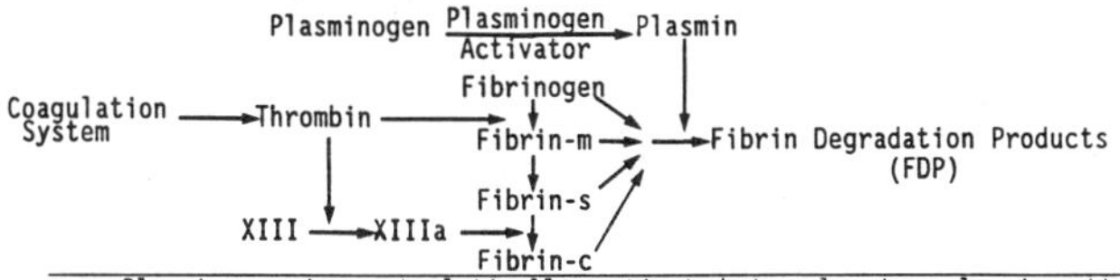

Plasminogen is proteolytically activated to plasmin; plasmin attacks fibrinogen and fibrin to produce fibrin degradation products(FDP). Urokinase is a pharmacologic activator of plasminogen, directly stimulating the conversion of plasminogen to plasmin. Plasmin is a protease which digests fibrin and fibrinogen to produce fibrin degradation products(FDP). FDP inhibit thrombin's conversion of fibrinogen to fibrin and thereby become circulating anticoagulants themselves. Plasmin also hydrolyzes prothrombin, factors V, VIII, and XII, the first component of complement and prekallikrein.

Both urokinase and streptokinase are equally effective in reperfusing occluded coronary arteries in patients with acute myocardial infarction; however, streptokinase cost much less than urokinase. Urokinase may be used if streptokinase resistance is high or when a second course of treatment is required; furthermore, urokinase is nonantigenic and does not cause allergic reactions as does streptokinase.

UROKINASE (Cont.)
DOSAGE FORMS: Inj: 5,000; 9,000; 250,000IU.
DOSAGE: Urokinase is administered IV, intracoronary and intra-arterial; dosage is given in the next Table:

Dosage of Urokinase

Condition	Route	Dosage
Acute Myocardial Infarction	Intra-coronary	Add contents of 3 reconstituted vials to (750,000 IU) to 500ml of 5% dextrose in water(1500IU/ml). Give 2,500-10,000 units of heparin; perform angiograph; give urokinase 6,000IU/min(4ml/min of sol'n). Monitor by angiography at 15-min intervals. Average total dose necessary for lysis of coronary artery thrombi is 500,000 IU.
	IV	Investigational: 1.5 million units initially, then 1.5 million units over 90 minutes.
Pulmonary Embolism	IV	4,400IU/kg infused over a period of ten min. followed by continuous infusion of 4,400IU/kg per hour for 12 to 24 hrs. Then given heparin and later oral anticoagulants.
Occluded Intravenous Catheter		5,000IU/ml instilled by tuberculin syringe in amounts equal to the internal volume of the catheter. Attempt aspiration of clot and urokinase after 5-10 min. Repeat attempt to aspirate every 5 minutes until catheter is patent.

PHARMACOKINETICS: Onset: Immediate; Duration: 12 hrs. after discontinuation; Half-Life: 16 min.
ADVERSE EFFECTS: Bleeding is the most common adverse effect. Severe internal bleeding occurs occasionally; rarely cerebral hemorrhage occurs. Allergic reactions occur much less frequently than with streptokinase.
CONTRAINDICATIONS: Active internal bleeding, history of cerebrovascular accident, recent intracranial or intraspinal surgery or trauma, intracranial neoplasm, arteriovenous malformation intracranial aneurysm, known bleeding diathesis, severe uncontrolled hypertension.

Anaphylactoid reactions are rare.

MONITOR: The tests that are done to monitor thrombolytic therapy (streptokinase or urokinase) are given in the next Table; (Sharma, G.V.R.K. et al., N. Engl. J. Med. 306, 1268-1276, 1982):

Tests to Monitor Thrombolytic Activity

Tests	Comment
Euglobulin Lysis Time	Most sensitive test but is not available in most laboratories
Thrombin Time	Next most sensitive test
Partial Thromboplastin Time(PTT)	Less Sensitive
Prothrombin Time(PT)	Less sensitive
Fibrin Degradation Products(FDP)	Less sensitive

The timing of the tests is given in the next Table:

Timing of Testing and Objective

Before Therapy
- Detect and correct coagulation defects (by means of thrombin, partial thromboplastin, and prothrombin times)
- Determine base line or control for fibrinolysis (any of the above tests; euglobulin lysis time or fibrin(ogen) degradation products if patient has been receiving heparin)

Drug Therapy (3-4 hr after start)
- Use same test(s) used for establishing base line or control

After Therapy
- Use partial thromboplastin time if heparin therapy is to begin

Objective
- Ensure establishment of fibrinolytic state:
- Determine whether values have marked prolongation over control value

VALPROIC ACID

(Depakene, Depakote)

USES: Valproic acid is an **anticonvulsant;** uses are given in the next Table:

Uses of Valproic Acid
Absence (Petit Mal) Seizures (FDA approved)
Widely used for **Primary Generalized Tonic-Clonic, Myoclonic** and **Atonic Seizures,** and for patients with **Mixed Forms of Generalized Seizures** (Penry, J.K. ed., Am. J. Med. 84, suppl. 1A, 1988).
Partial Seizures (Dean, J.C. and Penry, J.K., Epilepsia 29, 140, 1988)

DOSAGE FORMS: Sol'n 250mg/5ml; Caps: 125mg (sprinkles) 250mg; Tabs; Enteric-Coated: 125, 250, 500mg.

DOSAGE: Valproic acid is administered orally or rectally. Valproic acid capsules should be swallowed whole, not chewed, in order to prevent local irritation of the mouth and throat. If GI irritation occurs, the drug may be administered with food. Rectal administration by retention enema; dilute syrup 1:1 with water. The drug is well absorbed by this route. Rectal and oral doses are are equivalent. Dosage is given in the next Table:

Patient	Dosage
Children or Adults	Initial Dose: 10-15mg/kg daily in 1-3 divided doses. Weekly Intervals: May increase dose by 5-10mg/kg daily until seizures are controlled or adverse effects prevent further increases in dosage. Maximum recommended dosage is 60mg/kg daily. The drug should be administered in 2 or more divided doses when the dosage exceeds 250mg daily. Usual maintenance: 30-60mg/kg daily.

PHARMACOKINETICS: Time to steady state: 2-4 days; Therapeutic level: 50-100 mg/liter.

ADVERSE EFFECTS: GI, liver, hematologic toxicity, leukopenia, red blood cell aplasia and thrombocytopenia; weight gain, transient alopecia, rash, tremor, headache and insomnia.

Common adverse effects include nausea and vomiting, which may be minimized by using enteric-coated formulation (Depakote) or by taking the drug with food.

Valproate can interfere with conversion of ammonia to urea and infrequently causes lethargy associated with increased blood ammonia concentrations (Eadie, M.J. et al., Med. Toxicol. 3, 85, 1988).

Pancreatitis can also occur, and interstitial nephritis has been reported (Lin, C-Y and Chiang, H., Nephron. 48, 43, 1988). The most severe adverse reaction is hepatotoxicity which may lead to acute hepatic failure and death; this is rare but liver function tests should be performed every two months for six months after starting valproate.

DRUG INTERACTIONS: Increases phenobarbital levels by 30-40%. There is a transient decrease in phenytoin levels which returns to previous levels in several weeks.

MONITOR: Therapeutic levels: 50-100 micrograms/ml. Measure liver function tests every 2 months for 6 months after starting therapy.

VANCOMYCIN

(Lyphocin, Vancocin, Vancoled)

USES: Vancomycin is active against most **gram-positive organisms** but generally not gram-negative organisms, fungi, or yeast. Activities of vancomycin are given in the next Table (Levine, J.F., Med. Clin. No. Am. 71, 1135-1145, Nov. 1987; Adams, H.B., Personal Comm.):

Activities of Vancomycin

	Gram-positive cocci			Gram-negative bacilli				Anaerobes	
	S. aureus	Streptococci	Strep. entero.	H. influenzae	PEcK	Other Enterics	Pseudomonas a.	B. fragilis	Res. Anaerobes
Vancomycin	4	4	4	▩	▩	▩	▩	▩	▩

4=best activity; 3=good activity; 2=some activity; ▩ =little or no activity; PEcK (Mnemonic)= P. mirabilis, E. coli, Klebsiella; Res.= Resident

Vancomycin is bactericidal against the gram-positive organisms: Staphylococcus aureus and Staphylococcus epidermidis, both methicillin-susceptible and methicillin-resistant, diphtheroids, hemolytic streptococci, pneumococci, clostridium and viridans streptococci. It is bacteriostatic against enterococcus (Levine, J.F., Med. Clin. No. Am. 71, 1135-1145, Nov. 1987).

Parenteral vancomycin is the **drug of choice** for **treatment of methicillin-resistant staphylococcal infections**; it can also be used to treat other gram-positive infections in patients allergic to penicillin. **Oral vancomycin** is the **drug of choice for C. difficile enterocolitis.**

Examples of conditions that have been successfully treated with vancomycin are listed in the next Table:

Examples of Conditions Treated with Vancomycin
Endocarditis
Osteomyelitis
Pneumonia
Septicemia
Soft-Tissue Infections

High-risk patients for staphylococcal infections are patients with diabetes mellitus, peripheral vascular disease or burn wounds, prosthetic valve endocarditis, infected CSF shunts and granulocytopenic children with cancer, hemodialysis patients, peritoneal dialysis patients.

IV vancomycin is used for prophylaxis of bacterial endocarditis in penicillin-allergic adults and children with congenital heart disease, rheumatic or other acquired valvular heart disease, prosthetic or graft heart valves, idiopathic hypertrophic subaortic stenosis or mitral valve prolapse who undergo dental procedures that are likely to cause gingival bleeding, minor upper respiratory tract surgery or instrumentation. IV vancomycin is also used for prophylaxis in penicillin-allergic adults and children undergoing GI, biliary, or genitourinary tract surgery or instrumentation who are at risk of developing enterococcal endocarditis.

DOSAGE FORMS: Caps: 125, 250mg; Oral Sol'n: 1g, 10g; Parenteral: 500mg, 1g.

VANCOMYCIN (Cont.)

DOSAGE: Vancomycin is administered by slow IV infusion (usually over 1 hour), or orally. Dosage is given in the next Table:

Dosage of Vancomycin

Condition	Age	Route	Dosage
Usual Use	Adult	IV	2 grams per day, given in divided doses every 6 or 12 hours and infused over a period of at least one hour.
	Children	IV	Usual: 30mg/kg daily in 3 divided doses. CNS inf: 45mg/kg daily in 3 divided doses
	Neonates:	IV	10mg/kg/dose; CNS inf: 15mg/kg/dose.
	<7d, <1kg		Every 24 hr. dosing.
	<7d, 1-2kg		Every 18 hr. dosing.
	<7d, >2kg		Every 12 hr. dosing.
	>7d, <1kg		Every 18 hr. dosing.
	>7d, 1-2kg		Every 12 hr. dosing.
	>7d, >2kg		Every 8 hr. dosing.
Pseudomembranous colitis caused by C. difficile	Adult	Oral	125-500mg every 6 hours for 7-10 days
	Children	Oral	40-50mg/kg daily in 4 divided doses for 7-10 days

The dosage must be decreased in patients with renal impairment; a nomogram is provided in the package insert.

ADVERSE EFFECTS: Rapid IV infusion of vancomycin may cause pruritis, flushing of the face, neck, and torso ("red neck" or "red man syndrome"). Rapid bolus injection can also cause pain and muscle spasms of the chest and back. Life-threatening hypotension and cardiac arrest have occurred. The effect of vancomycin is usually due to a decrease in strength of contraction of the heart (negative inotropic effect) and vasodilation effect produced, in part, by histamine release. The phenomena may be an anaphylactoid reaction. Steroids [eg, 125mg methylprednisolone and the antihistamine, diphenhydramine (25mg)] tend to counteract these effects. These reactions can be minimized in most patients if the drug is infused slowly (Southorn, P.A. et al., Mayo Clin. Proc. 6, 721-724, Sept. 1986; Levy, M. et al., Pediatr. 86, 572-580, 1990).

The incidence of nephrotoxicity, which is usually reversible, has become uncommon in recent years (Farber, B.F. and Moellering, R.C., Jr., Antimicrob. Agents Chemother. 23, 138, 1983). Ototoxicity is rare and may be irreversible; it is probably associated with very high serum concentrations. Both nephrotoxicity and ototoxicity may be increased by concurrent use of aminoglycosides (Sorrell, T.C. and Collignon, P.J., J. Antimicrob. Chemother. 16, 235, 1985). Other adverse effects include reversible neutropenia, drug fever, and allergic rashes and phlebitis after IV injection.

MONITOR: Therapeutic Levels: Peak: 25-40 micrograms/ml; Trough: <5-10 micrograms/ml.

VASOPRESSIN (Antidiuretic Hormone, ADH)
(Pitressin)

USES: Vasopressin is a polypeptide (9-amino acids) hormone secreted by the hypothalamus and stored in the posterior pituitary; exogeneous vasopressin elicits all the pharmacologic responses usually produced by endogenous vasopressin (antidiuretic hormone, ADH). Uses of vasopressin are given in the next Table:

Uses of Vasopressin
Diabetes Insipidus
Stimulate Peristalsis (eg, postoperative abdominal distension, dispel gas prior to abdominal radiographic procedures)-used rarely
Diagnostic Uses: Differentiate Nephrogenic, Psychogenic, and Neurohypophyseal Diabetes Insipidus
GI Hemorrhage

DOSAGE FORMS: Vasopressin Injection: 20 units/ml (aqueous).

DOSAGE: Vasopression injection may be administered IM, IV, subcutaneously or applied topically to the nasal mucosa. Vasopressin injection has also been administered by continuous IV or intra-arterial infusion in the management of GI hemorrhage. Dosage is given in the next Table:

Dosage of Vasopressin

Condition	Age	Route	Dosage
Diabetes Insipidus	Adults	IM or Subcut.	Vasopressin Injection: 5-10 units, 2-4 times daily; range of dosage, 5-60 units daily
	Children	IM or Subcut.	Vasopressin Injection: 2.5-10 units, 2-4 times daily
		Nose	Vasopressin Injection: Titrate dose to achieve control of thirst and urination
Abdominal Distention	Adults	IM	Vasopressin Injection:5 units initially; subsequent injections every 3-4 hours with doses increased to 10 units as necessary.
	Children	IM	Vasopressin Injection: Proportionately reduced doses
Abdominal Radiographs and Kidney Biopsy	Adults	Subcut.	Vasopressin Injection: 5-15 units at 2 hrs. and at 30 minutes prior to abdominal radiographs and kidney biopsy; enema may be given prior to first dose
GI Hemorrhage	Adults	IV or Intra-arterial	Vasopression Injection: Mix with 0.9% sodium chloride or 5% dextrose to a concentration of 0.1-1.0 unit/ml, administer 0.2-0.9 units/minute. Titrate to effect.

ADVERSE EFFECTS: Tremor, sweating, vertigo, abdominal discomfort, nausea, vomiting, urticaria, anaphylaxis.

Overhydration with hyponatremia may occur, especially in children.

Large doses may cause myocardial infarction or other vascular insufficiency, particularly with IV or intraarterial infusion. Patients given vasopressin by IV or intraarterial infusion are often treated simultaneously with nitroglycerin infusion to minimize the risk of myocardial ischemia.

VECURONIUM
(Norcuron)

USES: **Vecuronium Bromide** is a **competitive, nondepolarizing neuromuscular blocking agent** used mainly to produce skeletal muscle relaxation in conditions listed in the next Table:

Uses of Vecuronium Bromide
During Surgery after General Anesthesia has been Induced
Increase Pulmonary Compliance during Assisted or Controlled Respirations
Facilitate Endotracheal Intubation
Facilitate Mechanical Ventilation in Intensive Care Settings

Vecuronium has minimal cardiovascular side effects and is relatively short acting. Excretion depends on biliary elimination; atracurium may be preferred to vecuronium in patients with hepatic impairment.

DOSAGE FORMS: IV Injection: 10mg vials.

DOSAGE: Vecuronium bromide is given IV; dosages are the same for adults and children and are given in the next Table:

Dosage of Vecuronium Bromide

Route	Dosage
IV bolus	Initially, 0.08-0.1mg/kg followed by 0.01-0.015mg/kg every 30-60 minutes. Use higher doses for more prolonged effects.
IV infusion	Usual: 1 microgram/kg/minute (Range: 0.5-1.7 microgram/kg/min).

ADVERSE EFFECTS: Respiratory paralysis will occur; provisions for maintenance of oxygenation and ventilation must be available. Cardiovascular effects are usually minimal and transient. Histamine release does not occur. Patients receiving continuous IV infusion of vecuronium may have prolonged paralysis after discontinuation of drip unless level of myoneuronal blockade is assessed frequently. In patients maintained at 90% myoneuronal blockade, average recovery time is 28 minutes (Darrah, W.C. et al., Crit. Care Med. 17, 1297-1300, 1987).

VERAPAMIL
(Isoptin, Calan, Verelan)

USES: Verapamil is a **calcium-channel blocking drug;** uses are given in the next Table:

Uses Of Verapamil
Supraventricular Tachyarrhythmias: Management and Prevention
Control of Ventricular Rate in Patients with Atrial Flutter or Fibrillation
Angina: Prinzmetal Variant Angina; Unstable or Chronic
Hypertension
Nocturnal Leg Cramps (Preliminary Data)

Supraventricular Tachyarrhythmias: IV verapamil is currently the drug of choice for rapid conversion of reentrant paroxysmal supraventricular tachycardias (PSVT) in adults that is unresponsive to vagal stimulation (eg, Valsalva's maneuver), including PSVT associated with accessory bypass tracts (eg, Wolff-Parkinson-White or Lown-Ganong-Levine syndrome). In the majority of patients with PSVT, conversion to sinus rhythm is achieved within 10 minutes with IV verapamil. Adenosine may soon replace verapamil as the drug of choice for PSVT; in some centers, this has already occurred. Oral verapamil has been effective in preventing recurrent PSVT in some patients.

Control of Ventricular Rate in Patients with Atrial Flutter or Fibrillation: In patients with flutter or fibrillation, IV verapamil is used to temporarily control rapid ventricular rate, usually decreasing heart rate by at least 20%. The drug rarely converts atrial flutter or fibrillation to normal sinus rhythm.

Angina: The uses of verapamil in different types of angina are given in the next Table:

Uses of Verapamil in Angina

Angina	Verapamil
Prinzmetal Variant Angina	Oral calcium-channel blocking agents are drugs of choice
Unstable or Chronic Stable Angina Pectoris	As effective as beta-adrenergic blocking agents (eg, propranolol) and/or nitrates; verapamil may reduce frequency of attacks allowing a dec. in sublingual nitroglycerine dosage, and inc. patient's exercise tolerance.

Treatment of hypertension with verapamil is given in the next Table (The 1988 Report of the Joint National Committee on Detection, Evaluation, and Treatment of High Blood Pressure, Arch. Intern. Med. 148, 1023-1038, 1988):

Treatment of Hypertension with Verapamil

Step 1: Nonpharmacologic Approaches (see **HYPERTENSION**)
↓
Step 2: Verapamil (Usual Minimum, 120 mg/day; Usual Maximum, 480 mg/day)
Observe up to 6 months; if treatment ineffective then,
↓
Step 3: Add a second drug of a different class
or Increase the dosage of verapamil
or Substitute another drug
↓
Step 4: Add a third drug of a different class
or Substitute a second drug
↓
Step 5: Consider further evaluation and/or referral
or Add a third or fourth drug

"Step-Down": For patients with mild hypertension, after 1 year of control, consider decreasing or withdrawing verapamil and other hypotensive drugs.

Nocturnal Leg Cramps: Recurrent nocturnal leg cramps, unresponsive to quinine, were treated successfully with verapamil (8 patients, 7 responded). The dosage was as follows: single oral dose of 120mg of verapamil at night for 8 weeks; usually, no improvement occurred until approximately 6 days of verapamil. No adverse effects of any type were reported (Baltodano, N., Arch. Intern. Med. 148, 1969-1970, 1988).

Mechanism of Action: Verapamil is a calcium ion blocking agent; it acts on the slow (calcium) channel, blocking the influx of calcium ion. It acts on cardiac tissue and arterial smooth muscle cells.

VERAPAMIL (Cont.)

DOSAGE FORMS: Tabs: 40, 80, 120mg; Tabs(extended release): 180, 240mg; Caps(extended release): 120, 240mg; Injection: 2.5mg/ml

DOSAGE: Verapamil is usually administered IV in the management of supraventricular tachyarrhythmais; for IV administration, verapamil is given slowly as a direct injection over a period of not less than 2 minutes or, in geriatric patients, of not less than 3 minutes. Verapamil is administered orally in the management of Prinzmetal variant angina or unstable or chronic stable angina.

The dosage of verapamil is given in the next Table:

Dosage of Verapamil

Condition	Age	Route	Dosage
Supraventricular Tachyarrhythmias	Adults	IV	5-10mg (0.075-0.15mg/kg); if necessary give second dose, 10mg (0.15mg/kg), 30 minutes after initial dose.
	< 1 yr.	IV	0.1-0.2mg/kg; repeat in 30 min. if necessary, monitor ECG continously. Use with extreme caution; may cause apnea, bradycardia or hypotension.
	1-15 yrs.	IV	0.1-0.3mg/kg; do not exceed 5mg; repeat in 30 min. if necessary, repeat; do not exceed 10mg
Usual	Adults	Oral	40-120mg every 8 hrs.
	Children	Oral	4-10mg/kg daily in 3 divided doses (max: adult dose).
Angina: Prinzmetal Variant Angina; or Unstable or Chronic Angina Pectoris	Adults	Oral	80mg every 6-8 hrs; increase, as necessary, by 80mg increments at weekly intervals, or, in patients with unstable angina, at daily intervals until optimum control. Max therapeutic response, 24-48 hrs. Maintenance dose:240-480mg daily, given in 3 or 4 divided doses.
Nocturnal Leg Cramps	Adults	Oral	120mg of verapamil at night.

The dosage of verapamil in adults with renal and/or hepatic impairment is given in the next Table:

Dosage of Verapamil in Adult Patients with Renal and/or Hepatic Impairment

Condition	Route	Dosage
Supraventricular Tachyarrhythmias	IV	5-10mg (0.075-0.15mg/kg). If second IV dose essential, reduce dose and give 60-90 min. after initial dose and monitor(BP,P-R interval)
Angina	Oral	Reduce dosage up to 60-70%

ADVERSE EFFECTS: Constipation is the most common side effect; other side effects include headache, vertigo, weakness, nervousness, pruritis, flushing, rash and gastric disturbances.

Cardiovascular adverse effects include orthostatic hypotension, A-V block, A-V dissociation, pedal edema, pulmonary edema, and CHF.

Rebound angina is associated with sudden withdrawal of verapamil.

Other adverse effects have included hyperprolactinemia, galactorrhea and feelings of coldness and numbness.

. Infants are particularly prone to adverse electrophysiologic and hemodynamic effects on the myocardium including hypotension, sinus bradycardia and asystole. Appropriate monitoring capabilities, calcium, volume and other advanced cardiac life support measures should be readily available (Porter, C.J. et al., Pediatrics 71, 748-755, 1983).

CONTRAINDICATIONS: Sick sinus syndrome, second- or third-degree A-V block, cardiogenic shock, or advanced congestive heart failure except when cardiac failure is secondary to supraventricular tachyarrhythmia. Severe adverse reactions have occurred in some patients with hypertrophic cardiomyopathy. Other contraindications include hypotension and severe hepatic disease. Use with extreme caution or not at all in patients under 1 year of age.

PHARMACOKINETICS: Bioavailability: 20-35%; Metabolism: Liver; there are active metabolites; Half-Life: 6-12 hours (increased in cirrhosis); Protein-Binding: 90%; Urinary Excretion of Unchanged Drug: 3-4%.

VERAPAMIL (Cont.)

DRUG INTERACTIONS: Interactions of verapamil are given in the next Table:

Drug Interactions of Verapamil

Drug	Interactions
Beta-Blockers, eg, Propranolol Metoprolol, including Timolol Eyedrops, etc.	With IV verapamil, severe hypotension, bradycardia and asystole. With oral verapamil, severe hypotension, bradycardia, cardiac failure, and heart block. Do not use beta blockers and verapamil together if left ventricular function is compromised.
Digoxin	Digoxin levels increased 50-75%.
Oral Quinidine	WithIV verapamil, severe hypotension.
Rifampin and other Enzyme-Inducing Drugs	Bioavailability of verapamil is reduced.
Cimetidine	The clearance of verapamil may be reduced.
Antihypertensives	Additive lowering of blood pressure.
Theophylline	Levels are increased.
Cyclosporine	Levels are increased.
Dantrolene	Cardiovascular collapse with fatal hyperkalemia may occur.

Numerous other potential drug interactions exist; verapamil should be used with caution in patients taking any drug that is highly protein bound.

MONITOR: Continuous ECG monitoring during IV administration.

VIDARABINE

(Adenine Arabinoside, Ara-A, Vira-A)

USES: **Vidarabine** is a purine nucleoside. It is an **antiviral agent;** uses are given in the next Table:

Uses of Vidarabine

Herpes Zoster (Shingles, Zoster) caused by reactivated Varicella-Zoster infections in Immunocompromised Adults and Children
Varicella-Zoster (Chickenpox) Infections in Immunocompromised Patients
Herpes Simplex Infections
Ophthalmic Uses:
Herpes Simplex Keratitis and Keratoconjunctivitis
Vaccine Keratitis

Vidarabine is considered an alternative therapy in Herpes Zoster, Varicella-Zoster, and Herpes Simplex infections due to effectiveness, ease of administration, and relatively fewer side effects of acyclovir.

Herpes Zoster: When vidarabine is used in immunocompromised patients with varicella-zoster infections, there is reduced severity of acute pain, accelerated vesicle healing and cessation of new vesicle formation, reduced cutaneous dissemination of the infection and the frequency of zoster-related visceral complications (uveitis or keratitis, hepatitis, encephalitis, and peripheral neuropathy), and decreased duration of post-herpetic neuralgia.The drug is not effective in the treatment of encephalitis caused by varicella-zoster. Acyclovir is the drug of choice (Medical Letter 32, 73-78, August 10, 1990).

Varicella-Zoster (Chickenpox) Infections in Immunocompromised Patients: When used early in the treatment of patients with varicella-zoster infections, vidarabine reduces the rate of formation of new vesicle formation and defervescence of the infection, and reduces the frequency of infection-related visceral complications. Acyclovir is the drug of choice (Medical Letter 32, 73-78, August 10, 1990).

Herpes Simplex Infections: IV vidarabine is used in the treatment of encephalitis caused by herpes simplex virus; however, acyclovir is apparently more effective than vidarabine in the treatment of herpes simplex encephalitis.

Vidarabine is used in the treatment of mucosal, cutaneous, localized CNS, and disseminated herpes simplex infections in neonates. In neonates with localized skin, eye, or mouth infections, vidarabine therapy prevents severe ocular and neurologic sequalae; vidarabine reduced mortality of patients with localized CNS disease or disseminated disease.

Ophthalmic Uses: Vidarabine is used topically in the treatment of keratitis and keratoconjunctivitis caused by herpes simplex virus, types 1 and 2. Epithelial infections may show a response to treatment within 2-4 days and heal completely in 1-3 weeks.

Apparently, there is no significant difference between topical vidarabine, idoxuride or trifluridine in time required for complete epithelial healing or superficial herpetic keratitis. Topical vidarabine is effective in treating recurrent disease in patients intolerant of or resistant to topical trifluridine.

DOSAGE FORMS: Parenteral: 200mg/ml; Ophth. Oint.: 3%.

VIDARABINE (Cont.)

DOSAGE: Vidarabine is administered by IV infusion over a period of 12-24 hours using an in line membrane filter with a pore size of 0.45 micrometer or smaller; pre-warm IV fluid, maximum concentration 0.45mg/ml. Dosage is given in the next Table:

Dosage of Vidarabine

Condition	Age	Route	Dosage
Normal Renal Function			
Herpes Simplex Encephalitis	Adults & Children	IV	15mg/kg daily for 10 days.
	Neonates	IV	15-30mg/kg daily for 10-14 days.
Herpes Zoster	Adults & Children	IV	10mg/kg daily for 5 days.
Varicella-Zoster (Chickenpox)	Neonates	IV	10mg/kg daily for 5 days.
Renal Impairment			If glomerular filtrate rate(GFR) <10ml/min., give 75% of usual vidarabine dose.
Topical Ophthalmic Application			Apply 3% ointment inside the lower conjunctival sac, 5 times daily at 3-hour intervals. If no signs of improvement after 7 days, or if complete re-epithelization has not occurred by 21 days, discontinue and change therapy.

ADVERSE EFFECTS: Use with caution in renal and hepatic disease. Do not dilute in biologic or colloid fluids. Neurologic side effects include tremor, ataxia, peripheral neuropathy, and encephalopathy.

LABORATORY: Document HSV infection prior to therapy. Monitor hepatic and hematologic status.

VINCRISTINE
(Oncovin)

USES: Vincristine is an **antineoplastic drug.** Vincristine acts by binding to microtubular proteins, blocking formation of the mitotic spindle, thus preventing polymerization and causing metaphase arrest. Vincristine has been used extensively in combination regimens because of its relative lack of hematologic toxicity. Uses are given in the next Table:

Uses of Vincristine
Acute and Chronic Leukemias
Hodgkin's Disease
Non-Hodgkin's Lymphomas
Neuroblastoma
Rhabdomyosarcoma
Wilm's Tumor
Ewing's Sarcoma
Others: Breast Carcinoma; Small Cell Carcinoma of the Lung, Multiple Myeloma, Brain Medulloblastoma

DOSAGE FORMS: Inj.: 1mg/ml.

DOSAGE: Vincristine sulfates is administered only by IV injection. It may be injected into the tubing or sidearm of a free-flowing IV infusion or directly into a vein over about a 1-minute period. Prevent extravasation. Intrathecal administration causes death. Consult protocols for dosage and the method and sequence of administration. Usual dosage is given in the next Table:

Usual Dosage of Vincristine

Age	Dosage
Adults	$1.4mg/m^2$ once weekly (max. $2mg/m^2$)
Children, >1 year	$2mg/m^2$ once weekly
Children, <10kg or Body Surface Area <$1m^2$	0.05mg/kg once weekly

Reduce dosage by 50% in patients with hepatic impairment (direct bilirubin >3mg/dL).

VINCRISTINE (Cont.)
PHARMACOKINETICS: Half-Life: Triphasic: 0.077 hr. and 2.3 hr. and 85 hr.; Metabolism: Incompletely metabolized by liver; Elimination: Primary bile; 70% of dose is excreted in feces; 12% in urine; Distribution: Vincristine does not penetrate the central nervous system(CNS).
ADVERSE EFFECTS: The major toxicity of vincristine is peripheral neuropathy. Loss of the Achilles tendon reflex is usually the first sign of peripheral neuropathy. Mild sensory neuropathy is common but does not require discontinuance of the drug. Other and more serious manifestations include: paresthesias, loss of deep tendon reflexes, ataxia, foot drop and muscle wasting. The muscle groups most often involved are the dorsiflexors of the hands and wrist and the extensors of the feet.

Alopecia is found in 20-70% of patients. Constipation and abdominal pain occur frequently; treat with enemas and laxatives. SIADH occurs rarely.

VITAMIN K_1

(AquaMEPHYTON, Konakion, Mephyton, Phytonadione)

USES: This preparation is identical to naturally occurring vitamin K_1. Vitamin K_1 is responsible for the synthesis of the **blood coagulation factors** in the liver; these factors are listed in the next Table:

Blood Coagulation Factors Requiring Vitamin K_1	
II	**Prothrombin**
VII	**Proconvertin**
IX	**Christmas Factor or Plasma Thromboplastin Component**
X	**Stuart-Prower Factor**

Vitamin K_1 is used in the prevention and treatment of hypoprothrombinemia caused by vitamin K_1 deficiency; uses of vitamin K_1 are given in the next Table:

Uses of Vitamin K_1 in Hypoprothrombinemia
Anticoagulant-Induced Hypoprothrombinemia: Drug of choice for treatment of of moderate or severe hemorrhage caused by overdose of coumarin or indandion derivatives. Ingestion of superwarfarin compounds commonly used as rodenticides may require prolonged therapy.
Hemorrhagic Disease of the Newborn: Prophylaxis and treatment.
Neonatal Hemorrhage resulting from anticonvulsant therapy during pregnancy.
Hypoprothrombinemia from other Causes: Infants who are breast fed or receiving milk substitute formulas; prolonged hyperalimentation; malabsorption syndrome: sprue, celiac disease, ulcerative colitis, regional enteritis, cystic fibrosis, prolonged diarrhea, obstructive jaundice, internal biliary fistula, dysentery, extensive diarrhea.
Hypoprothrombinemia induced by certain Drugs: salicylates, sulfonamides, quinine, quinidine or broad-spectrum antibiotic therapy

Hemorrhagic Disease of the Newborn: The American Academy of Pediatrics recommends that vitamin K_1 (phytonadione) be routinely administered to infants at birth to prevent hemorrhagic disease of the newborn; some state regulations currently require vitamin K prophylaxis in neonates. Dietary sources of vitamin K are inadequate during the first 5-8 days of the neonatal period.
Breast-Fed Infants with Diarrhea: Breast-fed infants who develop diarrhea of longer than several days' duration should receive vitmain K_1 (phytonadione) prophylactically.

VITAMIN K_1 (Cont.)

DOSAGE FORMS: Oral(Mephyton): Tabs 5mg; IV(AquaMEPHYTON): 2, 10mg/ml; IM(Konakion): 2, 10mg/ml.

DOSAGE: Vitamin K_1 (phytonadione) is administered orally or parenterally; dosage is given in the next Table:

Dosage of Vitamin K_1 (Phytonadione)

Condition	Age	Route	Dosage
Anticoagulant-induced Hypoprothrombinemia	Adult Children	IM, Subcut.	2.5-10mg; if necessary, repeat in 6-8 hours after first parenteral dose. Follow PT and PTT.
	Infant	IM, Subcut.	1-2mg/dose every 4-8 hours as needed. Follow PT and PTT.
Bleeding Present or Immediately Threatening		Slow IV	10-50mg. Repeat every 4 hours as needed. Consider continuous infusion. Follow PT & PTT.
Hemorrhagic Disease of the Newborn, Prophylaxis and Treatment	Neonate	Subcut. or IM	0.5-1mg immediately after delivery and repeated if necessary 6-8 hours later; rarely, a repeat dose 4-7 days later is needed. IM route is preferred.
		Oral	Investigational; 0.5-1mg/dose, IM preferred (Lane, P.A. and Hathaway, W.E., J. Pediatr. 106, 351-359, 1985).
Treatment of Neonates whose Mothers Received Anticonvulsants during Pregnancy	Neonate		See dosage above; however, these infants may require larger doses or repeat doses
Hypoprothrombinemia from other causes, e.g., Malabsorption; Therapy with Broad-Spectrum Antibiotics, Drugs	Adult	Oral, or Subcut. or IM	2-25mg, depending on deficiency
	Infant	Oral, or Subcut. or IM	2mg
	Children	Oral, or Subcut. or IM	5-10mg
Prevention of Hypoprothrombinemia Assoc. with Vit. K Def. in Patients receiving Total Parenteral Nutrition or Prolonged Hyperalimentation	Adults	IM or IV	5-10mg once weekly; may be added to TPN.
	Children	IM or IV	2-5mg, once weekly; may be added to TPN
Breast-Fed Infants or Infants receiving Milk, Substitute Formulas whenever vit. K content of Diet is <100microgram/liter	Infants	Oral IM Subcut.	1mg
Prevention of Hypoprothrombinemia in Breast-Fed Infants with Diarrhea longer than several days duration	Infants	IM	1mg

ADVERSE EFFECTS: Use with caution in presence of severe hepatic disease. Large doses (>25mg) in newborn may cause hyperbilirubinemia. IV injection should not exceed 1mg/min. IV doses may be associated with flushing, dizziness, hypotension, anaphylaxis.

MONITOR: Follow prothrombin time.

WARFARIN

(Coumadin, Panwarfin)

USES: Warfarin (4-hydroxycoumarin) is an **anticoagulant** that is generally used for follow-up anticoagulant therapy after the effects of full-dose heparin therapy have been established and when long-term anticoagulant therapy is indicated. Uses of warfarin are given in the next Table:

Uses of Warfarin as an Oral Anticoagulant
Deep Venous Thrombosis (DVT)
Pulmonary Embolism
Ischemic Heart Disease, e.g., Following Acute Myocardial Infarction
Atrial Fibrillation (AF)
Artificial (Metal or Plastic) Aortic or Mitral Valve Prosthesis
Tissue Mitral Valves, especially if Atrial Fibrillation (AF) Persists
Questionable Uses:
Transient Ischemic Attacks-Use Antiplatelet Agents
Peripheral Vascular Disease

When warfarin is used for follow-up therapy after heparin, therapy with the two drugs is usually overlapped until an adequate response to warfarin is obtained as indicated by PT determinations. Heparin and coumarin are administered concurrently for 5-10 days after the desired prothrombin time (PT) is achieved. This overlap is recommended because antithrombogenic effects of warfarin may not occur until up to 7 days after initiation of therapy.

Deep Venous Thrombosis: A single episode should be treated with warfarin for 3-6 months. Patients with recurrent DVT require lifelong treatment. Dipyridamole should be given to those patients who also have decreased platelet survival time.

Ischemic Heart Disease: Warfarin has been given for 3-6 months following acute myocardial infarction to reduce the incidence of recurrent thromboembolism in selected patients (eg, patients with large anterior infarction) (Gunnar, R.M., et al., J. Amer. Coll. Cardiol. 16, 249-292, August, 1990).

Atrial Fibrillation: Long-term warfarin therapy has been used to reduce the risk of embolism in patients with atrial fibrillation due to mitral stenosis, chronic sinoatrial disease, congestive cardiomyopathy or thyrotoxicosis. Routine use of warfarin is not indicated in patients with mitral valve prolapse.

Artificial Aortic or Mitral Valve Prostheses: Lifelong use of warfarin is necessary for patients with artificial (metal, plastic) aortic or mitral valve prostheses.

Mechanism of Action: Warfarin acts by decreasing the synthesis of the vitamin K-dependent clotting factors, prothrombin, factor VII, factor IX, and factor X. Warfarin is a coumarin derivative with a structure similar to that of vitamin K. Warfarin blocks vitamin K-dependent gamma carboxylation of glutamate residues resulting in the production of modified factors VII, IX, X and prothrombin (II); these are inactive in promoting coagulation because the gamma carboxylation is essential for the Ca^{+2} binding required for the binding of the factors to phospholipid-containing membranes.

DOSAGE FORMS: Tabs: 1, 2, 2.5, 5, 7.5, 10mg.

DOSAGE and Prothrombin Time(PT): Warfarin is administered orally in a single, daily dose. Dosage and prothrombin time monitoring are given in the next Table:

Dosage of Warfarin and Prothrombin Time

Day	Dose(mg)	Prothrombin Time (PT)
One	15	Determine PT prior to start of Warfarin (Control values usually 12-15 seconds).
Two	10	PT (Little change expected)
Three	10	PT (Rise to 16 to 20 seconds).
Four	5 to 7.5 (maintenance dose)	PT stabilized at 16 to 20 seconds, 1.3-1.5 times control value. Monitor PT twice during second week and weekly until maintenance dose established. Evaluate PT monthly and more frequently in patients with impaired liver function, congestive heart failure or frequent diarrhea.

WARFARIN (Cont.)

PHARMACOKINETICS: Onset and Duration: Peak PT effect occurs in 36-72 hours and at least 5-7 days of warfarin are required before full therapeutic effect is achieved. Duration After Discontinuation of Warfarin: Duration after discontinuance of warfarin is dependent on resynthesis of vitamin K-dependent clotting factors II, VII, IX and X (about 4-5 days). Absorption: Completely absorbed orally; Protein Binding: 97%; Half-Life: 42 hours.

Warfarin acts by decreasing the synthesis of the vitamin K-dependent clotting factors, prothrombin, factor VII, factor IX, and factor X. After administration of an oral anticoagulant, the level of factor VII is the first to decrease followed by the level of factor IX, followed by factor X and then factor II. An increased sensitivity to warfarin is found in patients with diarrhea and abnormalities of the small intestine such as sprue.

DRUG INTERACTIONS: Drug interactions with oral anticoagulants are given in the next Table (The Medical Letter, 26, 11-14, 1984; Glenny, R.W., South. Med. J. 80, 1266-1276, Oct. 1987; Hyers, T.M., Chest 95, 37S-51S, 1989):

Drug Interactions with Warfarin

Contraindicated	May Potentiate Effect	May Inhibit Effect	Drugs Whose Action is Enhanced by Warfarin
Acetylsalicylic acid	Alcohol	Barbiturates	Phenytoin(Dilantin)
Indomethacin	Allopurinol	Corticosteroids	Chlorpropamide
Phenylbutazone	Amiodarone	Cholestyramine	Tolbutamide
Sulfinpyrazine (Anturane)	Anabolic steroids	Diuretics	?Glipizide
Dipyridamole (Persantine)	Antibiotics	Ethchlorvynol (Placidyl)	?Glyburide
	Cimetidine	Glutethimide (Doriden)	
	Clofibrate	Griseofulin	
	Co-trimoxazole	Haloperidol (Haldol)	
	Disopyramide	Hereditary resistance	
	Disulfiram (Antabuse)	High Vit. K diet	
	Erythromycin	Meprobamate	
	Ethacrynic acid	Oral contraceptives	
	Glucagon	Rifampin	
	Hepatic Disease	Uremia	
	Hypermetabolic States		
	Low Vit. K diet		
	Mefenamic acid (Ponstel)		
	Methylphenidate (Ritalin)		
	Metronidazole		
	NSAIDs		
	Phenylbutazone		
	Phenytoin		
	Quinidine		
	Quinine		
	Trimethoprim-sulfamethoxazole		

Warfarin and its interaction with aspirin, is a major cause of drug-induced hospitalization primarily due to hemorrhage.

ADVERSE EFFECTS: Hemorrhage is the most frequent complication of treatment; the frequency of major bleeding is 5% to 10%. Hemorrhage is treated with vitamin K_1 until PT decreases (see VITAMIN K_1).

A rare complication of warfarin therapy is skin and soft tissue necrosis (Scandling, J., Walker, B.K., South. Med. J. 73, 1470-1472, 1980). Necrosis usually occurs within 5-7 days of initiating therapy. Treatment should include vitamin K and heparin both for the original thrombotic condition and to limit the area of necrosis (McGehee, W.G., et. al., Ann. Intern. Med. 100, 59-60, 1984).

CONTRAINDICATIONS: Contraindications are the same as those for heparin. Special caution must be used in patients with liver disease or vitamin K deficiency.

For thrombophlebitis during pregnancy, heparin is the drug of choice because it does not cross the placenta; warfarin crosses the placenta and is teratogenic.

PARAMETERS TO MONITOR: Prothrombin time (PT)-see Dosage Table. Also monitor hematocrit, stool guaiac, urinalysis for hematuria. Also monitor for ecchymosis, hemoptysis and epistaxis.

ZIDOVUDINE

(Azidothymidine [AZT]; Retrovir)

USES: Zidovudine is used in the management of human immunodeficiency virus (HIV) infections; HIV is a retrovirus. Zidovudine is indicated for the management of symptomatic HIV infections (acquired immunodeficiency syndrome [AIDS] or advanced AIDS-related complex[ARC]) in certain adults with a history of Pneumocystis carinii pneumonia or an absolute helper/inducer (CD4, T4) T-cell count from peripheral blood of less than 200/mm^3 at the time therapy with the drug is initiated. Zidovudine is also effective in asymptomatic and mildly symptomatic HIV infected individuals with CD4 counts less than 500/mm^3 (Volberding, P.A., et al., N. Engl. J. Med. 322, 941-949, April, 1990; Fischl, M.D., et al., Ann. Intern. Med. 112, 727-737, May, 1990). Zidovudine has also been shown to be of benefit in children with HIV infection (Pizzo, P.A., et al., N. Engl. J. Med. 319, 889-896, 1988).

AZT is made by Burroughs Wellcome Company, based in the Research Triangle Park, N.C., under the brand name Retrovir (zidovudine).

Clinical Trial: In early 1986, a controlled double-blind trial involving 282 adults in 12 centers [85 AIDS and 60 ARC patients versus placebo (75 AIDS and 62 ARC patients)], using oral azidothymidine, was undertaken. AIDS patients were accepted into the study only if they had had their first episode of pneumocystis carinii pneumonia(PCP) within 120 days. The subjects were stratified according to numbers of T-cells with CD4 surface markers and were randomly assigned to receive either 250mg of AZT or placebo by mouth every four hours for a total of 24 weeks.

Nineteen placebo recipients and 1 AZT recipient died during the study. Opportunistic infections developed in 45 subjects receiving placebo, as compared with 24 receiving AZT.

Immunological Response: Although T-4 lymphocytes increased with AZT in both AIDS and ARC patients, in AIDS patients, T-4 lymphocytes fell to pretreatment levels even though AZT was continued; in ARC patients, the beneficial effect on T-4 cells was sustained. Skin-test anergy was partially reversed in 29% of subjects receiving AZT, as compared with 9 percent of those receiving placebo (Fischl, M.A., et al., N. Engl. J. Med. 317, 185-191, 1987).

These data demonstrate that AZT decreases mortality and frequency of opportunistic infections, improves immune status and improves general health in certain patients with AIDS and AIDS-related complex(ARC). Subsequent studies have demonstrated benefit in asymptomatic and mildly symptomatic patients with CD4 counts less than 500/mm^3, in pediatric patients, and in patients with neurologic disease or thrombycytopenia.

Long-Term Use of AZT: Preliminary data on long-term use of AZT are not encouraging. Initially, during the first six months, patients treated with AZT gain weight and produce increased numbers of T-4 cells; this probably reflects increased survival of T-4 cells rather than increased cell division. During the next six months, patients lose the weight they have gained and the T-4 cells they have gained. After 14 months of therapy, patients have a weight loss comparable to their weight when they first started medication and progression of disease is evident (Dickinson, G., presented at Interscience Conference on Antimicrobial Agents and Chemotherapy, Oct. 1987). It may be that therapy with AZT will have to be modified after initial therapy.

Mechanism of Action: HIV is a retrovirus; retroviruses are RNA viruses which must replicate through a DNA intermediate. Once inside the host T-4 helper/inducer lymphocytes, the virus transcribes its RNA into DNA through the enzyme reverse transcriptase; AZT acts by inhibiting the activity of this enzyme.

The chemical structure of AZT is illustrated in the next Figure:

Chemical Structure of Azidothymidine (AZT) (Retrovir; Zidovudine)

Thymidine — 3'-Azido-3'-Deoxythymidine(AZT)

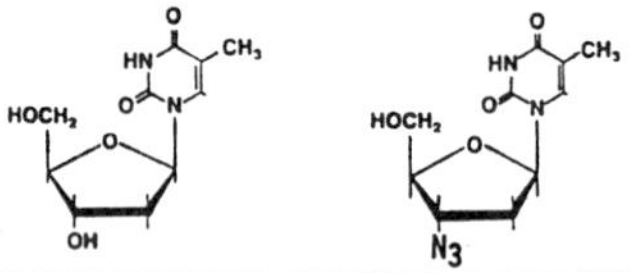

ZIDOVUDINE (Cont.)

AZT is a nucleoside analogue, modeled on the nucleoside thymidine; it was designed in the 1960's as an anticancer drug. At the sugar ring's 3' position, AZT has an azido (N_3) group instead of a hydroxyl group. Like thymidine, AZT is phosphorylated, as 5'-triphosphate, as illustrated in the next Figure; (Yarchoan, R. and Broder, S., N. Engl. J. Med. 316, 557-564, Feb 26, 1987):

Phosphorylation of Thymidine and AZT

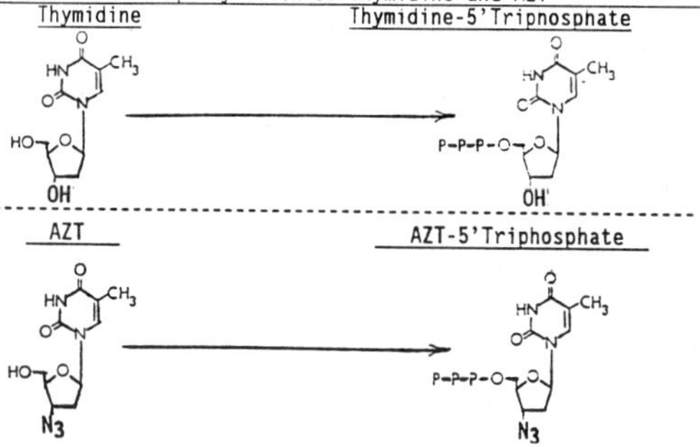

As the virus is preparing to invade the nucleus of the cell, AZT interferes with the synthesis of new DNA during reverse transcription by terminating the growth of the DNA chain as illustrated in the next Figure (Yarchoan,R. & Broder,S., N. Engl. J. Med. 316, 557-564, Feb. 26,1987):

Synthesis of DNA with Phosphorylated Thymidine and
Inhibition of DNA Synthesis with Phosphorylated AZT

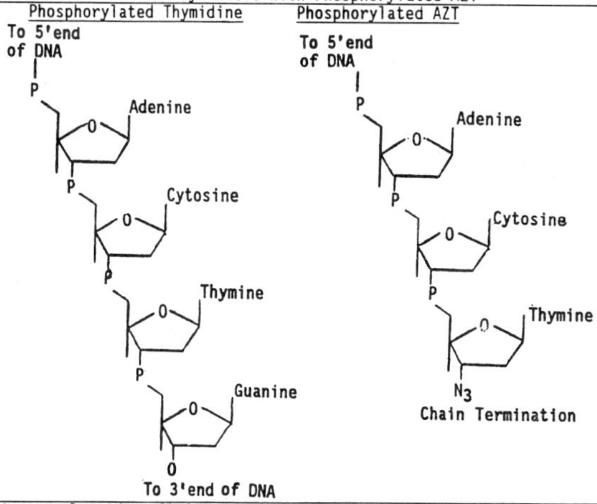

Incoming nucleotides find no attachment point and reverse transcription, that is, synthesis of DNA from an RNA template comes to a halt and, in this way, replication of HIV is blocked.

ZIDOVUDINE (Cont.)

DOSAGE FORMS: Caps: 100mg; Oral Solution: 50mg/5ml; Injection: 10mg/ml.

DOSAGE: The optimal dosage of AZT has not been determined. The recommended dose of AZT for asymptomatic adults is 100mg administered orally every 4 hours (500mg/day); some authors suggest an induction period with higher dose therapy (200mg every 4 hours for 1 month) particularly in symptomatic patients (Fischl, M.A., et al., NEJM 323, 1009-1014, October, 1990). The minimal effective dose has not yet been determined, but preliminary studies suggest that doses as low as 300mg daily may be effective (Collier, A.C., et al., NEJM 323, 1015-1021, October, 1990). The adult IV dose for symptomatic patients is 1-2mg/kg every 4 hrs 6 times daily.

Children (3 months to 12 years) should receive 180mg/m^2(max. 200mg/dose) orally every 6 hours (Medical Letter 32, 73-78, August 10, 1990). Pediatric IV dose is 0.5-1.8mg/kg/hr by continous infusion or 100mg/m^2 over 1 hr, 4 times daily.

Patients must take AZT for 4-6 weeks for it to be effective. AZT has little or no effect on the course of the disease during the first several weeks following initiation of the drug.

Dosage Adjustment: Anemia (hemoglobin, <7.5g/dl or reduction of >25% of baseline) and/or granulocytopenia (granulocyte count, <750/mm^2 or reduction of >50% from baseline) may require reduction in dosage.

ADVERSE EFFECTS: Adverse effects of AZT are given in the next Table; (Richman, D.D. et al., N. Engl. J. Med. 317, 192-197, July 23, 1987):

Adverse Effects of AZT
Bone Marrow Suppression
Anemia with Hemoglobin Levels <7.5g/dl
Neutropenia
Erythrocyte Macrocytosis
Nausea, Myalgia, Insomnia, Severe Headaches

Anemia often requires multiple red-cell transfusions. Erythropoietin is under investigation for treatment of AZT-induced anemia - see ERYTHROPOIETIN. Subjects who initially have low CD4 lymphocyte counts, low serum vitamin B12 levels, anemia or low neutrophil counts are more likely to have hematologic toxic effects.

Drug Interactions: Co-administration of zidovudine with other drugs metabolized by glucuronidation should be avoided because the combination may potentiate toxicity of either drug. Zidovudine recipients who also take acetaminophen have an increased incidence of granulocytopenia that appears to be related to the duration of acetaminophen use.

Ribavirin: When AZT and ribavirin are used in combination, ribavirin inhibits phosphorylation of AZT(Vogt,M.W. et al.,Science 235, 1376-1379, Mar.13, 1987).

Acyclovir: Severe incapacitating drowsiness and lethargy has been reported (Bach, M.C., N. Engl. J. Med. 316, No. 9, 547, Feb. 26, 1987).

PHARMACOKINETICS: G.I. Absorption: 60%; Half-Life: 1 hour; Metabolism: Liver (glucuronidation); Excretion: Kidney.

Cerebrospinal Fluid(CSF): Mean values in CSF are about 55% of plasma levels simultaneously measured 4 hours after dosing (Yarchoan, R. et al., Lancet 1, 575-580, 1986).

Laboratory Monitoring: Obtain complete blood count(CBC) prior to and every two weeks while the patient is treated with AZT.

The HIV core antigen concentration can be used to monitor the clinical response to AZT. Increases in the concentration of this antigen may correlate with clinical deterioration (Goudsmit, J. et al., Lancet 2, 177-180, 1986); HIV core antigen decreases in the serum of patients treated with AZT (Chaisson, R.E. et al., N. Engl. J. Med. 315, 1610-1611, 1986).

Costs of AZT: AZT is priced at about $5,500 a year wholesale, or $7,800 to $8,500 retail.

The costs of AZT are paid by the resources of the patient, insurance companies and Medicaid. When the resources of the patient are exhausted, patients may qualify for Medicaid. Medicaid is the public assistance program that in most states has agreed to cover the cost of AZT.

Research Projects: Research projects already underway or planned soon, designed to answer the following questions, are as follows:

(1) Whether lower doses of AZT are as effective as higher doses.
(2) Whether AIDS patients with Kaposi's sarcoma can benefit from a combination of AZT and interferon.
(3) Whether AZT is effective in post-exposure prophylaxis in HIV exposed individuals.
(4) Whether hemophiliacs, who have contracted AIDS through contaminated blood products, respond differently to AZT than patients who were exposed to AIDS from other means such as sexual intercourse.
(5) Whether AIDS patients show an even stronger response when they receive a combination of AZT and acyclovir, an anti-viral drug developed by Burroughs Wellcome for treatment of herpes.